TARGETED CANCER THERAPY

CURRENT CLINICAL ONCOLOGY™

Maurie Markman, MD, SERIES EDITOR

TARGETED CANCER THERAPY

Edited by

RAZELLE KURZROCK, MD, FACP

Department of Investigational Cancer Therapeutics,
Division of Cancer Medicine,
The University of Texas,
MD Anderson Cancer Center,
Houston, TX

MAURIE MARKMAN, MD

Department of Clinical Research,
The University of Texas,
MD Anderson Cancer Center,
Houston, TX

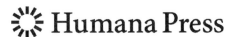 Humana Press

Editors
Razelle Kurzrock
Department of Investigational Cancer
Therapeutics, Division of Cancer Medicine
The University of Texas
MD Anderson Cancer Center
Houston, TX
rkurzroc@mdanderson.org

Maurie Markman
Department of Clinical Research
The University of Texas
MD Anderson Cancer Center
Houston, TX
mmarkman@mdanderson.org

Series Editor
Maurie Markman
Department of Clinical Research
The University of Texas
MD Anderson Cancer Center
Houston, TX
mmarkman@mdanderson.org

ISBN: 978-1-60327-423-4   e-ISBN: 978-1-60327-424-1

Library of Congress Control Number: 2007941656

Cover illustration: Figure 4, chapter 16, "Targeted Therapy of Sarcoma," by Joseph Ludwig and Jonathan C. Trent

Printed on acid-free paper

9 8 7 6 5 4 3 2 1

springer.com

Dedication

This book is dedicated to our courageous patients and their families engaged in the war against cancer.

Preface

Based on experience with a small number of cancers, it is now apparent that remarkable responses (without serious side effects) can be achieved by targeted therapy—that is, by using drugs that directly affect the molecular abnormality that characterizes a tumor. The era of personalized medicine in cancer has begun, and we believe that these early therapeutic successes represent just the tip of the iceberg. No longer a "one-size-fits-all" approach, the treatment of cancer is now increasingly being individualized based on an understanding of the underlying biologic mechanisms.

The limitations of chemotherapy, radiotherapy, and surgery are apparent and have been the impetus for developing targeted therapies. Novel emerging technologies in target identification, drug discovery, molecular markers, and imaging are rapidly changing the face of cancer. Personalized health planning, early diagnosis, and selecting optimal drugs for each patient with predictable side effects are developments that are directly in our sights. It is also becoming increasingly important to develop combinations of therapies and therapeutic modalities for treating cancer, as many cancers are complex and driven by more than one aberration. A primary objective is to design drug combinations that can overcome drug resistance. Cross talk among signaling pathways and parallel pathways that contribute to tumor pathogenesis is thought to contribute to single-agent resistance.

We are poised to change the landscape in oncology. The purpose of *Targeted Cancer Therapy* is to provide a state-of-the-art overview of where we are now in this process. We hope that the book will provide a foundation of knowledge in targeted cancer therapeutics that is useful to practicing and academic physicians, fellows, residents, and students, as well as basic scientists who are interested in the cancer field.

Razelle Kurzrock, MD, FACP
Maurie Markman, MD

Contents

Contributors

RAYMOND ALEXANIAN, MD • *Department of Lymphoma, UT MD Anderson Cancer Center, Houston, TX*

LUIS H. CAMACHO, MD, MPH • *Department of Investigational Cancer Therapeutics, UT MD Anderson Cancer Center, Houston, TX*

LAKSHMI CHINTALA, MD • *Department of Investigational Cancer Therapeutics, UT MD Anderson Cancer Center, Houston, TX*

JORGE CORTES, MD • *Department of Leukemia, UT MD Anderson Cancer Center, Houston, TX*

BARBARA S. CRAFT, MD • *Department of Investigational Cancer Therapeutics, UT MD Anderson Cancer Center, Houston, TX*

MICHAEL DAVIES, MD, PhD • *Department of Melanoma Medical Oncology, UT MD Anderson Cancer Center, Houston, TX*

ELIHU ESTEY, MD • *Department of Leukemia, UT MD Anderson Cancer Center, Houston, TX*

GUILLERMO GARCIA-MANERO, MD • *Department of Leukemia, UT MD Anderson Cancer Center, Houston, TX*

DON L. GIBBONS, MD, PhD • *Department of Hematology and Oncology (T/C), UT MD Anderson Cancer Center, Houston, TX*

DAVID HONG, MD • *Department of Investigational Cancer Therapeutics, UT MD Anderson Cancer Center, Houston, TX*

ELIAS JABBOUR, MD • *Department of Stem Cell Transplantation, UT MD Anderson Cancer Center, Houston, TX*

EDWARD F. JACKSON, MS, PhD • *Department of Imaging Physics, UT MD Anderson Cancer Center, Houston, TX*

ERIC JONASCH, MD • *Department of Genitourinary Medical Oncology, UT MD Anderson Cancer Center, Houston, TX*

HAGOP KANTARJIAN, MD • *Department of Leukemia, UT MD Anderson Cancer Center, Houston, TX*

MICHEAL J. KEATING, MD • *Department of Leukemia, UT MD Anderson Cancer Center, Houston, TX*

JERI KIM, MD • *Department of Genitourinary Medical Oncology, UT MD Anderson Cancer Center, Houston, TX*

KEVIN B. KIM, MD • *Department of Melanoma Medical Oncology, UT MD Anderson Cancer Center, Houston, TX*

SCOTT KOPETZ, MD • *Department of Gastrointestinal Medical Oncology, UT MD Anderson Cancer Center, Houston, TX*

VIKAS KUNDRA, MD, PhD • *Department of Diagnostic Radiology, UT MD Anderson Cancer Center, Houston, TX*

RAZELLE KURZROCK, MD, FACP • *Department of Investigational Cancer Therapeutics, Division of Cancer Medicine, UT MD Anderson Cancer Center, Houston, TX*

JOSEPH LUDWIG, MD • *Department of Sarcoma Medical Oncology, UT MD Anderson Cancer Center, Houston, TX*

MAURIE MARKMAN, MD, VP • *Department of Clinical Research, UT MD Anderson Cancer Center, Houston, TX*

STACY MOULDER, MD, MSCI • *Department of Breast Medical Oncology, UT MD Anderson Cancer Center, Houston, TX*

SUNIL PATEL, MD • *Department of Medical Oncology (T/C), UT MD Anderson Cancer Center, Houston, TX*

GARTH POWIS, PhD • *Department of Experimental Therapeutics, UT MD Anderson Cancer Center, Houston, TX*

ALFONSO QUINTÁS-CARDAMA, MD • *Department of Hematology and Oncology (T/C), UT MD Anderson Cancer Center, Houston, TX*

DAWID SCHELLINGERHOUT, MD • *Department of Diagnostic Radiology, UT MD Anderson Cancer Center, Houston, TX*

DAVID J. STEWART, MD, FRCPC • *Department of Thoracic Head/Neck Medical Oncology, UT MD Anderson Cancer Center, Houston, TX*

NIZAR TANNIR, MD • *Department of Genitourinary Medical Oncology, UT MD Anderson Cancer Center, Houston, TX*

JONATHAN C. TRENT, MD, PhD • *Department of Sarcoma Medical Oncology, UT MD Anderson Cancer Center, Houston, TX*

APOSTOLIA-MARIA TSIMBERIDOU, MD, PhD • *Department of Leukemia Research, UT MD Anderson Cancer Center, Houston, TX*

GAURI VARADHACHARY, MD, MBBS • *Department of Gastrointestinal Medical Oncology, UT MD Anderson Cancer Center, Houston, TX*

MICHAEL WANG, MD, MS • *Department of Lymphoma, UT MD Anderson Cancer Center, Houston, TX*

JOHN F. WARD, MD • *Department of Urology, UT MD Anderson Cancer Center, Houston, TX*

AMANDA WEDGWOOD, MSN, RN, CNS • *Department of Lymphoma, UT MD Anderson Cancer Center, Houston, TX*

SARAH J. WELSH, BM, BCh, PhD • *University of Oxford, Harris Manchester College, Oxford, UK*

JENNIFER WHELER, MD • *Department of Investigational Cancer Therapeutics, UT MD Anderson Cancer Center, Houston, TX*

ROBERT A. WOLFF, MD • *Department of Gastrointestinal Medical Oncology, UT MD Anderson Cancer Center, Houston, TX*

ANAS YOUNES, MD • *Department of Lymphoma, UT MD Anderson Cancer Center, Houston, TX*

YUHONG ZHOU, MD • *Department of Medical Oncology, Zhongshan Hospital, Fudan University, Shanghai, Peoples Republic of China*

AMADO J. ZURITA, MD • *Department of Genitourinary Medical Oncology, UT MD Anderson Cancer Center, Houston, TX*

1 Perspectives: *Bench to Bedside and Back*

Jennifer Wheler, MD *and Razelle Kurzrock,* MD, FACP

CONTENTS

ABSTRACT

Translational medicine has opened the gateway to the era of personalized medicine. No longer a "one size fits all" approach, the treatment of cancer is now based on an understanding of underlying biologic mechanisms and is increasingly being tailored to the molecular specificity of a tumor. Although oncology still functions within broad disease categories, the future will see an increasing shift to treatment based on the characteristics of an individual's tumor type. Interestingly, one of the first targeted therapies, all-*trans* retinoic acid in acute promyelocytic leukemia, was first demonstrated at the bedside with a subsequent return to the bench to elucidate its underlying basis. This was a translocation resulting in disruption of the retinoic acid receptor-α gene. Since then, a rigorous translational approach has led to other success stories, such as imatinib and dasatinib in Philadelphia-positive leukemias. With the discovery of novel biologic agents, future challenges lie in the investigation of optimal combinations and the identification of biomarkers that can provide both predictive and prognostic information. Genomics, proteomics, and the application of mathematical modeling are leading the way to biomarker discovery. Further elucidation of the cancer "stem cell hypothesis" will lead to treatment with combinations of agents used to

From: *Current Clinical Oncology: Targeted Cancer Therapy*
Edited by: R. Kurzrock and M. Markman © Humana Press, Totowa, NJ

target both early epigenetic mechanisms and downstream molecular events. With targeted agents that demonstrate increased efficacy and decreased toxicity, we are now approaching cancer as a chronic disease model. Personalized medicine, with a "bench to bedside and back" paradigm is poised to permanently alter the landscape for cancer management.

Key Words: Targeted therapy, Translational medicine, Bioinformatics, All-*trans* retinoic acid, GIST, Imatinib, Dasatinib, Epigenetics, Decitabine, Stem cell hypothesis

1. INTRODUCTION

We are in the midst of a revolution in the treatment of cancer. Translational medicine is leading the way into a new era of personalized medicine. Traditionally, there has been a gap between basic science and clinical medicine. Translational medicine fills this gap with a bidirectional approach linking the two. Scientific discovery is taken from the laboratory to the clinical setting, and clinical data are taken back to the laboratory. This model has been successfully adopted to identify targets in the preclinical setting, develop compounds based on these targets, and treat patients in clinical trials. Less acknowledged but just as important is the art of taking clinical observation back to the laboratory to clarify molecular pathways, resistance mechanisms, and genetic alterations.

During the past 20 years, this translational paradigm of "bench to bedside and back again" has enabled rapid progress in the elucidation of complex biologic mechanisms and the development of rational, targeted therapies. Key molecular processes—growth factor binding, signal transduction, gene transcription control, cell cycle checkpoints, apoptosis, angiogenesis—have emerged as potential targets. The development and regulatory approval of drugs such as rituximab, trastuzumab, imatinib, erlotinib, lapatinib, bevacizumab, and cetuximab have provided clinical validation for this molecularly targeted approach. These discoveries have radically changed the way cancer treatment is conceptualized. The historic "one size fits all" approach of treating cancer in the setting of broad tumor categories is being supplanted by the identification of specific targets and molecular subtypes, leading to a personalized approach to treatment based on a patient's unique tumor characteristics.

Targeted therapy is personalized therapy. To appreciate the novelty and success of the bench to bedside and back paradigm and the exponential growth in the field of translational medicine, it is helpful to contextualize this progress within a larger historical perspective. In the past, cancer treatments evolved from empiric observation and, not infrequently, chance observation. In 1942, the sinking of a U.S. battleship led to the recognition that mustard gas causes profound lymphoid and myeloid suppression. Following this accidental discovery, mustine (the prototype nitrogen mustard) was used to treat non-Hodgkin's lymphoma *(1)*. Since then, a majority of the more than 200 currently available cancer drugs were identified serendipitously from plants or fungi.

Translational medicine, fueled by the human genome project, has led to a bench to bedside approach to drug discovery. In revealing a vast amount of information about normal and malignant cells, the human genome project has provided a gateway to the current era of molecular medicine. The emerging fields of proteomics and genomics, bioinformatics and systems biology, and nuclear imaging and nanotechnology (among others) are providing the tools to mine and navigate these data. The development of rational drug therapy is now based on an understanding of the molecular genotypes and phenotypes of disease.

The histories behind the development of all-*trans* retinoic acid (ATRA), imatinib (Gleevec; Novartis, Cambridge, MA, USA), and decitabine (Dacogen; MGI Pharma/ SuperGen, Minneapolis, MN, USA) are different versions of the bench to bedside and back paradigm. Each story illustrates the importance and potential of a rigorous translational approach. The story of cancer stem cells is just beginning; however, it is already clear that the cancer stem cell hypothesis will further accelerate our understanding of carcinogenesis and lead to additional targeted therapies.

Translational medicine is the language that delineates and clarifies discoveries made at the bench so they can evolve into stories of clinical efficacy. We are currently authoring what might be conceptualized as the first chapter of personalized medicine. Subsequent chapters will describe combination therapies that target both the cancer stem cell for disease eradication and the downstream pathways for disease control and stabilization.

The bench to bedside and back paradigm of translational medicine has led to the discovery of therapies that have transformed the way cancer patients live. Although the ultimate goal is to prevent cancer entirely, a more immediate milestone is to transform cancer into a manageable disease. The language of translational medicine has enabled open communication and understanding between basic scientists and clinical researchers that will further refine targeted therapies to support a chronic disease model.

2. DEVELOPMENT OF ONE OF THE FIRST TARGETED THERAPIES: ALL-*TRANS* RETINOIC ACID AND THE BEDSIDE TO BENCH PARADIGM

With the exception of hormonal therapy for breast cancer, all-*trans* retinoic acid (ATRA) is one of the earliest examples of a successful targeted drug and serves as a model for developing novel biologic agents tailored to various other malignant tumors. The introduction of ATRA was a major breakthrough in the treatment of acute promyelocytic leukemia (APL). The molecular mechanism underlying ATRA-induced APL cell differentiation was not discovered until *after* the introduction of ATRA to the clinic. This discovery launched the first molecular marker used to diagnose and monitor minimal residual disease. ATRA exemplifies the success that can come from returning a compound from the clinical setting to the laboratory (bedside to bench) to enhance the understanding of disease and of a drug's activity. In recent years, ATRA in combination treatment has become an example of how systems-based synergistic targeted therapy is used to improve clinical outcomes.

Leukemia as a model for other disease types is being emulated in terms of molecular identification of subtypes and individualized treatment approaches. The responses of leukemia to therapies differ from one subtype to another; therefore, therapeutic strategies are disease pathogenesis-based and individualized. APL is a distinct subset of acute myeloid leukemia (AML), initially described in 1957 with case studies and characterized as the most malignant form of acute leukemia *(2)*. APL constitutes approximately 10% to 15% of all cases of AML.

ATRA was taken to the clinic before its specific mechanism, related to circumventing the impact of APL's aberrant PML-RAR (retinoic acid receptor) genotype was understood. ATRA was tested clinically based on the hypothesis that it could lead to the differentiation of immature leukemic cells. Until the late 1980s, the only effective treatment for APL was intensive chemotherapy, typically combining an anthracycline with cytosine arabinoside (AraC). During the late 1980s, investigators in China demonstrated that the vitamin A derivative ATRA could induce differentiation of HL-60, a cell line with promyelocytic features, as well as in fresh leukemic cells from patients. These preclinical studies led to the first clinical trial in 1986. This study of ATRA in 24 patients with APL demonstrated complete remission in all but one of the patients *(3)*. The remaining patient achieved a complete response (CR) when chemotherapy was added. A significant observation was the gradual terminal differentiation of malignant cells in the bone marrow. A second (French) study resulted in a CR in 14 of 22 patients through a differentiation effect of treatment *(4)*.

Consistent with our current paradigm of targeted therapy being more gentle and less toxic than past therapies, ATRA demonstrated less toxicity than conventional chemotherapy. The most severe associated side effect, retinoic acid syndrome (RAS), was rare. By its association with increased numbers of differentiated neutrophils secreting inflammatory cytokines, the RAS caused fever and respiratory distress followed by interstitial pulmonary infiltrates, weight gain, pleural or pericardial effusion, and renal failure. The incidence of RAS toxicity was minimized by the addition of cytotoxic therapy to ATRA.

Many subsequent randomized studies, internationally, confirmed the efficacy of ATRA for the treatment of APL. Studies demonstrated improved CR rates, decreased severe adverse effects compared to cytotoxic chemotherapy alone, and increased duration of remission *(5–7)*. Most patients treated with ATRA alone after demonstrating CR ultimately relapse, so the combination of ATRA and cytotoxic chemotherapy now constitutes front-line therapy for newly diagnosed APL.

The development of treatment approaches for APL serves as a paradigm for the design of rational therapies based on an oncogene-dependent pathway to PML-RARα *(8)*. APL is characterized by a distinct morphology of blast cells, an expansion and accumulation of leukemic cells that are thwarted at the promyelocytic stage of myelopoiesis. APL is cytogenetically associated in 95% of patients with reciprocal chromosomal translocations involving the retinoic acid receptor-α (RARα) gene on chromosome 17 [chromosomal translocation t(15;17)(q22;q21)]. The *PML* gene fuses with the *RARα* gene to form PML-RARα and RARα-PML chimeric genes with corresponding fusion oncoproteins. RARα is vital for granulocyte development *(9)*; and PML-RARα, the dysregulated RARα, plays a key role in the pathogenesis of APL. RARα –/– mice demonstrated accelerated granulopoiesis, indicating that this pathway can also function as a negative controller of granulocytic proliferation *(10)*. Heterodimerization of PML-RARα with *PML* confers a growth advantage, apoptosis resistance, and differentiation arrest of APL cells.

Further correlative investigations after these early clinical trials led to the discovery of one of the earliest validated biomarkers to predict response to treatment and as a harbinger of residual disease. Warrell and colleagues *(11)* showed that clinical response to ATRA in APL was associated with the expression of aberrant RARα nuclear receptor. The detection of this receptor demonstrated accuracy in its ability to detect residual leukemia in these patients. After entering CR, 75% to 90% of patients still have the PML-RARα fusion gene detected by reverse transcription polymerase chain reaction (RT-PCR) *(12)*.

Dependence on aberrant RARα oncoprotein expression for APL pathogenesis was subsequently further elucidated. RARα is a member of the nuclear hormone receptor superfamily and acts as a ligand-inducible transcriptional regulator. RARα requires heterodimerization with retinoid X receptor-α (RXRα) to bind retinoic acid response element (RARE) located in the promoter regions of the target genes. In APL cells, PML-RARα binds RARE through the DNA binding domain of RARα in a dominant manner. PML-RARα mediates transcriptional repression of *RARα* target genes by recruitment of co-repressors (CoR), histone deacetylase (HDAC), and DNA methyltransferase. This leads to a maturational block in myeloid differentiation, thought to be a first step of leukemogenesis.

By contrast, ATRA triggers the dissociation of the HDAC complex and recruitment of coactivators. ATRA also induces degradation of PML-RARα and activates normal RARα and PML, resulting in differentiation of APL cells. ATRA works by dissociating CoR from the PML-RARα oncoprotein and recruiting CoR to open the chromatin structure. The result is a conversion of PML-RARα from a transcription repressor to transcription activator *(13)*. ATRA also degrades the PML-RARα oncoprotein through a caspase-mediated cleavage pathway and proteosome-dependent degradation pathway. Simultaneously, RXR is released to reheterodimerize with RARα, leading to recovery of the RA pathway and granulocytic differentiation *(14,15)*. Degradation of PML-RARα also leads to relocalization of PML and the recovery of PML functions with subsequent growth arrest and apoptosis induction *(16,17)*.

In recent years, arsenic compounds, particularly arsenic trioxide (AS_2O_3), have shown success in the treatment of both primary cases and in relapsed and ATRA-resistant patients. During the 1990s, investigators in China reported that arsenic trioxide could induce a CR in patients with APL *(18)*. Functioning by a mechanism different from that of ATRA, arsenic can induce a CR rate of more than 80% in relapsed patients after treatment with ATRA. Trials in the United States showed molecular remission in more than 80% of relapsed APL patients, as measured by RT-PCR of marrow specimens for PML-RARα transcript. Currently, arsenic is considered a first-line therapy for relapsed APL patients. Because arsenic does not completely eradicate leukemic cells, the optimal postremission therapy remains undefined. Outcomes of autologous stem cell transplantation in patients with a second molecular remission after arsenic therapy have demonstrated a good success rate.

Elucidation of molecular mechanisms in the pathogenesis of APL and in the pharmacologic approaches has led to high CR rates with ATRA in combination with chemotherapy and as postremission consolidation treatment. The ATRA story introduced the concept of molecular target-based cancer treatment, which has been further developed by the tyrosine kinase inhibitor imatinib to treat chronic myelogenous leukemia (CML) successfully. Lessons learned from APL treatment inspire and increase our understanding of the complex biology of tumors and their mechanism-based diagnosis and treatment.

3. A MODEL OF BENCH TO BEDSIDE TARGETED DRUG DEVELOPMENT: THE STORY OF IMATINIB IN PHILADELPHIA-POSITIVE ACUTE LYMPHOBLASTIC LEUKEMIA, CHRONIC MYELOGENOUS LEUKEMIA, AND GASTROINTESTINAL STROMAL TUMORS

The success of imatinib in chronic myelogenous leukemia (CML) validated the hypothesis that a specific molecular understanding of cancer can directly affect cancer therapy. Imatinib demonstrated proof of the concept that major clinical benefit can be gained by targeting an oncogenic abnormality that drives a particular type of cancer in a particular subject population. It represents a notable example of how research at the "bench" translated to the "bedside" and then back again, can lead to the development of a successful molecular targeted therapy. The path leading to the U.S. Food and Drug Administration's (FDA) approval of imatinib for CML in 2001 and its subsequent development in gastrointestinal stromal tumors (GISTs) provided significant insight into the challenges of effectively translating targeted agents into use in the clinic.

The story behind the development of imatinib and its subsequent use in CML and GISTs illustrates fully the paradigm of bench to bedside and back. Whereas the mechanism of action of ATRA was discovered only after clinical efficacy was demonstrated in patients with APL, the mechanism of imatinib and its specific target were elucidated before it was transferred to the clinic. The theme of "kinase-dependent" cancers explains cancers whose growth is driven by a specific set of kinases. The distinct molecular abnormality underlying Philadelphia-positive leukemia is activation of ABL tyrosine kinase by a chromosome translocation *(19,20)*. Imatinib, a small-molecule tyrosine kinase inhibitor, is a direct inhibitor of BCR-ABL, KIT, and the platelet-derived growth factor receptor (PDGFR) alpha and beta. Imatinib binds competitively with ATP to BCR-ABL, blocking abnormal signaling and selectively inhibiting proliferation of BCR-ABL-positive cells.

The observation that imatinib inhibits other kinases, notably the oncoprotein c-Kit, led to another successful clinical translation of the drug for the treatment of GISTs. The basic science and subsequent clinical application followed by the return to the laboratory and reemergence in other treatment models serves as an example of how distinct molecular features of cancers can be used to select appropriate treatment. Both the successes and limitations of imatinib, notably de novo and acquired resistance patterns, provide guidance for the development of other molecular targeted therapies in cancer.

Just as APL demonstrates oncogene dependence on PML-RARα, CML requires the BCR-ABL oncogene for pathogenesis. CML is characterized by an overabundance of granulocytes, erythrocytes, and platelets in peripheral blood. The molecular hallmark of CML is the Philadelphia (Ph) chromosome, a reciprocal 9;22 translocation that generates the fusion oncogene bcr-abl. Since its identification in 1960, the Ph chromosome is now known to be present in more than 90% of CML cases *(21)*. The presence of the Ph chromosome in a hematopoietic stem cell leads to cytokine-independent cell growth and survival.

Imatinib created a revolution in the treatment of CML. CML typically has three progressive and distinct phases: a benign chronic phase, an accelerated phase, and a rapidly fatal blast crisis. Efficacy with imatinib treatment has been demonstrated in all three phases of the disease. Philadelphia-positive acute leukemias, which are notoriously resistant to chemotherapy, also bear a Bcr-Abl abnormality (p190$^{Bcr-Abl}$) *(19)* and respond to imatinib, albeit not as well as CML, which is characterized by a slightly different Bcr-Abl aberration (p210$^{Bcr-Abl}$). Before imatinib's discovery, treatment options were relatively limited, even for CML. Allogeneic bone marrow transplantation had good success rates; however, the need for a matched donor limited patient eligibility. Treatment for most patients initially consisted of hydroxyurea, busulfan or interferon-α. Intensive chemotherapy regimens also were used but were harsh and had little impact on survival.

3.1. Imatinib as a Model for Discovery of Approaches to Overcome Resistance

Resistance patterns significantly complicate the successful application of kinase inhibitors and other targeted therapies. The identification of CML resistance to imatinib is an example of how genomic and proteomic approaches can help identify both de novo and acquired resistance and help predict response to therapy. Investigation of resistance patterns to imatinib in CML led to the development of a successful second-generation tyrosine kinase inhibitor that overcomes resistance in some patients.

Defined as a relapse of disease in a patient who has been on continuous therapy after an initial response and first recognized in advanced-stage CML patients, acquired resistance also occurs in chronic-phase CML and GISTs. Some relapsed patients with CML have mutations in the ABL kinase domain that affects drug sensitivity *(22,23)*. In ABL, three mutations are most common. The emergence of imatinib-resistant kinase mutants in patients with CML prompted the development of second-generation inhibitors, such as dasatinib. Dasatinib targets the more conserved active form of the kinase and inhibits production of many of the imatinib-resistant mutants as well as other targets such as the nonreceptor tyrosine kinase Src *(24)*. Refinement of technologies, genotyping in particular, have led to the identification of resistant mutations.

Dasatinib is a compound that can successfully overcome acquired resistance in most CML patients. It was first reported to induce hematologic and cytogenetic remissions in a high percentage of imatinib-resistant CML patients in a Phase I trial *(25,26)*. With a potency of more than 300 times that of imatinib, dasatinib is an orally available, selective kinase inhibitor. It differs from imatinib in that it can bind to both the active and inactive conformations of the ABL kinase domain. Dasatinib also inhibits kinases such as Src, KIT, PDGFR, and others. There is only one known mutation of BCR-ABL against which dasatinib is not effective.

Results from a Phase I dose-escalation trial of dasatinib *(27)* demonstrated a complete hematologic response in 37 of 40 patients with chronic-phase CML. Major hematologic responses were seen in 31 of 44 patients with accelerated-phase CML, CML with blast crisis, or Ph-positive ALL. In these two phases, the rates of major cytogenetic response were 45% and 25%, respectively. At a median follow-up of more than 12 months, 95% of patients with chronic-phase disease had a durable response. At a median follow-up of 5 months, 82% of patients with accelerated-phase disease maintained this response. Consistent with preclinical data, all BCR-ABL genotypes with the exception of the T3151 mutation, demonstrated a response. The investigators concluded that dasatinib induces hematologic and cytogenetic responses in patients with CML or Ph-positive ALL who cannot tolerate or are resistant to imatinib.

Based on these results and on initial Phase II data, the FDA granted accelerated approval for dasatinib in June 2006 for patients with CML who demonstrated resistance or intolerance to prior therapy (including imatinib). Full approval was also granted for the treatment of adults with Ph+ ALL (Ph+ALL) with resistance or intolerance to prior therapy.

Recently published Phase II study results confirmed the beneficial effect of dasatinib in imatinib-resistant patients. Results of a randomized Phase II trial of dasatinib or high-dose imatinib for CML after failure of first-line imatinib demonstrated that, with a median follow-up of 15 months, complete hematologic responses were seen in 93% of patients receiving dasatinib versus 82% of patients receiving high-dose imatinib *(28)*. This difference was statistically significant ($p = 0.034$). Also significant was the improvement in cytogenetic response rate (RR) in patients treated with dasatinib (52%) versus those treated with high-dose imatinib (33%) ($p = 0.023$). Patients treated with dasatinib had significantly better molecular RRs and progression-free survival (PFS).

Findings from these studies highlight the importance of genotyping BCR-ABL to predict which patients will respond to treatment. The effectiveness of dasatinib in patients with imatinib-resistant disease also underscores the persistent role of BCR-ABL in disease activity and the need to define further the mechanisms of resistance and the therapies that target this pathway. In the future, genotyping will likely be performed on all CML patients. Genotyping allows the identification, a priori, of patients who will not respond to conventional treatment.

Further studies are needed to determine the role of other abnormalities in resistance. For instance, recent data from our laboratory suggest that some patients with advanced CML demonstrate down-regulation of the loss of Bcr-Abl expression *(29)*.

3.2. Mathematical Modeling as a Tool for Discovery

A quantitative understanding of cancer biology requires devising a mathematical framework that can describe fundamental principles underlying tumor initiation and progression. Tumorigenesis is governed by principles that explain evolution: mutation and selection. An example of the application of mathematical modeling to help streamline the acquisition of knowledge about molecular mechanisms is one developed for evaluating resistant populations in leukemia. A formula has been derived to calculate the probability of resistance by considering an exponentially growing leukemic stem cell population that produces resistant leukemic cells *(30)*. These calculations might be helpful for determining when imatinib therapy ought to be combined with other therapies, provide an accurate prognosis for the disease, and direct future efforts. This model may offer predictive power regarding the course the disease is likely to take.

The interactions between targeted agents and cancer cells is still not well understood. A mathematical approach can help augment molecular biology discoveries. For example, imatinib can be studied using a mathematical model of signaling events in CML cells. Models can elucidate the effects of imatinib on autophosphorylation of the BCR-ABL oncoprotein and subsequent signaling to predict a minimal concentration for drug efficacy. One such model demonstrates that cellular drug clearance mechanisms decrease the value of imatinib in blast crisis cells *(31)*. Michor and colleagues also designed a mathematical model to evaluate the kinetics of CML during treatment with imatinib *(32)*.

A mathematical approach can be applied to the complex interactions among molecular pathways. The possible combinations and permutations are so vast that the traditional methodical, labor-intensive approach of in vitro and in vivo experimentation cannot solve the problems of optimal drug targeting, delivery, and finding effective combinations in an efficient manner. In the future, mathematical modeling and other systems biology approaches will likely be the most feasible way to identify hypotheses that can then be efficiently tested preclinically and entered into early trial design.

3.3. GIST and the Development of Targeted Therapy

The discovery that the c-*kit* gene drives malignant activity in GISTs was exploitable by treatment with imatinib. The success of the treatment of GIST with imatinib provides another example of how biomarker identification predicts clinical response. Once again, the theme of "oncogene dependence" explains an underlying pathogenic mechanism and rationale for clinical evaluation of a targeted drug.

In February 2002, imatinib received accelerated approval by the FDA for use in patients with KIT-positive unresectable or metastatic GISTs. The approval was based on the RR observed in open-label, multinational studies *(33,34)*. Imatinib was subsequently demonstrated to prolong PFS in patients with GISTs *(35)*.

GISTs were rarely diagnosed until around the year 2000, when they became a focus of research. Prefiguring this increased interest was the finding during the late 1990s that gain-of-function mutations of the receptor tyrosine kinase KIT play a major role in the pathogenesis of GISTs. Previously classified as leiomyomas, leiomyosarcomas, and leiomyoblastomas, the term GIST was first used in 1983 *(36)* to describe gastrointestinal nonepithelial neoplasms that lacked the characteristics of smooth muscle cells. Historically, GISTs have been associated with a poor prognosis. The rates of recurrence after surgical resection are high as 90% *(37)*, with a 5-year overall survival (OS) ranging between 28% and 42% *(38)*. GISTs are highly radiation-resistant and chemoresistant. RRs to single-agent or combination chemotherapy have ranged from none to 9% in the presence of metastatic disease *(39–43)*. A combination trial using mesna, doxorubicin, ifosfamide, and dacarbazine reported an objective RR of 22% *(44)*, but these results have been questioned.

Preclinical evidence showed that most GISTs demonstrated gain-of-function mutations in the *KIT* (c-*kit*) proto-oncogene *(45)*. Constitutive activation of KIT in GISTs leads to uncontrolled cell proliferation and resistance to apoptosis *(46)*. GISTs also commonly demonstrate mutations of PDGFRα kinase. Imatinib's known mechanism of inhibition of the tyrosine kinases KIT and PDGFRα provided a rationale for its clinical evaluation in GIST.

In 2000, imatinib was administered for the first time to a GIST patient in a compassionate use setting. In this patient with advanced, heavily pretreated GIST, a dramatic radiographic, metabolic, and symptomatic response was observed at a dose of 400 mg daily *(47)*. The choice of dose was based on evidence of efficacy at this dose level in patients with CML as well as laboratory prediction of effective levels. The patient's liver lesions decreased to less than 25% of the initial tumor burden after 8 months of therapy. Toxicities were minimal. This patient remained in remission for several years before the disease recurred.

Based on the dramatic response in this GIST patient and a solid preclinical rationale (as well as a dearth of effective treatment options), several clinical trials were undertaken. Studies demonstrated that 75% to 90% of patients with advanced GISTs treated with imatinib had a clinical benefit *(33,35,48)*. Several large, randomized, Phase III studies demonstrated prolonged PFS and OS in patients with advanced GISTs *(49,51)*. Imatinib is now the standard of care in patients with metastatic or unresectable disease and has led to prolonged disease-free and OS.

The *KIT* gene encodes the KIT protein, which is the transmembrane receptor for the cytokine stem cell factor. KIT's intracytoplasmic domain functions as a tyrosine kinase. The c-*kit* proto-oncogene product CD117 (KIT) is a transmembrane protein receptor for the growth factor known as stem cell factor (SCF, or Steel factor) *(52)*. CD117 is a more specific marker for GIST than CD34, and it is expressed on 85% to 100% of GIST samples *(53)*. KIT is both a diagnostic marker and a therapeutic target. The malignant behavior of most GISTs can be explained by constitutive activation of KIT. After Hirota and colleagues initially identified the c-*kit* gain-of-function mutations *(45)*, another c-*kit* gene mutation was identified that causes constitutive activation of the ligand *(54)*. More than 100 gain-of-function mutations for c-*kit* have been identified in GISTs *(55,56)*.

These mutations have subsequently been evaluated as both prognostic and predictive markers. The presence of any *kit* mutation has been demonstrated to be an independent prognostic factor, indicating poor prognosis for patients with a localized GIST *(57)*. For example, patients with exon 11 mutations were found to have a 5-year PFS rate of 89% compared to 40% for patients with mutations at other exon sites ($p = 0.03$) *(58)*, thus establishing the presence of an exon 11 mutation as an independent predictor of survival. In the largest series to date, Heinrich and associates *(59)* evaluated 324 tumors of patients enrolled in a Phase II study for *kit* mutations and corresponding response to imatinib. *Kit* mutations were identified in 280 (86.4%) tumors. The presence of exon 11 mutations corresponded to a 67% objective RR, whereas exon 9 mutations corresponded to a 40% objective RR; the absence of any identifiable mutation was associated with a 39% partial RR ($p = 0.0022$.) Time-to-treatment failure was significantly longer for patients with exon 11 mutations compared to any other mutational status (576 days for exon 11 mutations, 308 days for exon 9 mutations, 251 days for no mutation; $p = 0.00112$). Patients with exon 11 mutations also demonstrated a trend toward increased OS compared to other mutations. The authors of this significant study concluded that *kit* mutational status could be used as a predictor of clinical response in patients with GISTs.

Despite high RRs and long duration of response in patients with GISTs treated with imatinib, resistance typically develops after a year of treatment. This acquired resistance is characterized by secondary mutations in the KIT or PDGFRα kinases, gene amplification, or loss of target kinase expression (49,60,61). Approximately 20% of GIST patients have de novo resistance to imatinib.

In January 2006, sunitinib (Sutent) received approval for the treatment of patients with imatinib-refractory (or intolerant) GISTs. Sunitinib is a small-molecule tyrosine kinase inhibitor. It inhibits vascular endothelial growth factor receptors (VEGFRs) types 1 and 2, PDGFRα and PDGFRβ, c-Kit, and the FLT3 and RET kinases. Compared to imatinib, sunitinib demonstrates greater potency against the c-Kit and PDGF kinases and additional inhibition of VEGFR2 and PDGFRβ. This activity may explain its efficacy in imatinib-resistant disease (62,63).

FDA approval was based on an international, randomized, double-blind, placebo-controlled trial of sunitinib in patients with GIST who had disease progression during prior imatinib treatment or who were intolerant of imatinib (64). The study randomized patients to receive sunitinib or placebo, and all patients received best supportive care. Patients who were randomized to placebo were allowed to cross over to receive sunitinib at the time of progression. At the time of the prespecified interim analysis, there was a statistically significant advantage for sunitinib over placebo regarding both time to progression (TTP) and PFS. The median TTP was 27 weeks for patients treated with sunitinib compared to 6 weeks for patients receiving placebo.

This study of sunitinib in GISTs is a good example of how novel targeted therapies may have a cytostatic rather than a cytotoxic effect. Whereas a significant improvement in TTP was noted in patients receiving sunitinib versus placebo, the RR for patients treated with sunitinib was only 7%. Biologic therapies may delay progression (and stabilize disease) without inducing any significant shrinkage in the tumor burden. This underscores a few key issues in the drug development process. Likely due in large part to the high cost associated with the clinical trials, compounds that fail to demonstrate significant activity, defined as an objective response, in the Phase I setting often do not progress further in development to Phase II trials. RR continues, therefore, to be an important endpoint, in a realistic sense, even if it is not necessarily stated as a primary objective in the Phase I trials. Despite a modest objective response, the approval of sunitinib for GISTs was enabled because of its orphan tumor status. For a lack of better therapies, sunitinib was approved because it improved PFS. In fact, because of the crossover design of the study, a valid OS endpoint will never be realized. Similarly, when many of the novel biologic agents are administered as single agents they may be effective only in terms of disease stabilization. For these agents, the challenge will be finding the right combination to further increase efficacy.

4. WHAT IS OLD IS NEW AGAIN: DECITABINE AND THE DAWN OF EPIGENETICS

Increasingly, attention is being focused on epigenetic changes to explain the pathogenesis of cancer. Epigenetic changes are important in both the primary growth of a tumor and the metastatic dissemination and survival of tumor cells (65). Although still in its infancy, epigenetics is an area of intense research. In contrast to genetic mutations that result in permanent alterations in primary DNA sequences, epigenetic mechanisms of gene expression involve reversible alterations in chromatin structure without changes in the primary nucleotide sequence *(66)*. The epigenetic mechanisms that are currently best understood are DNA methylation and histone acetylation, which lead to inactivation of transcription and silencing of tumor suppressor genes.

Hypermethylation inhibits the activation of promoter regions on DNA and subsequently the transcription of tumor suppressor genes. This area presents a rational target for therapy. Epigenetic therapy consists of reversing the silencing of these critical genes. The azacitidine class of drugs, including 5-azacitidine and 5-aza-2-deoxycytidine (decitabine), reverses DNA methylation and therefore prevents inactivation of tumor suppressor genes. The story of the development of these drugs spans more than 40 years and illustrates how the bench to bedside and back paradigm can be successfully implemented. First synthesized during the 1960s *(67)*, the azacitidine family was shown to have activity in hematologic malignancies. It was not until more than 20 years later, however, that the mechanism of action was understood.

Epigenetic changes caused by DNA methylation lead to gene silencing and subsequent malignant transformation. Promoter hypermethylation can inactivate transcription, and genome-wide hypomethylation leads to genomic instability. Both epigenetic phenomena are present in cancer. The potential reversibility of DNA methylation makes this a logical target for cancer treatment. When the promoter region of DNA is methylated, gene expression is inhibited. Transcriptional methylation is mediated by the recruitment of transcription repressors that are part of a large complex, HDACs *(68,69)*. Histone lysine methylation can result in either activation or repression of transcription. Histone modifications therefore promote or prevent binding of proteins and protein complexes that drive particular regions of the genome into active transcription or repression.

The azacitidine and the HDAC inhibitor classes of molecules exploit the epigenetic mechanisms of DNA methylation and histone modification. During the early 1990s, studies of 5-azacitidine in myelodysplastic syndrome (MDS), compared to best standard of care, resulted in improved response, quality of life, and OS *(70–72)*. In 2004, 5-azacitidine received FDA approval for the treatment of MDS.

Decitabine has demonstrated efficacy in leukemias and other hematologic malignancies and has had a low RR in solid tumors *(73)*. Initially shown to have antileukemic activity *(74)*, decitabine was subsequently studied in MDS, AML, and CML patients. Responses were seen for each of these diseases *(75–78)*. In May 2006, the FDA approved decitabine for the treatment of MDS. The approval was based in part on a Phase III trial of MDS patients at medium to high risk of developing AML. Results showed that the addition of decitabine to supportive therapy yielded a significant increase in overall RR compared with supportive therapy alone (17% vs. 0%; $p < 0.001$; CR, 9%; PR, 8%). The median time to response was 93 days, with a median duration of 288 days. Among decitabine-treated patients who had undergone two or more treatment cycles, the overall RR was 21%. Benefit in the form of hematologic improvement was observed in an additional 13% of patients compared with 7% in the supportive care group. Treatment with decitabine did not significantly delay the median time to AML or death.

The uncertainties that remain in terms of decitabine's exact mechanism of action highlight the need for ongoing translational studies from the bedside back to the bench. Although preventing DNA promoter hypermethylation is a rational strategy, it is possible that drugs that prevent methylation could also produce unwanted effects. Decitabine is a cytosine analogue that inhibits DNA methyltransferases (DNMTs), reverses methylation, and can reactivate silenced genes *(79)*. DNA methylation status is determined by a complex mechanism involving interaction among various DNMTs and other enzymes (e.g., HDACs). Decitabine becomes incorporated into DNA and inhibits DNA methylation. It may, however, have more than one mechanism of action. It leads to reactivation of genes that were previously silenced through its demethylation activity, and it may also exert an effect through a cytotoxic pathway. High concentrations of decitabine incorporated into DNA can inhibit DNA synthesis and lead to cell cycle arrest. Low concentrations of decitabine incorporated into DNA in place of cytosine can trap DNA methyltransferases and then lead to DNMT degradation without cell cycle arrest. DNA replication without DNMTs leads to global and gene-specific hypomethylation. Because global hypomethylation can increase the activation of specific genes (e.g., oncogenes), the off-target effects remain controversial and uncertain.

Over the years, decitabine has been studied in escalating doses to the maximum tolerated dose even though in vitro studies demonstrated that optimal methylation occurred at lower doses *(80)*. Not until 2004 was decitabine shown to be more efficacious at a lower dose of 15 mg/m^2, although no correlation was made with DNA methylation after therapy *(81)*. Other recent clinical trials also showed that lower doses have a better response with less toxicity *(82,83)*. In solid tumors, however, higher doses may be desirable to produce a cytostatic effect.

Analysis of molecular response in tumor tissues following exposure to chromatin remodeling agents may enable us to identify novel mechanisms pertaining to cancer epigenetics and design more efficacious regimens. Discoveries in laboratory techniques and assays since the early 1990s have refined the quantification of DNA methylation. Better assays have enabled measurement of global hypomethylation changes before and after administration of decitabine. Hypermethylation of repetitive sequences called long interspersed nucleotide elements (LINE) can be a good pharmacodynamic surrogate of decitabine's hypomethylating activity but not necessarily a biologic surrogate of clinical activity. Results from correlative studies in clinical trials, taken together, provide proof-of-concept that decitabine acts by hypomethylation in hematologic malignancies. Further studies will be undertaken to assess the possibility that decitabine may induce responses in ways other than demethylation.

In contrast to the significant activity of decitabine demonstrated in hematologic malignancies, it produced only limited activity in early Phase II trials of solid tumors (including melanoma, colorectal, head and neck, renal cell, testicular, and ovarian cancers) *(84)*. The difference in clinical activity between hematologic and solid tumors may be explained by several discrete factors, including differences in drug penetration, drug conversion, and the speed of cell cycles. Most of the early clinical trials of decitabine in solid tumors probably did not use high enough dose levels of the drug, and responses were typically evaluated too soon (after only two courses). Subsequent studies showed activity between two to five courses of treatment. Future studies in solid tumors need to incorporate pharmacodynamic endpoints and correlative epigenetic analyses, and they must wait until after completion of three cycles before evaluating patients for response (to assess the objective response accurately).

Further preclinical research since these initial studies has demonstrated a potential benefit of decitabine in solid tumors. The study of epigenetic mechanisms in thoracic oncology, for example, is an area of intense interest and research. In preclinical studies, decitabine is being evaluated for a possible role in increasing the immunogenicity of tumor cells. Decitabine leads to increased expression of the cancer testis antigens (CTAs) NY-ESO-1 and MAGE-3 CTA and restored p16, RASSF1A, and TFPI-2 expression in cultured tissue from thoracic malignancies. CTAs comprise a group of immunogenic tumor-associated antigens that are not expressed in normal tissue (except in male germline cells and placenta). After treatment with decitabine, cancer cells, but not normal human bronchial epithelial cells, can be recognized by cytotoxic T lymphocytes (CTLs) specific for NY-ESO-1 *(85)*.

These preclinical data led to a Phase I proof of concept study *(86)* designed to demonstrate that decitabine exposure can result in CTAs and tumor suppression gene modulation. Although there were no objective clinical responses, disease stabilization was noted in 4 of 25 evaluable patients in this study. One patient remained on study for 10 months, and one remained on study for 1 year before disease progression. Results from correlative studies on tissue biopsies from these patients confirmed previous in vitro studies and the initial hypothesis. Up-regulated mRNA and protein expression of the CTAs NY-ESO-1 and MAGE-3 and p16 were shown in a significant number of patients. The immune response to CTAs is limited in thoracic oncology patients. Conceivably, the up-regulated expression of these antigens could lead to the development of effective immunotherapy strategies.

Induction/repression of gene expression were also studied in an exploratory analysis with decitabine. Although the sample size was limited and did not permit robust statistical outcomes, the feasibility of comprehensive gene expression profiling was demonstrated. The use of RNA amplified from laser-captured tumor cells (from fine-needle aspirations) indicated that exposure to decitabine modulates global gene expression patterns in these thoracic malignancies. Notably, the genes that were induced by decitabine were generally repressed in lung cancers compared to their expression in normal epithelial cells. Conversely, genes that were repressed by decitabine treatment were generally overexpressed by lung cancer cells compared to cells in the normal adjacent tissue.

The rationale for evaluating combinations of epigenetic mechanisms is exemplified by combining DNMT inhibitors with HDAC inhibitors, which leads to a synergistic activation of gene expression. In vitro studies have explored this hypothesis *(87)*, and clinical studies are underway. The DNMT inhibitor azacitidine was evaluated in combination with phenyl-butyrate, an HDAC inhibitor, and showed efficacy in myeloid neoplasms *(88)*. Combining decitabine with valproic acid in patients with AML and MDS resulted in an RR of 22% *(89)*. These studies support further trials of chromatin remodeling agents for cancer immunotherapy, including administration with HDAC inhibitors or recombinant NY-ESO-1 or MAGE-3 protein vaccines and/or infusion of tumor antigen-recognizing CTLs *(90)*.

Decitabine has been in development for four decades. A rigorous translational approach, with studies that continually return from the clinic to the laboratory, has led to the discovery of several key mechanisms of action, including the reactivation of silenced genes and the activation of immunomodulatory genes. Further studies are needed to elucidate other downstream mechanisms that are not yet completely understood. Decitabine's use in solid tumors was initially disappointing, but it is increasingly apparent that it has possible benefit, particularly in combination treatment. Translational medicine continues to generate a greater understanding of its potential use. Epigenetic mechanisms present the hope of being an even more robust source of therapeutic targets than those provided by genetic permutatons.

5. NEW MODEL OF CARCINOGENESIS: CANCER STEM CELL HYPOTHESIS

Research in both hematologic and solid malignancies has demonstrated that only a small percentage of cancer cells have the capacity to form new tumors. Despite a clonal origin, evidence shows that the tumor cell population is, in fact, heterogeneous in terms of capacity for proliferation and differentiation *(91)*. The cancer stem cell hypothesis could explain this heterogeneity. This hypothesis speculates that only a small percentage of cells in the tumor, called cancer stem cells, are able to proliferate and self-renew. Prior to consideration of the role of stem cells, the cancer model was based on unregulated growth attributed to acquired genetic events. Such events result in activation of genes promoting proliferation, silencing of genes that inhibit proliferation, and altered function of genes responsible for programmed cell death.

It was first suggested more than 40 years ago that CML arises from a transformed hematopoietic stem cell. This theory was based on the observation that granulocytes and red blood cells (RBCs) from patients with CML had a common cell of origin *(91)*. Stem cells were isolated a decade and a half ago (with isolated CML stem cells showing expansion ex vivo). More than a decade ago, hematopoietic stem cells from patients with AML or CML generated leukemia in vivo when injected into NOD/SCID mice. More recently, cancer stem cells that are distinct from differentiated cells comprising the bulk of the tumor have been identified in MDS, multiple myeloma, and brain, breast, and lung cancers. The significance of these cancer stem cells is not yet known.

The stem cell hypothesis may help explain the failure of imatinib therapy to cure CML. Whereas imatinib is toxic to differentiated CML progenitor cells, CML stem cells may be resistant to the drug. Hematopoietic stem cells are largely quiescent and typically express high levels of ATP-binding cassette transporters, including the multidrug resistance genes. In CML stem cells, the *BCR-ABL* gene may be silent. It is possible that CML stem cells survive for years even if *BCR-ABL* activity is completely inhibited. The rapid responses seen in patients with CML when imatinib is administered may be explained by imatinib's activity against differentiated CML progenitor cells that constitute most of the leukemia. Not being able to cure CML even with such potent activity is consistent with this hypothesis of stem cell resistance to imatinib. By contrast, the slow, durable responses that were seen occasionally with CML patients treated with interferon (IFN) are explained by data showing activity of IFN against the rare CML stem cells.

Therapy aimed at BCR-ABL activity in CML is an example of a target-directed approach for anticancer therapy. However, drugs that target cancer-specific pathways may not be the ultimate answer. Many cancers, even at the initial diagnosis, have probably already acquired multiple oncogenic mutations that are capable of driving tumor growth. Targeting only one mechanism may have a limited effect. Even a response to therapy may not ultimately predict OS because the response reflects only the targeting of differentiated cells versus stem cells with clonogenic potential.

Properties that are shared with normal stem cells seem to be responsible for cancer stem cell resistance to many therapeutic agents. Targets that share properties with normal stem cells, therefore, may have particularly strong anticancer potential. Examples of these targets include signaling pathways such as Notch, Wnt, and Hedgehog, which are important for the generation and maintenance of normal stem cells during embryonic development. Considering pathways that are involved in the development of normal stem cells raises the question of how it would be possible to develop agents without significant toxicity profiles. Several hypotheses have been offered to explain how normal stem cells may be protected. Normal stem cells have cell cycle checkpoints that can protect them from cellular damage. The stage of differentiation may also constitute a therapeutic ratio; or in other words, the stem cells that engender cancer might not be the most primitive tissue stem cells *(92)*.

Logical too is the possibility of further progress by using therapeutic combinations that lead to both disease stabilization and eradication of cancer stem cells (for potential cure). This paradigm has not been explored adequately in combination studies; however, the emergence in recent years of a rich literature on cancer stem cells, as well as the elucidation of pathways involved with stem cell differentiation will likely lead to future combination trials.

Traditional response criteria measure tumor bulk and may not reflect changes in cancer stem cells. Dramatic responses may occur, but they are unlikely to be maintained over the long term if rare cancer stem cells responsible for maintaining disease are not targeted as well. Standard response criteria may potentially overestimate or underestimate treatment effect on cancer stem cells. It is important to develop validated biomarkers so the potential benefit of biologic agents can be realized before they are abandoned for lack of single-agent, cytotoxic activity.

6. LOOKING FORWARD: THE FUTURE OF TRANSLATIONAL MEDICINE

Personalized medicine has arrived, but this is just the beginning. Further innovation in technologies will contribute to this revolution in drug development. Among the most important aspects of improved drug development will be the identification of pharmacodynamic biomarkers, validating effective early surrogates of tumor response, and the predictive reclassification of disease. Molecular phenotyping prior to selecting a drug is now in widespread use.

The realization of a vision of personalized medicine is complex. Targeted therapies are emerging from our knowledge of the human genome and the use of sophisticated bioinformatics. Targeted imaging agents will be used to deliver therapy. Drug resistance will become more predictable. Newly identified biomarkers will allow earlier measurement of drug effects. Traditional disease categories will continue to be eroded as genetic profiling enables more targeted therapy. Treatment with more selective and less toxic therapies will further redefine the paradigm of cancer as one of a chronic disease model.

It is likely that during the next decade we will focus on eliciting more information from smaller and smaller pieces of tumor tissue. Molecular histopathology will be a core discipline. Eventually, developments in functional imaging and perhaps serum proteomics will drive non-tissue-based methods of obtaining the same information.

Translational medicine has created a language that is used for effective communication between clinical researchers and basic scientists. No longer perceived as a gap, this space between the bench and the bedside is now a robust, interdisciplinary meeting place. The stories behind the development of early targeted therapies—including ATRA, imatinib, and decitabine—provide models and lessons for ongoing discoveries. As the language of translational medicine evolves, the bench to bedside and back paradigm will transform cancer medicine.

REFERENCES

1. Goodman LS, Wintrobe MM, Dameshek W, et al. Nitrogen mustard therapy: use of methyl-bis(beta-chloroethyl)amine hydrochloride and tris(beta-chloroethyl)amine hydrochloride for Hodgkin's disease, lymphosarcoma, leukemia, and certain allied and miscellaneous disorders. JAMA 1946;105:475–6. Reprinted in JAMA 1984;251:2255–61.
2. Hillestad LK. Acute promyelocytic leukemia. Acta Med Scand 1957;159:189–94.

3. Fenaux P, Chevret S, Guerci A, et al. Long-term follow-up confirms the benefit of all-trans retinoic acid in acute promyelocytic leukemia. Leukemia 2000;14:1371–7.

4. Tallman MS, Andersen JW, Schiffer CA, et al. All-trans-retinoic acid in acute promyelocytic leukemia. N Engl J Med 1997;337:1021–8.

5. Zhou GB, Zhao WL, Wang ZY, et al. Retinoic acid and arsenic for treating acute promyelocytic leukemia. PLoS Med 2005;2:e12.

6. Warrell RP Jr, de The H, Wang ZY, et al. Acute promyelocytic leukemia. N Engl J Med 1993;329:177–89.

7. Wang ZY. Ham-Wasserman lecture: treatment of acute leukemia by inducing differentiation and apoptosis hematology. Am Soc Hematol Educ Program 2003;1–13.

8. Weinstein, IB. Cancer: addiction to oncogenes—the Achilles heal of cancer. Science 2002;297:63–4.

9. Tsai S, Collins SJ. A dominant negative retinoic acid receptor blocks neutrophil differentiation at the promyelocyte stage. Proc Natl Acad Sci U S A 1993;90:7153–7.

10. Labrecque J, Allan D, Chambon P, et al. Impaired granulocytic differentiation in vitro in hematopoietic cells lacking retinoic acid receptors alpha1 and gamma. Blood 1998;92:607–15.

11. Warrell RP Jr, Frankel SR, Miller WH, et al. Differentiation therapy of acute promyelocytic leukemia with tretinoin (all-trans-retinoic acid). N Engl J Med 1991;324:1385–93.

12. Avvisati G, Lo Coco F, Mandelli F. Acute promyelocytic leukemia: clinical and morphologic features and prognostic factors. Semin Hematol 2001;38:4–12.

13. Collins SJ. Acute promyelocytic leukemia: relieving repression induced remission. Blood 1998;91:2631–3.

14. Nervi C, Ferrara FF, Fanelli M, et al. Caspases mediate retinoic acid-induced degradation of the acute promyelocytic leukemia PML/RARalpha fusion protein. Blood 1998;92:2244–51.

15. Zhu J, Gianni M, Kopf E, et al. Retinoic acid induces proteasome-dependent degradation of retinoic acid receptor alpha (RARalpha) and oncogenic RARalpha fusion proteins. Proc Natl Acad Sci USA 1999;96:14807–12.

16. Zhu J, Shi XG, Chu HY, et al. Effect of retinoic acid isomers on proliferation, differentiation and PML relocalization in the APL cell line NB4. Leukemia 1995;9:302–9.

17. Salomoni P, Pandolfi PP. The role of PML in tumor suppression. Cell 2002;108:165–70.

18. Shen ZX, Chen GQ, Ni JH, et al. Use of arsenic trioxide (As$_2$O$_3$) in the treatment of acute promyelocytic leukemia (APL). II. Clinical efficacy and pharmacokinetics in relapsed patients. Blood 1997;89:3354–60.

19. Kurzrock R, Shtalrid M, Romero P, et al. A novel C-abl protein product in Philadelphia-positive acute lymphoblastic leukaemia. Nature 1987;325:631–5.

20. Tibes R, Trent J, Kurzrock R. Tyrosine kinase inhibitors and the dawn of molecular cancer therapeutics. Annu Rev Pharmacol Toxicol 2005;45:357–84.

21. Shepherd P, Suffolk R, Halsey J, et al. Analysis of molecular breakpoint and m-RNA transcripts in a prospective randomized trial of interferon in chronic myeloid leukaemia: no correlation with clinical features, cytogenetic response, duration of chronic phase, or survival. Br J Haematol1995;89:546–54.

22. Gorre M, Mohammed M, Ellwood K, et al. Clinical resistance to STI-571 cancer therapy caused by BCR-ABL gene mutation or amplification. Science 2001;293:876–80.

23. Shah NP, Nicoll JM, Nagar B, et al. Multiple BCR-ABL kinase domain mutations confer polyclonal resistance to the tyrosine kinase inhibitor imatinib (ST1571) in chronic phase and blast crisis chronic myeloid leukemia. Cancer Cell 2002;2:1117.

24. Shah NP, Tran C, Lee FY, et al. Overriding imatinib resistance with a novel ABL kinase inhibitor. Science 2004;305:399–401.

25. Sawyers CL, Kantarjian H, Shah N, et al. Dasatinib (BMS-354825) in patients with chronic myeloid leukemia (CML) and Philadelphia-chromosome positive acute lymphoblastic leukemia (Ph+ ALL) who are resistant or intolerant to imatinib: update of a phase I study. Presented at the American Society of Hematology 47th Annual Meeting, 2005. Abstract 38.

26. Sawyers CL, Shah NP, Kantarjian HM, et al. Hematologic and cyogenetic responses in imatinib-resistant chronic phase chronic myeloid leukemia patients treated with the dual SRC/ABL kinase inhibitor BMS-354825: results from a phase I dose escalation study. Presented at the American Society of Hematology 46th Annual Meeting, 2005. Abstract 128.

27. Talpaz M, Shah NP, Kantarjian H, et al. Dasatinib in imatinib-resistant Philadelphia chromosome-positive leukemias. N Engl J Med 2006;35:2531–41.

28. Kantarjian H, Pasquini R, Hamerschlak N, et al. Dasatinib or high-dose imatinib for chronic-phase chronic myeloid leukemia after failure of first-line imatinib: a randomized phase-2 trial. Blood 2007;109:5143–50.

29. Kurzrock R, Talpaz M, Li L, et al. Distinct biological impact of dephosphorylation vs downregulation of p210Bcr-Abl: implications for imatinib mesylate response and resistance. Leuk Lymphoma 2006;47:1651–64.

30. Abbott LH, Michor F, Mathematical models of targeted cancer therapy. Br J Cancer 2006;95:1136–41.

31. Charusanti P, Hu X, Chen L, et al. A mathematical model of BCR-ABL autophosphorylation signaling through the CRKL pathway, and Gleevec dynamics in chronic myeloid leukemia. Discrete Continuous Dynam Syst Ser B 2004;4:99–114.
32. Michor F, Hughes TP, Iwasa Y, et al. Dynamics of chronic myeloid leukemia. Nature 2005;435:1267–70.
33. Demetri GD, von Mehren M, Blanke CD, et al. Efficacy and safety of imatinib mesylate in advanced gastrointestinal stromal tumors. N Engl J Med 2002;347:472–80.
34. Dagher R, Cohen M, Williams G, et al. Approval summary: imatinib mesylate in the treatment of metastatic and/or unresectable malignant gastrointestinal stromal tumors. Clin Cancer Res 2002;8:3034–8.
35. Verweij J, Casali P, Zalcberg J, et al. Progression-free survival in gastrointestinal stromal tumours with high-dose imatinib: randomised trial. Lancet 2004:364:1127–34.
36. Mazur MT, Clark HB. Gastric stromal tumors: reappraisal of histogenesis. Am J Surg Pathol 1983;7:507–19.
37. Ng EH, Pollock RE, Munsell MF, et al. Prognostic factors influencing survival in gastrointestinal leiomyosarcomas: implications for surgical management and staging. Ann Surg 1992;215:68–77.
38. Pierie JP, Choudry U, Muzikansky A, et al. The effect of surgery and grade on outcome of gastrointestinal stromal tumors. Arch Surg 2001;136:383–9.
39. Plaat BE, Hollema H, Molenaar WM, et al. Soft tissue leiomyosarcomas and malignant gastrointestinal stromal tumors: differences in clinical outcome and expression of multidrug resistance proteins. J Clin Oncol 2000;18:3211–20.
40. Ryan DP, Puchalski T, Supko JG, et al. A phase II and pharmacokinetic study of ecteinascidin 743 in patients with gastrointestinal stromal tumors. Oncologist 2002;7:531–8.
41. Edmonson JH, Marks RS, Buckner JC, et al. Contrast of response to dacarbazine, mitomycin, doxorubicin, and cisplatin (DMAP) plus GM-CSF between patients with advanced malignant gastrointestinal stromal tumors and patients with other advanced leiomyosarcomas. Cancer Invest 2002;20:605–12.
42. Trent JC, Beach J, Burgess MA, et al. A two-arm phase II study of temozolomide in patients with advanced gastrointestinal stromal tumors and other soft tissue sarcomas. Cancer 2003;98:2693–9.
43. De Pas T, Casali PG, Toma S, et al. Gastrointestinal stromal tumors: should they be treated with the same systemic chemotherapy as other soft tissue sarcomas? Oncology 2003;64:186–8.
44. Antman K, Crowley J, Balcerzak SP, et al. An intergroup phase III randomized study of doxorubicin and dacarbazine with or without ifosfamide and mesna in advanced soft tissue and bone sarcomas. J Clin Oncol 1993;11:1276–85
45. Hirota S, Isozaki K, Moriyama Y, et al. Gain-of-function mutations of c-kit in human gastrointestinal stromal tumors. Science 1998;279:577–80.
46. Tuveson DA, Willis NA, Jacks T, et al. STI571 inactivation of the gastrointestinal stromal tumor c-KIT oncoprotein: biological and clinical implications. Oncogene 2001;20:5054–8.
47. Joensuu H, Roberts PJ, Sarlomo-Rikala M, et al. Effect of the tyrosine kinase inhibitor ST1571 in a patient with a metastatic gastrointestinal stromal tumor. N Engl Med 2001;344:1052–6.
48. Van Oosterom AT, Judson I, Verweij J, et al. Safety and efficacy of imatinib (STI571) in metastatic gastrointestinal stromal tumours: phase I study. Lancet 2001;358:1421–3.
49. Van Glabbeke M, Verweij J, Casali PG, et al. Initial and late resistance to imatinib in advanced gastrointestinal stromal tumors is predicted by different prognostic factors: a European Organisation for Research and Treatment of Cancer–Italian Sarcoma Group–Australasian Gastrointestinal Trials Group Study. J Clin Oncol 2005;23:5795–804.
50. Rankin C, Mehren MV, Blanke C. Dose effect of imatinib in patients with metastatic GIST: phase III sarcoma group study S0033. J Clin Oncol 2004;22(suppl):819s. Abstract 9005.
51. Verweij J, Casali P, Zalcberg J, et al. Progression-free survival in gastrointestinal stromal tumours with high-dose imatinib: randomised trial. Lancet 2004;364:1127–34.
52. Williams DE, Eisenman J, Baird A, et al. Identification of a ligand for the c-kit proto-oncogene. Cell 1990;63:167–74.
53. Sarlomo-Rikala M, Kovatich AJ, Barusevicius A, et al. CD117: a sensitive marker for gastrointestinal stromal tumors that is more specific than CD34. Mod Pathol 1998;11:728–34.
54. Nakahara M, Isozaki K, Hirota S, et al. A novel gain-of-function mutation of c-kit gene in gastrointestinal stromal tumors. Gastroenterology 1998;115:1090–5.
55. Moskaluk CA, Tian Q, Marshall CR, et al. Mutations of c-kit JM domain are found in a minority of human gastrointestinal stromal tumors. Oncogene 1999;18:1897–902.
56. Hirota S, Nishida T, Isozaki K, et al. Gain-of-function mutation at the extracellular domain of KIT in gastrointestinal stromal tumors. J Pathol 2001;193:505–10.
57. Kim TW, Lee H, Kang YK, et al. Prognostic significance of c-kit mutation in localized gastrointestinal stromal tumors. Clin Cancer Res 2004;10:3076–81.

58. Singer S, Rubin BP, Lux ML, et al. Prognostic value of KIT mutation type, mitotic activity, and histologic subtype in gastrointestinal stromal tumors. J Clin Oncol 2002;20:3898–905.

59. Heinrich MC, Shoemaker JS, Corless CL, et al. Correlation of target kinase genotype with clinical activity of imatinib mesylate in patients with metastatic GI stromal tumors (GISTs) expressing KIT. Proc Am Soc Clin Oncol 2005;23:7. Abstract 7.

60. De Jong FA, Verweij J. Role of imatinib mesylate (Gleevec/Glivac) in gastrointestinal stromal tumors. Expert Rev Anticancer Ther 2003;3:757–66.

61. Weisberg E, Griffin JD. Resistance to imatinib (Glivec): update on clinical mechanisms. Drug Resist Update 2003;6:231–8.

62. Miller KD, Burstein HJ, Elias AD, et al. Phase II study of SU11248, a multi-targeted receptor tyrosine kinase inhibitor (TKI), in patients with previously treated metastatic breast cancer (MBC). J Clin Oncol 2005;23:19s. Abstract 3001.

63. Chen H, Isozaki K, Kinoshita K, et al. Imatinib inhibits various types of activating mutant kit found in gastrointestinal stromal tumors. Int J Cancer 2003;105:130–5.

64. Goodman VL, Rock EP, Dagher R, et al. Approval summary: sunitinib for the treatment of imatinib refractory or intolerant gastrointestinal stromal tumors and advanced renal cell carcinoma. Clin Cancer Res 2007;13:1367–73.

65. Chen W, Cooper TK, Zahnow CA, et al. Epigenetic and genetic loss of Hic1 function accentuates the role of p53 in tumorigenesis. Cancer Cell 2004;6;387–98.

66. Esteller M. Epigenetics provides a new generation of oncogenes and tumour-suppressor genes. Br J Cancer 2006;94:179–83.

67. Pliml J, Sorm F. Synthesis of 2'-deoxy-D-ribofuranosyl-5-azacytosine. Coll Czech Chem Commun 1964;29:2576–7.

68. Fujita N, Takebayashi S, Okumura K, et al. Methylation-mediated transcriptional silencing in euchromatin by methyl-CpG binding protein MBD1 isoforms. Mol Cell Biol 1999;19z:6415–26.

69. Hendrich B, Abbott C, McQueen H, et al. Genomic structure and chromosomal mapping of the murine and human Mbd1, Mbd2, Mbd3, and Mbd4 genes. Mamm Genome 1999;10:906–12.

70. Kornblith AB, Herndon JE, Silverman LR, et al. Impact of azacytidine on the quality of life of patients with myelodysplastic syndrome treated in a randomized phase III trial: a Cancer and Leukemia Group B study. J Clin Oncol 2002;20:2441–52.

71. Silverman LR, Demakos EP, Peterson BL, et al. Randomized controlled trial of azacitidine in patients with the myelodysplastic syndrome: a study of the cancer and leukemia group B. J Clin Oncol 2002;20:2429–40.

72. Silverman LR, Holland JF, Weinberg RS, et al. Effects of treatment with 5-azacytidine on the in vivo and in vitro hematopoiesis in patients with myelodysplastic syndromes. Leukemia 1993;7:21–9.

73. Aparicio A, Eads CA, Leong LA, et al. Phase I trial of continuous infusion 5-aza-2'-deoxycytidine. Cancer Chemother Pharmacol 2003;51:231–9.

74. Sorm F, Vesely J. Effect of 5-aza-2'-deoxycytidine against leukemic and hemopoietic tissues in AKR mice. Neoplasma 1968;15:339–43.

75. Wijermans P, Lübbert M, Verhoef G, et al. Low-dose 5-aza-2'-deoxycytidine, a DNA hypomethylating agent, for the treatment of high-risk myelodysplastic syndrome: a multicenter phase II study in elderly patients. J Clin Oncol 2000;18:956–62.

76. Kantarjian H, Oki Y, Garcia-Manero G, et al. Results of a randomized study of 3 schedules of low-dose decitabine in higher-risk myelodysplastic syndrome and chronic myelomonocytic leukemia. Blood 2007;109:52–7.

77. Kantarjian H, Issa JP, Rosenfeld CS, et al. Decitabine improves patient outcomes in myelodysplastic syndromes: results of a phase III randomized study.Cancer 2006;106:1794–803.

78. Kantarjian HM, O'Brien S, Cortes J, et al. Results of decitabine (5-aza-2' deoxycytidine) therapy in 130 patients with chronic myelogenous leukemia. Cancer 2003;98:522–8.

79. Issa JP. Decitabine. Curr Opin Oncol 2003;15:446–51.

80. Driscoll JS, Marquez VE, Plowman J, et al. Antitumor properties of 2(1H)-pyrimidinone riboside (zebularine) and its fluorinated analogues. J Med Chem 1991;34,3280–4.

81. Issa JP, Garcia-Manero G, Giles FJ, et al. Phase 1 study of low-dose prolonged exposure schedules of the hypomethylating agent 5-aza-2'-deoxycytidine (decitabine) in hematopoietic malignancies. Blood 2004;103:1635–40.

82. Issa JP, Gharibyan V, Cortes J, et al. Phase II study of low-dose decitabine in patients with chronic myelogenous leukemia resistant to imatinib mesylate. J Clin Oncol 2005;23:3948–56.

83. Lubbert M, Daskalakis M, Kunzmann R, et al. Nonclonal neutrophil responses after successful treatment of myelodysplasia with low-dose 5-aza-2'-deoxycytidine (decitabine). Leuk Res 2004;28:1267–71.

84. Aparicio A, Weber JS. Review of the clinical experience with 5-azacytidine and 5-aza-2'-deoxycytidine in solid tumors. Curr Opin Invest Drugs 2002;3:627–33.

85. Weiser T, Guo ZS, Ohnmacht GA, et al. Sequential 5-aza-2'-deoxycytidine-depsipeptide FR901228 treatment induces apoptosis preferentially in cancer cells and facilitates their recognition by cytolytic T lymphocytes specific for NY-ESO-1. J Immunother 2001;24:151–61.

86. Schrump DS, Fischette MR, Nguyen DM, et al. Phase I study of decitabine-mediated gene expression in patients with cancers involving the lungs, esophagus, or pleura. Clin Cancer Res 2006;12:5777–85.

87. Cameron EE, Bachman KE, Myöhänen S, et al. Synergy of demethylation and histone deacetylase inhibition in the re-expression of genes silenced in cancer. Nat Genet 1999;21:103–7.

88. Gore SD, Baylin S, Sugar E, et al. Combined DNA methyltransferase and histone deacetylase inhibition in the treatment of myeloid neoplasms. Cancer Res 2006;66:6361–9.

89. Garcia-Manero G, Kantarjian HM, Sanchez-Gonzalez B, et al. Phase 1/2 study of the combination of 5-aza-2'-deoxycytidine with valproic acid in patients with leukemia. Blood 2006;108:3271–9.

90. Rudek MA, Zhao M, He P, et al. Pharmacokinetics of 5-azacitidine administered with phenylbutyrate in patients with refractory solid tumors or hematologic malignancies. J Clin Oncol 2005;23:3906–11.

91. Jordan CT. Cancer stem cell biology: from leukemia to solid tumors. Curr Opin Cell Biol 2004;16:708–12.

92. Bedi A, Zehnbauer BA, Collector MI, et al. BCR-ABL gene rearrangement and expression of primitive hematopoietic progenitors in chronic myeloid leukemia. Blood 1993;81:2898–902.

2 Targeted Therapy in Acute Myelogenous Leukemia

Elihu Estey, MD

CONTENTS

ABSTRACT

This chapter explores the antiacute myelogenous leukemia effects of various targeted therapies. It discusses combinations of targeted therapies with each other and particularly with chemotherapy. The extent to which a "targeted therapy's" target is known a priori and the adequacy of relevant trial designs are discussed along with the relevance of new criteria for response, which patients are candidates for targeted therapy, and the appropriateness of conventional statistical methodology. The utility of identifying the "maximum tolerated" dose and emphasis on single-arm, Phase II trials followed by large randomized trials versus alternative methods such as a focus on the "optimal biologic" dose, more adaptive single-arm designs, and smaller randomized trials are also covered.

Key Words: Acute myelogenous leukemia, Targeted therapy, ATRA and arsenic trioxide gemtuzumab, FLT-3 inhibitors, Farnesyl transferase inhibitors, Epigenetic-acting agents, Clinical trial design

1. INTRODUCTION

The only therapy known to produce long-term survival of patients with acute myelogenous leukemia (AML) is "chemotherapy," generally containing cytosine arabinoside (ara-C). Such therapy is itself targeted; that is, if there were no selectivity of a given chemotherapy for

From: *Current Clinical Oncology: Targeted Cancer Therapy*
Edited by: R. Kurzrock and M. Markman © Humana Press, Totowa, NJ

malignant cells vis à vis their normal counterparts, disease remission and prolonged survival would not occur. For the purposes of this discussion, targeted therapy refers to a treatment that is less toxic to normal cells than chemotherapy, particularly cells in the bone marrow, oral cavity, gastrointestinal epithelia, and lung. Because damage to those cells is usually responsible for treatment-related death (TRD) in patients with AML, rates of TRD are typically lower with targeted therapy than with chemotherapy. However, a reduction in TRD from the use of targeted therapy is obviously insufficient to improve long-term outcome in AML unless accompanied by an anti-AML effect that is, at worst, only slightly less and, at best, considerably greater than that seen after chemotherapy.

This chapter explores the extent to which the desired anti-AML effects have been observed with various targeted therapies. It discusses combinations of targeted therapies with each other and, particularly, with chemotherapy. Discussion of the latter is topical because several targeted agents—e.g., gemtuzumzab ozogamycin (a recombinant, humanized anti-CD33 monoclonal antibody), midostaurin (a synthetic indolocarbazole protein kinase C, or PKC, inhibitor), and lestaurtinib (an orally bioavailable indolocarbazole derivative with antineoplastic properties)—are seemingly most effective when given in conjunction with chemotherapy. Interspersed throughout the chapter are informal discussions of several general issues (e.g., the extent to which a "targeted therapy's" target is known a priori, the adequacy of relevant trial designs). The chapter concludes with a more formal consideration of these and other issues that have come to the forefront consequent to the use of targeted therapy. They include the relevance of new criteria for response (e.g., complete response with incomplete platelet recovery, and hematologic improvement), which patients are candidates for targeted therapy, and the appropriateness of conventional statistical methodology, such as identification of the "maximum tolerated" dose and emphasis on single-arm, Phase II trials followed by large randomized trials versus alternative methods (e.g., focus on the "optimal biologic" dose, more adaptive single-arm designs, and smaller randomized trials).

2. ATRA AND ATO IN APL

Targeted therapy's most striking success has come from administration of all-*trans* retinoic acid (ATRA), arsenic trioxide (ATO), and particularly ATO + ATRA to treat acute promyelocytic leukemia (APL). The original rationale for treating APL with ATRA was its in vitro activity as a "differentiating agent *(1)*". This ability was found to be paralleled clinically by a clinical remission (CR) rate of 80% to 90% in untreated APL, with the CR (< 5% abnormal promyelocytes and blasts in the marrow, platelet and neutrophil counts > 100,000 and 1000/μl, respectively) not preceded by marrow aplasia but by differentiation of promyelocytes into myelocytes/metamyelocytes and eventually neutrophils. In 20% of cases there is a substantial increase (e.g., to > 50,000) in the number of circulating mature myeloid cells, often accompanied by fever, effusions, edema, and lung infiltrates, constituting an "APL differentiation syndrome" (APLDS, previously "ATRA syndrome" but now recognized to occur after ATO as well) *(2)*. The pathogenesis of the APLDS is thought to involve ATRA-mediated up-regulation of CD38 on the surface of blood cells and subsequent binding of these cells to epithelial cells with consequent cytokine release. Binding seems to involve interaction between CD38 and CD31, the latter found on the surface of epithelial cells. Steroids are highly effective in the treatment of APLDS.

Remissions induced and maintained by single-agent ATRA are transient, typically lasting only several months. This observation motivated combining ATRA with chemotherapy.

Early trials randomly assigned untreated patients to chemotherapy without ATRA or to induction therapy with ATRA followed by chemotherapy once the patient was in CR. These trials found that ATRA, while having little effect on the CR rate, substantially increased relapse-free survival (RFS). For example, Fenaux et al. reported a probability of relapse 1 year after attainment of CR at 40% ± 12% in patients given ATRA + daunorubicin + ara-C (DA) vs. 19% ± 8% in patients given DA, thus prompting early termination of the trial (3). Subsequent randomized trials suggested that ATRA should be combined with chemotherapy, both at diagnosis and during postremission therapy (4). This approach is now standard therapy for untreated APL and can be expected to cure > 90% of patients who present with a white blood cell (WBC) count < 10,000 and 70% to 80% of patients presenting with higher WBC counts (5).

Given for prolonged periods, ATRA induces its own metabolism with decreased serum tretinoin concentrations despite a constant ATRA dose. This decline was hypothesized to account for resistance to single-agent ATRA and led to the design of a liposomal preparation that could be given by vein with the intent of circumventing "first-pass" hepatic metabolism. Indeed, Estey et al. found that 10 of 34 untreated patients [29%, 95% confidence interval (CI) 15%–47%] given liposomal ATRA monotherapy remained in CR for a median 4.5 years (range 3.0–5.5 years), a result that seemed unlikely had patients received monotherapy with oral ATRA and suggesting that APL was curable with targeted therapy (6). However, although liposomal ATRA undoubtedly produced increased areas under the curve (AUC) of serum tretinoin concentration versus time, the relation between the AUC and the response to liposomal ATRA was not systematically explored. Nonetheless, it was clear that some patients had substantial remissions despite relatively low AUCs and vice versa.

Clinical results with ATRA were already apparent when an explanation became available for its ability to differentiate APL cells but not, at least clinically, other types of AML cells (1). In particular, in more than 95% of cases, APL results from a chromosomal translocation, t(15; 17). This translocation produces a fusion protein PML/RARα, the gene for PML being located on chromosome 15 and the gene for RARα on chromosome 17. The PML-RARα protein is an aberrant form of the normal retinoic acid receptor (RARα) that, unlike RARα, attracts "co-repressor" complexes that interfere with gene transcription. The preferential binding of PML-RARα to DNA results in a "dominant negative" effect in which normal RARα (from the remaining normal chromosome 17 moiety) can no longer facilitate transcription of genes involved in promyelocytic differentiation. Pharmacologic doses of ATRA release co-repressor complexes and lead to degradation of PML-RARα, resulting in resumption of transcription. Zhou et al. identified missense mutations in the ATRA-binding domain of PML-RARα (7) that were associated with resistance to ATRA. Hence, resistance to ATRA may occur both pharmacologically and through mutations in ATRA's target, PML-RARα.

Trials of ATO in APL were largely inspired by arsenic's role in traditional Chinese medicine. Chinese investigators randomly assigned untreated patients to receive ATRA, ATO, or ATO + ATRA. Once in CR, these patients were treated with chemotherapy plus the original induction regimen (8). There was a sevenfold reduction in PML-RARα transcript number at the time of CR in the ATRA group, a 32-fold reduction in the ATO group, and a 119-fold reduction in the ATO + ATRA group, which also produced the highest RFS rate. Matthews et al. reported a 86% CR rate in 72 untreated patients given single-agent ATO, a rate similar to that expected with single-agent ATRA, as well as, at a median follow-up of 25 months, an 87% ± 5% probability of RFS at 3 years, a decidedly higher response rate than expected with ATRA ATRA *(9)*. These results clearly indicate that ATO is effective than ATRA in untreated APL.

Like the Chinese investigators, Estey et al. combined ATO + ATRA in untreated patients *(10)*. These patients were divided into low risk (WBC count < 10,000, 41 patients) and high risk. Unlike the Chinese, other agents [here, gemtuzumab ozogamycin (GO), Mylotarg] were given to low-risk patients only if a polymerase chain reaction (PCR)-based test for PML-RARα remained, or reverted to, positive (molecular relapse) after treatment with ATO + ATRA. High-risk patients received ATO + ATRA + GO for induction and in CR. The most interesting results were in the low-risk patients (Fig. 1). Of the 41 patients, 38 went into CR; and, strikingly, with a median follow-up of 1.5 years, none of the 38 has had a molecular or hematologic relapse, thus requiring continued GO or anthracyclines. Ten patients have been followed in CR for 1 to 2 years, eight for 2 to 3 years, and five for 3 to 4 years. At least in the past, the probability of relapse of APL patients declined sharply once the patients had been in CR for 2 years—in contrast to CML where relapses (e.g., after imatinib) occurred over a longer period of time.

Accordingly, it seems fair to say that the combination of ATO + ATRA serves as perhaps the best example of the potential of targeted therapy in leukemia. The Italian Cooperative Group GIMEMA is currently randomizing low-risk patients under age 70 to ATO + ATRA or ATRA + chemotherapy. Older patients are receiving ATO + ATRA; these patients have had a 15% to 20% TRD rate with postremission chemotherapy.

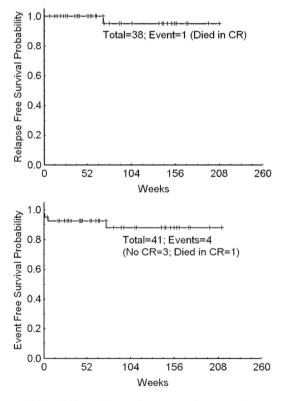

Fig. 1. a Relapse-free survival in 38 low-risk patients entering complete response (CR) after arsenic trioxide (ATO) plus all-trans retinoic acid (ATRA): ATO + ATRA. **b** Event-free survival in 41 low-risk patients given ATO + ATRA. PS, performance status; B2M, β_2-microglobulin.

The most notable toxicity of ATO + ATRA is the APLDS, although, bearing in mind the somewhat vague criteria for its diagnosis, the incidence does not appear different than seen after ATRA or ATO when used alone. A distinctive toxicity of ATO is cardiac arrhythmia, usually atrial in origin, for which African Americans appear to have a predilection (11). It should be noted that long-term toxicities of ATO + ATRA are less defined than those following ATRA + chemotherapy. Nonetheless, depending on results of the GIMEMA trial, there is a possibility that ATO + ATRA will become standard treatment, at least for low-risk patients, particularly those > age 60.

3. AGENTS TARGETING CD33

About 85% of cases of AML are "CD33 positive," meaning that the surface antigen CD33 is present on > 20% of a patient's blast cells. The apparent lack of CD33 expression on nonhematopoietic cells spurred interest in drugs that target CD33.

3.1. Lintuzumab

Lintuzumab is a humanized, recombinant anti-CD33 monoclonal antibody unlinked to a toxin. It is an effective anti-APL agent, although its use in APL has been superseded by the use of gemtuzumab (see below). For example, lintuzumab produced polymerase chain reaction (PCR) "negativity" in 11 of 22 patients with APL who remained PCR-"positive" in hematologic clinical remission (CR) following chemotherapy (12). Its success in APL seems plausibly explained by the fact that most APL promyelocytes express large amounts of CD33 on their surface. In contrast, lintuzumab's effectiveness in more common types of AML, which are less "CD33-positive" than APL and in which the AML stem cell is thought to be CD33-negative, has been more difficult to demonstrate. In particular, Feldman et al. randomized 191 patients with AML in their first relapse after a CR that had lasted less than 1 year or who had not entered CR following chemotherapy ± lintuzumab (13). Patients who entered CR initially assigned. The study had 80% power at a two-sided α level of 0.05 to detect an improved CR rate from the expected 20% with chemotherapy to 40% with addition of lintuzumab. CR rates were 29% (27/94) in the arm with lintuzumab versus 23% (22/97) in the arm without ($p = 0.41$), with an exact 95% confidence interval (CI) for the true difference in CR rates [–0.20, 0.08], a more useful post hoc statistic than "power," indicating that a difference of 12% was as beneficial as no difference. There was no difference in survival (median 5 months in each arm). However, given the low CR rates, a difference would have been difficult to demonstrate. Thus, lintuzumab might be more productively explored in patients with untreated AML (as has been done with gemtuzumab), where higher CR rates would be expected, as well as in patients in CR, a topic to which I return later. Plans for a trial in untreated patients are in progress.

3.2. Gemtuzumab Ozogamycin (Mylotarg)

Gemtuzumab (GO) consists of an anti-CD33 monoclonal antibody that is linked to an intercalating agent, calicheamycin. As with lintuzumab, GO's signal success as a single agent has been in APL, reflecting both the high density of CD33 expression in APL noted earlier and the APL cell's lack of the multidrug resistance gene protein (MDR1), responsible for expelling drugs such as calicheamycin from cells. As suggested by an M. D. Anderson trial, the effectiveness of GO + ATRA in low-risk, untreated APL patients is probably similar to that of ATO + ATRA(14) (Fig. 2). In patients with high-risk APL, the GO + ATO + ATRA

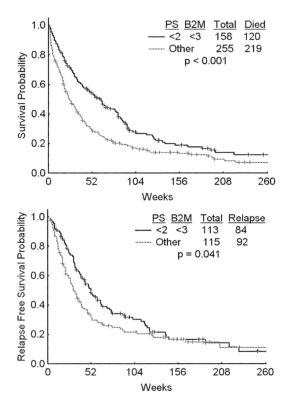

Fig. 2. Survival and relapse-free survival probabilities according to performance status and serum β_2-migroglubulin level in patients age ≥ 60 years given standard regimens at M. D. Anderson over the last decade. The data suggest that although standard therapy might be appropriate for the better group it is not the optimal therapy for the worse one.

combination appears the most effective of those we investigated, for example, producing a CR rate of 15 of 19 (79%) versus 18 of 28 (64%) for a standard chemotherapy + ATRA induction regimen (exact 95% CI for the true difference [–0.46, 0.15] consistent with a true difference of 30% being as plausible as no difference); differences in event-free survival are similar but are confounded because only the GO + ATO + ATRA group received ATRA in CR. The U.S. Intergroup (SWOG + CALGB + ECOG) trial is currently investigating GO + ATO + ATRA in high-risk, untreated APL patients. GO has also been used to treat APL during molecular relapse after ATRA + chemotherapy. For example, Lo Coco et al. reported that 14 of 16 such cases achieved molecular remission after receiving GO, with 8 of the 16 patients being in at least a second relapse, and that survival was prolonged if patients were treated at molecular, in contrast to hematologic, relapse relapse *(15)*. The latter observation is confounded by that the interval from molecular relapse to death is longer than the interval from hematologic relapse to death even without treatment. Nonetheless, given the minimal toxicity of GO in APL, pretrial benefit/risk ratios would not putatively be the same were patients in molecular relapse to be randomized between immediate treatment with GO and delaying treatment until hematologic relapse. Hence, it is difficult to advocate such a trial; instead, patients in molecular relapse of APL are candidates for ATO or GO.

Like lintuzumab, single-agent GO seems much less effective in other types of AML. The U.S. Food and Drug Administration (FDA) approved GO for use in patients age ≥ 60 years with relapsed AML largely on the basis of a study of 142 patients, median age 61 years, in their first relapse after a minimum duration of a first CR months *(16)*. The CR rate was 16%; no data for survival survival in all 142 patients were provided. An additional 14% of patients had bone marrow with <5% blasts and neutrophil counts >1000 cells/mm^3 (marrow and neutrophil criteria for CR), together with a platelet count of 30,000 to 100,000/mm^3, which, although obviating the need for platelet transfusions, was below the 100,000/mm^3 required for a designation of CR. The response in these patients was deemed CRp; and although the longer time needed to achieve CRp than CR or the possibility that CR and CRp patients differed with regard to important covariates that influence survival (e.g., duration of first CR, performance status), were not taken into account, survival appeared similar for CR and CRp patients. Additionally, although myelosuppression was similar to that seen with standard chemotherapy and the incidence of severe (grade 3–4) hyperbilirubinemia was relatively high (23%), the rates of severe infection (28%), mucositis (4%), and nausea/vomiting (11%) were relatively low; and treatment was often in an outpatient setting. Subsequently, hyperbilirubinemia following GO was often found to result from a sinusoidal obstructive syndrome (SOS), formerly hepatic venoocclusive disease caused by the presence of CD33 on sinusoidal cells *(17)*. Development of the syndrome was of particular concern given that SOS also complicates allogeneic stem cell transplant (SCT), a procedure that might be used after GO, particularly if a CR or CRp followed use of the latter. However, Wadleigh et al. found that if more than 3 to 4 months elapsed between GO and SCT the incidence of SOS was reduced (9/10 in patients receiving SCT <3.5 months after GO vs. 0/4 in patients given transplants >3.5 months after GO) *(18)*.

The FDA approval has almost certainly increased the number of patients receiving GO regardless of age. However, the absence of randomized trials has made it difficult to know if GO is preferable to more standard regimens, particularly those containing ara-C. This issue was examined in a multivariate analysis in which treatment (ara-C-containing as given at M.D. Anderson 128 patients vs. GO 128 patients in the multicenter trial that led to FDA approval), duration of the first CR, age, and cytogenetics were examined as potential predictors of response. Leopold et al. found that GO appeared superior to ara-C in patients with first CR durations of less than a 1 year, particularly if at age >75 years, whereas ara-C demonstrated superiority in patients with longer CR durations, particularly if age <45 years *(19)*. The observation that GO was more effective in one prognostic group and ara-C in another suggests that the drugs may be qualitatively different, providing a rationale for combining them, as described below. Such combinations would seem of particular use given that neither standard ara-C-containing regimens nor single-agent GO is adequate treatment for relapsed AML. The same appears true in older patients with untreated AML. Accordingly, Estey et al. found that after accounting for prognosis and effects due to a lack of randomization the probability was <1% (abnormal cytogenetics) and 15% (normal cytogenetics) that survival was longer if GO (51 patients age >65), rather than idarubicin + ara-C (31 similarly aged patients), was given as the initial treatment *(20)*. Using the conventional 9 mg/m^2 dose on days 1 and 15 schedule, Amadori et al. reported a CR + CRp rate of 17% (95% CI 8%–32%) in 40 patients age ≥60 years *(21)*. Hence, despite the attention given GO-induced SOS, this author believes that single-agent GO's principal shortcoming is that it is no more effective than standard chemotherapy.

However, observing the modicum of single-agent activity prompted several groups to combine standard therapy with GO after identifying GO doses that seem to be associated with little risk of adding to the toxicity of standard therapy or of SOS, typically 3 mg/m^2 on day 1. Most notably, Burnett et al. randomized 1115 untreated patients age <60 years to various standard chemotherapies ± GO 3 mg/m^2 on day 1 *(22)*. CR rates were similar (85%). Although with a median follow-up of 15 months, there has been no difference in deaths during CR, relapse was reduced in the GO group, resulting in improved ($p = 0.008$) RFS; specifically 3-year RFS rates were 40% with and 51% without GO. The beneficial effect of GO was seen principally in patients with favorable or intermediate cytogenetics, in whom there was also a trend for longer survival. There was also more mucositis in the GO arm, suggesting that the effect of GO merely reflected administration of "more chemotherapy." Arguing against this possibility, however, the effect of GO was similar with DA/standard dose ara-C ("3+7") and with FLAG-Ida [fludarabine/cytarabine/granulocyte colony stimulating factor (G-CSF)/idarubicin], a regimen that uses higher ara-C doses. The Burnett et al. results are the most striking yet obtained with any new agent in untreated AML, and U.S. groups are attempting to reproduce these results. Korean investigators have also reported favorable results with 3+7 + GO combinations in older patients compared to historical controls given 3+7 *(23)*.

4. IODINE-131 ANTI-CD45 ANTIBODY

Expression of CD45 is limited to myeloid and lymphoid cells. However, because CD45 is found on both malignant and normal cells, it is most readily targeted in conjunction with SCT, the objective being to reduce the risk of relapse, which constitutes the primary cause of failure after SCT. Pagel et al. added iodine-131-labeled anti-CD45 antibody to a busulfan + cyclophosphamide (BuCy) preparative regimen and, after accounting for prognosis, found that the risk of death in the 59 patients thus treated was 65% (95% CI 0.39–1.08, $p = 0.09$) of that seen in 509 previous patients given BuCy alone *(24)*. This result is likely to encourage a randomized trial comparing BuCy ± iodine-131/anti-CD45 antibody.

5. FLT3 INHIBITORS

FLT3 is tyrosine kinase (TK). The gene coding for FLT3 demonstrates two types of mutation: those that affect the gene's length through "internal tandem duplications" (ITDs) and point mutations that affect the TK activation loop *(25)*. Both make FLT3 TK constitutively active, with a resulting survival and/or proliferative advantage conferred on the mutant cells. Development of drugs that inhibit aberrant FLT3 TK was encouraged by the unfavorable effect on RFS seen in patients with FLT3 ITD (but not point mutations), most of whom have a normal karyotype and would be otherwise considered to belong to an intermediate-prognosis group group *(26–28)*. The effect on the status of FLT3 is, however, altered by the presence or absence of aberrations in the NPM, CEBPA, and MLL genes and by overexpression or underexpression of BAALC and ERG *(29)*. Furthermore, in approximately one in five cases, a discordance has been noted between FLT3 status (aberrant or wild type) at diagnosis and at relapse, suggesting that FLT3 does not play a crucial role in AML pathogenesis *(30)*.

As with GO, FLT3 inhibitors appear to be much more effective when used in combination with standard chemotherapy than when used alone. Midostaurin (PKC412) and lestaurtinib (CEP-701) are the inhibitors that have received most attention; each is generally taken orally for 21 to 28 days per cycle. Stone et al. reported one CR among 10 patients with relapsed disease (duration of prior CR not specified), seven with refractory AML (never in CR), and three with untreated AML given single-agent midostaurin *(31)*; each of the 20 patients had a FLT3 ITD or point mutation. Similarly, none of 29 untreated patients given single-agent lestaurtinib because of age >70 years (25 patients) or age 60 to 70 years with performance status > 2 or significant heart disease (4 patients) achieved CR (although 3 of 5 patients with a FLT3 ITD or point mutation had a transient decrease in blasts versus 5 of 22 patients with wild-type FLT3) FLT3) *(32)*. In contrast, a combination of midostaurin 3+7 in untreated patients produced a CR rate of 11 of 12 patients if a FLT3 aberration was present and 18 of 26 patientsif it was not *(33)*. Assuming an 80% CR rate in patients with 3+7 alone, the probability of observing ≥ 11 CRs in 12 patients is 28% (i.e., $p = 0.28$). Nonetheless, these results have prompted the U.S. Intergroup to undertake a soon-to-be-initiated large randomized trial of 3+7 $\pm$ midostaurin in untreated patients with FLT3 ITDs or point muations; such a trial will take several years to complete. Similarly, the British NCRI (formerly the Medical Research Council) will compare 3+7 $\pm$ lestaurtinib in untreated patients.

Determining which patients are likely to respond to a given targeted therapy has importance for specific patients and for evaluation of specific targeted agents, as can be seen from the debate about whether and which patients with wild-type FLT3 should be eligible for trials of FLT3 inhibitors. Levis et al. assessed the relation between a clinical response to midostaurin or lestaurtinib and the ability of plasma taken as soon as 2 days after treatment begins to inhibit FLT3 compared to the inhibitory activity of pretreatment plasma *(34)*. Altogether, 11 of 16 patients whose plasma inhibitory activity (PIA) was at least 85% showed a clinical response versus 0 of 8 with PIA <85%. In principle, results from the PIA assay could be used either to increase the dose of a FLT3 inhibitor or withdraw patients from a trial of such an inhibitor. Using cell lines and primary samples from patients, the authors found that lestaurtinib was both more cytotoxic than midostaurin and less specific for FLT3, a property it shared with a metabolite of midostaurin, CGP52412. These results suggest that the "off-target effects" of targeted therapy must be considered when planning trials with these agents.

6. FARNESYL TRANSFERASE INHIBITORS

Protein farnesylation, a chemical reaction catalyzed by protein farnesyl transferase (FT), has important roles in membrane association and protein–protein interactions among various eukaryotic proteins. The development of FT inhibitors (FTIs) is instructive regarding the dangers of assuming a mechanism of action for a "targeted therapy." RAS is a substrate for farnesylation, and RAS mutations occur in 10% to 20% of patients with AML *(35)*. Hence, FTIs were initially viewed as "RAS inhibitors." However, there is little to indicate a higher response rate to FTIs in patients with RAS mutations. In fact, although many proteins are substrates for farnesylation, the ones critical to FTI's effects are unknown. Indeed, the association between inhibition of FT and response to FTI is somewhat tenuous. Thus, although Lancet et al. (described two paragraphs below) noted a response in 7 of 43 versus 0 of 16 ($p = 0.11$) according to whether farnesylation was inhibited, mononuclear cells rather than blasts per se were used to assay FT inhibition.

Tipifarnib, the principal FTI studied in AML patients, has been administered in relapsed/refractory and untreated disease. Harousseau et al. found that 6 of 135 patients with relapsed AML (50% in first relapse, median duration of first CR not provided) and 3 of 117 with refractory AML given tipifarnib 600 mg orally twice daily for 21 days in 4-week cycles achieved CR; an additional 2 patients achieved CRp *(36)*. Questions have arisen about the need to treat this number of patients before concluding that the drug was not particularly active in this setting. Answers to such questions depend on the desired response rate, which in turn depends on the response rate in some control groups given more standard therapies. However, not infrequently, trials of targeted therapy do not specify a formal, even historical, control group, making it difficult to judge their clinical utility.

Lancet et al. gave tipifarnib 600 mg twice daily by mouth to 158 patients with untreated AML judged to be poor candidates for standard therapy because they were either age ≥ 65 years, had "unfavorable" cytogenetics, had an antecedent hematologic disorder, or had received prior cytotoxic therapy for another disease. The CR rate was 14%, and median survival was 5.3 months months *(37)*. To estimate how these results might compare those seen with standard therapy, Estey et al. (unpublished) compared survival times between 140 of the 158 patients in the above-mentioned Lancet et al. trial who were age ≥ 65 years and untreated patients age ≥ 65 years treated at M. D. Anderson (MDA) with intermediate-dose ara-C + idarubicin (IA) ($n = 124$ patients) or + agents other than idarubicin (XA) ($n = 49$ patients). Because there was no randomization between tipifarnib and IA or XA, comparisons were confounded by center effects (five centers in the tipifarnib trial versus MDA). This motivated use of Bayesian sensitivity analyses accounting for hypothetical between-center effects as well as age, performance status, cytogenetics, and whether AML was de novo or secondary. These analyses suggested that although the odds were 7:1 that use of tipifarnib was associated with shorter survival than use of IA or XA it was nonetheless plausible (95% credible interval for relative risk included 1.0) that survival with tipifarnib was in fact longer than with IA or XA. From a purely medical perspective, the magnitude of the difference in survival was sufficiently small that a case could be made for use of tipifarnib, given its greater convenience.

Of course, this type analysis ignores the obvious point that tipifarnib (or other targeted therapies) will be used in combination even if ineffective as single agents when compared to standard therapy. Nonetheless, I believe that single-arm trials administering experimental therapies to patients with AML should include interim comparison of survival times with those obtainable with other therapies, including other experimental therapies. This can forestall situations where large numbers of patients are given relatively ineffective treatments. Randomized Phase II trials to avoid treatment-trial confounding may be desirable.

7. EPIGENETIC THERAPY

7.1. Hypomethylating Agents (Azacitidine and Decitabine)

7.1.1. STANDARD DOSES

Azacitidine has been used in the treatment of hematologic malignancies for almost 40 years. In 1976, Von Hoff et al. reported that the drug produced a response rate of 36% and a CR rate of 20% in patients with previously treated AML *(38)*; and in the early 1990s, Silverman et al. described activity in myelodysplasia (MDS) *(39)*. Resurgence of interest in azacitidine and the related drug decitabine (DAC) has paralleled realization of the importance of "epigenetics" in cancer *(40)*. Epigenetics refers to changes that affect gene expression (e.g., during fetal development). One such change involves the methylation status of CpG-rich sequences in the genome. Specifically, hypermethylation leads to inhibition of gene expression. Hypermethylation is functionally equivalent to a genetic mutation because it is permanent, being passed from mother to daughter cells. Various putative tumor suppressor genes have been demonstrated to be hypermethylated in MDS *(41)*, thus presumably being silenced and enabling development of the disease. Shen et al. noted that methylation levels of different genes in MDS varied from 7% to 70%, correlated with each other, and predicted survival time of patients with MDS independently of the International Prognostic Scoring System (IPSS) score (42). Both DAC and azacitidine inhibit DNA methyltransferase, thus preventing a methylated gene from being passed to daughter cells at cell division. Unlike azacitidine, DAC is not incorporated into RNA, only into DNA; in fact, azacitidine's entry into DNA, and thus its ability to inhibit DNA methyltransferases, results from its intracellular conversion to DAC. Because it is not incorporated into RNA, DAC has 10-fold greater demethylating activity than azacitidine at equimolar concentrations.

Most experience with azacitidine and DAC has been in MDS patients. However, because the distinction between AML and high-risk MDS (e.g., with 10%–20% blasts) is malleable, it is reasonable to think that some of the high-risk MDS results may be applicable to AML. Based on randomized trials comparing the drug to supportive care, both azacitidine and DAC have been approved by the FDA for treatment of MDS. In the azacitidine trial (92 patients of median age 67 given supportive care versus 99 median age 69 given azacitidine), patients in the supportive care group who after 4 months remained transfusion-dependent, developed worsening cytopenia or a more advanced FAB classification stage were given azacitidine 75 mg/m^2 subcutaneously daily on 7 consecutive days, with cycles to begin on days 1, 29, 57, and 85. Approximately 46% of the patients had high-risk MDS, and substantial numbers of these had AML, using the currently accepted $\geq 20\%$ blast criterion (43,44). The "response rate" was 47% in the azacitidine arm versus 17% in the supportive care arm. However, 77% of the azacitidine-induced responses were "hematologic improvement" (HI, as defined by Cheson et al. (45)), such that the CR rate was 10%. While HI was associated with a decreased need for transfusion and a corresponding increase in quality of life, the median survival time among patients with high-risk FAB subtypes (primarily RAEB or RAEB-t) was 18 months for patients randomized to azacitidine versus 13 months for patients randomized to supportive care. These results were essentially unchanged when considering only patients with 20% to 30% blasts (i.e., AML). Although the ability to cross over to azacitidine decreased the difference in survival between supportive care and azacitidine, such a crossover would of course be done in clinical practice. It is of interest that although the median survival time among high-risk MDS patients randomized to azacitidine is similar to that reported by the EORTC after administration of low-dose ara-C to similarly aged patients (46), use of the former drug is undoubtedly much more widespread, at least in the United States.

The DAC trial included 89 patients given DAC and 81 given supportive care (47). In both groups the median age was 70 years, and about 70% of patients had high-risk MDS, with 25% of these patients having 20% to 30% blasts. DAC was given at 15 mg/m^2 every 8 hours for 3 days IV, repeated every 6 weeks. Using similar definitions, response rates were somewhat lower than those seen with azacitidine; and as with azacitidine, most responses were less than a CR. Decitabine produced beneficial effects regarding the need for transfusions and the quality of life. However, as with azacitidine, these effects were more impressive than those on survival. Indeed, although results were not categorized by risk group, DAC did not improve survival compared to supportive care. Although both DAC and azacitidine produced statistically significant delays in time to AML or death (i.e., "progression-free survival") (with medians of 12.0 months, DAC vs. 6.8 months, supportive care, in high-risk patients), I believe that progression-free survival is considerably less important than survival; after all, patients presumably care little about whether they die with or without "AML", and the definition of AML is itself arbitrary.

7.1.2. Low-Dose DAC

Two confounding factors in any analysis of the effects of azacitabine and DAC are the number of courses administered and the interval between courses. In the Silverman et al. study, 50% of patients needed at least three courses before a response was observed, and 25% of responses, or at least best responses, were seen between course 5 and course 17 *(43,44)*. A similar phenomenon occurs with DAC. Hence, it might be contended that the outcome with DAC, rather than supportive care, would have been better had more than 52% of patients received more than two courses, especially given that 40% of the patients receiving fewer than three courses had neither disease progression nor adverse events.

These considerations have prompted the use of "low-dose DAC." Thus, the drug's cytotoxic and hypomethylating effects are distinct, with the latter more relevant for response. Use of higher doses increases the cytotoxic, but not the hypomethylating, effect; and a reduction of cytotoxicity (e.g., by use of lower doses) can prolong the period over which patients can receive DAC, thus maximizing demethylation.

Data in support of these hypotheses were published by Yang et al., *(48)* who compared patients with CML given 500 to 900 mg/m^2 over 5 days using single doses of 50 to 90 mg/m^2 ("high doses") and patients with AML given 25 to 100 mg/ m over 5 days using single doses of 5 to 20 mg/m^2 ("low doses"). At 2 to 4 and 5 to 8 days after beginning treatment, total DNA methylation decreased to the same extent in both high-dose and low-dose groups. Although increasing amounts of demethylation were observed as the dose increased from 5 to 20 mg/m^2, demethylation was similar at the 20 and 90 mg/m^2 doses. There was no relation between demethylation and response in the high-dose study, but responders showed more demethylation than nonresponders in the low-dose study. Such a result might be expected if response was related to cytotoxicity as well as demethylation at the higher doses but only to demethylation at the lower doses. As the authors noted, attempts to draw conclusions are made more difficult by the facts that demethylation may not correlate with reexpression of a gene, and that the latter may not correlate with the presence of the relevant protein and by the confounding between diagnosis and dose (only CML patients received the higher doses). It is also possible that the cells studied before and after treatment had intrinsic differences in methylation status, with the former being more heavily methylated;that is, the data may have reflected "passive," rather than "active," demethylation; specifically, although patients did not differ regarding blast counts before treatment and when studied after treatment, it is plausible that the original blasts were replaced by rapidly cycling blasts that differed in methylation status. Arguing against passive demethylation is the observation that administration of cytotoxic chemotherapy to patients with ALL did not lead to demethylation.

The "plateau" in demethylation at 20 mg/m^2 led to a trial of low-dose DAC in high-risk MDS. In this trial 95 patients were randomized among 20 mg/m^2 IV daily × 5 days, 10 mg/m^2 subcutaneously twice daily for 5 days, and 10 mg/m^2 IV daily × 10 days, with randomization unbalanced so as to favor the arm with the higher CR rates at the time when a patient presented *(49)*. Two-thirds of the patients had high-risk high-risk MDS, with the remainder having low-risk MDS. The CR rate was 34% and was highest (25/64, 39%) in the 20 mg/m^2 IV daily × 5 arm; CR was seen in 11 of 37 in patients with high-risk MDS. With a median follow-up of 9 months, the median survival was about 18 months. In contrast to previous results, there was no correlation between total demethylation and response, but the CR group more often had reexpression of the p15^{INK4B} gene, which serves to block progression through the cell cycle and thus may be considered a "tumor suppressor."

Table 1
Comparison of Low-Dose and High-Dose Decitabine

Parameter	Low-dose decitabine (95 patients) (49)	High-dose decitabine (89 patients) (47)
CR rate	34%	9%
IPSS Int ≥ 2	66%	69%
AML (20–30% blasts)	0	16%
Median age	65 years	70 years
Dose per course	100 mg/m^2	135 mg/m^2
Time between courses	6 weeks	4 weeks
Patients receiving <3 courses	11%	48%
Median no. of courses	6–9	3
Median no. of courses to CR	3	Not stated

CR, complete response; IPSS, international prognostic scoring system; AML, acute myelogenous leukemia.

The most notable aspect of this "low-dose" trial is the considerably higher CR rate than was reported with "high-dose" DAC in the DAC versus supportive care trial (Table 1). The characteristics of the two groups appear similar (noting that the response rate in patients with AML on the high-dose study was similar to the response rate of patients without AML). Nonetheless, it would be of interest to perform a multivariate analysis asking whether, after accounting for various potential prognostic factors, treatment (low-dose vs. high-dose) affected the probability of CR, although such an analysis would of course not exclude the possibility of selection bias.

Any superiority of low-dose DAC over high-dose DAC may have less to do with differences in dose (100 mg/m^2 vs. 135 mg/m^2 per course) than to differences in the number of courses administered and the interval between courses (Table 1). This of course begs the question of how many courses of DAC should be given in the absence of response. Data from M. D. Anderson patients with high-risk MDS or AML suggest that there are diminishing returns after a fifth such course (Table 2).

Currently there is little experience with low-dose DAC (20 mg/m^2 daily days 1–5) in AML, although Schiller et al. (50), using this dose every 4 weeks, reported a CR in 3 of 27 patients (+ 4 patients with CR with incomplete blood count recovery) in patients who were age ≥60 years (median age 69 years) and not considered candidates for standard therapy; 8 patients received fewer than cycles but only because of death, progression, or choice.

Table 2
Response Rate on Each Course (*n* = 14) of Decitabine

Parameter	1	2	3	4	5	6	7	8	9	10	11	12	13	14
Patients receiving course	97	76	50	33	24	18	13	7	7	6	6	5	5	4
Patients receiving course who achieved CR on course	7%	20%	20%	15%	13%	6%	0	0	0	0	17%	0	0	0

7.2. Hypomethylating Agents + Histone Deacetylase Inhibitors

The binding of histone deacetylase (HDAC)-containing protein complexes to methylated CpG islands leads to removal of acetate groups from histone molecules in the adjacent chromatin. Deacetylation of histones leads to chromatin condensation, a configuration that blocks transcription *(51)*. Accordingly, various histone deacetylase inhibitors (HDACis) have been developed to, as with hypomethylating agents, reactivate transcription (e.g., of tumor suppressor genes). Eighteen human HDACs are known and fall into one of four classes *(51)*. As defined by their chemistry, there are six HDACi classes. Different HDACis affect different HDACs; for example, valproic acid (VPA) inhibits class I and class IIa HDACs, and vorinostat (formerly suberoylanilide hydroxamic acid, or SAHA) inhibits class I and class 2 HDACs. Whether inhibition of particular HDACs is more important than inhibition of others is unknown.

VPA's activity and tolerable toxicity in MDS led to its combination with DAC, 15 mg/m^2 daily × 10 days days *(52)*. Three doses of VPA (20, 35, or 50 mg/kg/day the same days as DAC) were studied, with most of the patients receiving the 50 mg/kg dose after it was identified as safe (the principal side effect was a 20% incidence of grade 3 to 4 somnolence). In total, 38 of the 53 patients had relapsed AML; 4 of the 38 responded (CR or CRp), whereas a response in patients with untreated high-risk MDS or AML—all considered poor candidates for standard therapy primarily because of age—was seen in 7 of 12 patients. Although histone acetylation was more frequent at the 50 mg/kg dose, acetylation was unrelated to the VPA levels or the response. Although patients with less baseline p15^{INK4B} methylation were more likely to respond, p15^{INK4B} reactivation was unrelated to response, with both observations contrasting with those made during the aforementioned low-dose DAC trial. Explanations for these discrepancies include (1) statistical (i.e., direct relations exist but could not be detected because of the small sample sizes); (2) the use of an HDACi in one study but not in the other; (3) the effects on epigenetic phenomena are outweighed by the effect of the status of "downstream pathways"; and (4) epigenetic modulation is unrelated to response, with the findings reported in the low-dose DAC study representing chance observations.

Although DAC + VPA clearly has "activity," its benefit relative to other therapies (e.g., single-agent, low-dose DAC) is unclear. Consequently, the principal M. D. Anderson study for patients age ≥ 60 years with untreated AML or high-risk MDS is randomization between DAC ± VPA.

7.3. Epigenetic-Acting Drugs as Sensitizers to Other Therapies

Epigenetic-acting drugs seem to sensitize AML cells to various agents; they include ara-C (azacitidine), idarubicin (vorinostat), and GO (azacitidine). Sensitization to ara-C putatively reflects azacitidine's ability to induce deoxycitidine kinase, required for phosphorylation of ara-C to the active ara-CTP *(53)*. Idarubicin and vorinostat appear synergistic, possibly because the latter can facilitate binding of idarubicin to DNA. Sensitization to GO may result from azacitidine's ability to up-regulate expression of the protein kinase Syk, which is related to the in vitro response to GO *(54)*. These observations have led to M. D. Anderson trials of azacitidine and ara-C and of idarubicin + vorinostat in relapsed AML, and A Southwest Oncology Group (SWOG) trial will investigate the azacitidine + GO combination in older patients with untreated AML.

7.4. Antagonists of BCL-2 and MDR1

Large randomized trials in older patients of 3+7 ± genasense, a drug thought to enhance chemotherapy-induced apoptosis by antagonizing BCL-2, and of 3+7 ± zosuquidar, postulated to overcome the effect of MDR1, which promotes extrusion of idarubicin, have failed to show a benefit in the experimental arm arm (55,56). A prior study of 3+7 ± the MDR1 antagonist PSC833 in a similar population was stopped before accrual was complete in part because of more death in the PSC arm, pointing out the real possibility that an investigational arm can be worse than standard treatment treatment (57).

7.5. Aurora Kinase Inhibitors

Aurora kinases A, B, and C play an essential role in the formation and operation of the mitotic spindle and are overexpressed in many cancers. The aurora kinase inhibitor VX-680 has been shown to reduce colony formation by AML blasts taken from patients and to reduce AML development in nude mice (58,59). Use of these drugs in AML will be of considerable interest.

7.6. Immune System Modulators

To date, there has been a strong relation between response to new drugs and response to standard drugs. This suggests that investigating new agents in remission after standard therapy (i.e., after the latter has had at least some success) might be useful. With agents that modulate the immune system, the remission setting is particularly attractive. For example, after randomizing 320 patients with a median age of 55 years, 78% of whom were less than 3 months from completion of consolidation therapy and 260 of whom were in their first CR, Brune et al. reported that leukemia-free survival was superior in patients assigned to the combination of histamine dihydrochloride and interleukin-2 rather than no treatment treatment (60). Although this study can be criticized < 10% of patients had unfavorable karyotypes and because survival was unaffected (i.e., results were similar to those often seen in studies randomizing patients to maintenance with standard chemotherapy or no maintenance), it is likely that other immune modulators will also be investigated in patients in CR, some under the hypothesis that there are AML-associated antigens that can be selectively targeted.

Perhaps the best-studied AML-associated antigens are proteinase 3 (PRTN3) and Wilms' tumor antigen 1 (WT-1). PRTN3 is a serine protease expressed in the azurophilic granules of myeloid leukemia cells (CML and AML) at two- to fivefold the amount found in normal myeloid cells; PRTN3 may be important in maintaining the AML phenotype (61). Molldrem et al. have identified PR1, an HLA–A2-binding 9 amino acid derived from PRTN3, as a myeloid leukemia-associated cytotoxic T lymphocyte (CTL) antigen finding PR1-specific high-avidity CTL in 11 of 12 patients with CML responding to interferon versus none of seven patients without a response (62). They suggested that failure of myeloid leukemia patients to develop an immune response to their disease spontaneously resulted from overexpression of PRTN3, leading to apoptosis of PR1-specific high-avidity CTL (63). Vaccination with PR1 has been studied under the hypothesis that it might increase PR1 immunity if done when the number of AML blasts had been reduced (e.g., following chemotherapy). Clinical responses have resulted after PR1 vaccination of patients with AML (64) and have occurred only in patients in whom there was at least a twofold increase in the number of PR1-specific CTLs; in contrast, there was no relation between

Table 3
Partial List of Targeted Therapies

Drug	Class	No. of patients	CR rate (responses <CR)	Effect on survival	Comment
Tipifarnib (37)	Farnesyl transferase inhibitor	158 (median age 74)	14% (9%)	Median 5.3 months	Being compared to supportive care alone in European study
Tipifarnib + etoposide (75)	Farnesyl transferase inhibitor	60 (age ≥ 70, median age 77)	21% (20%)	Not stated	Phase I-II study
Decitabine (76)	Hypomethylating agent	29 (median age 72)	14% (17%)	Median 7.5 months	Being combined with HiDACs (see text)
Lestuarinib (32)	FLT3 inhibitor	27 (median age 73)	0% (11%)	Not stated	Results similar to those with PKC312
PKC 412 + 3+7 (33)	FLT3 inhibitor	38 (age <60)	11/12 with ITD; 18/26 without ITD 85% ± GO	Not stated	Randomized trial in progress
Gemtuzumab ozogamycin (GO) (22)	Anti-CD33 antibody attached to toxin	1115 (age <60; randomized to 3+7, 3+7 + etoposide, or FLAG-ida each ± GO		At 3 years: 53% + GO, 46% – GO; GO least effective with adverse cytogenetics	DFS at 3 years: 51% +, 40% –GO; GO least effective with adverse cytogenetics
Genasense (55)	BCL2 antagonist	503 (age >60); randomized to 3+7 ± genasense	48% with genasense, 52% without genasense	None (at 1 year: 36% with gensense, 40% without genasense)	
Zosuquidar (56)	MDR1 anatagonist	422 (age >60, median age 67 randomized to 3+7 ± zosuquidar	Not stated	None; (median survival times were 7.7 months with and 9.4 months without zosuquidar)	

response and the number of CTLs directed against the "control" antigen PP65. An immune response was indeed more common in patients who had minimal residual, rather than overt, disease when beginning vaccination. An ongoing trial is randomly assigning patients age > 50 years with AML in remission after completion of consolidation therapy to either PR1 vaccine or discontinuation of therapy. Like PR-1, WT-1 is overexpressed in AML blasts and induces spontaneous HLA-A2 restricted CTLs (65). Vaccination with WT-1 has also produced clinical responses in AML, with the responses paralleled by decreased levels of WT-1 mRNA (66). The future is likely to see identification of AML-associated antigens that bind to other HLA types and use of AML-antigen-specific CTLs obtained from normal volunteers, expanded ex vivo, and then administered to patients.

Table 3 a summary of results when some of the targeted therapies discussed in this chapter are used for remission induction.

8. GENERAL ISSUES

8.1. Which Patients Are Candidates for Targeted Therapies?

We previously argued that patients in remission after standard chemotherapy might well receive targeted therapies. The reasons are (1) their documented sensitivity to therapy; (2) the observation that patients who are sensitive to one therapy are more likely to be sensitive to another; (3) their minimal residual disease status; and (4) their high risk of relapse if continued on the therapy that produced a remission. This risk approaches 50% at 6 months from remission date in patients with abnormalities involving more than three chromosomes, thus providing a counterargument to the belief that such patients have "no active disease to follow."

There is increasing use of targeted therapies in untreated, especially older, patients rather than patients in relapse. As outcome with standard chemotherapy is clearly unsatisfactory in many untreated older patients, the heterogeneity of AML makes it useful to attempt to identify subgroups of untreated older patients for whom standard induction therapy might be reasonable reasonable (67). One possibility is to use cytogenetics purpose, considering patients without the abnormalities noted in the previous paragraph as possible candidates. If it is not feasible to delay induction therapy to await cytogenetic results, patients can be divided into those with a performance status of 0 or 1 and a serum β_2-microglobulin level < 3.0 mg/L and those with either a performance status of 2 or with a serum β_2-microglobulin level > 2.9 mg/L. Over the last decade at M. D. Anderson, the CR rate for the latter patient category is only 45%, whereas the transplant-related mortality (TRM) rate is 24% with a median survival of only 6 months (68). Hence, these patients seem to be appropriate candidates for targeted treatment. In contrast, patients with performance status < 2 and serum β_2-microglobulin level < 3 mg/L had a 72% CR rate and only a 9% TRM rate. Nonetheless, their median survival is still only 14 months (Fig. 3), reflecting the transient nature of most of these CRs. With the data suggesting that induction therapy can influence CR duration duration, (69) it seems plausible that some patients in group might prefer targeted therapy and some standard induction therapy given the possibility that investigational therapy produces worse results than standard therapy.

Regardless of specific recommendations, any choice of therapy in older patients must refer to the observations of Sekeres et al., (70) who noted that 74% of older patients that their chances of cure with standard chemotherapy were at least 50%; in contrast, 85% of their physicians estimated this chance to be < 10%. Although the most plausible cause of this discrepancy is patients' natural tendency to believe what they want to believe, there may also be gaps in communication between physicians and patients.

8.2. New Response Criteria

For many years, the response to induction therapy for AML was classified as CR or no CR. Essentially all patients who are alive in CR 3 years after treatment with AML—thus being considered "potentially cured"—have obtained a CR. Furthermore, it is known that, after accounting for time needed to achieve CR, patients who obtain CR live longer than those who do not. Recently, responses less than CR have recently been recognized. An example is CRp (i.e., CR with incomplete platelet recovery). Attaining CRp suggests that a treatment is more "active" than if, despite survival time sufficiently long to observe CR or CRp, neither response occurred ("resistant"). However, it is also important to assess whether CRp conveys clinical benefit (i.e., lengthens survival relative to resistance). This appears to be the case *(71)*, and the same appears to be the case with HI *(45,72)*, but there is less information regarding "marrow CR" (i.e., bone marrow with <5% blasts but with minimum requirements for the neutrophil and/or platelet count).

8.3. Clinical Trial Design

8.3.1. MAXIMUM TOLERATED DOSE VS. OPTIMUM BIOLOGIC DOSE

There are two approaches to determining the appropriate dose of a targeted therapy. With the first approach, this dose is defined as the "maximum tolerated dose" (MTD), and the second emphasizes identification of a dose that produces a biologic effect thought relevant to the therapy's mechanism of action; the latter dose, called the "optimum biologic dose" (OBD), is often lower than the MTD. Although a focus on the OBD is attractive, it may be based in many cases on an overly optimistic belief that a targeted therapy's mechanism of action is known. It might be interesting in at least some Phase II trials to compare response rates with the MTD and the OBD.

8.3.2. LARGER VS. SMALLER TRIALS AND THE 5% SIGNIFICANCE LEVEL

Typically, a targeted therapy is compared with a more standard therapy in a trial whose sample size is computed with the objective of identifying a relatively modest improvement (e.g., 3 months in median survival). It seems fair to inquire whether trials should be concerned with detecting larger, more medically significant, differences, thus requiring fewer patients per treatment arm. The desirability of large sample sizes inherently rests on an assumption that progress in the treatment of AML in the elderly (e.g., age >60 years) can be made only gradually and in small steps; accordingly, clinical trials must be designed to have adequate power to identify small differences. It is not clear whether recent history in other leukemias supports this assumption. Thus, ATRA or arsenic trioxide in untreated APL, 2-chlorodeoxyadenosine in hairy cell leukemia, and interferon or imatinib in chronic phase CML are examples demonstrating that advances in treatment often occur in one large step rather than in many smaller ones. Compounding the problem is the nearly universal use of type 1 (false-positive) and type 2 (false-negative) error rates of 5% and 20%, respectively. In my opinion *(73)*, this policy pays little attention to differences between diseases. Thus, these rates are sensible when studying a new drug in a disease where standard treatment is reasonably good and thus where the principal concern is to prevent use of a falsely promising drug that might usurp standard therapy. In contrast, AML in the elderly is a disease for which there is no satisfactory treatment, so there may be more reason to protect against a false-negative result than a false-positive result. If so, it would be more logical to accept a type 1 error of 20% and a type 2 error of only 5%. Although not subscribing to this view, I see no more reason to protect against a false-positive than a false-negative result in clinical trials on AML of the elderly. Thus, it might be reasonable to specify type 1 and type 2 errors of 20% each. The point is that type 1 and type 2 error rates should not be taken as constants.

Enrolling fewer patients on each trial permits a larger number of treatments to be investigated. This ability is useful because a preclinical rationale is an imperfect predictor of clinical success. If preclinical rationale cannot yet replace empiricism, we should be interested in examining a larger number of therapies. Thus, rather than randomizing 240 patients between a standard and an investigational induction regimen, we might be better served by randomizing the same 240 patients among a standard and three investigational induction regimens. It is true that such trials would be nominally "underpowered." However, this argument ignores the false-negative rate inherent in the selection of which investigational regimen to study. For example, if there are three potential regimens that could be investigated and if preclinical rationale is, as argued above, a poor predictor of clinical results, limiting ourselves to one regimen in effect potentially entails a false-negative rate of 67%. Simply put, the most egregious false-negative result may be when a treatment is not studied at all *(74)*.

REFERENCES

1. Scaglioni P, Pandolfi P. The theory of APL revisited. Curr Top Immunol Microbiol 2007;313:85–100.
2. Tallman M, Sanz M, Lo Coco F. Tricks of the trade for the appropriate management of newly diagnosed acute promyelocytic leukemia. Blood 2005;105:3019–25.
3. Fenaux P, Le Deley MC, Castaigne S, et al. Effect of all transretinoic acid in newly diagnosed acute promyelocytic leukemia: results of a multicenter randomized trial; European APL 91 Group. Blood 1993;82:3241–9.
4. Fenaux P, Chastang C, Chevret S, et al. A randomized comparison of all transretinoic acid (ATRA) followed by chemotherapy and ATRA plus chemotherapy and the role of maintenance therapy in newly diagnosed acute promyelocytic leukemia; the European APL Group. Blood 1999;94:1192–200.
5. Sanz M, Martin G, Gonzalez M, et al. Risk-adapted treatment of acute promyelocytic leukemia with all-trans-retinoic acid and anthracycline monochemotherapy: a multicenter study by the PETHEMA group. Blood 2004;103:1237–43.
6. Estey E, Koller C, Tsimberidou AM, et al. Potential curability of newly diagnosed acute promyelocytic leukemia without use of chemotherapy: the example of liposomal all-trans retinoic acid. Blood 2005;105:1366–7.
7. Zhou DC, Kim SH, Ding W, et al. Frequent mutations in the ligand-binding domain of PML-RARalpha after multiple relapses of acute promyelocytic leukemia: analysis for functional relationship to response to all-trans retinoic acid and histone deacetylase inhibitors in vitro and in vivo. Blood 2002;99:1356–63.
8. Shen ZX, Shi ZZ, Fang J, et al. All-trans retinoic acid/As_2O_3 combination yields a high quality remission and survival in newly diagnosed acute promyelocytic leukemia. Proc Natl Acad Sci U S A 2004;101:5328–35.
9. Matthews V, George B, Lakshmi K et al. Single-agent arsenic trioxide in the treatment of newly diagnosed acute promyelocytic leukemia: durable remissions with minimal toxicity Blood 2006;107;2627–32.
10. Estey E, Garcia-Manero G, Ferrajoli A, et al. Use of all-trans retinoic acid plus arsenic trioxide as an alternative to chemotherapy in untreated acute promyelocytic leukemia. Blood 2006;107; 3469–73.
11. Patel SP, Garcia-Manero G, Ferrajoli A, et al. Cardiotoxicity in African-American patients treated with arsenic trioxide for acute promyelocytic leukemia. Leuk Res 2006;30:362–3.
12. Jurcic JG, DeBlasio T, Dumont L, et al. Molecular remission induction with retinoic acid and anti-CD33 monoclonal antibody HuM195 in acute promyelocytic leukemia. Cancer Res 2000;6:372–80.
13. Feldman EJ, Brandwein J, Stone R, et al. Phase III randomized multicenter study of a humanized anti-CD33 monoclonal antibody, lintuzumab, in combination with chemotherapy, versus chemotherapy alone in patients with refractory or first-relapsed acute myeloid leukemia. J Clin Oncol 2005;23:4110–6.
14. Estey E, Giles F, Beran M, et al. Experience with gemtuzumab ozogamycin ("mylotarg") and all-trans retinoic acid in untreated acute promyelocytic leukemia. Blood 2002;99;4222–4.

15. Lo Coco F, Cimino G, Breccia M, et al. Gemtuzumab ozogamicin (Mylotarg) as a single agent for molecularly relapsed acute promyelocytic leukemia. Blood 2004;104;1995–9.

16. Sievers EL, Larson RA, Stadtmauer EA, et al. Efficacy and safety of gemtuzumab ozogamicin in patients with CD33-positive AML in first relapse. J Clin Oncol 2001;19:3244–54.

17. Giles FJ, Kantarjian HM, Kornblau SM, et al. Mylotarg (gemtuzumab ozogamicin) therapy is associated with hepatic venoocclusive disease in patients who have not received stem cell transplantation. Cancer 2001;92:406–13.

18. Wadleigh M, Richardson PG, Zahrieh D, et al. Prior gemtuzumab ozogamicin exposure significantly increases the risk of veno-occlusive disease in patients who undergo myeloablative allogeneic stem cell transplantation. Blood 2003;102:1578–82.

19. Leopold LH, Berger MS, Cheng SC, et al. Comparative efficacy and safety of gemtuzumab ozogamicin monotherapy and high-dose cytarabine combination therapy in patients with acute myeloid leukemia in first relapse. Clin Adv Hematol Oncol 2003;1:220–5.

20. Estey EH, Thall PF, Giles FG, et al. Gemtuzumab ozogamycin with or without interleukin 11 in patients 65 years of age or older with untreated AML or high-risk MDS: comparison with idarubicin plus high-dose continuous infusion cytosine arabinoside. Blood 2002;99:4343–9.

21. Amadori S, Suciu S, Stasi R, et al. Gemtuzumab ozogamycin as single-agent treatment for frail patients age 61 years of age and older with acute myeloid leukemia: final results of AML-15B, a phase 2 study of the European Organization for Research and Treatment of Cancer and Gruppo Italiano Malattie Ematologiche dell' Adulto Leukemia groups. Leukemia 2005;19:1768–73.

22. Burnett A, Kell W, Goldstone A et al. The addition of gemtuzumb ozogamycin to induction chemotherapy for AML improves disease-free survival without extra toxicity: preliminary analysis of 1,115 patients in the MRC AML 15 trial. Blood 2006;108(11):8. Abstract 13.

23. Eom K-S, Kim H-J, Min C-K, et al. Gemtuzumab ozogamycin in combination with attenuated doses of standard induction chemotherapy can successfully induce complete remission without increasing toxicity in patients with newly-diagnosed AML age 55 or older. Blood 2006;108(11):561. Abstract 1982.

24. Pagel JM, Appelbaum FR, Eary JF, et al. ^{131}I-anti-CD45 antibody plus busulfan and cyclophosphamide before allogeneic hematopoietic cell transplantation for treatment of acute myeloid leukemia in first remission. Blood 2006;107:2184–91.

25. Fröhling S, Scholl C, Gilliland DG, et al. Genetics of myeloid malignancies: pathogenetic and clinical implications. J Clin Oncol 2005;23:6285–95.

26. Whitman SP, Archer KJ, Feng L, et al. Absence of the wild-type allele predicts poor prognosis in adult de novo acute myeloid leukemia with normal cytogenetics and the internal tandem duplication of FLT3: a Cancer and Leukemia Group B study. Cancer Res 2001;61:7233–9.

27. Yanada M, Matsuo K, Suzuki T, et al. Prognostic significance of FLT3 internal tandem duplication and tyrosine kinase domain mutations for acute myeloid leukemia: a meta-analysis. Leukemia 2005;19:1345–9.

28. Mead A, Linch D, Hills R, et al. Favourable prognosis associated with FLT3 tyrosine kinase domain mutations in AML in contrast to the adverse outcome associated with internal tandem duplications. Blood 2005;106. Abstract 334.

29. Mrojek K, Marcucci G, Paschka P, et al. Clinical relevance of mutations and gene-expression changes in adult acute myeloid leukemia with normal cytogenetics: are we ready for a prognostically prioritized molecular classification? Blood 2007;109:431–48.

30. Kottaridis PD, Gale RE, Langabeer SE, et al. Studies of FLT3 mutations in paired presentation and relapse samples from patients with acute myeloid leukemia: implications for the role of FLT3 mutations in leukemogenesis, minimal residual disease detection, and possible therapy with FLT3 inhibitors. Blood 2002;100:2393–8.

31. Stone R, DeAngelo D, Klimek V, et al. Patients with acute myeloid leukemia and an activating mutation in FLT3 respond to a small-molecule FLT3 tyrosine kinase inhibitor, PKC412. Blood 2005;105:54–60.

32. Knapper S, Burnett A, Littlewood T, et al. A phase 2 trial of the FLT3 inhibitor lestaurtinib (CEP701) as first-line treatment for older patients with acute myeloid leukemia not considered fit for intensive chemotherapy. Blood 2006;108:3262–70.

33. Stone R, Fischer T, Paquette R, et al. Phase 1b study of PKC412, an oral flt3 kinase inhibitor, in sequential and simultaneous combinations with daunorubicin and cytarabine induction and high-dose cytarabine consolidation in newly-diagnosed adult patients with AML under age 61. Blood 2006;108(11):50a. Abstract 157.

34. Levis M, Brown P, Smith BD, et al. Plasma inhibitory activity (PIA): a pharmacodynamic assay reveals insights into the basis for cytotoxic response to FLT3 inhibitors. Blood 2006;108:3477–83.

35. Beaupre D, Kurzrock R. RAS and leukemia: from basic mechanisms to gene-directed therapy. J Clin Oncol 1999;7:1071–9.

36. Harousseau JL, Lancet JE, Reiffers J, et al. A phase 2 study of the oral farnesyltransferase inhibitor tipifarnib in patients with refractory or relapsed acute myeloid leukemia. Blood 2007;109:5151–6.
37. Lancet J, Gojo I, Gotlib J, et al. A phase 2 study of the farnesyltransferase inhibitor tipifarnib in poor-risk and elderly patients with previously untreated acute myelogenous leukemia. Blood 2007;109:1387–94.
38. Von Hoff DD, Slavik M, Muggia FM. 5-Azacytidine: a new anticancer drug with effectiveness in acute myelogenous leukemia. Ann Intern Med 1976;85:237–45.
39. Silverman LR, Holland JF, Weinberg RS, et al. Effects of treatment with 5-azacytidine on the in vivo and in vitro hematopoiesis in patients with myelodysplastic syndromes. Leukemia 1993;7(suppl 1):21–9.
40. Egger G, Liang G, Aparicio A, et al. Epigenetics in human disease and prospects for epigenetic therapy. Nature 2004;429:457–63.
41. Boumber YA, Kondo Y, Chen X, et al. RIL, a LIM gene on 5q31, is silenced by methylation in cancer and sensitizes cancer cells to apoptosis. Cancer Res 2007;67:1997–2005.
42. Shen L, Kantarjian H, Saba H, et al. CpG island methylation is a poor prognostic factor in myelodysplastic syndrome patients and is reversed by decitabine therapy: results of a phase III randomized study. Blood 2005;106:790a. Abstract.
43. Silverman LR, Demakos EP, Peterson BL, et al. Randomized controlled trial of azacitidine in patients with the myelodysplastic syndrome: a study of the Cancer and Leukemia Group B. J Clin Oncol 2002;20:2429–40.
44. Silverman LR, McKenzie DR, Peterson BL, et al. Further analysis of trials with azacitidine in patients with myelodysplastic syndrome: studies 8421, 8921, and 9221 by the Cancer and Leukemia Group B. J Clin Oncol 2006;24:3895–903.
45. Cheson BD, Greenberg PL, Bennett JM, et al. Clinical application and proposal for modification of the International Working Group (IWG) response criteria in myelodysplasia. Blood 2006;108:419–25.
46. Zwierzina H, Suciu S, Loeffler-Ragg J, et al. Low-dose cytosine arabinoside (LD-AraC) vs LD-AraC plus granulocyte/macrophage colony stimulating factor vs LD-AraC plus interleukin-3 for myelodysplastic syndrome patients with a high risk of developing acute leukemia: final results of a randomized phase III study (06903) of the EORTC Leukemia Cooperative Group. Leukemia 2005;19:1929–33.
47. Kantarjian H, Issa JP, Rosenfeld CS, et al. Decitabine improves patient outcomes in myelodysplastic syndromes: results of a phase III randomized study. Cancer 2006;106:1794–803.
48. Yang AS, Doshi KD, Choi SW, et al. DNA methylation changes after 5-aza-2'-deoxycytidine therapy in patients with leukemia. Cancer Res 2006;66:5495–503.
49. Kantarjian H, Oki Y, Garcia-Manero G, et al. Results of a randomized study of 3 schedules of low-dose decitabine in higher-risk myelodysplastic syndrome and chronic myelomonocytic leukemia. Blood 2007;109:52–7.
50. Casten A, Schiller G, Larsen J, et al. Phase 2 study of low-dose decitabine for the front-line treatment of older patients with acute myeloid leukemia. Blood 2006;108. Abstract 1984.
51. Bolden JE, Peart MJ, Johnstone RW. Anticancer activities of histone deacetylase inhibitors. Nat Rev Drug Discov 2006;5:769–84.
52. Garcia-Manero G, Kantarjian HM, Sanchez-Gonzalez B, et al. Phase 1/2 study of the combination of 5-aza-2'-deoxycytidine with valproic acid in patients with leukemia. Blood 2006;108:3271–9.
53. Kong XB, Tong WP, Chou TC, et al. Induction of deoxycytidine kinase by 5 dyacytidine in ML-60 cell line resistant to anabnosylcytosine. Mol Pharmacol 1991;39:250–7.
54. Balaian L, Ball ED. Cytotoxic activity of gemtuzumab ozogamicin (Mylotarg) in acute myeloid leukemia correlates with the expression of protein kinase Syk. Leukemia 2006;20:2093–101.
55. Marcucci G, Moser B, Blum W, et al. A phase III randomized trial of intensive induction and consolidation chemotherapy +/− genasense (oblimersen sodium;G3139), a pro-apoptotic Bcl-2 antisense oligonucleotide in untreated acute myeloid leukemia patients >60 years old: a Cancer and Acute Leukemia Group B study. Presented at ASCO 2007.
56. Cripe L, Li X, Litzow M, et al. A randomized placebo-controlled, double-blind trial of the MDR modulator Zosuquidar during conventional induction and post-remission therapy for patients >60 years of age with newly-dignosed acute myeloid leukemia or high-risk myelodysplastic syndrome. Blood 2006;108(11):129a. Abstract 423.
57. Baer MR, George SL, Dodge RK, et al. Phase 3 study of the multidrug resistance modulator PSC-833 in previously untreated patients 60 years of age and older with acute myeloid leukemia: Cancer and Leukemia Group B study 9720. Blood 2002;100:1224–32.
58. Doggrell S. Dawn of aurora kinase inhibitors as anticancer drugs. Expert Opin Invest Drugs 2004;13:1199–201.
59. Gautschi O, Mack P, Davies A, et al. Aurora kinase inhibitors: a new class of targeted drugs in cancer. Clin Lung Cancer 2006;8:93–8.

60. Brune M, Castaigne S, Catalano J, et al. Improved leukemia-free survival after postconsolidation immunotherapy with histamine dihydrochloride and interleukin-2 in acute myeloid leukemia: results of a randomized phase 3 trial. Blood 2006;108:88–96.

61. Molldrem JJ. Vaccination for leukemia. Biol Blood Marrow Transpl 2006;12:13–8.

62. Molldrem JJ, Lee PP, Wang C, et al. Evidence that specific T lymphocytes may participate in the elimination of chronic myelogenous leukemia. Nat Med 2000;6:1018–23.

63. Molldrem JJ, Lee PP, Kant S, et al. Chronic myelogenous leukemia shapes host immunity by selective elimination of high-avidity leukemia-specific T cells. J Clin Invest 2003;111:639–47.

64. Qazilbash M, Wieder E, Rios R, et al. Vaccination with the PR1 leukemia-associated antigen can induce complete remission in patients with myeloid leukemia. Blood 2004;104. Abstract 259.

65. Azuma T, Makita M, Ninomiya K, et al. Identification of a novel WT-1-derived peptide which induces human leukocyte antigen-A24-restricted anti-leukaemia cytotoxic T lymphocytes. Br J Haematol 2002;116:601–3.

66. Keilholz U, Scheibenbogen C, Letsch A, et al. WT1-peptide vaccination shows high immunogenicity and clinical activity in patients with acute myeloid leukemia. Blood 2005;106:122a. Abstract.

67. Estey E. Acute myeloid leukemia and myelodysplastic syndrome in older patients. J Clin Oncol 2007;25:1908–15.

68. Tsimberidou A-M, Kantarjian H, O'Brien S, et al. Prognostic significance of β_2-microglobulin levels in acute myeloid leukemia. Blood 2006;108(11):240a. Abstract.

69. Estey E, Dohner H. Acute myeloid leukemia. Lancet 2006;368:1894–907.

70. Sekeres MA, Stone RM, Zahrieh D, et al. Decision-making and quality of life in older adults with AML or advanced MDS. Leukemia 2004;18:809–16.

71. Estey E, Garcia-Manero G, Giles F, et al. Clinical relevance of CRp in untreated AML. Blood 2005;106. Abstract 541.

72. Yanada M, Huang X, Garcia-Manero G, et al. Effect of hematologic improvement on survival in patients given targeted therapy as initial treatment of acute myeloid leukemia or high risk myelodysplastic syndrome. Br J Haematol 2007;138:555–7.

73. Estey E. Clinical trials in AML of the elderly: should we change our methodology? Leukemia 2004;18:1772–4.

74. Estey E, Thall P. New designs for phase 2 clinical trials. Blood 2003;102:442–8.

75. Karp J, Feldman E, Morris L, et al. Active oral regimen for elderly adults with newly-diagnosed AML: phase 1 trial of oral tipifarnib combined with oral etoposide for adults age 70 who are not candidates for traditional cytotoxic chemotherapy. Blood 2006;108(11):130a. Abstract 426.

76. Lubbert M, Ruter B, Schmid M, et al. Continued low-dose decitabine is an active first-line treatment of older AML patients: first results of a multicenter phase II study. Blood 2005;106:527a. Abstract 1852.

3 Targeted Therapy in Breast Cancer

Barbara S. Craft, MD *and Stacy Moulder,* MD, MSCI

CONTENTS

INTRODUCTION
MOLECULAR MECHANISMS INVOLVED FOR BREAST CANCER
   GROWTH AND PATIENT SURVIVAL
TARGETED THERAPIES FOR THE TREATMENT OF BREAST CANCER
FUTURE DIRECTION OF TARGETED THERAPY FOR BREAST CANCER
REFERENCES

ABSTRACT

Targeted drugs are active as single agents for the treatment of breast cancer and offer the opportunity to reverse resistance to chemotherapy and hormonal therapy. Targeted therapies have been established for the treatment of advanced breast cancer and are now demonstrating benefit in the adjuvant arena. This review summarizes the results of several trials involving the use of targeted therapy for the treatment of breast cancer and discusses future directions for breast cancer therapy.

Key Words: Breast cancer, Biologic therapy, Targeted therapy, Adjuvant therapy, Metastatic disease

1. INTRODUCTION

Even with advances in screening for early detection, aggressive therapy for localized disease, and treatment for metastatic disease, breast cancer continues to be a major health problem. It was projected that in 2007 an estimated 178,480 American women would be diagnosed with breast cancer and that 40,460 women would die from the disease *(1)*.

Once the diagnosis of breast cancer is established, treatment depends on the disease stage and pathologic features, such as receptor status and tumor grade. Stage IV breast cancer is also known as advanced or metastatic disease and represents tumor metastasis to organ systems outside the breast and adjacent lymph nodes. Advanced breast cancer carries a median survival of approximately 2 years after documentation of metastasis. Disease response has been demonstrated with various chemotherapy agents (Table 1); however, in

From: *Current Clinical Oncology: Targeted Cancer Therapy*
Edited by: R. Kurzrock and M. Markman © Humana Press, Totowa, NJ

Table 1
Active Chemotherapy Agents for the Treatment
of Breast Cancer

	Response Rate (%)
Anthracyclines	
Doxorubicin	10–50%
Epirubicin	13–48%
Liposomal doxorubicin	10–50%
Microtubule Stabilizers	
Docetaxel	18–68%
Paclitaxel	16–62%
Nab-paclitaxel	33–48%
Ixabepilone	12–57%
Other Active Agents	
Capecitabine	20–35%
Vinorelbine	25–50%
Gemcitabine	12–37%
Cisplatin/Carboplatin	9–51%

randomized trials, reductions in tumor size have not always correlated with improvement in progression-free or overall survival. Although no clinical trial has ever demonstrated improved survival with chemotherapy over best supportive care in patients with advanced breast cancer, several randomized trials have demonstrated a modest prolongation of survival when newer therapy regimens were compared with older, inferior regimens (2–4). As such, treatment for most patients with advanced breast cancer is considered palliative in nature, although durable complete remissions have been achieved in a small number of patients (< 5%) (5).

Fortunately, most patients diagnosed with breast cancer are treated for localized disease. In this group of patients, prognosis is heavily dependent on the number of axillary lymph nodes involved, the size of the primary tumor, and the pathologic features of the primary tumor (histologic grade, hormone receptor status, HER2 status, presence or absence of lymphovascular invasion). Most patients with localized breast cancer undergo surgical resection of the primary tumor (mastectomy or breast-conserving surgery) and evaluation of the ipsilateral axillary nodal basin (sentinel lymph node biopsy and/or complete axillary node dissection). After definitive surgery, patients may undergo radiation therapy to the remaining breast tissue/chest wall and draining lymph nodes to reduce the risk of local recurrence. Systemic adjuvant therapy may also be recommended for patients with significant risk of disseminated disease based on unfavorable characteristics of the primary tumor or the presence of lymph node involvement. Adjuvant therapy has been demonstrated to reduce the risk of breast cancer recurrence by 30% to 50% (6,7).

Approximately 20% to 25% of patients with breast cancer present with locally advanced (stage IIb or III) disease. If left untreated after surgical resection, approximately 80% of these women develop metastatic breast cancer (8). The use of chemotherapy or hormonal therapy prior to surgical resection (neoadjuvant therapy) is often a feasible option in this group of patients. Several rationales exist to support the use of neoadjuvant chemotherapy. First, most patients (~80%) have either a complete response (CR) or partial (PR) response in the primary tumor (9). By decreasing the size of the primary tumor, patients may require a less extensive operative procedure, and in some cases tumors may be "down-staged" from inoperable to operable. Second, the effects of treatment are directly observed, and therapy can be altered based on tumor response, which results in less patient exposure to the toxicity of ineffective therapy. Finally, neoadjuvant therapy in patients with locally advanced disease provides the unique opportunity to obtain tissue for research before and after therapy to correlate tumor response with molecular parameters.

Since the 1980s, breast cancer mortality rates have declined overall, most notably in patients less than 70 years of age. This decrease has been attributed, in part, to earlier diagnosis using screening mammography; however, the more aggressive use of adjuvant and neoadjuvant therapy has also played a role in the decrease (10).

Clinical trials have demonstrated benefit for targeted therapy in the treatment of both advanced and localized breast cancer. Such success has generated continued excitement about the development of additional targeted agents in breast cancer for reasons that include the ability to tailor therapy to select patients whose tumors express targets of interest, reduced systemic toxicity, and synergistic effects in combination with cytotoxic therapy.

2. MOLECULAR MECHANISMS INVOLVED FOR BREAST CANCER GROWTH AND PATIENT SURVIVAL

2.1. Hormone Receptors

Beatson's 1896 publication documenting breast cancer regression after oophorectomy offered the first hint of cancer cell dependence on endogenous signaling pathways but was limited by lack of an identified target (11). The discovery of the estradiol/estrogen receptor (ER) and progesterone receptor (PR) signaling pathways later led to the development of medical therapies that have become the cornerstone for the treatment of patients with hormone receptor positive breast cancer.

Both ER and PR are dimeric proteins that, upon ligand activation, complex with co-activator and co-repressor proteins and eventually regulate gene expression (12). Multiple isoforms exist for both ER and PR and allow for variations in ligand recognition, dimerization, and differential regulation of target genes (13). Two subunits of ER, ERα and ERβ, are encoded by distinct genes that are differentially expressed in cancer cell compared to normal tissue. Conformational changes that affect receptor signaling occur after ligand binding and are dependant upon interaction of ligand (or drug) with the ligand-binding pocket.

2.2. Receptor Tyrosine Kinases

Extracellular signals that influence cancer cell growth, survival, and differentiation are initiated through activation of receptor tyrosine kinases (RTKs). These proteins are localized in the cell membrane and contain a ligand binding extracellular domain, an anchoring transmembrane domain and a kinase domain that contains the ATP binding site necessary for receptor activation. RTKs activate signaling pathways by altering the phosphorylation state of a broad range of downstream target proteins (Fig. 1).

2.2.1. HUMAN EPIDERMAL GROWTH FACTOR FAMILY OF RECEPTORS

The human epidermal growth factor (HER) family of receptors consists of four RTKs with similar homology, HER1 (also referred to as epidermal growth factor receptor, or EGFR), HER2, HER3, and HER4. Upon ligand binding, the receptors form either homodimers with like receptors or heterodimers with other members of the family. Heterodimer formation

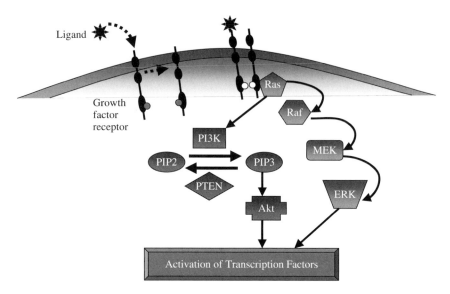

Fig. 1. Simplified presentation of signal transduction pathways.

increases the affinity for ligand and augments signaling effects that lead to changes in cellular proliferation, angiogenesis, and apoptosis *(14,15)*. HER2 lacks a known ligand but partners with the other members of the family to enhance ligand-induced signaling. Overexpression of HER2 also results in ligand-independent homodimer formation in preclinical models. HER2 overexpression occurs in 15% to 30% of patients with breast cancer and correlates with a poor prognosis and decreased survival *(16,17)*.

Other members of the HER family of receptors have been evaluated as potential targets for the treatment of breast cancer. Preclinical experiments demonstrated that HER1/EGFR "specific" small-molecule tyrosine kinase inhibitors (TKIs) induce the formation of inactive HER1/HER2 heterodimers and inhibit heregulin-mediated growth in breast cancer cell lines *(18)*. Thus, in cells that overexpress HER2 and also exhibit HER1/EGFR, inhibitors of HER1/EGFR can sequester HER2 from functional interactions with other signaling partners such as HER3 and HER4 *(19)*. In addition, co-expression of both HER1/EGFR and HER2 has been associated with enhanced cell transformation in preclinical models and a more aggressive clinical course in patients with breast cancer *(20)*.

2.2.2. VASCULAR ENDOTHELIAL GROWTH FACTOR RECEPTORS

The vascular endothelial growth factor (VEGF) pathway consists of various ligands (VEGF-A, VEGF-B, VEGF-C, VEGF-D, VEGF-E) and RTKs: VEGFR-1 (FLT1), VEGFR-2 (FLK/KDR), and VEGFR-3 (FLT4) *(21)*. Ligand and/or receptor overexpression have been documented in many common malignancies, including breast cancer, and are considered essential for angiogenesis *(22,23)*. Activation of VEGFR-1 results in endothelial cell differentiation and increased migration *(24)*. Activation of the VEGF pathway results in endothelial cell differentiation, proliferation and migration *(24,25)*. VEGFR-2 and VEGFR-3 also affect vascular permeability and lymphangiogenesis *(26)*. Angiogenesis is required for breast cancer growth, invasion, and metastasis; and clinical observations have linked increased tumor microvessel density (a measure of angiogenesis) with increased risk of recurrence and decreased overall survival in patients with breast cancer *(27–29)*.

2.2.3. Insulin-like Growth Factor Receptors

Type I insulin-like growth factor receptor, (IGF1R) is a heterotetrameric protein consisting of two polypeptide chains, each containing an extracellular α and β subunit *(30)*. Peptides such as insulin-like growth factor I (IGF-I) and IGF-II bind to the ligand-binding domain within the α subunit, leading to activation of the tyrosine kinase found in the β subunit. IGF1R shares similar homology with the insulin receptor (IR), and hybrid IGF1R/IR complexes can be expressed and demonstrate higher ligand binding affinity for IGF-II *(31)*.

Human breast cancers express higher levels of IGF-I, IGF-II, IGF1R, and IR compared with normal breast tissue *(32,33)*. In preclinical models, alteration of IGF expression or activity induces proliferation, cell migration and evasion of apoptosis in both normal mammary cells, and breast cancer cell lines *(34)*. In addition, inhibition of IGF1R suppresses growth and induces apoptosis in breast cancer xenograft models *(35,36)*.

2.3. Key Signaling Pathways for Breast Cancer

Coordination of signaling cascades from the cell membrane to the nucleus involves the activation of kinases as well as a variety of molecules known as scaffolding, docking, or adaptor proteins *(37)*. Although inhibitors of ER and RTKs have been most extensively studied for the treatment of patients with breast cancer, the downstream signaling cascades activated by these receptors contain numerous potential targets for anticancer therapy, and inhibitors of these pathways are in early clinical development.

2.3.1. Mitogen-Activated Protein Kinase Pathways

Transduction of growth factor signaling from cell surface RTKs to the nucleus occurs via activation of intracellular kinases in the MAPK family of kinases (Erk1/2, JNK1-3, p38 kinases) *(38,39)*. Mitogen-activated protein kinases (MAPKs) play a crucial role in cancer cell survival and proliferation through phosphorylation of transcription factors, cytoskeletal proteins, and other protein kinases. RTK activation leads to activation of RAS/RAF, which then activates MAPK kinases (MEKs), which phosphorylate downstream MAPKs (Fig. 1). MAPK pathway activity is markedly increased in HER2-overexpressing cell lines, and inhibition of MAPK signaling results in reduction of heregulin-induced S-phase entry and decreased proliferation in human breast cancer cell lines *(40,41)*. In addition, 25% to 50% of human breast cancers express elevated levels of activated ERK1/2 independent of HER2 expression *(42)*.

2.3.2. Phosphoinositol 3′OH Kinase/AKT Pathway

Also involved in cellular signaling and important for suppression of apoptosis is the phosphoinositol 3′OH kinase (PI3K)/AKT pathway. This pathway can be activated by several cell surface receptors (ER, HER family, IGF1R) and oncogenic RAS *(43)*. Activated PI3K catalyzes production of phosphatidylinositol 3,4,5 triphosphate (PIP3), which in turn activates AKT/protein kinase B (PKB). Activated AKT has multiple substrates, including upstream activators of the mammalian target of rapamycin (mTOR). Thus, signaling through this pathway regulates mTOR, which functions in cytoskeleton organization, response to oxidative stress, protein synthesis, and cell cycle progression *(44)*.

HER2-overexpressing tumors demonstrate a high level of PI3K/AKT activity, mostly due to heterodimerization with HER3 *(45)*. Additionally, mutations in the *PI3KCA* gene have been detected in 25% of breast cancers, and the introduction of expression vectors for such mutations transforms human mammary epithelial cells grown in culture *(46,47)*.

Phosphatase and tensin homologue deleted in chromosome 10 (PTEN) dephosphorylates PIP3 and antagonizes PI3K function (Fig. 1). Gene deletions and inactivating mutations reduce PTEN activity but are rare (< 5%) in breast cancers. Low PTEN levels have, however, been described in 26% to 30% of breast cancers and were associated with a higher incidence of lymph node metastasis and a worse prognosis *(48,49)*.

3. TARGETED THERAPIES FOR THE TREATMENT OF BREAST CANCER

3.1. Modulation of Estrogen Receptor Signaling

Selective estrogen response modulators (SERMs) structurally resemble estrogens, put upon binding to estrogen receptors, exert functionally different effects in normal tissue and cancer cells. They function as ER agonists in some tissues but oppose the action of estrogen in others. For many decades, the SERM tamoxifen was the gold standard for treating both pre- and postmenopausal patients with hormone receptor-positive breast cancer. Response rates to tamoxifen range from 16% to 56% in patients with metastatic breast cancer, with a median time to progression of approximately 6 months *(50–52)*.

In the adjuvant setting, 5 years of tamoxifen administration has resulted in a 47% mean decrease in the annual odds of recurrence and a 26% mean decrease in the annual odds of death in both pre- and postmenopausal women. Tamoxifen also decreases the incidence of new primary breast cancer by almost 50% *(7)*. These effects of tamoxifen were independent of a patient's sex, age, and menopausal status but were absolutely dependent on ER/PR expression, as measured by immunohistochemistry *(53)*. ER response modulation with tamoxifen or raloxifene has also demonstrated value in the prevention of breast cancer in women at moderate to high risk of developing the disease *(54,55)*. Whereas tamoxifen acts as an estrogen antagonist in breast tissue, it has partial agonist activity in other tissues. Such dichotomy results in an increased risk of endometrial cancer and thromboembolic disease but an improvement in bone health and reduced cholesterol levels in postmenopausal women.

In postmenopausal women, inhibitors of aromatase, the enzyme that converts androgenic substrates to estrogens, have been effective for the treatment of hormone receptor-positive breast cancer in both localized and advanced settings. Unlike SERMs, aromatase inhibitors (AIs) block the estrogen/ER pathway without agonist activity in normal tissue *(56)*. AIs demonstrated improved efficacy when compared to tamoxifen as a first-line treatment of women with ER-positive and/or PR-positive metastatic breast cancer and were quickly moved into the adjuvant arena *(51,52,57)*.

The Arimidex, Tamoxifen, Alone or in Combination (ATAC) trial was a double-blind, multicenter trial in postmenopausal women with surgically treated, localized breast cancer whose tumors were either known ER/PR-positive or in whom receptor status was unknown. Patients were randomized to receive anastrozole 1 mg by mouth daily, tamoxifen 20 mg by mouth daily, or the combination. A significant improvement in disease-free survival (DFS) with was seen in the group of women receiving anastrozole, along with a superior time to recurrence and fewer contralateral recurrences compared to tamoxifen *(58)*. Additional studies of AIs as primary adjuvant therapy or following tamoxifen have shown similar benefit, as demonstrated in Table 2. To date, no firm conclusions can be drawn regarding the preferential use of AIs as first-line therapy versus their use as sequential therapy following tamoxifen. In addition, adjuvant studies to determine the benefit of ovarian ablation and aromatase inhibition in premenopausal women are ongoing. The role of aromatase inhibitors for the prevention of breast cancer also remains undefined.

Table 2
Adjuvant Endocrine Therapy Trials

Trial	Study arms	No.	Follow-up	DFSHR (p)	OSHR (p)
ATAC (58)	A× 5 years	3125	68	0.87	0.97
	T× 5 years	3116	months	(0.01)	(0.07)
	A+T× 5 years[a]	3125			
NCIC-MA 17 (105)	T× 5 years →	2583	30	0.58(<0.001)	0.82
	L× 5years		months		(0.3)
	T× 5years → P	2587			
	× 5 years				
IES (106)	T× 2–3 years	2380	31	0.73	0.83
	→ E× 2–3 years		months	(0.0001)	(0.08)
		2362			
	T× 5 years				
BIG 198 (107)	L ×5 years	4003	26	0.81	
	or		months	(0.003)	
	L × 2 years →				
	T × 3 years				
	T × 5 years	4007			
	or				
	T × 2 years →				
	L × 3 years				

DFSHR, disease-free survival hazard ratio; OSHR, overall survival hazard ratio; A, arimidex; T, tamoxifen; L, letrozole; P, placebo; E, exemestane
[a]This arm stopped at early analysis due to lack of benefit

Fulvestrant is an ER antagonist with no known agonist activity (pure antiestrogen) that down-regulates both the ERs and PRs (59–61). Fulvestrant has been shown to be as efficacious as anastrozole in patients with tamoxifen-refractory metastatic breast cancer. It is approved as a second-line agent for metastatic breast cancer in postmenopausal women after progression on endocrine therapy.

Interestingly, modulation of the ER pathway using targeted agents with diverse mechanisms of action has resulted in differing toxicity profiles. For example, the ATAC trial demonstrated that anastrozole was associated with a lower incidence of hot flashes, vaginal bleeding, endometrial cancer, cerebrovascular ischemic events, and thromboembolic events but demonstrated a higher incidence of musculoskeletal pain and bone fractures compared to tamoxifen. In addition, trials in the metastatic setting demonstrated a response to aromatase inhibitors in patients with tamoxifen-refractory disease (and vice versa), suggesting that a single pathway can be successfully targeted by multiple agents with differing mechanisms of action and that the side effects of such agents do not necessarily share similarity (62).

3.2. Targeting the HER Signaling Pathway

3.2.1. TARGETING THE HER SIGNALING PATHWAY USING ANTIBODY THERAPY

Trastuzumab (Herceptin) is a recombinant humanized monoclonal antibody against the extracellular domain of HER2. Trastuzumab inhibits cancer cell proliferation, induces apoptosis, and reduces tumor-induced angiogenesis in preclinical breast cancer models (63).

The exact mechanism of trastuzumab activity remains unknown; however, preclinical data suggest that the drug induces antibody-mediated cytotoxicity as well as sequesters HER2 and prevents interactions with other members of the HER family.

Trastuzumab has demonstrated activity as a single agent (PR=24%–35%) in patients with metastatic breast cancer whose tumors overexpress HER2 *(64–66)*. Phase I trials initially investigated weekly administration (4 mg/kg loading dose, followed by 2 mg/kg weekly maintenance doses), but later pharmacokinetic studies suggested that an alternative dosing schedule (8 mg/kg loading followed by 6 mg/kg every-3-weeks) was feasible. The q-3 week dosing schedule was similar in efficacy and toxicity compared to weekly dosing, but offered increased easy of administration and fewer patient visits for therapy *(67)*.

Trastuzumab also augments the effects of chemotherapy. A pivotal trial randomized 469 women with previously untreated HER2-overexpressing metastatic breast cancer to chemotherapy alone (either doxorubicin/epirubicin and cyclophosphamide or paclitaxel) or chemotherapy plus trastuzumab *(4)*. Disease response rate, median duration of response, and overall survival were all improved in patients who received chemotherapy with trastuzumab.

Although earlier phase trials did not demonstrate significant cardiac toxicity with single-agent trastuzumab, a higher rate of congestive heart failure (CHF) was noted in patients treated with trastuzumab. When compared to the antracycline/trastuzumab arm, the incidence of CHF was less in patients receiving paclitaxel/trastuzumab. Upon further analysis of time to disease progression, death, or cardiac dysfunction, the median time to undesired clinical outcome was still in favor of combination therapy with trastuzumab. Based upon the results of this randomized trial, other trastuzumab based chemotherapy regimens have been investigated for the treatment of patients with HER2 overexpressing metastatic breast cancer (Table 3).

Trastuzumab has also been used as adjuvant therapy to reduce the risk of recurrence in patients with localized breast cancer *(68,69)*. The interim results of several large randomized trials of adjuvant trastuzumab have been reported (Table 4).

The Herceptin Adjuvant (HERA) [Breast International Group (BIG) 01-01] trial, was an open-label, Phase III trial designed to evaluate the effectiveness of adjuvant trastuzumab administered after completion of adjuvant systemic chemotherapy *(70)*. This study randomized patients who had completed adjuvant chemotherapy to undergo observation alone, a regimen of trastuzumab administered every 3 weeks for 1 year, or a regimen that included the same schedule of trastuzumab for 2 years. At the 12-month follow-up, there was an improvement in DFS as well as the time to distant recurrence in patients with

Table 3
Chemotherapy Drugs Commonly Combined
with Trastuzumab

Drug(s)	Response Rate
Paclitaxel (+/− carboplatin)	36–77%
Docetaxel (+/− platinum)	58–79%
Navelbine	40–86%
Gemcitabine (+/− carboplatin)	36–44%
Capecitabine	60–76%

Table 4
Current Adjuvant Trials Evaluating Trastuzumab

Trial	Study arms	No.	Median follow-up (months)	DFS(%)	HR(p)	OS(%)	HR (p)
HERA (70)	→ obs	1698	24	74		90	
	Any chemo → Tq3w × 1 year	1703		81	0.63 (<0.0001)	92	0.63 (0.0051)
	→ Tq3w × 2 years						
NSABP B-31 with	AC × 4 → P × 4	1679	24	67		87	
NCCTG N9831 (71)	AC × 4 → P × 4 + Tqw × 1 year	1672		85	0.48 (<0.0001)	91	0.67 (0.02)
FinHer (72)	D or V → FEC	116	36	78		90	
	D or V + Tqw → FEC	115		89	0.42 (0.01)	96	0.41 (0.07)
BCIRG 006 (74)	AC × 4 → D × 4	1073	23	73			
	AC × 4 → D × 4 → Tq3w × 1 year	1074		84	0.49 (<0.0001)		
	D/C/Tqw × 6 → Tq3w × 1 year	1075		80	0.61 (0.0002)		

AC, doxorubicin/cyclophosphamide; P, paclitaxel; T, trastuzumab; D, docetaxel; C, carboplatin; V, vinorelbine; FEC, fluorouracil/ epirubicin/cyclophosphamide; Tqw, 4 mg/kg loading dose followed by 2 mg/kg/week; Tq3w, 8 mg/kg loading dose followed by 6 mg/kg every 3 weeks received adjuvant trastuzumab. To date, the optimal duration of trastuzumab administration (1 year versus 2 years) remains undefined.

The North Central Cancer Treatment Group (NCCTG) N9831 and National Surgical Adjuvant Breast and Bowel Project (NSABP) B-31 trials shared a similar study design and have thus been reported in a joint analysis. After a median follow-up of 24 months, a significant reduction in risk of disease recurrence and improvement in DFS was seen in patients receiving trastuzumab. Overall survival was also significantly improved for the trastuzumab arm, 91.4% versus 86.6% in the control arm ($p = 0.015$) *(71)*.

Although the Finland Herceptin (FinHer) trial was designed to evaluate the effects of adjuvant docetaxel versus vinorelbine followed by 5-fluorouracil, epirubicin and cyclophosphamide (FEC), it included a small subset of 232 patients with HER2-positive disease who were also randomized to either chemotherapy alone or 9 weekly treatments of trastuzumab given concurrently with docetaxel or vinorelbine *(72)*. Despite the shorter duration of therapy, improvement in DFS was similar to that observed in the other adjuvant trials that administered trastuzumab for 1 year. Such results call into question the optimal duration of trastuzumab needed to demonstrate clinical benefit in the adjuvant setting. Moreover, due to the prolonged half-life of trastuzumab, it is likely that therapeutic concentrations of the drug were present when patients received subsequent epirubicin. Thus, the combined treatment with an anthracycline cannot be excluded as the reason that a shorter duration of therapy showed similar benefit as in the studies that used extended administration of trastuzumab *(72)*.

Of further interest, the FinHer study demonstrated an improvement in left ventricular ejection fraction in patients receiving adjuvant trastuzumab despite the combined anthracycline and trastuzumab exposure. A similar cardiac toxicity profile was also seen in a small neoadjuvant study combining epirubicin with trastuzumab in patients with HER2-overexpressing locally advanced breast cancer *(73)*.

The Breast Cancer International Research Group (BCIRG) trial alternatively questioned the role for anthracyclines in the adjuvant setting for patients with HER2-overexpressing breast cancer. Patients enrolled in the control arm received doxorubicin-cyclophosphamide (AC) followed by docetaxel. Patients treated in the trastuzumab-containing arms received either AC followed by docetaxel with trastuzumab or docetaxel and platinum (carboplatin or cisplatin) with trastuzumab *(74)*. This study demonstrated that 1 year of trastuzumab improved the DFS compared to adjuvant chemotherapy alone, however, longer follow-up is needed to determine if anthracyclines are necessary for the treatment of HER2-positive breast cancer.

Other antibodies that target HER2 are at earlier stages in clinical development. Pertuzumab (2C4) is a monoclonal antibody that binds to HER2 on a different epitope than trastuzumab. It blocks heterodimer formation, which results in decreased intracellular signaling *(75)*. Phase II trials investigating pertuzumab are currently accruing patients with metastatic breast cancer.

Planned or ongoing clinical trials are underway to determine the benefit of antibodies against EGFR in combination with irinotecan *(15)* or in combination with carboplatin for the treatment of ER-, PR-, and HER2-negative (triple negative) metastatic breast cancer.

3.2.2. TARGETING THE HER SIGNALING PATHWAY USING SMALL-MOLECULE INHIBITORS

Lapatinib (Tykerb) is a small-molecule TKI that targets both HER1 (EGFR) and HER2. In preclinical models, lapatinib inhibited growth and induced apoptosis in HER1 (EGFR)/HER2 overexpressing breast cancer cell lines *(76,77)*. Phase I studies have demonstrated responses for lapatinib both as a single agent (6%) and combined with trastuzumab (26%) *(78,79)*. A randomized Phase III trial demonstrated improved efficacy for the combination of capecitabine and lapatinib compared to single-agent capecitabine in patients with HER2-positive metastatic breast cancer who had received prior anthracyclines, taxanes, and trastuzumab *(80)*. Lapatinib has also demonstrated clinical responses when administered with paclitaxel in patients with inflammatory breast cancer *(81)*. Large randomized Phase III trials are currently in progress to determine the role of lapatinib in combination with paclitaxel or in combination with paclitaxel and trastuzumab as first-line therapy for patients with HER2-overexpressing metastatic breast cancer *(82)*. The use of lapatinib for the adjuvant treatment of breast cancer has yet to be defined.

In contrast to lapatinib, oral TKIs that exclusively target HER1 (EGFR) have demonstrated little single-agent activity in heavily pretreated breast cancer patients *(83,84)*. To date, no studies have demonstrated an improved response rate or time to progression with the combination of HER1 (EGFR) inhibitors and chemotherapy for the treatment of breast cancer *(86–89)*. In addition, the combination of the small-molecule TKI gefitinib with trastuzumab resulted in a lower response rate and worse median time to progression than would be expected with trastuzumab alone *(85)*.

Canertinib (CI-1033) is an oral TKI that irreversibly inhibits the entire HER family of receptors. In Phase I trials, it was well tolerated and evidence of stable disease was seen, prompting current Phase II trials *(90)*.

3.3. Targeting VEGF for the Treatment of Breast Cancer

Bevacizumab (Avastin) is a recombinant, humanized antibody against VEGF. The drug has demonstrated single-agent response rates of 6.7% to 17.0% in breast cancer patients with previously treated metastatic disease *(91)*. When given in combination with capecitabine as a second- to third-line therapy for metastatic breast cancer, bevacizumab did not significantly improve DFS, although a doubling in response rate was seen *(91,92)*. However, patients who received bevacizumab in combination with paclitaxel as first-line therapy for metastatic breast cancer had improved response rates and DFS compared to patients receiving paclitaxel alone *(93)*. These results suggest that earlier exposure to biologic compounds may be necessary for maximum efficacy. It is also feasible that not all chemotherapeutic agents are equally synergistic with biologic agents; thus, careful consideration of the drug's mechanism of action and preclinical demonstration of synergy should be considered prior to implementation of clinical trials investigating combination therapy.

The role of bevacizumab in combination with dose-dense adriamycin plus cytoxan (AC) followed by paclitaxel as adjuvant therapy in patients with node-positive breast cancer is currently under investigation. Bevacizumab has also been tested in combination with neoadjuvant chemotherapy for the treatment of patients with inoperable and inflammatory breast cancer *(94,95)* In addition, a Phase II study combining bevacizumab and trastuzumab has been reported, with a response rate exceeding 50% in the absence of chemotherapy *(96)*.

Small-molecule TKIs that target angiogenesis have demonstrated mixed results in patients with metastatic breast cancer. ZD6474 (inhibits VEGFR-2, EGFR, FDFR-1, RET) demonstrated no objective clinical response and no effect on tumor perfusion as measured by dynamic contrast-enhanced (DCE) MRI, but sunitinib (inhibits VEGF, PDGF, KIT, FLT3) demonstrated activity in patients with heavily pretreated advanced breast cancer *(97,98)*.

Completion of ongoing clinical trials is needed to establish the role of these agents in combination with chemotherapy.

3.4. Other Targeted Drugs for Breast Cancer Therapy

Farnesyltransferase (FTase) catalyzes the thiol-ester attachment of a farnesyl moiety onto proteins such as Ras and can be specifically targeted to inhibit the posttranslational processing necessary for membrane localization of such signaling proteins *(99)*. FTIs have demonstrated single-agent activity (~25% clinical benefit rate) in patients with advanced breast cancer and are now being evaluated in the neoadjuvant setting in combination with chemotherapy *(100,101)*.

Several mTOR inhibitors are also being studied for the treatment of metastatic breast cancer. Temsirolimus has demonstrated a response rate of 9.2% in heavily pretreated patients *(102)*. A randomized Phase II study investigated letrozole ± Temsirolimus in patients with ER-positive and/or PR-positive metastatic breast cancer. The addition of Temsirolimus resulted in an improved DFS versus letrozole alone, although a larger follow-up Phase III trial failed to show benefit *(103,104)*. Phase I/II studies of everolimus in combination with chemotherapy or trastuzumab are ongoing in patients with metastatic breast cancer.

4. FUTURE DIRECTION OF TARGETED THERAPY FOR BREAST CANCER

Inhibition of the complex signaling networks responsible for breast cancer growth, survival, and resistance to chemotherapy has demonstrated early success but remains a daunting challenge for drug development. Further insight into the mechanism of action of targeted agents and their effects on downstream signaling is needed to exploit maximally their role in breast cancer therapy.

In addition, although targeted agents were anticipated to have fewer systemic effects, clinical trials have demonstrated significant toxicity, including diarrhea, hypertension, and CHF in a significant number of patients treated with these agents. As such, continued research should include molecular predictors to identify patient populations likely to benefit from these drugs. As an example, HER2 expression was identified as a predictive marker for response prior to initiation of clinical trials with anti-HER2 therapies. These assays proved vital to drug development as trastuzumab would likely have been discarded owing to inadequate activity in an unselected patient population.

Significant effort has been spent in the development of small-molecule inhibitors and antibodies against IGF1R *(34)*. Most of these agents are in early phase development as single agents and have not undergone combination studies with chemotherapy or endocrine therapy. Agents targeting B-RAF, aurora kinases, Src, and PDGF are also in early clinical development and may play a key role in the treatment of breast cancer.

With a growing knowledge base of signaling networks, the multitude of novel biologic agents entering the clinical arena will present challenges for developing and incorporating targeted agents into standard systemic therapy regimens. It is also likely that combinations of agents, blocking several steps in cellular pathways, will prove most efficacious for the treatment of select populations of patients. Preclinical models must be improved to determine which drugs or combinations should proceed forward into clinical development for the treatment of breast cancer to utilize limited clinical resources rationally. Although there are many challenges to consider, targeted therapies have demonstrated substantial benefit for patients with breast cancer, and continued development of these agents should ultimately lead to improvement in quality of life and reduced mortality for these patients.

REFERENCES

1. Jemal A, Siegel R, Ward E, et al. Cancer statistics, 2007. CA Cancer J Clin 2007;57:43–66.
2. Nabholtz JM, Senn HJ, Bezwoda WR, et al. Prospective randomized trial of docetaxel versus mitomycin plus vinblastine in patients with metastatic breast cancer progressing despite previous anthracycline-containing chemotherapy; 304 Study Group. J Clin Oncol 1999;17:1413–24.
3. Bishop JF, Dewar J, Toner GC, et al. Initial paclitaxel improves outcome compared with CMFP combination chemotherapy as front-line therapy in untreated metastatic breast cancer. J Clin Oncol 1999;17:2355–64.
4. Slamon DJ, Leyland-Jones B, Shak S, et al. Use of chemotherapy plus a monoclonal antibody against HER2 for metastatic breast cancer that overexpresses HER2. N Engl J Med 2001;344:783–92.
5. Greenberg PA, Hortobagyi GN, Smith TL, et al. Long-term follow-up of patients with complete remission following combination chemotherapy for metastatic breast cancer. J Clin Oncol 1996;14:2197–205.
6. Polychemotherapy for early breast cancer: an overview of the randomised trials; Early Breast Cancer Trialists' Collaborative Group. Lancet 1998;352:930–42.
7. Tamoxifen for early breast cancer: an overview of the randomised trials; Early Breast Cancer Trialists' Collaborative Group. Lancet 1998;351:1451–67.
8. Mauriac L, Durand M, Avril A, et al. Effects of primary chemotherapy in conservative treatment of breast cancer patients with operable tumors larger than 3 cm: results of a randomized trial in a single centre. Ann Oncol 1991;2:347–54.
9. Perloff M, Lesnick GJ, Korzun A, et al. Combination chemotherapy with mastectomy or radiotherapy for stage III breast carcinoma: a Cancer and Leukemia Group B study. J Clin Oncol 1988;6:261–9.
10. Berry DA, Cronin KA, Plevritis SK, et al. Effect of screening and adjuvant therapy on mortality from breast cancer. N Engl J Med 2005;353:1784–92.
11. Beatson CT. On treatment of inoperable cases of carcinoma of the mamma: suggestions for a new method of treatment with illustrative cases. Lancet 1896;2:104–7.
12. Smith DF, Toft DO. Steroid receptors and their associated proteins. Mol Endocrinol 1993;7:4–11.
13. Pennisi E. Differing roles found for estrogen's two receptors. Science 1997;277:1439.
14. Atalay G, Cardoso F, Awada A, et al. Novel therapeutic strategies targeting the epidermal growth factor receptor (EGFR) family and its downstream effectors in breast cancer. Ann Oncol 2003;14:1346–63.
15. Hobday TJ, Perez EA. Molecularly targeted therapies for breast cancer. Cancer Control 2005;12:73–81.
16. Menard S, Fortis S, Castiglioni F, et al. HER2 as a prognostic factor in breast cancer. Oncology 2001;61(suppl 2):67–72.
17. Ross JS, Fletcher JA. The HER-2/neu oncogene in breast cancer: prognostic factor, predictive factor, and target for therapy. Stem Cells 1998;16:413–28.
18. Moulder SL, Yakes FM, Muthuswamy SK, et al. Epidermal growth factor receptor (HER1) tyrosine kinase inhibitor ZD1839 (Iressa) inhibits HER2/neu (erbB2)-overexpressing breast cancer cells in vitro and in vivo. Cancer Res 2001;61:8887–95.
19. Arteaga CL, Ramsey TT, Shawver LK, et al. Unliganded epidermal growth factor receptor dimerization induced by direct interaction of quinazolines with the ATP binding site. J Biol Chem 1997;272:23247–54.
20. Nicholson S, Sainsbury JR, Halcrow P, et al. Expression of epidermal growth factor receptors associated with lack of response to endocrine therapy in recurrent breast cancer. Lancet 1989;1:182–5.
21. Ferrara N, Gerber HP, LeCouter J. The biology of VEGF and its receptors. Nat Med 2003;9:669–76.
22. Fan F, Wey JS, McCarty MF, et al. Expression and function of vascular endothelial growth factor receptor-1 on human colorectal cancer cells. Oncogene 2005;24:2647–53.
23. Schneider BP, Sledge GW Jr. Drug insight: VEGF as a therapeutic target for breast cancer. Nat Clin Pract Oncol 2007;4:181–9.
24. Fong GH, Rossant J, Gertsenstein M, et al. Role of the Flt-1 receptor tyrosine kinase in regulating the assembly of vascular endothelium. Nature 1995;376:66–70.
25. Dvorak HF. Vascular permeability factor/vascular endothelial growth factor: a critical cytokine in tumor angiogenesis and a potential target for diagnosis and therapy. J Clin Oncol 2002;20:4368–80.
26. Stacker SA, Caesar C, Baldwin ME, et al. VEGF-D promotes the metastatic spread of tumor cells via the lymphatics. Nat Med 2001;7:186–91.
27. Weidner N, Semple JP, Welch WR, et al. Tumor angiogenesis and metastasis?correlation in invasive breast carcinoma. N Engl J Med 1991;324:1–8.
28. Brem SS, Gullino PM, Medina D. Angiogenesis: a marker for neoplastic transformation of mammary papillary hyperplasia. Science 1977;195:880–2.
29. Weinstat-Saslow DL, Zabrenetzky VS, VanHoutte K, et al. Transfection of thrombospondin 1 complementary DNA into a human breast carcinoma cell line reduces primary tumor growth, metastatic potential, and angiogenesis. Cancer Res 1994;54:6504–11.

30. Ullrich A, Bell JR, Chen EY, et al. Human insulin receptor and its relationship to the tyrosine kinase family of oncogenes. Nature 1985;313:756–61.
31. Pandini G, Vigneri R, Costantino A, et al. Insulin and insulin-like growth factor-I (IGF-I) receptor overexpression in breast cancers leads to insulin/IGF-I hybrid receptor overexpression: evidence for a second mechanism of IGF-I signaling. Clin Cancer Res 1999;5:1935–44.
32. Bonneterre J, Peyrat JP, Beuscart R, et al. Prognostic significance of insulin-like growth factor 1 receptors in human breast cancer. Cancer Res 1990; 50:6931–5.
33. Peyrat JP, Bonneterre J, Beuscart R, et al. Insulin-like growth factor 1 receptors in human breast cancer and their relation to estradiol and progesterone receptors. Cancer Res 1988; 48:6429–33.
34. Sachdev D, Yee D. Inhibitors of insulin-like growth factor signaling: a therapeutic approach for breast cancer. J Mamm Gland Biol Neoplasia 2006;11:27–39.
35. Arteaga CL, Kitten LJ, Coronado EB, et al. Blockade of the type I somatomedin receptor inhibits growth of human breast cancer cells in athymic mice. J Clin Invest 1989;84:1418–23.
36. Salatino M, Schillaci R, Proietti CJ, et al. Inhibition of in vivo breast cancer growth by antisense oligodeoxynucleotides to type I insulin-like growth factor receptor mRNA involves inactivation of ErbBs, PI-3K/Akt and p42/p44 MAPK signaling pathways but not modulation of progesterone receptor activity. Oncogene 2004;23:5161–74.
37. Pawson T, Scott JD. Signaling through scaffold, anchoring, and adaptor proteins. Science 1997;278:2075–80.
38. Greulich H, Erikson RL. An analysis of Mek1 signaling in cell proliferation and transformation. J Biol Chem 1998;273:13280–8.
39. Tibbles LA, Woodgett JR. The stress-activated protein kinase pathways. Cell Mol Life Sci 1999;55:1230–54.
40. Janes PW, Daly RJ, deFazio A, et al. Activation of the Ras signalling pathway in human breast cancer cells overexpressing erbB-2. Oncogene 1994; 9:3601–8.
41. Fiddes RJ, Janes PW, Sivertsen SP, et al. Inhibition of the MAP kinase cascade blocks heregulin-induced cell cycle progression in T-47D human breast cancer cells. Oncogene 1998;16:2803–13.
42. Xing C, Imagawa W. Altered MAP kinase (ERK1,2) regulation in primary cultures of mammary tumor cells: elevated basal activity and sustained response to EGF. Carcinogenesis 1999;20:1201–8.
43. Carraway H, Hidalgo M. New targets for therapy in breast cancer: mammalian target of rapamycin (mTOR) antagonists. Breast Cancer Res 2004;6:219–24.
44. Asnaghi L, Bruno P, Priulla M, et al. mTOR: a protein kinase switching between life and death. Pharmacol Res 2004;50:545–9.
45. Holbro T, Beerli RR, Maurer F, et al. The ErbB2/ErbB3 heterodimer functions as an oncogenic unit: ErbB2 requires ErbB3 to drive breast tumor cell proliferation. Proc Natl Acad Sci U S A 2003;100:8933–8.
46. Bachman KE, Argani P, Samuels Y, et al. The PIK3CA gene is mutated with high frequency in human breast cancers. Cancer Biol Ther 2004;3:772–5.
47. Kang S, Bader AG, Vogt PK. Phosphatidylinositol 3-kinase mutations identified in human cancer are oncogenic. Proc Natl Acad Sci U S A 2005;102:802–7.
48. Perren A, Weng LP, Boag AH, et al. Immunohistochemical evidence of loss of PTEN expression in primary ductal adenocarcinomas of the breast. Am J Pathol 1999;155:1253–60.
49. Tsutsui S, Inoue H, Yasuda K, et al. Reduced expression of PTEN protein and its prognostic implications in invasive ductal carcinoma of the breast. Oncology 2005;68:398–404.
50. Ingle JN, Ahmann DL, Green SJ, et al. Randomized clinical trial of diethylstilbestrol versus tamoxifen in postmenopausal women with advanced breast cancer. N Engl J Med 1981;304:16–21.
51. Bonneterre J, Buzdar A, Nabholtz JM, et al. Anastrozole is superior to tamoxifen as first-line therapy in hormone receptor positive advanced breast carcinoma. Cancer 2001;92:2247–58.
52. Mouridsen H, Gershanovich M, Sun Y, et al. Phase III study of letrozole versus tamoxifen as first-line therapy of advanced breast cancer in postmenopausal women: analysis of survival and update of efficacy from the International Letrozole Breast Cancer Group. J Clin Oncol 2003;21:2101–9.
53. Hortobagyi GN. Opportunities and challenges in the development of targeted therapies. Semin Oncol 2004;31:21–7.
54. Fisher B, Costantino JP, Wickerham DL, et al. Tamoxifen for prevention of breast cancer: report of the National Surgical Adjuvant Breast and Bowel Project P-1 Study. J Natl Cancer Inst 1998;90:1371–88.
55. Vogel VG, Costantino JP, Wickerham DL, et al. Effects of tamoxifen vs raloxifene on the risk of developing invasive breast cancer and other disease outcomes: the NSABP Study of Tamoxifen and Raloxifene (STAR) P-2 trial. JAMA 2006;295:2727–41.
56. Smith IE, Dowsett M. Aromatase inhibitors in breast cancer. N Engl J Med 2003;348:2431–42.
57. Buzdar A. An overview of the use of non-steroidal aromatase inhibitors in the treatment of breast cancer. Eur J Cancer 2000;36(suppl 4):S82–4.

58. Howell A, Cuzick J, Baum M, et al. Results of the ATAC (arimidex, tamoxifen, alone or in combination) trial after completion of 5 years' adjuvant treatment for breast cancer. Lancet 2005;365:60–2.

59. Howell A, Pippen J, Elledge RM, et al. Fulvestrant versus anastrozole for the treatment of advanced breast carcinoma: a prospectively planned combined survival analysis of two multicenter trials. Cancer 2005;104:236–9.

60. Howell A, Robertson JF, Quaresma Albano J, et al. Fulvestrant, formerly ICI 182,780, is as effective as anastrozole in postmenopausal women with advanced breast cancer progressing after prior endocrine treatment. J Clin Oncol 2002;20:3396–403.

61. Osborne CK, Pippen J, Jones SE, et al. Double-blind, randomized trial comparing the efficacy and tolerability of fulvestrant versus anastrozole in postmenopausal women with advanced breast cancer progressing on prior endocrine therapy: results of a North American trial. J Clin Oncol 2002;20:3386–95.

62. Thurlimann B, Hess D, Koberle D, et al. Anastrozole ('Arimidex') versus tamoxifen as first-line therapy in postmenopausal women with advanced breast cancer: results of the double-blind cross-over SAKK trial 21/95—a sub-study of the TARGET (Tamoxifen or 'Arimidex' Randomized Group Efficacy and Tolerability) trial. Breast Cancer Res Treat 2004;85:247–54.

63. Emens LA, Davidson NE. Trastuzumab in breast cancer. Oncology (Williston Park) 2004;18:1117–28; discussion 1131–2, 1137–8.

64. Smith IE. Efficacy and safety of Herceptin in women with metastatic breast cancer: results from pivotal clinical studies. Anticancer Drugs 2001;12(suppl 4):S3–10.

65. Vogel CL, Cobleigh MA, Tripathy D, et al. Efficacy and safety of trastuzumab as a single agent in first-line treatment of HER2-overexpressing metastatic breast cancer. J Clin Oncol 2002;20:719–26.

66. Cobleigh MA, Vogel CL, Tripathy D, et al. Multinational study of the efficacy and safety of humanized anti-HER2 monoclonal antibody in women who have HER2-overexpressing metastatic breast cancer that has progressed after chemotherapy for metastatic disease. J Clin Oncol 1999;17:2639–48.

67. Baselga J, Carbonell X, Castaneda-Soto NJ, et al. Phase II study of efficacy, safety, and pharmacokinetics of trastuzumab monotherapy administered on a 3-weekly schedule. J Clin Oncol 2005;23:2162–71.

68. Osoba D, Burchmore M. Health-related quality of life in women with metastatic breast cancer treated with trastuzumab (Herceptin). Semin Oncol 1999;26:84–8.

69. Osoba D, Slamon DJ, Burchmore M, et al. Effects on quality of life of combined trastuzumab and chemotherapy in women with metastatic breast cancer. J Clin Oncol 2002;20:3106–13.

70. Smith I, Procter M, Gelber RD, et al. 2-year follow-up of trastuzumab after adjuvant chemotherapy in HER2-positive breast cancer: a randomised controlled trial. Lancet 2007;369:29–36.

71. Romond EH, Perez EA, Bryant J, et al. Trastuzumab plus adjuvant chemotherapy for operable HER2-positive breast cancer. N Engl J Med 2005;353:1673–84.

72. Joensuu H, Kellokumpu-Lehtinen PL, Bono P, et al. Adjuvant docetaxel or vinorelbine with or without trastuzumab for breast cancer. N Engl J Med 2006;354:809–20.

73. Buzdar AU, Ibrahim NK, Francis D, et al. Significantly higher pathologic complete remission rate after neoadjuvant therapy with trastuzumab, paclitaxel, and epirubicin chemotherapy: results of a randomized trial in human epidermal growth factor receptor 2-positive operable breast cancer. J Clin Oncol 2005;23:3676–85.

74. Slamon D, Eiermann W, Robert N, et al. Phase III randomized trial comparing doxorubicin and cyclophosphamide followed by docetaxel (ACT) with doxorubicin and cyclophosphamide followed by docetaxel and trastuzumab (ACTH) with docetaxel, carboplatin and trastuzumab (TCH) in HER2 positive early breast cancer patients: BCIRG 006 study. Breast Cancer Res 2005;94:S5.

75. Agus DB, Gordon MS, Taylor C, et al. Phase I clinical study of pertuzumab, a novel HER dimerization inhibitor, in patients with advanced cancer. J Clin Oncol 2005;23:2534–43.

76. Rusnak DW, Lackey K, Affleck K, et al. The effects of the novel, reversible epidermal growth factor receptor/ErbB-2 tyrosine kinase inhibitor, GW2016, on the growth of human normal and tumor-derived cell lines in vitro and in vivo. Mol Cancer Ther 2001;1:85–94.

77. Xia W, Mullin RJ, Keith BR, et al. Anti-tumor activity of GW572016: a dual tyrosine kinase inhibitor blocks EGF activation of EGFR/erbB2 and downstream Erk1/2 and AKT pathways. Oncogene 2002;21: 6255–63.

78. Burris HA 3rd, Hurwitz HI, Dees EC, et al. Phase I safety, pharmacokinetics, and clinical activity study of lapatinib (GW572016), a reversible dual inhibitor of epidermal growth factor receptor tyrosine kinases, in heavily pretreated patients with metastatic carcinomas. J Clin Oncol 2005;23:5305–13.

79. Storniolo A, Burris, H, Pegram, M et al. A phase I, open-label study of lapatinib (GW572016) plus trastuzumab; a clinically active regimen. Proc Am Soc Clin Oncol 2005;23:559. Abstract.

80. Geyer CE, Forster J, Lindquist D, et al. Lapatinib plus capecitabine for HER2-positive advanced breast cancer. N Engl J Med 2006;355:2733–43.

81. Cristofanilli M, Boussen H, Baselga J, et al. A phase II combination study of lapatinib and paclitaxel as a neoadjuvant therapy in patients with newly diagnosed inflammatory breast cancer (IBC). Breast Cancer Res Treat 2006;100(suppl 1).

82. Moy B, Goss PE. Lapatinib: current status and future directions in breast cancer. Oncologist 2006;11: 1047–57.

83. Baselga J, Albanell J, Ruiz A, et al. Phase II and tumor pharmacodynamic study of gefitinib in patients with advanced breast cancer. J Clin Oncol 2005;23:5323–33.

84. Von Minckwitz G, Jonat W, Fasching P, et al. A multicentre phase II study on gefitinib in taxane- and anthracycline-pretreated metastatic breast cancer. Breast Cancer Res Treat 2005;89:165–72.

85. Arteaga CL, O'Neil A, Moulder SL, et al. A phase i-ii study of combined blockade of the erB receptor network with trastuzumab and gefitinib (Iressa) in patients (pts) with HER2-overexpressing metastatic breast cancer (met br ca). Presented at the 27th Annual San Antonio Breast Cancer Symposium, San Antonio, TX, December 2004. Abstract 24.

86. Ciardiello F, Troiani T, Caputo F, et al. Phase II study of gefitinib in combination with docetaxel as first-line therapy in metastatic breast cancer. Br J Cancer 2006;94:1604–9.

87. Fountzilas G, Pectasides D, Kalogera-Fountzila A, et al. Paclitaxel and carboplatin as first-line chemotherapy combined with gefitinib (IRESSA) in patients with advanced breast cancer: a phase I/II study conducted by the Hellenic Cooperative Oncology Group. Breast Cancer Res Treat 2005;92:1–9.

88. Grahm D, Hillman D, Hobday T, et al. N0234: phase II study of erlotinib (OSI-774) plus gemcitabine as first- or second-line therapy for metastatic breast cancer (MBC). Presented at the 2005 ASCO Annual Meeting.

89. Guarneri V, Fressoldati A, Ficarra G, et al. Final results of a phase II, double blind, placebo controlled, randomized trial of preoperative chemotherapy + gefitinib with biomarker evaluation in operable breast cancer. Ann Oncol 2006;17(suppl 9).

90. Allen LF, Eiseman IA, Fry DW, et al. CI-1033, an irreversible pan-erbB receptor inhibitor and its potential application for the treatment of breast cancer. Semin Oncol 2003;30:65–78.

91. Cobleigh MA, Langmuir VK, Sledge GW, et al. A phase I/II dose-escalation trial of bevacizumab in previously treated metastatic breast cancer. Semin Oncol 2003;30:117–24.

92. Miller KD, Chap LI, Holmes FA, et al. Randomized phase III trial of capecitabine compared with bevacizumab plus capecitabine in patients with previously treated metastatic breast cancer. J Clin Oncol 2005;23:792–9.

93. Miller KD, Jea G. E2100: a randomized phase III trial of paclitaxel versus paclitaxel plus bevacizumab as first-line therapy for locally recurrent or metastatic breast cancer: ASCO annual meeting proceedings. J Clin Oncol 2005;23:16S.

94. Overmoyer B, Silverman P, Leeming R, et al. Phase II trial of neoadjuvant docetaxel with or without bevacizumab in patients with locally advanced breast cancer. J Clin Oncol 2004 2004;22:727.

95. Wedam SB, Low JA, Yang SX, et al. Antiangiogenic and antitumor effects of bevacizumab in patients with inflammatory and locally advanced breast cancer. J Clin Oncol 2006;24:769–77.

96. Pegram M, Chan D, Dichmann RA, et al. Phase II combined biological therapy targeting the oncogene and the vascular endothelial growth factor using trastuzumab (T) and Bevacizumab (B) in the first-line treatment of HER2-amplified breast cancer. Breast Cancer Res Treat 2006;100:S28–9.

97. Miller KD, Burstein HJ, Elias AD, et al. Phase II study of SU11248, a multitargeted receptor tyrosine kinase inhibitor (TKI), in patients (pts) with previously treated metastatic breast cancer (MBC). J Clin Oncol 2005;23:563.

98. Miller KD, Trigo JM, Wheeler C, et al. A multicenter phase II trial of ZD6474, a vascular endothelial growth factor receptor-2 and epidermal growth factor receptor tyrosine kinase inhibitor, in patients with previously treated metastatic breast cancer. Clin Cancer Res 2005;11:3369–76.

99. Ohkanda J, Knowles DB, Blaskovich MA, et al. Inhibitors of protein farnesyltransferase as novel anticancer agents. Curr Top Med Chem 2002;2:303–23.

100. Sparano JA, Moulder S, Kazi A, et al. Targeted inhibition of farnesyltransferase in locally advanced breast cancer: a phase I and II trial of tipifarnib plus dose-dense doxorubicin and cyclophosphamide. J Clin Oncol 2006;24:3013–8.

101. Johnston SR, Hickish T, Ellis P, et al. Phase II study of the efficacy and tolerability of two dosing regimens of the farnesyl transferase inhibitor, R115777, in advanced breast cancer. J Clin Oncol 2003;21:2492–9.

102. Chan S, Scheulen ME, Johnston S, et al. Phase II study of temsirolimus (CCI-779), a novel inhibitor of mTOR, in heavily pretreated patients with locally advanced or metastatic breast cancer. J Clin Oncol 2005;23:5314–22.

103. Chollet P, Abrial C, Tacca O, et al. Mammalian target of rapamycin inhibitors in combination with letrozole in breast cancer. Clin Breast Cancer 2006;7:336–8.

104. Baselga J, Fumoleau P, Gil M, et al. Phase II three-arm study of CCI-779 in combination with letrozole in postmenopausal women with locally advanced or metastatic breast cancer: preliminary results. Proc Annu Meeting Am Soc Clin Oncol 2004;22:(14S):544. Abstract.
105. Ingle JN, Tu D, Pater JL, et al. Duration of letrozole treatment and outcomes in the placebo-controlled NCIC CTG MA.17 extended adjuvant therapy trial. Breast Cancer Res Treat 2006;99:295–300.
106. Coombes RC, Kilburn LS, Snowdon CF, et al. Survival and safety of exemestane versus tamoxifen after 2–3 years' tamoxifen treatment (Intergroup Exemestane Study): a randomised controlled trial. Lancet 2007;369:559–70.
107. Monnier A. The evolving role of letrozole in the adjuvant setting: first results from the large, phase III, randomized trial BIG 1–98. Breast 2006;15(suppl 1):S21–9.

4 Targeted Therapy in Chronic Lymphocytic Leukemia

*Apostolia-Maria Tsimberidou, MD, PhD
and Michael J. Keating, MD*

CONTENTS

INTRODUCTION
MOLECULAR MECHANISMS PERTINENT TO DISEASE
TARGETED THERAPIES
FUTURE DIRECTIONS IN MOLECULAR THERAPEUTICS
REFERENCES

ABSTRACT

Chronic lymphocytic leukemia (CLL) is characterized by a monoclonal population of mature, activated B lymphocytes. It is a heterogeneous disorder with a variable clinical course. Although in recent years the introduction of chemoimmunotherapeutic combinations such as fludarabine, cyclophosphamide, and rituximab (FCR) has induced response rates of 95% in previously untreated patients and increased the rates of failure-free survival, CLL remains incurable for many patients. However, a better understanding of the molecular basis of CLL has led to the development of several novel therapeutic strategies that target molecular pathways. These targeted therapies inhibit signaling pathways involved in growth and proliferation in CLL cells. Among the targeted therapies being investigated in CLL are the following: monoclonal antibodies against CD52 (alemtuzumab), CD20 (rituximab, ofatumumab), CD23 (lumiliximab), and CD40 (HCD122); agents that target molecular pathways, such as cyclin-dependent kinase inhibitors (flavopiridol); peptidase inhibitors (talabostat); Bcl-2-targeting agents (antisense oligonucleotide, oblimersen; small molecule inducing apoptosis, gossypol); heat shock protein 90 inhibitors that target 70-kDa zeta-associated protein (17-AAG, CNF2024); immunomodulating agents (lenalidomide; immunostimulatory oligonucleotides CpG); hypomethylating agents (decitabine; valproic acid); antiangiogenic agents (bevacizumab); and gene therapies. This chapter reviews the use of targeted therapies as single agents and in combination with chemotherapy for CLL.

Key Words: CLL, Prognosis, Therapy, Targeted, Phase I, Fludarabine, Alemtuzumab, Rituximab, Lenalidomide, Gene therapy

From: *Current Clinical Oncology: Targeted Cancer Therapy*
Edited by: R. Kurzrock and M. Markman © Humana Press, Totowa, NJ

1. INTRODUCTION

Chronic lymphocytic leukemia (CLL) is characterized by a progressive accumulation of monoclonal CD5+ B cells in bone marrow, lymphoid tissue, and peripheral blood. CLL lymphocytes express HLA-DR, pan-B antigens (CD19 and CD20), CD5, CD23, weak surface immunoglobulins (IgM or IgM and IgD), and either κ or λ light chain-bearing B cells *(1)*.

B-cell CLL is the most common type of leukemia in the Western world. In 2001, the age-adjusted incidence of CLL in the United States was 4.6 per 100,000 persons *(2)*. According to the Surveillance, Epidemiology, and End Results (SEER) program of the National Cancer Institute, the age-adjusted incidence rate was 3.8 per 100,000 persons per year from 2000 to 2003 *(3)*. The American Cancer Society estimated that 10,020 people (6280 men, 3740 women) would be diagnosed with CLL in 2006 and that 4660 men and women would die from the disease *(3)*.

The clinical course of CLL varies widely and is associated with prolonged survival (Fig. 1) Treatment of CLL is usually deferred until indications for therapeutic intervention are present *(4)*. Combination therapy with nucleoside analogues and rituximab has led to improved outcomes of CLL, but chemotherapy causes myelosuppression and other toxicities. Therefore, there is interest in eliminating the use of chemotherapy for CLL. Targeted therapies that inhibit signaling pathways for growth and proliferation of cancer cells, such as molecularly targeted drugs, monoclonal antibodies, and gene therapies, are being investigated as alternatives or adjuvants to chemotherapy for CLL.

In this chapter, we review the characteristics and molecular mechanisms of CLL and focus on targeted therapeutic strategies and future directions.

1.1. Current Therapies

In recent years, the development of new therapeutic strategies has led to stepwise improvements in clinical outcomes in CLL (Fig. 2). For several decades, the alkylating agent chlorambucil was the standard of care for CLL *(5)*. In two randomized trials, chlorambucil was shown to slow disease progression but not to prolong survival (Table 1) *(5)*.

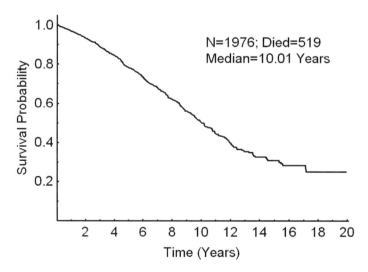

Fig. 1. Overall survival among 1976 patients with chronic lymphocyic leukemia (CLL) treated at M. D. Anderson Cancer Center from 1985 to 2005.

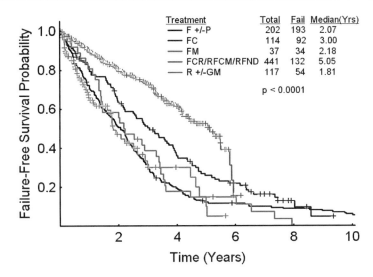

Fig. 2. Failure-free survival by regimen in patients with CLL who required therapy. C, cyclophosphamide; D, dexamethasone; F, fludarabine; GM, granulocyte-macrophage colony-stimulating factor; P, prednisone; R, rituximab; N, novantrone (mitoxantrone); M, mitoxantrone.

In another randomized study comparing chlorambucil with fludarabine, response rates and remission duration were superior with fludarabine therapy *(6)*. Single-agent fludarabine induces response in 70% to 80% of untreated patients and in 45% to 55% of patients with relapsed CLL *(6,7)*. For fludarabine treatment, with or without prednisone (F ± P) *(8–10)*, response rates are 79% in untreated patients and 52% in previously treated patients *(10)*. We found that fludarabine and cyclophosphamide combination therapy is even more effective, inducing overall responses of 88% in untreated patients and 39% [complete response (CR), 3%] in patients with fludarabine-refractory disease *(11)*; similar results have been reported by other investigators *(12,13)*.

The superiority of fludarabine and cyclophosphamide combination therapy was also shown in a randomized study comparing single-agent fludarabine with fludarabine plus cyclophosphamide combination therapy in patients younger than 65 years with untreated advanced CLL *(14)* and in another Phase III trial comparing fludarabine plus cyclophosphamide with single-agent fludarabine in patients with untreated CLL (US Intergroup Trial E2997) (Table 1) *(15)*. Finally, superior results with fludarabine and cyclophosphamide compared with fludarabine alone or chlorambucil were shown in the preliminary analysis of the CLL4 trial (United Kingdom) *(16)*.

On the basis of the observation that rituximab enhances the cytotoxicity of both fludarabine and cyclophosphamide, Keating et al. combined rituximab with fludarabine and cyclophosphamide (FCR) in the treatment of CLL. FCR induced a CR in 70% and partial response (PR) in 25% of untreated patients with CLL *(17)*; and the overall response rate was 73% (CR 32%) in patients with relapsed or refractory CLL *(18)*. With fludarabine and mitoxantrone (FM) combination therapy, the response rate was 83% (CR 20%) in untreated patients, but the addition of mitoxantrone to fludarabine did not significantly increase the CR rate beyond what is achieved with single-agent fludarabine *(19)*. Fludarabine, cyclophosphamide, and mitoxantrone (FCM) has induced a response rate of 78% (CR 50%) in resistant or relapsed CLL *(20)*. FCM and rituximab combination therapy with pegfilgrastim support has also been highly effective as a frontline therapy *(21)*. Among 29 patients evaluable for response at 3

Table 1
Selected Frontline Therapies for CLL

Study	Regimen and schedule	No. of patients	OR(%)	CR(%)	Median PFS	Median survival	Comments
O'Brien, 1993 (10)	Fludarabine, IV, 30 mg/m²/d × 5 d q + prednisone, PO, 30 mg/m² × 5 d q 28 d	95	79	63 (CR+ nodular PR)	TTP, 30 months in PR; NR in CR	78% at 2 years	
Keating, 1998 (7)	Fludarabine, IV, 25–30 mg/m²/d × 5 d q. 28 d or fludarabine, IV, 30 mg/m²/d + prednisone, PO, 40 mg/m² × 5 d q 28 d	71 & 103	80 & 77	38 & 23	TTP in responders, 31 months	63 months	
Dighiero, 1998 (5)	A. Chlorambucil 0.1 mg/kg/d (vs. no Rx) B. Chlorambucil 0.3 mg/kg/day + prednisone 40mg/m² × 5 days (vs. no Rx)	A. 301 (vs. 308) B. 460 (vs. 466)	A. 76 B. 69	A. 45 B. 28	A. 60% (vs. 55%) $p = 0.03$ B. 73% (vs. 67%) $p < 0.001$	At 7 yrs A. 70% (vs. 68%) $p = 0.74$ B. 78% (vs. 73%) $p = 0.16$	2 randomized trials; response assessed in 95% (A) and 96% (B) of patients who remained alive at 9 months
Rai, 2000 (6)	Fludarabine (IV, 25 mg/m²/d × 5 d q 28 d) vs. chlorambucil (PO, 40 mg/m² q 28 d) vs. fludarabine (20 mg/m² × 5 d q 28 d) plus chlorambucil (20 mg/m² q 28 d)	170 vs. 181 vs. 123	63 vs. 37, ($p < 0.001$) vs. 61	20 vs. 4, (p < 0.001) vs. 20	20 vs. 14 vs. NR months ($p < 0.001$)	66 vs. 56 vs. 55 months ($p = 0.21$)	Randomized; combination arm: early discontinuation

Study	Regimen						Comments
O'Brien, 2001 (11)	Fludarabine 30 mg/m²/d × 3 d plus cyclophosphamide 300–500 mg/m²/d × 3 d q 28 d	34	88	35	TTP, 72% at 2 years	82% at 2 years	
Lundin, 2002 (52)	Alemtuzumab, SC, 30 mg thrice weekly × 18 weeks (starting dose 3 mg)	41	87	19	TTF, not reached, 18⁺ (7–44⁺) months	NR	OR, 81% of intent-to-treat
Hainsworth, 2003 (64)	Rituximab 375 mg/m² weekly × 4	44	51	4	19 months	NR	
Byrd, 2003 (99)	Fludarabine 25 mg/m²/d × 5 d q 28 d + concurrent rituximab 375 mg/m² day 1 × 6 courses followed by 4 weekly doses of rituximab vs. fludarabine 25 mg/m²/d × 5d q 28 d × 6 courses + sequential rituximab (× 4) consolidation	51 vs. 53	90 vs. 77	47 vs. 28	PFS at 2 years, 70% each arm	92% vs. 98%	Randomized
Keating, 2005 (17)	Fludarabine 25 mg/m²/d × 3 d, cyclophosphamide 250 mg/m²/d × 3 d, and rituximab 375 mg/m² of q. 28d	224	95	70	TTF, 88% at 2 years	92% at 2 years	

(Continued)

Table 1
(Continued)

Study	Regimen and schedule	No. of patients	OR(%)	CR(%)	Median PFS	Median survival	Comments
Eichhorst, 2006 (14)	Fludarabine (25 mg/m²/d × 5 d) vs. fludarabine (30 mg/m m²/d × 3 d) plus cyclophosphamide (250 mg/m²/d × 3 d) q 28 d	182 vs. 180	83 vs. 94, p = 0.001	7 vs. 24, p < 0.001	20 vs. 48 months (p = 0.001)	81% vs. 80% at 3 yrs (p = 0.74)	Randomized
Flinn, 2007 (15)	Fludarabine 25 mg/m²/d × 5 d vs. cyclophosphamide 600 mg/m² day 1 + fludarabine 20 mg/m²/d × 5 d q 28 d	137 vs. 141	60 vs. 74, p = 0.01	5 vs. 23, p < 0.001	19 vs. 32 months (p < 0.001)	80% vs. 79% at 2 yrs (p = 0.69)	Randomized
Kay, 2007 (22)	Pentostatin 2 mg/m², cyclophosphamide 600 mg/m², and rituximab 375 mg/m² day 1 q 21 d × 6	65	91	41	33 months	NR	

CR, complete remission; d, day; NR, not reported; OR, overall response; PFS, progression-free survival; PR, partial remission; Rx, treatment; TTF, time to failure; TTP, time to progression months, the overall response rate was 97% (CR 41%) *(22)*. The Cancer and Leukemia Group B (CALGB) has explored fludarabine with concurrent or sequential rituximab therapy and demonstrated that concurrent rituximab is associated with higher rates of response (Table 1). Recently, other investigators reported favorable results with pentostatin, cyclophosphamide, and rituximab (PCR) combination therapy in untreated CLL (Table 1) *(22)*. A randomized Phase III study comparing FCR with PCR in untreated and previously treated CLL is ongoing.

The FCR therapy has been used in combination with the monoclonal antibody alemtuzumab (CFAR) in previously treated CLL *(23)*. CFAR consists of cyclophosphamide 250 mg/m^2 on days 3 to 5, fludarabine 25 mg/m^2 on days 3 to 5, intravenous alemtuzumab 30 mg on days 1, 3, and 5, and rituximab 375 to 500 mg/m^2 on day 2, every 4 weeks. CFAR induced responses in 65% of patients (CR 24%). With a median follow-up of 12 months, the median time to disease progression was 26 months and the median survival was 19 months *(23)*.

Another regimen with significant antileukemic activity in relapsed or refractory CLL is oxaliplatin, fludarabine, cytarabine, and rituximab (OFAR) combination therapy *(24)*. The OFAR regimen consists of oxaliplatin 25 mg/m^2/day, days 1 to 4; fludarabine 30 mg/m^2, days 2 and 3; cytarabine 1 g/m^2, days 2 and 3; rituximab 375 mg/m^2, day 3; and pegfil-grastim 6 mg, day 6, every 4 weeks. The overall response rate was 50% for patients with Richter's syndrome and 36% for patients with heavily pretreated fludarabine-refractory CLL. Responses included 7 of 19 (37%) patients with 17p deletion, 2 of 6 (33%) patients with 11q deletion, 4 patients with trisomy 12, and 2 of 5 (40%) patients with 13q deletion *(24)*.

1.2. Prognosis

The Rai and Binet systems have been used extensively for the clinical staging of patients with CLL *(25,26)*. More recently, chromosomal abnormalities such as 17p and 11q deletion *(27,28)*, 6q deletion *(29)*, mutations in the *p53 (30)* or ataxia telangiectasia (*ATM*) gene *(31)*, the mutational status of the immunoglobulin heavy chain variable gene (*IgV*$_H$) *(32)*; expression of 70-kDa zeta-associated protein (ZAP-70) *(33–35)*, CD38 *(36)*, or soluble CD23 *(37)*; high thymidine kinase level *(38)*; older age *(39,40)*; and high β_2-microglobulin level *(41,42)* have been identified as prognostic factors in CLL. A unique micro-RNA signature composed of 13 genes has also been associated with disease progression in CLL *(43)*.

In a retrospective analysis of 2189 patients with CLL or small lymphocytic lymphoma who were seen at The University of Texas M. D. Anderson Cancer Center from 1985 to 2005, independent factors predicting shorter survival were the presence of a 17p or 6q deletion, age ≥60 years, albumin < 3.5 g/dl, β_2-microglobulin ≥ 2 mg/L *(41,42)*, creatinine ≥ 1.6 mg/dl, hepatomegaly, hemoglobin < 11 g/dl, male sex, platelet count < 100 × 10^9/L, and absolute lymphocyte count ≥ 30 × 10^9/L *(44)*. Although new markers such as ZAP-70 and *IgV*$_H$ mutational status are being validated in clinical trials, their use is currently limited mainly because the follow-up period for the patients tested is too short. As more effective treatment strategies become available over time and with the use of risk-adapted therapies in ongoing clinical trials, the value of prognostic factors may change.

2. MOLECULAR MECHANISMS PERTINENT TO DISEASE

Chronic lymphocytic leukemia is currently viewed as two entities, both originating from antigen-stimulated mature B lymphocytes, which either escape death through the intercession of external signals or die by apoptosis *(45)*. IgV_H mutations have recently been identified in CLL. IgV_H genes, which are at least 98% homologous to the germline sequence in patients with CLL, are independently associated with a more aggressive clinical course compared to immunoglobulin molecules that have undergone somatic mutations (< 98% homology to the germline sequence) *(32,46,47)*. The marker CD38, which modulates intracellular signaling and crosslinking of CD38, exerts inhibitory action in normal mature B cells. CD38 expression in CLL has been associated with a worse prognosis *(48)* but this observation has not been confirmed in our series. The antiapoptotic protein BCL-2 is elevated in CLL, resulting in the accumulation of CLL cells. Hypermethylation of the promoter region of the *bcl-2* gene has been associated with high levels of BCL-2 protein *(49)*.

The *p53* gene, located at chromosome region 17p, is known to exert tumor suppression. Deletions in this chromosome locus have been shown to promote prolonged cell survival and accelerated cell proliferation, which are associated with advanced-stage disease and transformed CLL *(50)*. The *ATM* gene, located at chromosome region 11q22-23, is also considered to be a tumor suppressor gene. CLL associated with 11q22-23 deletion presents with extensive lymphadenopathy. Deletion of chromosome 6q may also be an initial event in leukemogenesis probably owing to the absence of an unidentified recessive tumor suppressor gene *(29)*.

MicroRNAs are a new class of genes that are normally made by cells and regulate the functions of many genes. In CLL, micro-RNAs are dysregulated at the transcriptional/posttranscriptional level. The micro-RNA genes *miR-15a* and *miR-16-1*, located at 13q14.3, are reportedly frequently deleted and/or down-regulated in patients with B-cell CLL. These genes negatively regulate *Bcl-2* at a posttranscriptional level, and this repression is thought to induce apoptosis *(51)*. The micro-RNA genes *miR-15* and *miR-16* are natural antisense Bcl-2 interactors and therefore could be used in the treatment of Bcl-2-overexpressing tumors *(51)*.

A unifying hypothesis for the development, growth, and evolution of CLL has been proposed. *(45)* According to this hypothesis, stimulatory and growth signals from the microenvironment allow the CLL cells to escape apoptosis and proliferate. These signals are delivered by B-cell and other receptors and by direct contact with stromal cells. The B-cell receptor permits binding of autoantigens and maintains the capacity to transmit stimulatory signals to the cell nucleus, mainly in cells with unmutated CLL B-cell receptors *(45)*.

3. TARGETED THERAPIES

3.1. Alemtuzumab

Alemtuzumab (Campath-1H), an anti-CD52 humanized monoclonal antibody, has been extensively investigated in CLL. It has significant antileukemic activity, which is high in the blood, bone marrow, and spleen and low in lymph nodes. The Food and Drug Administration (FDA) has approved alemtuzumab for patients with B-cell CLL who have been treated with alkylating agents and for whom fludarabine therapy has failed.

As a first-line therapy, alemtuzumab administered subcutaneously three times weekly for 18 weeks induced a response rate of 87% (CR 19%) and clearance of CLL cells from the blood and CR or nodular PR rates in the bone marrow of 95% and 66%, respectively *(52)*. The response rate in lymph nodes was 87% (CR 29%). The most noteworthy adverse events were transient injection site reactions (90% of patients) and cytomegalovirus reactivation (10%), which responded to ganciclovir therapy *(52)*. Alemtuzumab has mainly been investigated in relapsed or refractory CLL (Table 2) In a pivotal multicenter clinical trial, intravenous alemtuzumab induced responses in 33% of patients with relapsed or refractory B-cell CLL who had been exposed to alkylating agents and in whom fludarabine therapy had failed (Table 2) *(53)*. The median time to response was 1.5 months, and the median time to disease progression was 9.5 months for responders. Grade 3 or 4 infections were reported in 27% of patients but in only 10% of responders *(53)*.

Other Phase II clinical trials have demonstrated that alemtuzumab therapy produces favorable clinical outcomes (Table 2) *(54,55)*, including the eradication of minimal residual disease (MRD) in some patients *(56)*. In a study of alemtuzumab in 91 patients with previously treated CLL, eradication of MRD from the blood and bone marrow, defined as less than 1 CLL cell in 10^5 normal cells and detected by flow cytometry, occurred in 20% of patients and was associated with longer treatment-free and overall survival *(56)*. However, 47% of patients with MRD-negative remissions had MRD again at 28 months *(56)*. In another study, 41 patients were treated with alemtuzumab at doses of 10 to 30 mg, 3 times weekly, for 4 weeks *(57)*. Infection prophylaxis was also administered during therapy and for 2 months after treatment. Alemtuzumab produced an overall response rate of 46%, and 38% of patients achieved eradication of MRD, as detected by polymerase chain reaction (PCR) testing for the specific immunoglobulin heavy-chain rearrangement. With a median follow-up of 18 months, the median time to disease progression had not been reached in responders. Notably, 30% of patients developed infections, including reactivation of cytomegalovirus in nine patients, and three patients developed Epstein-Barr virus-positive large cell lymphoma *(57)*.

Because of its eradication of MRD, alemtuzumab has been explored as consolidation therapy in CLL *(58,59)*. A Phase II study demonstrated that subcutaneous alemtuzumab was effective and well tolerated in patients with CLL who had responded to fludarabine induction therapy and that subsequent peripheral blood stem cell transplantation was feasible *(59)*. In particular, 34 patients < 65 years of age were treated with alemtuzumab at 10 mg, 3 times weekly, for 6 weeks. The CR rate improved from 35% after fludarabine induction to 79% after alemtuzumab consolidation; and 56% of patients achieved molecular remission, as assessed by the polyclonality of the immunoglobulin heavy chain. Although cytomegalovirus reactivation occurred in 18 patients, it was successfully treated with ganciclovir *(59)*.

Published data suggest that alemtuzumab may be more effective in CLL with *p53* mutations or deletions *(55)*. Among 36 patients with fludarabine-refractory CLL treated with alemtuzumab, response rates were higher in patients with *p53* mutations and/or deletions (40%; 6/15) compared with others (19%; 4/19), and the median response duration for this subset of patients was 8 months (range 3–17 months) *(55)*.

These studies demonstrate the clinical activity of alemtuzumab in CLL. However, opportunistic infections require close monitoring and aggressive administration of prophylaxis against cytomegalovirus with ganciclovir or foscarnet and against *Pneumocystis carinii* pneumonia and DNA viruses.

3.2. Rituximab

Rituximab (IDEC-C2B8) is a chimeric antibody that binds to the B-cell surface antigen CD20. Although highly effective in follicular lymphoma, with an overall response rate of

Table 2
Selected Published Results of Targeted Therapies in Previously Treated CLL

Investigator, year	Regimen and schedule	No. of patients	Fluadarabine refractory(%)[a]	OR (%)	CR (%)	Median PFS (months)	Median survival (months)	Comments
Osterborg, 1997 (100)	Alemtuzumab, 30 mg thrice weekly × 12 weeks	29	N/A	42	4	Remission duration, 12	NR	3 Patients had prior fludarabine
Keating, 2002 (53)	Alemtuzumab 30 mg thrice weekly × 12 weeks	93	48	33	2	5	16	
Rai, 2002 (54)	Alemtuzumab, 30 mg thrice weekly × 16 weeks	24	71	33	0	7	28	
Lozanski, 2004 (55)	Alemtuzumab, 30 mg thrice weekly × 12 weeks	36	81	31	6	Remission duration, 10	NR	Response, 40% (6/15) if p53 mutations/deletions vs. 19% (4/21) if other
Moreton, 2005 (56)	Alemtuzumab, 30 mg thrice weekly until maximum response	91	50	53	35	MRD(-), NR; MRD(+), 20; PR, 13	MRD(-), not reached; MRD(+), 41; PR, 30	20% of patients achieved MRD negativity

Reference	Treatment						Comments
O'Brien, 2001 (61)	Rituximab, escalating dose 375–2250 mg/m² weekly × 4 weeks	40	53	36	0	8	80% at 1 year	Survival data include 10 patients with other lymphoid malignancies
Byrd, 2001 (62)	Rituximab, 100-375 mg/m² thrice weekly × 4 weeks	33	52	52 (45%, intent-to-treat)	3	In responders, 11	NR	6 patients. were previously untreated
Huhn, 2001 (63)	Rituximab, 375 mg/m² weekly × 4 weeks	30	77	25 (23%, intent-to-treat)	0	16	NR	
Faderl, 2003 (68)	Alemtuzumab (30 mg thrice weekly × 4-8 weeks) + concurrent rituximab (375 mg/m² weekly × 4 weeks)	32	54	63	6	6	11	Survival data include 15 patients with other lymphoid malignancies

(Continued)

Table 2
(Continued)

Investigator, year	Regimen and schedule	No. of patients	Fludarabine refractory(%)[a]	OR (%)	CR (%)	Median PFS (months)	Median survival (months)	Comments
Chanan-Khan, 2006 (73)	Lenalidomide, 25 mg/d PO × 21 d q 28 d	45	51	47	9	81% at 1 year	NR	
Byrd, 2007 (85)	Flavopiridol, 60–80 mg/m^2 weekly × 46 weeks	42	83	45	0	In responders, 13	NR	

O'Brien, 2005 (88)	Oblimersen sodium 3 mg/kg/d × 5 d (c.1) or × 7 d (subsequently) q 3 weeks	26	69	8	0	NR	NR	Phase II results are reported
O'Brien, 2007 (89)	Fludarabine (25 mg/m²/d, days 1-3) plus cyclophosphamide (250 mg/m²/d, days 1–2) with vs. without oblimersen sodium (3 mg/kg/d ? days ?3 to day 3	120 vs. 121	57 vs. 59	17% vs. 7% (p = 0.25)	9 vs 0. 3 (p = 0.03)	Time to progression, 6 vs. 9 (NS)	34 vs. 33	Survival benefit with three-drug arm in fludarabine-sensitive patients (p = 0.05)

[a]Fludarabine refractory CLL is defined as CLL with no response to fludarabine or progression within 6 months of treatment
CR, complete remission; d, day; MRD, minimal residual disease; NR, not reported; NS, not significant (difference); OR, overall response; PFS, progression-free survival; PR, partial remission

60%, single-agent rituximab has inferior clinical activity in small lymphocytic lymphomas (overall response rate 13%) *(60)*. Rituximab has clinical activity in B-cell CLL; but compared with its activity in follicular lymphoma, it is less effective in clearing disease from the bone marrow, and the response duration is short *(61–64)*. Single-agent rituximab induces responses in 23% to 45% (CR 0%–3%) of previously treated patients (Table 2) *(61–63)*. A Phase II study demonstrated a dose-response relation, as response rates increased with increasing rituximab dose *(61)*. Response rates (all PRs) increased from 22% at doses of 500 to 825 mg/m^2 to 43% at doses of 1000 to 1500 mg/m^2 to 75% at the highest dose of 2250 mg/m^2 (p = 0.007) *(61)*. In another study, rituximab was administered at 375 mg/m^2 weekly for 4 consecutive weeks as a first-line therapy in CLL and was repeated at 6-month intervals *(64)*. Overall, 44 patients were treated, and the response rate after the first course of rituximab was 51% (CR 4%); after completion of one or more additional courses (28 patients), the overall response rate was 58% (CR 9%). However, the progression-free survival duration of 18.6 months was inferior to that reported with first-line plus maintenance rituximab in patients with follicular lymphoma *(64)*. Rituximab has been used in combination with granulocyte-macrophage colony-stimulating factor (GM-CSF) on the basis of in vitro *(65)* and clinical data in indolent lymphoma showing increased antitumor activity when combined with GM-CSF *(66)*. This regimen resulted in a 79% response rate (CR 36%) in patients with indolent lymphoma *(66)*; but in those with CLL who were ≥ 70 years of age, the response rates were 61% (CR 7%) *(67)*.

3.3. Alemtuzumab and Rituximab

Alemtuzumab has been evaluated in combination with rituximab in relapsed/refractory CLL *(68,69)*. In our institution, concurrent alemtuzumab and rituximab therapy induced responses in 63% of patients (Table 2). The most common toxicities were infections and infusion-related reactions. Cytomegalovirus antigenemia was noted in 27% of the patients, but only 15% were symptomatic and required therapy *(68)*.

3.4. Ofatumumab

Ofatumumab (HuMax CD20), a monoclonal antibody, which targets a different epitope of CD20 than that targeted by rituximab, is thought to kill rituximab-resistant cells (Table 3) *(70)*. In a Phase I/II clinical trial, ofatumumab was administered as an intravenous infusion once weekly for 4 weeks in 33 patients with relapsed/refractory CLL. At the maximum tolerated dose, ofatumumab induced a nodular PR or PR in 46% of patients. The most common toxicities were infusion reactions *(71)*. These results led to an ongoing international study of ofatumumab for patients with CLL who failed treatment with fludarabine and alemtuzumab or who failed fludarabine and were intolerant to or ineligible to receive alemtuzumab.

3.5. Lenalidomide

Immunomodulating drugs such as lenalidomide are thought to exert their antileukemic activity via pleiotropic immunomodulatory mechanisms. These agents decrease the production of cytokines, including tumor necrosis factor-α (TNFα), vascular endothelial growth factor, and interleukin-6 *(71,72)*. Lenalidomide also modulates an immune effector cell response through activation of T cells and natural killer cells and directly induces apoptosis in tumor cells *(73)*. Phase II clinical trials demonstrated that lenalidomide is

Table 3
Selected Targeted Therapies for CLL

Drug	Target	Route of adminis-tration	Overall response in previously treated CLL(%)	Key toxicities	Ongoing/planned use	Comments
Alemtuzumab	CD52	IV, SC	31–53 (CR, 0–35)	Immunosup-pression CMV reactivation	Combination with cytotoxics (e.g., CFAR)MRD eradication17p deletion	CMV monitoring and prophylaxis; activity in CLL with 17p deletion
Rituximab	CD20	IV	52–77 (CR, 0–3)	Infusion-related events	Combination with cytotoxics or other targeted therapies	
Ofatumumab (HuMax-CD20)	CD20 novel epitope	IV	46 (CR, 0)	Infusion-related events	Phase III pivotal study in relapsed CLL after fludarabine failurePhase II in combination with fludarabine, cyclophos-phamide in untreated CLL	HuMax-20 kills rituximab-resistant cells and fresh CLL cells expressing low levels of CD20

(Continued)

Table 3
(Continued)

Drug	Target	Route of adminis-tration	Overall response in previously treated CLL(%)	Key toxicities	Ongoing/planned use	Comments
Lenalidomide	Immunomodulatory down-regulation of cytokines (e.g., TNF, VEGF, IL-6)Activation of immune effector cells	PO	32–47 (CR 5–9)	Fatigue, thrombocy-topenia, neutropenia	Ongoing phase II in relapsed/refractory CLL Phase II–III study of two lenalidomide dose regimens in relapsed or refractory CLL	
Lumiliximab	CD23	IV	0 (decrease in ALC and lympha-denopathy)	Headache, GI	Ongoing phase II/III randomized international study of FCR with or without lumiliximab	It may enhance activity of FCR
Flavopiridol	Cyclin-dependent kinase; p53 independent	IV	45%	Hyperacute tumor lysis syndrome	Ongoing phase II in previously treated CLLOngoing phase I as consolidation after cytoreductive therapy	Other phase I or II studies are ongoing to optimize dose and schedule

Agent	Target	Route	Response	Toxicity	Clinical trials	Notes
Oblimersen	BCL-2	IV	8% (0)	Cytokine release syndrome, fatigue, GI	Ongoing phase I-II in combination with rituximab in previously treated CLL	Phase III randomized trial of FC ± oblimersen demonstrated superior rates of CR and nodular CR(89)
Gossypol	Bcl-2 homology 3 of BCL-2 antagonists	PO	0 (decrease in ALC and lymphadenopathy in untreated CLL, phase 1)	GI, fatigue, neutropenia	Ongoing Phase I as single agent in lymphoproliferative disorders; Ongoing phase I-II in combination with rituximab in relapsed/refractory CLL	Gossypol+ rituximab, PR 42%
CNF1010(17-AAG)	Heat shock protein 90	IV	Too early		Phase 1 in ZAP-70-positive CLL Phase 1, 17-AAG ± rituximab in relapsed CLL	
CNF 2024	Heat shock protein 90	PO	Too early		Ongoing Phase I in relapsed CLL	

ALC, absolute lymphocyte count; CFAR, cyclophosphamide/fludarabine/alemtuzumab/rituximab; CMV, cytomegalovirus; CR, complete remission; FC, fludarabine, cyclophosphamide; FCR, fludarabine/cyclophosphamide/rituximab; GI, gastrointestinal; IL, interleukin; MRD, minimal residual disease; PR, partial remission; TNF, tissue necrosis factor; VEGF, vascular endothelial growth factor; ZAP, zeta-associated protein clinically active in CLL *(73,74)*. Among 43 patients, most of whom had advanced or fludarabine-refractory CLL, treatment with lenalidomide at 25 mg orally on days 1 through 21 of a 28-day cycle induced a response rate of 47% *(73)*. In our institution, lenalinomide was administered starting at 10 mg daily for 28 days, followed by titration upward in 5-mg increments every 28 days to a maximum daily dose of 25 mg *(74)*. At 3 months, the response rate was 32% (CR 5%; nodular PR 5%) *(74)*. Adverse events included fatigue, thrombocytopenia, neutropenia, and gastrointestinal toxicities *(73,74)*.

Lenalidomide in combination with rituximab is currently being investigated in relapsed or refractory CLL.

3.6. Vaccines and Gene Therapy

Active immunotherapy strategies, such as vaccines, expanded and activated T cells, and allogeneic stem cell transplantation are also being investigated in CLL. CLL is considered ideal for vaccine development because of the availability of CLL cells in the peripheral blood and their expression of markers that can be targeted for immune recognition *(75)*. CLL cells can be stimulated to express immune co-stimulatory molecules via ligation of CD40 by CD154. The co-stimulatory molecules, such as CD80, CD86, and adhesion molecules, allow CLL cells to stimulate T cells against leukemia-associated antigens. In a Phase I clinical trial, autologous CLL cells were transduced to express murine CD154. The treatment was well tolerated, and it increased the absolute T-cell and the leukemia-specific T-cell counts and reduced lymphocyte counts and lymphadenopathy *(75)*. In another Phase I trial, a new replication-defective adenovirus encoding a humanized, functional, membrane-stable CD154 molecule (ISF35) that efficiently transduces CLL B cells was used *(76)*. A single dose of ISF35-transduced autologous leukemia cells was administered (1×10^8, 3×10^8, or 1×10^9). In four reported patients, transduction efficiency ranged from 49% to 77%, viability of transduced cells was 92% to 95%, the ISF35-transduced CLL cells were induced to express CD95, and acute absolute lymphocyte count reductions were noted *(76)*.

Tumor-specific antigenicity of unique antigenic determinants [idiotype (Id)] of the immunoglobulin expressed in a given B-cell malignancy led to Phase I-II clinical trials of recombinant idiotype-keyhole limpet hemocyanin (rId-KLH) immunizations in follicular lymphoma. This strategy was shown to elicit specific anti-idiotypic responses in patients with follicular lymphoma who had responded to their initial course of chemotherapy *(77–79)*. With a median follow-up of 5.3 years from the last dose of chemotherapy given before vaccine treatment, the median disease-free and overall survival durations of patients mounting an anti-idiotype immune response were significantly longer than those for patients who did not mount an immune response. Improved disease-free and overall survivals were also observed in patients who mounted a specific immune response compared to those who did not *(78)*. In a subsequent study in patients with follicular lymphoma, GM-CSF as an adjuvant to rId-KLH immunization was shown to be safe and effective in generating specific anti-idiotypic responses *(80)*. These results led to an ongoing Phase I-II clinical trial of rId-KLH with GM-CSF in patients with early-stage, untreated CLL *(81)*.

3.7. Lumiliximab

Lumiliximab (IDEC-152) is an immunoglobulin G (IgG)-1 macaque-human anti-CD23 monoclonal antibody. In a Phase I study in patients with CLL, single-agent lumiliximab was administered at doses ranging from 125 mg/m^2 weekly to 500 mg/m^2 thrice weekly, for 4 weeks *(82)*. Lumiliximab-induced adverse events were headache, constipation, nausea, and cough. A decrease in lymphocyte counts was noted in 91% (42/46) of all patients and in 59% of patients with baseline lymphadenopathy; but no confirmed responses were noted *(82)*. On the basis of these observations, a Phase I-II study of lumiliximab and FCR combination therapy was initiated in relapsed CD23+ B-cell CLL. Lumiliximab was administered at 375 mg/m^2 or 500 mg/m^2 in combination with FCR every 4 weeks *(83)*. No dose-limiting toxicity was noted for lumiliximab, and the 500 mg/m^2 dose was used in the Phase II portion of the study. Among 31 patients evaluable for response after three or more cycles of therapy, the overall response rate was 68% (CR 42%, PR 10%, unconfirmed PR 16%). It is thought that this combination may enhance the activity of FCR in progressive CLL after prior therapy *(83)*. When these results were compared with early data for FCR alone, it appeared that the addition of lumiliximab to FCR increased the CR rate from 25% to 48%. However, more patients in the early FCR study had advanced Rai stage disease (50% vs. 22%) and were rituximab-naive (88% vs. 40%). These results led to an ongoing multicenter, global, randomized study of lumiliximab and FCR versus FCR alone *(84)*.

3.8. Flavopiridol

Flavopiridol (alvocidib) is a broad cyclin-dependent kinase inhibitorthat induces apoptosis in leukemic cell lines andin human CLL cells in vitro *(85)*. Its activity is p53 independent, and it also decreases the expression of the proteins Mcl-1 and XIAP, which mediate resistance to apoptosis in CLL cells. When administered as a continuous infusion, flavopiridol had no activity; but the response rate was 11% when it was given as an 1-hour bolus in patients with recurrent CLL *(86)*. When administered in three cohorts (cohort 1: 30 mg/m^2 loading dose followed by 30 mg/m^2 4-hour infusion; cohort 2: 40 mg/m^2 loading dose followed by40 mg/m^2 4-hour infusion; and cohort 3: cohort 1 dose for treatments1 to 4, then a 30 mg/m^2 loading dose followed by a 50 mg/m^2 4-hour infusion), flavopiridol resulted in a 45% PR rate, with a median duration that exceeded 12 months *(85)*. Responses were noted in patients with genetically high-risk disease, including 42% of patients with del(17p13.1)and 72% of patients with del(11q22.3). The dose-limiting toxicity was hyperacute tumor lysis syndrome. This study suggests that flavopiridol can be used for elimination of MRD after cytoreductive therapy *(85)*.

3.9. Talabostat

Talabostat is an oral small-molecule inhibitor of dipeptidyl peptidases, such as CD26 and fibroblast activation protein, which is expressed in bone marrow, lymph nodes, and the stroma of solid tumors and induces cytokine and chemokine expression in lymph nodes and the spleen *(87)*. Based on its enhancement of the activity of rituximab in patients with B-cell malignancies, talabostat and rituximab combination therapy was explored in a Phase II study in patients with CLL who had failed fludarabine and/or rituximab therapy. Rituximab was administered at 375 mg/m^2 on days 1, 8, 15, and 22; and talabostat was given at 300 µg orally twice daily for 6 days following each rituximab infusion. The overall response rate was 22% (8/36 patients), and the median response duration was 5 months. Toxicities were similar to those associated with rituximab alone, with the exception of edema, which occurred in 25% of patients *(87)*.

3.10. Oblimersen

Oblimersen sodium (Genasense, G3139) is a Bcl-2 antisense oligonucleotide *(88)*. In a Phase I study of pretreated CLL, oblimersen induced a PR in 8% (2/26) of patients and resulted in the reduction of organomegaly, lymphadenopathy, or lymphocyte counts in several patients. The most common adverse events were a cytokine release syndrome, fatigue, night sweats, and gastrointestinal symptoms *(88)*. In a Phase III study, patients with relapsed or refractory CLL were randomized to receive fludarabine plus cyclophosphamide, with or without oblimersen sodium (Table 2) *(89)*. The three-drug combination resulted in higher rates of CR and nodular PR (17%) compared with fludarabine and cyclophosphamide (7%) ($p = 0.025$) *(89)*.

3.11. Gossypol

Gossypol (AT-101) is a small molecule that mimics the inhibitory Bcl-2 homology 3 (BH3) domain of endogenous antagonists of the Bcl-2 family antiapoptotic proteins Bcl-2, Bcl-$_{XL}$, Bcl-$_W$, and Mcl-1 *(90)*. Gossypol induces apoptosis and enhances the cytotoxicity of rituximab in CLL cells. In a Phase II study, gossypol and rituximab combination therapy was investigated in patients with relapsed/refractory CLL *(91)*. Gossypol was administered at 30 mg/day for 21 or 28 days for three 28-day cycles. Rituximab was administered at 375 mg/m^2 on days 1, 3, 5, 8, 15, 22, 29, 31, 33, 40, 57, 59, and 61. Preliminary results demonstrated that gossypol and rituximab induced a PR in 42% (5/12) of patients, with improved lymphocyte counts, splenomegaly, and/or lymph node size. The most frequent toxicities were gastrointestinal effects, fatigue, and neutropenia. The study is ongoing, with different gossypol schedules being tested in an attempt to improve activity and reduce toxicity *(91)*.

3.12. Obatoclax

Obatoclax (GX15-070) is a synthetic small molecule that inhibits the binding of the antiapoptotic properties of Bcl-2, Bcl-$_{XL}$ and Bcl-$_W$, and Mcl-1 to the proapoptotic proteins Bax and Bak, which is believed to reinstate programmed cell death in transformed cells. In a Phase I trial in CLL, the main adverse events were drowsiness and euphoria *(92)*. Although the clinical activity of this agent was limited (one unconfirmed PR and seven cases of stable disease among 15 patients), improvement in thrombocytopenia was noted in some patients with baseline cytopenia *(92)*.

3.13. Heat Shock Protein 90 Inhibitors

Heat shock protein 90 (Hsp90) is a ubiquitous molecular chaperone that is necessary for the expression and activity of the tyrosine kinase ZAP-70,*(93)* which is expressed aberrantly in 45% of patients with B-cell CLL, particularly those with unmutated B-cell receptor genes, and has been associated with an adverse prognosis *(34)*. In vitro studies demonstrated that the Hsp90 inhibitor 17-allyl-amino-demethoxy-geldanamycin (17-AAG) induces ZAP-70 degradation and apoptosis in CLL lymphocytes *(93)*. Another Hsp90 inhibitor, CNF2024 (CF1983 mesylate), is currently being investigated in patients with relapsed CLL or intolerance to purine analogue-based therapy (Table 3).

3.14. Targeted Therapies in Advanced Experimental Trials

Ongoing clinical trials are exploring targeted therapies as single agents or in combination with chemotherapy and a monoclonal antibody *(94)*. For instance, FCR has been combined with the vascular endothelial growth factor (VEGF)-specific antibody bevacizumab or with GM-CSF. Other agents being investigated include the tyrosine kinase inhibitor dasatinib

(BMS-354825); the Bcl-2 synthesis inhibitor SPC2996; an anti-CD40 monoclonal antibody, HCD122; the immunostimulatory oligonucleotide CpG; green tea extract; a nonaddictive derivative of opium, noscapine; the selective inhibitor of cyclin-dependent kinases (CDK) 2, 3, and 7, SNS-032; the immunotoxin CAT-8015; an oral small-molecule oxindole kinase inhibitor of FMS-like tyrosine kinase 3, tyrosine kinase receptor KIT, VEGF receptors, and platelet-derived growth factor receptors, sunitinib (SU11248); and an inhibitor of the mammalian target of rapamycin (mTOR) kinase, temsirolimus (CCI-779). Additional agents being studied include bryostatin I in combination with rituximab; a proteasome inhibitor, bortezomib, in combination with fludarabine, with or without rituximab; the immunotoxin LMB-2; a multikinase inhibitor, sorafenib; the bifunctional alkylating agent bendamustine combined with rituximab; bendamustine and mitoxantrone; combination therapy with the hypomethylating agents decitabine and valproic acid; the Hsp90 inhibitor 17-AAG, with or without rituximab; the histone deacetylase inhibitor MGCD0103 (MG-0103); the VEGF receptor-2 tyrosine kinase inhibitor AZD2171; fludarabine and thalidomide in newly diagnosed CLL; fludarabine with or without alemtuzumab; fludarabine and cyclophosphamide, with or without alemtuzumab; and cyclophosphamide and rituximab followed by vaccine therapy (94). Purine analogues that are being developed include the cytosine nucleoside analogue azacytidine; nelarabine (506U78), a prodrug of the deoxyguanosine (dGuo) analogue 9-β-D-arabinofuranosyl guanine, which has shown clinical activity in 7% of patients with fludarabine-refractory CLL; (95) forodesine hydrochloride (BCX-1777), a potent inhibitor of purine nucleoside phosphorylase (96), which is undergoing Phase I testing; and clofarabine (2-chloro-2-deoxy-fluoro-ß-D-arabinofuranosyladenine), a nucleoside analogue that has shown cytoreduction in relapsed CLL and is being investigated in Phase I testing (97).

4. FUTURE DIRECTIONS IN MOLECULAR THERAPEUTICS

The indolent clinical behavior of CLL has often led to the approach of deferring treatment in asymptomatic patients until indications for therapeutic intervention are present. However, the presence of poor prognostic features, even in asymptomatic patients, may warrant close monitoring or even early therapeutic intervention should the patient and/or physician be uncomfortable with deferring therapy. In recent years, a better understanding of the pathogenetic mechanisms of CLL has led to the identification of biologic markers, such as 17p deletions/p53 mutations, unmutated IgV$_H$, expression of ZAP-70 and CD38, and other factors that are associated with a poor prognosis. Although the prognostic significance of some markers, such as CD38, has not been confirmed in all series, other markers, such as 17p deletions (27), have an established adverse effect on prognosis. Patients with such genomic aberrations should be considered for investigational therapies that include agents with promising antileukemic activity, such as alemtuzumab or oxaliplatin, fludarabine, cytarabine, and rituximab combination therapy.

The development of targeted therapies is an area of great interest because these agents have a specific mechanism of action and therefore are associated with less toxicity compared with standard chemotherapy. However, as CLL is characterized by molecular diversity, it is likely that multiple targeted therapies will be needed to control the disease. Although the available targeted therapies have limited activity as single agents, patients with CLL appear to benefit from combinations of therapies, such as monoclonal antibodies, and cytotoxic chemotherapy (Fig. 2). Several new prognostic markers are being validated in clinical trials *(30,31,36–38,43)*, and the consensus is that until these results become available treatment decisions outside of clinical trials should conform to the National Cancer Institute-sponsored Working Group criteria *(98)*. The continuing identification of molecular pathways that drive the CLL clone in individual patients and further development of therapies that target these pathways will lead to optimal, personalized risk therapies in CLL.

REFERENCES

1. Muller-Hermelink HK, Catovsky D, Montserrat E, et al. Chronic lymphocytic leukemia/small lymphocytic lymphoma. In: Jaffe ES, Stein H, Wardiman JW (eds) Tumors of Haematopoietic and Lymphoid Tissues. World Health Organization Classification of Tumors. Lyon: IARC Press; 2001. p. 127–30.
2. U.S. Cancer Statistics Working Group. United States Cancer Statistics: 2001 Incidence and Mortality. Washington, DC: Department of Health and Human Services, Centers for Disease Control and Prevention, and National Cancer Institute; 2001.
3. Surveillance Epidemiology and End Results: Chronic Lymphocytic Leukemia. Washington, DC: National Cancer Institute. Accessed April 30, 2007 at http://seer.cancer.gov/statfacts/html/clyl.html/.
4. Rai K, Patel DV. Chronic lymphocytic leukemia. In: Hoffman R, Benz EJ, Shattil SJ, et al (eds) Hematology: Basic Principles and Practice. 3rd edition. Philadelphia: Churchill Livingstone; 2000. p. 1350–63.
5. Dighiero G, Maloum K, Desablens B, et al. Chlorambucil in indolent chronic lymphocytic leukemia; French Cooperative Group on Chronic Lymphocytic Leukemia. N Engl J Med 1998;338:1506–14.
6. Rai KR, Peterson BL, Appelbaum FR, et al. Fludarabine compared with chlorambucil as primary therapy for chronic lymphocytic leukemia. N Engl J Med 2000;343:1750–7.
7. Keating MJ, O'Brien S, Lerner S, et al. Long-term follow-up of patients with chronic lymphocytic leukemia receiving fludarabine regimens as initial therapy. Blood 1998;92:1165–71.
8. Keating MJ, Kantarjian H, O'Brien S, et al. Fludarabine: a new agent with marked cytoreductive activity in untreated chronic lymphocytic leukemia. J Clin Oncol 1991;9:44–9.
9. Keating MJ, O'Brien S, Kantarjian H, et al. Long-term follow-up of patients with chronic lymphocytic leukemia treated with fludarabine as a single agent. Blood 1993;81:2878–84.
10. O'Brien S, Kantarjian H, Beran M, et al. Results of fludarabine and prednisone therapy in 264 patients with chronic lymphocytic leukemia with multivariate analysis-derived prognostic model for response to treatment. Blood 1993;82:1695–700.
11. O'Brien SM, Kantarjian HM, Cortes J, et al. Results of the fludarabine and cyclophosphamide combination regimen in chronic lymphocytic leukemia. J Clin Oncol 2001;19:1414–20.
12. Flinn IW, Byrd JC, Morrison C, et al. Fludarabine and cyclophosphamide with filgrastim support in patients with previously untreated indolent lymphoid malignancies. Blood 2000;96:71–5.
13. Hallek M, Schmitt B, Wilhelm M, et al. Fludarabine plus cyclophosphamide is an efficient treatment for advanced chronic lymphocytic leukaemia (CLL): results of a phase II study of the German CLL Study Group. Br J Haematol 2001;114:342–8.
14. Eichhorst BF, Busch R, Hopfinger G, et al. Fludarabine plus cyclophosphamide versus fludarabine alone in first-line therapy of younger patients with chronic lymphocytic leukemia. Blood 2006;107:885–91.
15. Flinn IW, Neuberg DS, Grever MR, et al. Phase III trial of fludarabine plus cyclophosphamide compared with fludarabine for patients with previously untreated chronic lymphocytic leukemia: US Intergroup Trial E2997. J Clin Oncol 2007;25:793–8.
16. Catovsky D, Richards S, Hillmen P. Early results from LRF CLL4: a UK multicenter randomized trial. Blood 2005;106:212a. Abstract 716.
17. Keating MJ, O'Brien S, Albitar M, et al. Early results of a chemoimmunotherapy regimen of fludarabine, cyclophosphamide, and rituximab as initial therapy for chronic lymphocytic leukemia. J Clin Oncol 2005;23:4079–88.
18. Wierda W, O'Brien S, Wen S, et al. Chemoimmunotherapy with fludarabine, cyclophosphamide, and rituximab for relapsed and refractory chronic lymphocytic leukemia. J Clin Oncol 2005;23:4070–8.
19. Tsimberidou AM, Keating MJ, Giles FJ, et al. Fludarabine and mitoxantrone for patients with chronic lymphocytic leukemia. Cancer 2004;100:2583–91.
20. Bosch F, Ferrer A, Lopez-Guillermo A, et al. Fludarabine, cyclophosphamide and mitoxantrone in the treatment of resistant or relapsed chronic lymphocytic leukaemia. Br J Haematol 2002;119:976–84.
21. Faderl S, Wierda WG, O'Brien S, et al. Fludarabine, cyclophosphamide, mitoxantrone plus rituximab as frontline therapy for CLL: results of a phase 2 study. Blood 2006;108:803a. Abstract 2836.

22. Kay NE, Geyer SM, Call TG, et al. Combination chemoimmunotherapy with pentostatin, cyclophosphamide, and rituximab shows significant clinical activity with low accompanying toxicity in previously untreated B chronic lymphocytic leukemia. Blood 2007;109:405–11.

23. Wierda WG, O'Brien S, Faderl S, et al. Combined cyclophosphamide, fludarabine, alemtuzumab, and rituximab, an active regimen for heavily treated patients with CLL. Blood 2006;108:14a. Abstract 31.

24. Tsimberidou AM, Wierda WG, O'Brien S, et al. Combination of oxaliplatin, fludarabine, cytarabine, and rituximab in Richter's syndrome and fludarabine-refractory chronic lymphocytic leukemia. Blood 2006;108:799a. Abstract 2825.

25. Rai KR, Sawitsky A, Cronkite EP, et al. Clinical staging of chronic lymphocytic leukemia. Blood 1975;46:219–34.

26. Binet JL, Auquier A, Dighiero G, et al. A new prognostic classification of chronic lymphocytic leukemia derived from a multivariate survival analysis. Cancer 1981;48:198–206.

27. Dohner H, Stilgenbauer S, Benner A, et al. Genomic aberrations and survival in chronic lymphocytic leukemia. N Engl J Med 2000;343:1910–6.

28. Grever MR, Lucas DM, Dewald GW, et al. Comprehensive assessment of genetic and molecular features predicting outcome in patients with chronic lymphocytic leukemia: results from the US Intergroup Phase III Trial E2997. J Clin Oncol 2007;25:799–804.

29. Cuneo A, Rigolin GM, Bigoni R, et al. Chronic lymphocytic leukemia with 6q- shows distinct hematological features and intermediate prognosis. Leukemia 2004;18:476–83.

30. El Rouby S, Thomas A, Costin D, et al. p53 gene mutation in B-cell chronic lymphocytic leukemia is associated with drug resistance and is independent of MDR1/MDR3 gene expression. Blood 1993;82:3452–9.

31. Austen B, Powell JE, Alvi A, et al. Mutations in the ATM gene lead to impaired overall and treatment-free survival that is independent of IGVH mutation status in patients with B-CLL. Blood 2005;106:3175–82.

32. Oscier DG, Gardiner AC, Mould SJ, et al. Multivariate analysis of prognostic factors in CLL: clinical stage, IGVH gene mutational status, and loss or mutation of the p53 gene are independent prognostic factors. Blood 2002;100:1177–84.

33. Crespo M, Bosch F, Villamor N, et al. ZAP-70 expression as a surrogate for immunoglobulin-variable-region mutations in chronic lymphocytic leukemia. N Engl J Med 2003;348:1764–75.

34. Rassenti LZ, Huynh L, Toy TL, et al. ZAP-70 compared with immunoglobulin heavy-chain gene mutation status as a predictor of disease progression in chronic lymphocytic leukemia. N Engl J Med 2004;351:893–901.

35. Orchard JA, Ibbotson RE, Davis Z, et al. ZAP-70 expression and prognosis in chronic lymphocytic leukaemia. Lancet 2004;363:105–11.

36. Hamblin TJ, Orchard JA, Ibbotson RE, et al. CD38 expression and immunoglobulin variable region mutations are independent prognostic variables in chronic lymphocytic leukemia, but CD38 expression may vary during the course of the disease. Blood 2002;99:1023–9.

37. Reinisch W, Willheim M, Hilgarth M, et al. Soluble CD23 reliably reflects disease activity in B-cell chronic lymphocytic leukemia. J Clin Oncol 1994;12:2146–52.

38. Hallek M, Langenmayer I, Nerl C, et al. Elevated serum thymidine kinase levels identify a subgroup at high risk of disease progression in early, nonsmoldering chronic lymphocytic leukemia. Blood 1999;93:1732–7.

39. Montserrat E, Gomis F, Vallespi T, et al. Presenting features and prognosis of chronic lymphocytic leukemia in younger adults. Blood 1991;78:1545–51.

40. Molica S, Brugiatelli M, Callea V, et al. Comparison of younger versus older B-cell chronic lymphocytic leukemia patients for clinical presentation and prognosis: a retrospective study of 53 cases. Eur J Haematol 1994;52:216–21.

41. Keating MJ, Lerner S, Kantarjian H, et al. The serum β_2-microglobulin level is more powerful than stage in predicting response and survival in chronic lymphocytic leukemia. Blood 1995: 86:606a. Abstract.

42. Hallek M, Wanders L, Ostwald M, et al. Serum beta(2)-microglobulin and serum thymidine kinase are independent predictors of progression-free survival in chronic lymphocytic leukemia and immunocytoma. Leuk Lymphoma 1996;22:439–47.

43. Calin GA, Ferracin M, Cimmino A, et al. A MicroRNA signature associated with prognosis and progression in chronic lymphocytic leukemia. N Engl J Med 2005;353:1793–801.

44. Tsimberidou AM, McLaughlin P, O'Brien S, et al. A prognostic score for chronic lymphocytic leukemia and small lymphocytic lymphoma: analysis of 2189 patients. Blood 2006;108:788a. Abstract 2783.

45. Chiorazzi N, Rai KR, Ferrarini M. Chronic lymphocytic leukemia. N Engl J Med 2005;352:804–15.

46. Damle RN, Wasil T, Fais F, et al. Ig V gene mutation status and CD38 expression as novel prognostic indicators in chronic lymphocytic leukemia. Blood 1999;94:1840–7.

47. Hamblin TJ, Davis Z, Gardiner A, et al. Unmutated Ig V(H) genes are associated with a more aggressive form of chronic lymphocytic leukemia. Blood 1999;94:1848–54.

48. Zupo S, Rugari E, Dono M, et al. CD38 signaling by agonistic monoclonal antibody prevents apoptosis of human germinal center B cells. Eur J Immunol 1994;24:1218–22.

49. Hanada M, Delia D, Aiello A, Stadtmauer E, et al. bcl-2 gene hypomethylation and high-level expression in B-cell chronic lymphocytic leukemia. Blood 1993;82:1820–8.

50. Hall PA, Lane DP. Tumor suppressors: a developing role for p53? Curr Biol 1997;7:R144–7.

51. Calin GA, Croce CM. Genomics of chronic lymphocytic leukemia microRNAs as new players with clinical significance. Semin Oncol 2006;33:167–73.

52. Lundin J, Kimby E, Bjorkholm M, et al. Phase II trial of subcutaneous anti-CD52 monoclonal antibody alemtuzumab as first-line treatment for patients with B-cell chronic lymphocytic leukemia. Blood 2002;100:768–73.

53. Keating MJ, Flinn I, Jain V, et al. Therapeutic role of alemtuzumab in patients who have failed fludarabine: results of a large international study. Blood 2002;99:3554–61.

54. Rai KR, Freter CE, Mercier RJ, et al. Alemtuzumab in previously treated chronic lymphocytic leukemia patients who also had received fludarabine. J Clin Oncol 2002;20:3891–7.

55. Lozanski G, Heerema NA, Flinn IW, et al. Alemtuzumab is an effective therapy for chronic lymphocytic leukemia with p53 mutations and deletions. Blood 2004;103:3278–81.

56. Moreton P, Kennedy B, Lucas G, et al. Eradication of minimal residual disease in B-cell chronic lymphocytic leukemia after alemtuzumab therapy is associated with prolonged survival. J Clin Oncol 2005;23:2971–9.

57. O'Brien SM, Kantarjian HM, Thomas DA, et al. Alemtuzumab as treatment for residual disease after chemotherapy in patients with chronic lymphocytic leukemia. Cancer 2003;98:2657–63.

58. Wendtner CM, Ritgen M, Schweighofer CD, et al. Consolidation with alemtuzumab in patients with chronic lymphocytic leukemia in first remission—experience on safety and efficacy within a randomized multicenter phase III trial of the German CLL Study Group. Leukemia 2004;18:1093–101.

59. Montillo M, Tedeschi A, Miqueleiz S, et al. Alemtuzumab as consolidation after a response to fludarabine is effective in purging residual disease in patients with chronic lymphocytic leukemia. J Clin Oncol 2006;24:2337–42.

60. McLaughlin P, Grillo-Lopez AJ, Link BK, et al. Rituximab chimeric anti-CD20 monoclonal antibody therapy for relapsed indolent lymphoma: half of patients respond to a four-dose treatment program. J Clin Oncol 1998;16:2825–33.

61. O'Brien SM, Kantarjian H, Thomas DA, et al. Rituximab dose-escalation trial in chronic lymphocytic leukemia. J Clin Oncol 2001;19:2165–70.

62. Byrd JC, Murphy T, Howard RS, et al. Rituximab using a thrice weekly dosing schedule in B-cell chronic lymphocytic leukemia and small lymphocytic lymphoma demonstrates clinical activity and acceptable toxicity. J Clin Oncol 2001;19:2153–64.

63. Huhn D, von Schilling C, Wilhelm M, et al. Rituximab therapy of patients with B-cell chronic lymphocytic leukemia. Blood 2001;98:1326–31.

64. Hainsworth JD, Litchy S, Barton JH, et al. Single-agent rituximab as first-line and maintenance treatment for patients with chronic lymphocytic leukemia or small lymphocytic lymphoma: a phase II trial of the Minnie Pearl Cancer Research Network. J Clin Oncol 2003;21:1746–51.

65. Venugopal P, Sivaraman S, Huang XK, et al. Effects of cytokines on CD20 antigen expression on tumor cells from patients with chronic lymphocytic leukemia. Leuk Res 2000;24:411–5.

66. McLaughlin P, Liu N, Poindexter N, et al. Rituximab plus GM-CSF for indolent lymphoma. In: Proceedings of the 9th International Conference on Malignant Lymphomas; Lugano, Switzerland. Ann Oncol 2005:15(suppl 5):68. Abstract 104.

67. Ferrajoli A, O'Brien S, Faderl S, et al. The combination of rituximab and GM-CSF in elderly patients with chronic lymphocytic leukemia. J Clin Oncol 2006;24(18S):361s. Abstract 6602.

68. Faderl S, Thomas DA, O'Brien S, et al. Experience with alemtuzumab plus rituximab in patients with relapsed and refractory lymphoid malignancies. Blood 2003;101:3413–5.

69. Nabhan C, Patton D, Gordon LI, et al. A pilot trial of rituximab and alemtuzumab combination therapy in patients with relapsed and/or refractory chronic lymphocytic leukemia. Leuk Lymphoma 2004;45:2269–73.

70. Coiffier B, Tilly H, Pedersen LM, et al. HuMax CD20 fully human monoclonal antibody in chronic lymphocytic leukemia: early results from an ongoing phase I/II clinical trial. Blood 2005;106:135a. Abstract 448.

71. Harris R, Viza D, Todd R, et al. Detection of human leukaemia associated antigens in leukaemic serum and normal embryos. Nature 1971;233:556–7.

72. Mitsiades CS, Mitsiades N. CC-5013 (Celgene). Curr Opin Invest Drugs 2004;5:635–47.

73. Chanan-Khan A, Miller KC, Musial L, et al. Clinical efficacy of lenalidomide in patients with relapsed or refractory chronic lymphocytic leukemia: results of a phase II study. J Clin Oncol 2006;24:5343–9.

74. Ferrajoli A, O'Brien S, Faderl S, et al. Lenalidomide induces complete and partial responses in patients with relapsed and treatment-refractory chronic lymphocytic leukemia. Blood 2006;108:153. Abstract 305.

75. Wierda WG, Cantwell MJ, Woods SJ, et al. CD40-ligand (CD154) gene therapy for chronic lymphocytic leukemia. Blood 2000;96:2917–24.

76. Wierda WG, O'Brien SM, Aguillon RA, et al. Membrane-stable, humanized CD154 gene therapy for patients with CLL. Blood 2006;108:596a. Abstract 2104.

77. Kwak LW, Campbell MJ, Czerwinski DK, et al. Induction of immune responses in patients with B-cell lymphoma against the surface-immunoglobulin idiotype expressed by their tumors. N Engl J Med 1992;327:1209–15.

78. Hsu FJ, Caspar CB, Czerwinski D, et al. Tumor-specific idiotype vaccines in the treatment of patients with B-cell lymphoma—long-term results of a clinical trial. Blood 1997;89:3129–35.

79. Kwak LW, Young HA, Pennington RW, et al. Vaccination with syngeneic, lymphoma-derived immunoglobulin idiotype combined with granulocyte/macrophage colony-stimulating factor primes mice for a protective T-cell response. Proc Natl Acad Sci U S A 1996;93:10972–7.

80. Bendandi M, Gocke CD, Kobrin CB, et al. Complete molecular remissions induced by patient-specific vaccination plus granulocyte-monocyte colony-stimulating factor against lymphoma. Nat Med 1999;5:1171–7.

81. A phase 1/2 study to evaluate the feasibility and tolerability of treatment of previously untreated B-cell chronic lymphocytic leukemia patients with recombinant idiotype conjugated to klh (Id-KLH) administered with GM-CSF: Genitope Corporation. Accessed April 30, 2007 at http://www.genitope.com/tr2011.html/.

82. Byrd JC, O'Brien S, Flinn I, et al. Safety and efficacy results from a phase I trial of single-agent lumiliximab (anti-CD23 antibody) for chronic lymphocytic leukemia. Blood 2004;104:686a. Abstract 2503.

83. O'Brien S, Byrd JC, Kipps TJ, et al. Lumiliximab with fludarabine, cyclophosphamide, and rituximab for patients with relapsed chronic lymphocytic leukemia. J Clin Oncol 2006;24(18S):360s. Abstract 6597.

84. Byrd JC, Castro J, O'Brien S, et al. Comparison of results from a phase 1/2 study of lumiliximab (anti-CD23) in combination with FCR for patients with relapsed CLL with published FCR results. Blood 2006;108:14a. Abstract 32.

85. Byrd JC, Lin TS, Dalton JT, et al. Flavopiridol administered using a pharmacologically derived schedule is associated with marked clinical efficacy in refractory, genetically high-risk chronic lymphocytic leukemia. Blood 2007;109:399–404.

86. Byrd JC, Peterson BL, Gabrilove J, et al. Treatment of relapsed chronic lymphocytic leukemia by 72-hour continuous infusion or 1-hour bolus infusion of flavopiridol: results from Cancer and Leukemia Group B study 19805. Clin Cancer Res 2005;11:4176–81.

87. Khan KD, O'Brien S, Rai KR, et al. Phase II study of talabostat and rituximab in fludarabine/rituximab-resistant or refractory patients with CLL. J Clin Oncol 2006;24(18S):360s. Abstract 6598.

88. O'Brien SM, Cunningham CC, Golenkov AK, et al. Phase I to II multicenter study of oblimersen sodium, a Bcl-2 antisense oligonucleotide, in patients with advanced chronic lymphocytic leukemia. J Clin Oncol 2005;23:7697–702.

89. O'Brien S, Moore JO, Boyd TE, et al. Randomized phase III trial of fludarabine plus cyclophosphamide with or without oblimersen sodium (Bcl-2 antisense) in patients with relapsed or refractory chronic lymphocytic leukemia. J Clin Oncol 2007;25:1114–20.

90. Becattini B, Kitada S, Leone M, et al. Rational design and real time, in-cell detection of the proapoptotic activity of a novel compound targeting Bcl-X(L). Chem Biol 2004;11:389–95.

91. Castro JE, Olivier LJ, Robier AA, et al. A phase II, open label study of AT-101 in combination with rituximab in patients with relapsed or refractory chronic lymphocytic leukemia. Blood 2006;108:803a. Abstract 2838.

92. O'Brien S, Kipps TJ, Faderl S, et al. A phase I trial of the small molecule pan-bcl-2 family inhibitor GX15–070 administered intravenously (IV) every 3 weeks to patients with previously treated chronic lymphocytic leukemia. Blood 2005;106:135a. Abstract 446.

93. Castro JE, Prada CE, Loria O, et al. ZAP-70 is a novel conditional heat shock protein 90 (Hsp90) client: inhibition of Hsp90 leads to ZAP-70 degradation, apoptosis, and impaired signaling in chronic lymphocytic leukemia. Blood 2005;106:2506–12.

94. Chronic lymphocytic leukemia. Washington, DC: National Library of Medicine, U.S. National Institutes of Health. Accessed April 30, 2007 at http://clinicaltrials.gov/.

95. Pilot study of pharmacodynamic investigation of treatment with 506U78 combined with fludarabine in refractory leukemics. Accessed April 30, 2007 at http://ctr.gsk.co.uk/Summary/nelarabine/I_PGAA1005.pdf/.

96. Balakrishnan K, Nimmanapalli R, Ravandi F, et al. Forodesine, an inhibitor of purine nucleoside phosphorylase, induces apoptosis in chronic lymphocytic leukemia cells. Blood 2006;108:2392–8.

97. Gandhi V, Plunkett W, Bonate PL, et al. Clinical and pharmacokinetic study of clofarabine in chronic lymphocytic leukemia: strategy for treatment. Clin Cancer Res 2006;12:4011–7.
98. Binet JL, Caligaris-Cappio F, Catovsky D, et al. Perspectives on the use of new diagnostic tools in the treatment of chronic lymphocytic leukemia. Blood 2006;107:859–61.
99. Byrd JC, Peterson BL, Morrison VA, et al. Randomized phase 2 study of fludarabine with concurrent versus sequential treatment with rituximab in symptomatic, untreated patients with B-cell chronic lymphocytic leukemia: results from Cancer and Leukemia Group B 9712 (CALGB 9712). Blood 2003;101:6–14.
100. Osterborg A, Dyer MJ, Bunjes D, et al. Phase II multicenter study of human CD52 antibody in previously treated chronic lymphocytic leukemia: European Study Group of CAMPATH-1H Treatment in Chronic Lymphocytic Leukemia. J Clin Oncol 1997;15:1567–74.

5 Targeted Therapy in Chronic Myeloid Leukemia

Elias Jabbour, MD, Jorge Cortes, MD, and Hagop Kantarjian, MD

Contents

Abstract

The successful introduction of the tyrosine kinase inhibitors (TKIs) has revolutionized the outcome of patients with chronic myeloid leukemia (CML). Imatinib mesylate therapy induced high rates of complete cytogenetic and major molecular responses and improved survival for patients with CML. A small proportion of patients in chronic phase CML and more patients in advanced phases are resistant to imatinib or develop resistance during treatment through *BCR-ABL*-dependent and *BCR-ABL*-independent mechanisms. Novel, more potent TKIs can overcome imatinib resistance, including dasatinib (a potent dual Src and Bcr-Abl inhibitor), nilotinib (a selective potent Bcr-Abl inhibitor), bosutinib and INNO406 (both Src-Abl inhibitors), among others. Other approaches are exploring combination therapy, agents affecting various oncogenic pathways, and immune modulation. This chapter reviews some of these targeted therapies, particularly those for which clinical data are already available.

Key Words: Chronic myeloid leukemia, Tyrosine kinase inhibitor, Resistance, BCR-ABL

From: *Current Clinical Oncology: Targeted Cancer Therapy*
Edited by: R. Kurzrock and M. Markman © Humana Press, Totowa, NJ

1. INTRODUCTION

Chronic myeloid leukemia (CML) is an uncommon disease. Its incidence is low, but its prevalence is increasing. In the United States, approximately 4500 new cases of CML are diagnosed annually *(1)*. The median age at diagnosis is 55 years. With an estimated survival rate of 90% at 5 years and an annual mortality rate of 2%, the prevalence of CML in 20 years may reach 200,000 to 300,000 cases in the United States.

The cytogenetic hallmark of CML is the Philadelphia chromosome (Ph), created by a reciprocal translocation between chromosomes 9 and 22 (t[9;22][q34;q11]). The molecular consequence of this translocation is the generation of a *BCR-ABL* fusion oncogene, which in turn translates into a Bcr-Abl oncoprotein. This most frequently has a molecular weight of 210 kDa (p210$^{Bcr/Abl}$) and has increased tyrosine kinase activity. Such activity is essential for its transforming capability by activating multiple signal transduction pathways, including Ras/Raf/mitogen-activated protein kinase (MAPK), phosphatidylinositol 3 kinase, STAT5/Janus kinase (JAK), and Myc. Bcr-Abl oncoprotein activity leads to uncontrolled cell proliferation and reduced apoptosis, resulting in the malignant expansion of the bone marrow-derived pluripotent stem cells *(2,3)*.

CML normally progresses through three clinically recognized phases. Around 90% of patients are diagnosed during the typically indolent chronic phase, which is followed by an accelerated phase and a terminal blastic phase *(2)*. Although progression through all stages is most common, 20% to 25% of patients progress directly from the chronic to the blastic phase. The mechanisms behind CML disease progression are not fully understood. The criteria for the CML accelerated phase and the CML blastic phase are defined hematologically based on blast cell and progenitor cell counts *(2)*. The time course for progression can be extremely variable. As patients progress through the phases, cytogenetic abnormalities may be detected in addition to Ph chromosome perturbation (termed clonal evolution). Mutations and deletions in specific genes may also occur (e.g., *p53*, *p16/INK4a*, and *RB*) *(4–6)*.

Historically, CML was treated with busulfan or hydroxyurea, and typically had a poor prognosis *(2–7)*. Busulfan and hydroxyurea controlled the hematologic manifestations of the disease but did not delay disease progression. Treatment with interferon-α (IFNα) produced complete cytogenetic responses in 5% to 25% of patients with CML chronic phase and improved survival compared with previous treatments (5-year survival rates: IFNα 57% vs. chemotherapy 42%; $p < 0.00001$) *(8)*. Combining IFNα with cytarabine (a DNA synthesis inhibitor) produced additional benefits *(9,10)*. Hematopoietic stem cell transplantation (SCT) is curative in CML, but it is indicated after imatinib failure because it carries a significant risk of mortality. The 5-year survival with IFNα/imatinib was significantly superior to allogeneic SCT *(11)*.

Imatinib mesylate, a potent and selective Bcr-Abl tyrosine kinase inhibitor (TKI), is now established frontline standard therapy in CML. A complete cytogenetic response to imatinib can be achieved in 50% to 60% of patients in the chronic phase after failing IFNα *(12,13)* therapy and in more than 80% of those receiving imatinib as first-line therapy *(14,15)*. Responses are durable in most patients treated for early chronic phase CML, particularly among those who achieve major molecular responses (e.g., ≥ 3-log reduction in transcript levels) *(16,17)*.

Despite the excellent results with imatinib in CML, resistance occurs at an annual rate of approximately 4% in newly diagnosed CML and more often in advanced disease *(18,19)*.

Several approaches may overcome or prevent the development of imatinib resistance, including the use of new, more potent TKIs (20).

Here we review the most current information regarding targeted therapy in CML and detail the results of frontline therapy and of therapy with the novel TKIs.

2. IMATINIB: FRONTLINE THERAPY FOR CML

Imatinib mesylate (Gleevec/Glivec; Novartis, Basel, Switzerland), an orally available small-molecule TKI, was the first therapy designed to target selectively the causative *BCR-ABL* oncogene in CML (21). Imatinib also inhibits other signaling proteins, including platelet-derived growth factor receptor (PDGFR) and Kit (22). Imatinib acts by binding to the inactive form of Bcr-Abl oncoprotein, preventing a conformational switch to its active form, thus preventing Bcr-Abl autophosphorylation and blocking signal transduction.

The prospective International Randomized Trial of Interferon plus cytarabine versus Imatinib [STI-571] (IRIS) study of 1106 patients with newly diagnosed CML in the chronic phase established the superiority of imatinib 400 mg daily over IFNα and low-dose cytarabine. The complete hematologic response rates were 95% versus 55%; the complete cytogenetic response rates were 76% versus 15%; and the 18-month progression-free survival (PFS) rates were 97% versus 91% ($p < 0.001$). The molecular response rates were also significantly better, with estimated 12-month major molecular response rates of 40% versus 2% (14). Based on the results of these studies, imatinib became the standard first-line therapy for newly diagnosed CML (14,23).

A 5-year update of the IRIS study continued to show positive results (24). A total of 382 patients remained on imatinib frontline therapy. The cumulative complete hematologic response, major cytogenetic response, and complete cytogenetic response rates were 98%, 92%, and 87%, respectively. The 5-year incidence of complete cytogenetic response was 69%. The estimated 5-year event-free survival rate was 83%; only 6.3% of patients have so far progressed to accelerated and blastic phases. The overall annual progression rate declined to 0.9% during the fifth year of therapy, compared with 1.5%, 4.8%, and 7.5%, respectively, during the previous 3 years, suggesting that disease progression may be diminished in the following years. The estimated 5-year survival rate was 89%; excluding non-CML deaths, it was 95%. The intensity of the cytogenetic response after 12 and 18 months of imatinib therapy correlated with survival without transformation. The estimated 5-year survival rate in patients not achieving a major cytogenetic response at 12 months was significantly less (81%) than those who achieved major cytogenetic response (complete 97%, partial 93%; $p < 0.001$). At 18 months of therapy, the estimated 5-year survival rate for patients achieving a complete cytogenetic response was significantly better than in those who did not achieve complete cytogenetic response (99% vs. 90%; $p < 0.001$) (24). There was continuous improvement in the molecular response rate: The rate of major molecular response improved from 53% at 1 year to 80% at 4 years of therapy ($p < 0.001$) (24).

2.1. Survival Advantage

The IRIS study did not document a survival advantage because of its crossover design. However, comparisons with historic studies confirmed the long-term survival superiority of first-line imatinib therapy in newly diagnosed CML. In a retrospective study, the estimated 5-year survival rate for imatinib was 88%, compared with 63% for IFN-based therapies ($p = 0.00001$) (25). A second study compared long-term survival rates among patients originally randomized to imatinib in the IRIS trial with patients in the CML study *(26)*. The estimated 3-year survival rate with imatinib in the IRIS trial was 92% compared with 84% for IFNα plus cytarabine. Imatinib has also demonstrated a survival advantage in patients with advanced-phase CML. In a Phase II study of patients in late CML chronic phase after failing previous IFNα therapy, the 5-year overall survival rate was 79% *(13)*. After 48 months, survival rates in Phase II trials, including patients with CML-accelerated phase or CML-blastic phase treated with imatinib 600 mg/day, were 45% and 12%, respectively *(12,27–30)*.

2.2. Long-Term Safety

Most adverse events with imatinib therapy were of mild to moderate severity. Treatment was discontinued for adverse events in 3% to 5% of patients *(14,26,28,29)*. Grade 3 to 4 hematologic toxicities were moderate and included neutropenia in 3% to 48% and anemia and thrombocytopenia in 5% to 42%. Recently, imatinib was reported to be associated with cardiotoxicity and congestive heart failure, although this toxicity is rare *(31)*. Among 1276 patients treated at a single institution, 22 (1.8%) patients (median age 70 years) were identified as having symptoms that could be attributed to congestive heart failure *(32)*; 8 were considered possibly or probably related to imatinib. Eighteen patients had previous medical conditions predisposing to cardiac disease: congestive heart failure (6 patients), diabetes mellitus (6 patients), hypertension (10 patients), coronary artery disease (8 patients), arrhythmia (3 patients), and cardiomyopathy (1 patient). Of the 22 patients, 11 continued imatinib therapy with dose adjustments and management for the congestive heart failure symptoms with no further complications.

2.3. Imatinib Dose Schedules

The optimal dose of imatinib has not been established. In the dose-finding Phase I study, the maximum tolerated dose was not identified. Because of the good responses obtained at a dose of 300 to 400 mg daily, particularly in patients in the chronic phase, and because the blood concentration of imatinib at 400 mg daily was consistently higher than that required to inhibit 50% of Bcr-Abl tyrosine kinase activity in vitro *(33,35)*, that dose was chosen for subsequent studies. Imatinib 600 mg daily was more effective than 400 mg for patients in accelerated phase or blastic phase disease *(28,29)*. Treatment of late chronic phase CML patients with imatinib 400 mg twice daily after IFNα failure resulted in a complete cytogenetic response rate of 90%, compared to 48% in history-matched controls treated with standard dose therapy. In addition, 56% of patients had a major molecular response, including 41% with undetectable levels *(35)*. The toxicity profile was similar to that of imatinib 400 mg, although there was a higher rate of grade 3 to 4 myelosuppression. In patients with both prior hematologic and cytogenetic resistance to 400 mg of imatinib daily, increasing the dose to 800 mg resulted in a complete hematologic response rate of 65% and a complete cytogenetic response rate of 18% *(36)*. Several Phase II studies, using high-dose imatinib in patients with previously untreated CML in the chronic phase, have documented higher rates of complete cytogenetic response (up to 95%) and of molecular responses, particularly at the level of a 4-log or greater reduction in transcript levels *(25,37–39)*. When compared to history-matched cohorts of patients treated with the standard dose, patients treated with high-dose imatinib had higher rates of complete cytogenetic response (91% vs. 76%, $p = 0.002$); these occurred earlier, with 88% achieving this response after 6 months of therapy versus 56% with the standard dose ($p < 0.00001$). The cumulative incidences of major molecular response and complete molecular response were significantly better with high-dose imatinib *(40)*. Progression-free and transformation-free survivals were also better with high-dose imatinib ($p = 0.02$ and $p = 0.005$, respectively). Results from ongoing randomized studies will determine if the positive results obtained with high-dose imatinib translates into prolonged progression-free and/or overall survival.

2.4. Monitoring Response to Imatinib Therapy and Minimal Residual Disease

Because most patients achieve a complete cytogenetic response with imatinib, realizing a molecular response has become the endpoint of anti-CML strategies and has led to redefining the therapeutic goals for CML. The IRIS trial showed that reducing the level of BCR-ABL transcripts by 3 logs or more below a standard baseline value correlated with PFS *(17)*. In addition, one study reported that achieving a major molecular response within the first 12 months of therapy was predictive of durable cytogenetic remission *(16)*. The lack of consistency in reporting BCR-ABL transcript levels has been a source of debate. A recent consensual proposal suggests harmonizing the differing methodologies for measuring BCR-ABL transcripts by using a conversion factor whereby individual laboratories can express BCR-ABL transcript levels on internationally agreed scales: Results can then be converted by comparing the analysis of standardized reference samples with a value of 0.1% corresponding to major molecular response in all laboratories *(41)*. For practical purposes, a major molecular response can be defined as a reduction of BCR-ABL/ABL transcripts to 0.1% or less *(41)*. After a patient has achieved a complete cytogenetic response, a reverse transcriptase polymerase chain reaction (RT-PCR) can be performed every 3 to 6 months and a routine cytogenetic analysis every 12 months. This latter study may detect clonal evolution and chromosomal abnormalities occurring in normal metaphases.

2.5. Imatinib Resistance

Despite the evident benefits of imatinib over prior treatments, some patients may be intrinsically resistant to imatinib, whereas others may acquire resistance with continuing therapy *(42)*. The estimated 2-year incidence of resistance is 80% in the blastic phase, 40% to 50% in the accelerated phase, and 8% to 10% in the chronic phase *(30)*. Annual relapse rates of 4% have been reported in newly diagnosed patients in the chronic phase *(18,19,42)*. The IRIS trial showed that the risk of progression from chronic phase to accelerated phase is associated with the degree of cytogenetic response: The annual rate of progression was 2% in patients with a partial cytogenetic response at 18 months and 0.2% in those with a complete cytogenetic response at 18 months *(24)*.

Multiple mechanisms of resistance to imatinib have been identified. Two of the best characterized are increased expression of Bcr-Abl kinase via gene amplification and mutations in the *BCR-ABL* fusion gene affecting drug-binding or kinase activity *(18)*. The latter is a dominant and well understood mechanism of acquired resistance *(18,43)*. Mutations disrupt critical contact points between imatinib and Bcr-Abl or induce a transition from the inactive to the active configuration, to which imatinib is unable to bind. Thus, the trend toward increasing imatinib resistance in late-phase CML is consistent with the higher rates of *BCR-ABL* point mutations in these patients *(44–47)*. The number of *BCR-ABL* mutations detected in patients with resistant CML has steadily increased. Not all mutations have the same biochemical and clinical properties: Some *BCR-ABL* mutations result in a highly resistant phenotype in vitro, whereas others are relatively sensitive and resistance may be overcome by imatinib dose increase *(18,48–50)*. The T315I mutation and some mutations affecting the so-called P-loop of Bcr-Abl confer a greater level of resistance to imatinib and to the novel TKIs *(43)*. Other mechanisms of resistance, such as overexpression or amplification of the Bcr-Abl message and/or protein, clonal evolution, and expression of the P-glycoprotein (Pgp), may influence patient outcome *(51–53)*.

2.6. Overcoming Imatinib Resistance

Several approaches have been investigated to overcome or prevent the development of resistance to imatinib. These include (1) high-dose imatinib; (2) new, more potent TKIs, which would also be less susceptible to mutation-induced mechanisms of resistance; (3) imatinib combinations; and (4) non-TKI approaches. The first of the newer-generation TKIs, dasatinib (Sprycel; BMS-354825), an orally bioavailable dual Bcr-Abl and Src inhibitor, has been recently approved by the U.S. Food and Drug Administration (FDA) for the treatment of CML after imatinib failure. Nilotinib (Tasigna; AMN-107) is another oral more potent and selective Bcr-Abl inhibitor awaiting approval. Bosutinib and others are in advanced clinical trials. Other strategies include vaccines and investigational approaches.

3. DASATINIB

Dasatinib, a dual inhibitor of SRC and ABL kinases, has been approved by the FDA for use in patients with imatinib-resistant and imatinib-intolerant CML. In preclinical evaluations, dasatinib showed activity against 18 of 19 imatinib-resistant BCR-ABL mutants lines *(54)*. The exception was a line carrying the T315I mutant. In preclinical models, dasatinib is about 300 times more potent than imatinib.

In a Phase I dose-escalation study, dasatinib demonstrated significant activity in patients with imatinib-resistant and imatinib-intolerant chronic phase CML, with a complete hematologic response rate of 92% and a major cytogenetic response rate of 45% *(55)*. Consistent with preclinical results, two patients with the T315I mutant failed to respond to dasatinib. This study also demonstrated significant activity against CML in advanced phases, including major hematologic responses in 31 of 44 patients with CML-accelerated phase, CML-blastic phase, or Ph-positive acute lymphoblastic leukemia (ALL).

Results from a Phase II study of dasatinib 70 mg orally twice daily in patients with chronic phase CML who had either imatinib resistance ($n = 288$) or intolerance ($n = 99$) showed, after a median follow-up of 15 months, that 80% of patients intolerant of imatinib achieved a major cytogenetic response (75% complete), whereas only 52% of patients resistant to imabinib achieved a major cytogenetic response (40% complete) *(56)*. In another Phase II study, patients with chronic phase CML after resistance to standard dose imatinib (400–600 mg/day) were randomized (2:1) to dasatinib 70 mg twice daily ($n = 101$) or high-dose imatinib ($n = 49$) *(57)*. With a median follow-up of 15 months, 35% of patients treated with dasatinib achieved a complete cytogenetic response compared to 16% of patients treated with high-dose imatinib. The difference in response rates was most evident in patients with failure on imatinib 600 mg daily (major cytogenetic response rates 49% vs. 24%) but not in patients with failure on imatinib 400 mg a day (major cytogenetic response rates 58% vs. 53%). PFS was better with dasatinib (estimated 12-month rates 94% vs. 70%; $p < 0.0001$). Dasatinib has also shown activity in CML-accelerated phase and CML-blastic phase patients after imatinib failure. Preliminary results from the first 174 patients treated in CML-accelerated phase showed a major hematologic response in 64% of patients (complete in 45%); major cytogenetic response was achieved in 48% *(58)*. The complete hematologic response rates in patients with CML-blastic phase and Ph-positive ALL were 27% and 35%,

Table 1
Results of Dasatinib Phase II Studies in CML and Ph-positive ALL Post-imatinib Failure

Disease phase	No.	Hematologic response (%)		Cytogenetic response (%)	
		Major	Complete	Major	Complete
Chronic	387		91	58	49
Accelerated	174	64	45	37	28
Myeloid blastic	157	50	27	38	31
Ph-positive ALL	46	51	33	57	54
Chronic-randomized					
Dasatinib	101		92	48	35
High-dose imatinib	49		82	33	16

CML, chronic myeloid leukemia; ALL, acute lymphoid leukemia; Ph, Philadelphia chromosome; CHR, complete hematologic response; HR, hematologic response

respectively; the major cytogenetic response rates were 38% (31% complete) and 57% (54% complete), respectively (Table 1) *(59,60)*.

Pooled safety analysis of all six studies showed that dasatinib was well tolerated. Most drug-related serious adverse events were managed with dose interruptions or reductions. Myelosuppression was the most common reason for dose reductions or interruptions. Grade 3 to 4 thrombocytopenia, neutropenia, and anemia were reported in 50% to 60% of patients in the chronic phase. Nonhematologic adverse events were mild to moderate. Pleural effusions were observed in 5% to 35%; they were severe in 3% to 15%. They are managed with treatment interruptions/dose reductions, steroids, and diuretics.

3.1. Optimizing Dose and Schedule

The initial Phase I trial of dasatinib had shown similar hematologic responses and cytogenetic responses rates at total daily doses of 100 mg and 140 mg daily in both twice-daily and once-daily schedules. Side effects appeared to be lower with lower doses and single-dose daily schedules. Based on these observations, 662 patients with CML-chronic phase after imatinib failure were randomized to four treatment arms: (1) dasatinib 100 mg once daily ($n = 166$); (2) dasatinib 50 mg twice daily ($n = 166$); (3) dasatinib 140 mg once daily ($n = 163$); or (4) dasatinib 70 mg twice daily ($n = 167$) *(61)*. With a minimum follow-up of 6 months, there was no difference in efficacy in the four arms: Complete hematologic response rates varied between 87% and 93%, major cytogenetic response rates between 54% and 59%, and complete cytogenetic response rates between 42% and 45%. In contrast, patients receiving dasatinib 100 mg once daily had fewer pleural effusions ($p = 0.028$), less anemia ($p = 0.032$), less neutropenia ($p = 0.035$), and less thrombocytopenia ($p = 0.001$) than those receiving the three other dose schedules *(61)*. In patients with advanced stage disease, dasatinib 140 mg once daily was equivalent in activity to 70 mg twice daily with a significantly lower incidence of pleural effusion ($p = 0.024$) *(62)*.

3.2. Frontline Therapy

In a Phase II study of newly diagnosed CML-chronic phase, 24 patients received dasatinib 100 mg once daily or 50 mg twice daily. The complete cytogenetic response rates at 6 and

9 months were 73% and 95%, respectively, which is better than results with historical data in patients treated with standard-dose and high-dose imatinib *(63)*.

4. NILOTINIB

Nilotinib is an orally administered derivative of imatinib in clinical development. It inhibits BCR-ABL with a 30- to 50-fold greater potency than imatinib *(64)*. Like imatinib, nilotinib binds Bcr-Abl in its inactive conformation. Nilotinib inhibited the activity of 32 of 33 mutant forms of BCR-ABL detected in imatinib-resistant patients. Nilotinib was not active against the T315I mutant type *(65–68)*.

In a Phase I dose-escalation study, nilotinib was evaluated in 119 patients with imatinib-resistant and imatinib-intolerant CML in various phases or with Ph-positive ALL *(69)*. Among 12 patients with CML-chronic phase, 11 achieved a complete hematologic response and 9 a cytogenetic response (6 complete). Nilotinib also demonstrated activity against advanced disease. Among 46 patients with active CML-accelerated phase, 21 achieved a complete hematologic response and 9 returned to the chronic phase. Altogether, 22 patients with CML-accelerated phase achieved cytogenetic responses, including 9 major and 6 complete. Among 24 patients in myeloid CML-blastic phase, 2 achieved complete hematologic response and 6 returned to the chronic phase. Among nine patients with lymphoid CML-blastic phase, one achieved a marrow response, and two returned to chronic phase. Seven patients each with myeloid (29%) or lymphoid (22%) CML-blastic phase achieved a cytogenetic response with nilotinib. Nilotinib doses of 400 mg and 600 mg twice daily produced the best responses. At the dose of 400 mg twice daily, grade 3 or 4 nonhematologic adverse events included pruritus (3%), increased total and unconjugated bilirubin (3%), increased lipase (9%), and increased liver enzyme levels (3%). The incidence of grade 3 or 4 thrombocytopenia was 25%, and the incidences of grade 3 or 4 anemia and neutropenia were less than 10%.

Results from the Phase II pivotal trials were recently reported *(70–72)*. A total of 282 patients with CML-chronic phase after imatinib failure were treated with nilotinib 400 mg twice daily. The complete hematologic response rate was 74%, the major cytogenetic response rate was 52%, and the complete cytogenetic response rate was 34%. The estimated 1-year survival rate was 95%. Side effects were modest, including grade 3 to 4 myelosuppression in 20% to 30%; no pleural effusions were observed. Response rates were similar in patients with imatinib resistance versus intolerance and in patients with or without mutations *(70)*. The activity of nilotinib in CML-accelerated and CML-blastic phase after imatinib failure were also encouraging, although the response rates were lower and the response durations shorter (Table 2) *(71,72)*. Among 64 patients in accelerated phase, the hematologic response rate was 59%, and the major cytogenetic rate was 36%. Among 130 patients in blastic phase and Ph-positive ALL, the complete hematologic response rate was 11%.

4.1. Frontline Therapy

In preliminary results from 14 patients with newly diagnosed CML treated with nilotinib 400 mg twice daily *(73)*, a major cytogenetic response was observed in all patients at 3 months (complete in 13 and partial in 1); the complete cytogenetic response rate was 100% in all evaluable patients at 6 months (*n* = 13) and 9 months (*n* = 11). Major molecular response rates at 6 and 9 months were significantly higher with nilotinib compared with historic data with standard-dose and high-dose imatinib *(73)*.

Table 2
Results of Nilotinib Phase II Studies in CML and Ph-positive ALL Post-Imatinib Failure

| Disease | No. | Complete hematologic response (%) | Cytogenetic response (%) | |
			Major	Complete
CML				
Chronic	280	74	52	34
Accelerated	64	25	36	22
Blastic	96	13	NR	NR
ALL, Ph-positive	34	6	NR	NR

NR, no response.

5. BOSUTINIB (SKI606)

Bosutinib (SKI606) is an orally available dual Src/Abl inhibitor that is 30 to 200 times more potent than imatinib. It has minimal inhibitory activity against c-Kit and PDGFR (and is therefore expected to produce less myelosuppression and pleural effusions). In a Phase I/II study of 69 patients with CML treated after imatinib failure, the complete hematologic response rate among 48 patients in the chronic phase was 84%, and the cytogenetic response rate was 81%, (major 52%, complete 33%) *(74)*. The median at the study follow-up was short. Grade 3 to 4 toxicities were minimal, including skin rashes in 6% and thrombocytopenia in 6%. Mild to moderate diarrhea was common at the Phase II dose selected of 500 mg orally daily.

6. INNO-406

INNO-406 is an orally available, dual Abl/Lyn kinase inhibitor that is up to 55-times more potent than imatinib in Bcr-Abl cell lines. INNO-406 demonstrates specific Src kinase activity against Lyn kinase. In an ongoing Phase I study, INNO-406 was well tolerated in patients at a dose of 240 mg/day, with encouraging evidence of clinical activity in imatinib-resistant and nilotinib-intolerant patients, with 6 of 14 patients (43%) showing evidence of response *(75)*.

7. OTHER AGENTS

MK0457 is an aurora kinase inhibitor with selective inhibitory activity against T315I mutant CML. In a preliminary experience involving 11 patients with CML-advanced phase and T315I mutations, MK0457 given at 8 to 32 mg/m^2 hourly for 5 days induced responses in five patients: two complete cytogenetic responses and three partial minor cytogenetic responses *(76)*. Other aurora kinase inhibitors with potential activity against T315I mutant CML are AT9283 and KW2449. Other classes of agents that have shown reasonable activity against CML after imatinib failure include farnesyl transferase inhibitors (tipifarnib), decitabine, and homoharringtonine *(77–79)*.

8. IMMUNOTHERAPY AND RESIDUAL DISEASE

The observation of a graft-versus-leukemia effect following SCT suggests that immunotherapy aimed at CML is an approach worth investigating. Because the Bcr-Abl fusion protein represents a unique tumor-specific antigen, vaccination using peptides based on the BCR-ABL junction point may be useful, especially for reducing residual disease levels after maximal responses to imatinib have been achieved *(80,82)*. Two recent clinical studies of vaccination using peptides derived from the Bcr-Abl fusion region have demonstrated that patients develop a functional immune response to these peptides *(82,83)*. In one study, vaccination of nine patients who had achieved stable but incomplete cytogenetic responses (median Ph-positive level 10%) on imatinib resulted in an improved cytogenetic response, including a complete cytogenetic response, in five patients. Three patients also achieved a complete molecular response.

9. CONCLUSION AND FUTURE PERSPECTIVES

Targeted therapy with TKIs has significantly improved the prognosis for patients with CML, particularly those in the chronic phase. Emergence of resistance in a small proportion of patients with newly diagnosed CML underlines the complex interactions in CML pathophysiology and the need to improve therapy. Current and future studies are exploring the role of the new TKIs (dasatinib, nilotinib, bosutinib) as frontline therapy in CML to reduce or prevent emergence of resistance due to mutations or other mechanisms. Long-term treatment of CML may require a combination of TKIs and possibly compounds with other mechanisms of action, both conventional and targeted. As understanding of the molecular biology of the Ph chromosome, the *BCR-ABL* gene, and Bcr-Abl kinase increases, evaluation of treatment options will become more accurate, as will timing the administration of the various modalities. In addition to measuring drug efficacy this will ultimately allow us to direct therapies to specific patient subgroups.

REFERENCES

1. Jemal A, Siegel R, Ward E, et al. Cancer statistics, 2006. CA Cancer J Clin 2006;56:106–30.
2. Faderl S, Talpaz M, Estrov Z, et al. The biology of chronic myeloid leukemia. N Engl J Med 1999;341:164–72.
3. Goldman JM, Melo JV. Chronic myeloid leukemia—advances in biology and new approaches to treatment. N Engl J Med 2003;349:1451–64.
4. Lionberger JM, Wilson MB, Smithgall TE. Transformation of myeloid leukemia cells to cytokine independence by Bcr-Abl is suppressed by kinase-defective Hck. J Biol Chem 2000;275:18581–5.
5. Donato NJ, Wu JY, Stapley J, et al. BCR-ABL independence and LYN kinase overexpression in chronic myelogenous leukemia cells selected for resistance to STI571. Blood 2003;101:690–8.
6. Dai Y, Rahmani M, Corey SJ, et al. A Bcr/Abl-independent, Lyn-dependent form of imatinib mesylate (STI-571) resistance is associated with altered expression of Bcl-2. J Biol Chem 2004;279:34227–39.
7. Faderl S, Kantarjian HM, Talpaz M. Chronic myelogenous leukemia: update on biology and treatment. Oncology (Williston Park) 1999;13:169–80.
8. Chronic Myeloid Leukemia Trialists' Collaborative Group. Interferon alfa versus chemotherapy for chronic myeloid leukemia: a meta-analysis of seven randomized trials. J Natl Cancer Inst 1997;89:1616–20.
9. Guilhot F, Chastang C, Michallet M, et al. Interferon alfa-2b combined with cytarabine versus interferon alone in chronic myelogenous leukemia. French Chronic Myeloid Leukemia Study Group. N Engl J Med 1997;337:223–9.
10. Kantarjian HM, O'Brien S, Smith TL, et al. Treatment of Philadelphia chromosome-positive early chronic phase chronic myelogenous leukemia with daily doses of interferon alpha and low-dose cytarabine. J Clin Oncol 1999;17:284–92.
11. Hehlmann R, Pfirrmann M, Hochhaus A, et al. Randomized comparison of primary allogeneic stem cell transplantation and best available drug treatment in chronic myeloid leukemia. Blood 2006;108:427.
12. Kantarjian H, Sawyers C, Hochhaus A, et al. Hematologic and cytogenetic responses to imatinib mesylate in chronic myelogenous leukemia. N Engl J Med 2002;346:645–52.
13. Kantarjian HM, Cortes JE, O'Brien S, et al. Long-term survival benefit and improved complete cytogenetic and molecular response rates with imatinib mesylate in Philadelphia chromosome-positive chronic-phase chronic myeloid leukemia after failure of interferon-α. Blood 2004;104:1979–88.

14. O'Brien SG, Guilhot F, Larson RA, et al. Imatinib compared with interferon and low-dose cytarabine for newly diagnosed chronic-phase chronic myeloid leukemia. N Engl J Med 2003;348:994–1004.
15. Kantarjian H, Talpaz M, O'Brien S, et al. High-dose imatinib mesylate therapy in newly diagnosed Philadelphia chromosome-positive chronic phase chronic myeloid leukemia. Blood 2004;103:2873–8.
16. Cortes J, Talpaz M, O'Brien S, et al. Molecular responses in patients with chronic myelogenous leukemia in chronic phase treated with imatinib mesylate. Clin Cancer Res 2005;11:3425–32.
17. Hughes TP, Kaeda J, Branford S, et al. Frequency of major molecular responses to imatinib or interferon alfa plus cytarabine in newly diagnosed chronic myeloid leukemia. N Engl J Med 2003;349:1423–32.
18. Hochhaus A, Kreil S, Corbin AS, et al. Molecular and chromosomal mechanisms of resistance to imatinib (STI571) therapy. Leukemia 2002;16:2190–6.
19. Gambacorti-Passerini CB, Gunby RH, Piazza R, et al. Molecular mechanisms of resistance to imatinib in Philadelphia-chromosome-positive leukaemias. Lancet Oncol 2003;4:75–85.
20. Jabbour E, Cortes J, Giles F, et al. Current and emerging treatment options in chronic myeloid leukemia. Cancer 2007;109:2171–81.
21. Druker BJ, Tamura S, Buchdunger E, et al. Effects of a selective inhibitor of the Abl tyrosine kinase on the growth of Bcr-Abl positive cells. Nat Med 1996;2:561–6.
22. Beran M, Cao X, Estrov Z, et al. Selective inhibition of cell proliferation and BCR-ABL phosphorylation in acute lymphoblastic leukemia cells expressing Mr 190,000 BCR-ABL protein by a tyrosine kinase inhibitor (CGP-57148). Clin Cancer Res 1998 ;4:1661–72.
23. Kantarjian HM, Cortes JE, O'Brien S, et al. Imatinib mesylate therapy in newly diagnosed patients with Philadelphia chromosome-positive chronic myelogenous leukemia: high incidence of early complete and major cytogenetic responses. Blood 2003;101:97–100.
24. Druker BJ, Guilhot F, O'Brien S, et al. Five-year follow-up of patients receiving imatinib for chronic myeloid leukemia. N Engl J Med 2006;355:2408–17.
25. Kantarjian HM, Talpaz M, O'Brien S, et al. Survival benefit with imatinib mesylate versus interferon-α-based regimens in newly diagnosed chronic-phase chronic myelogenous leukemia. Blood 2006;108:1835–40.
26. Roy L, Guilhot J, Krahnke T, et al. Survival advantage from imatinib compared with the combination interferon-α plus cytarabine in chronic-phase chronic myelogenous leukemia: historical comparison between two phase 3 trials. Blood 2006;108:1478–84.
27. Gambacorti-Passerini C, Talpaz M, Sawyers C, et al. Five year follow-up results of a phase II trial in patients with late chronic phase CML treated with imatinib who are refractory/intolerant to interferon alfa. Blood 2005;107:317a.
28. Sawyers CL, Hochhaus A, Feldman E, et al. Imatinib induces hematologic and cytogenetic responses in patients with chronic myelogenous leukemia in myeloid blast crisis: results of a phase II study. Blood 2002;99:3530–9.
29. Talpaz M, Silver RT, Druker BJ, et al. Imatinib induces durable hematologic and cytogenetic responses in patients with accelerated phase chronic myeloid leukemia: results of a phase 2 study. Blood 2002;99:1928–37.
30. Silver RT, Talpaz M, Sawyers CL, et al. Four years of follow-up of 1027 patients with late chronic phase (L-CP), accelerated phase (AP), or blast crisis (BC) chronic myeloid leukemia (CML) treated with imatinib in three large phase II trials. Blood 2004;104:11a.
31. Kerkela R, Grazette L, Yacobi R, et al. Cardiotoxicity of the cancer therapeutic agent imatinib mesylate. Nat Med 2006;12:908–16.
32. Atallah E, Durand JB, Kantarjian H, et al. Congestive heart failure is a rare event in patients receiving imatinib therapy. Blood 2006;108. Abstract 246.
33. Peng B, Hayes M, Resta D, et al. Pharmacokinetics and pharmacodynamics of imatinib in a phase I trial with chronic myeloid leukemia patients. J Clin Oncol 2004;22:935–42.
34. Schmidli H, Peng B, Riviere GJ, et al. Population pharmacokinetics of imatinib mesylate in patients with chronic-phase chronic myeloid leukaemia: results of a phase III study. Br J Clin Pharmacol 2005;60:35–44.
35. Cortes J, Giles F, O'Brien S, et al. Result of high-dose imatinib mesylate in patients with Philadelphia chromosome-positive chronic myeloid leukemia after failure of interferon-α. Blood 2003;102:83–6.
36. Kantarjian H, Talpaz M, O'Brien S, et al. Dose escalation of imatinib mesylate can overcome resistance to standard-dose therapy in patients with chronic myelogenous leukemia. Blood 2003;101:473–5.
37. Hughes TP, Branford S, Matthews J, et al. Trial of higher dose imatinib with selective intensification in newly diagnosed CML patients in chronic phase. Blood 2003:102:31a.
38. Cortes J, Giles F, Salvado A, et al. High-dose (HD) imatinib in patients with previously untreated chronic myeloid leukemia (CML) in early chronic phase (CP): preliminary results of a multicenter community based trial. J Clin Oncol 2005; 23:564a.

39. Rosti G, Martinelli G, Castagnetti F, et al. Imatinib 800 mg: preliminary results of a phase II trial of the GIMEMA CML working party in intermediate Sokal risk patients and status-of-the-art of an ongoing multinational, prospective randomized trial of imatinib standard dose (400 mg daily) is high dose (800 mg daily) in high Sokal risk patients. Blood 2005; 106:320a.

40. Aoki E, Kantarjian H, O'Brien S, et al. High-dose (HD) imatinib provides better responses in patients with untreated early chronic phase (CP) chronic myeloid leukemia (CML). Blood 2006;108. Abstract 2143.

41. Hughes TP, Deininger MW, Hochhaus A, et al. Monitoring CML patients responding to treatment with tyrosine kinase inhibitors: review and recommendations for harmonizing current methodology for detecting BCR-ABL transcripts and kinase domain mutations and for expressing results. Blood 2006;108:28–37.

42. Shah NP. Loss of response to imatinib: mechanisms and management. Hematology Am Soc Hematol Educ Program 2005;183–7.

43. Gorre ME, Mohammed M, Ellwood K, et al. Clinical resistance to STI-571 cancer therapy caused by BCR-ABL gene mutation or amplification. Science 2001;293:876–80.

44. Branford S, Rudzki Z, Walsh S, et al. Detection of BCR-ABL mutations in patients with CML treated with imatinib is virtually always accompanied by clinical resistance, and mutations in the ATP phosphate-binding loop (P-loop) are associated with a poor prognosis. Blood 2003;102:276–83.

45. Jabbour E, Kantarjian H, Jones D, et al. Frequency and clinical significance of BCR-ABL mutations in patients with chronic myeloid leukemia treated with imatinib mesylate. Leukemia 2006;20:1767–73.

46. Soverini S, Martinelli G, Rosti G, et al. ABL mutations in late chronic phase chronic myeloid leukemia patients with up-front cytogenetic resistance to imatinib are associated with a greater likelihood of progression to blast crisis and shorter survival: a study by the GIMEMA Working Party on Chronic Myeloid Leukemia. J Clin Oncol 2005;23:4100–9.

47. Nicolini FE, Corm S, Le QH, et al. Mutation status and clinical outcome of 89 imatinib mesylate-resistant chronic myelogenous leukemia patients: a retrospective analysis from the French intergroup of CML (Fi(varphi)-LMC Group). Leukemia 2006;20:1061–6.

48. Von Bubnoff N, Schneller F, Peschel C, et al. BCR-ABL gene mutations in relation to clinical resistance of Philadelphia-chromosome-positive leukaemia to STI571: a prospective study. Lancet 2002;359:487–91.

49. Corbin AS, Buchdunger E, Pascal F, et al. Analysis of the structural basis of specificity of inhibition of the Abl kinase by STI571. J Biol Chem 2002;277:32214–9.

50. Azam M, Latek RR, Daley GQ, et al. Mechanisms of autoinhibition and STI-571/imatinib resistance revealed by mutagenesis of BCR-ABL. Cell 2003;112:831–43.

51. Gambacorti-Passerini C, Zucchetti M, Russo D, et al. Alpha1 acid glycoprotein binds to imatinib (STI571) and substantially alters its pharmacokinetics in chronic myeloid leukemia patients. Clin Cancer Res 2003;9:625–32.

52. Donato NJ, Wu JY, Stapley J, et al. Imatinib mesylate resistance through BCR-ABL independence in chronic myelogenous leukemia. Cancer Res 2004; 64:672–7.

53. Donato NJ, Wu JY, Stapley J, et al. BCR-ABL independence and LYN kinase overexpression in chronic myelogenous leukemia cells selected for resistance to STI571. Blood 2003;101:690–8.

54. Shah NP, Tran C, Lee FY, et al. Overriding imatinib resistance with a novel ABL kinase inhibitor. Science 2004;305:399–401.

55. Talpaz M, Shah NP, Kantarjian H, et al. Dasatinib in imatinib-resistant Philadelphia chromosome-positive leukemias. N Engl J Med 2006;354:2531–41.

56. Baccarani M, Kantarjian HM, Apperley JF, et al. Efficacy of dasatinib (SPRYCEL) in patients (pts) with chronic phase chronic myelogenous leukemia (CP-CML) resistant to or intolerant of imatinib: updated results of the CA180013 START-C phase II study. Blood 2006;108. Abstract 164.

57. Shah N, Pasquini R, Rousselot P, et al. Dasatinib (SPRYCEL) vs escalated dose of imatinib (im) in patients (pts) with chronic phase chronic myeloid leukemia (CP-CML) resistant to imatinib: results of the CA180–017 START-R randomized study. Blood 2006;108. Abstract 167.

58. Cortes J, Kim DW, Guilhot F, et al. Dasatinib (SPRYCEL) in patients (pts) with chronic myelogenous leukemia in accelerated phase (AP-CML) that is imatinib-resistant (im-r) or -intolerant (im-i): updated results of the CA180–005 START-A phase II study. Blood 2006;108. Abstract 2160.

59. Martinelli G, Hochhaus A, Coutre S, et al. Dasatinib (SPRYCEL) efficacy and safety in patients (pts) with chronic myelogenous leukemia in lymphoid (CML-LB) or myeloid blast (CML-MB) phase who are imatinib-resistant (im-r) or -intolerant (im-i). Blood 2006;108. Abstract 745.

60. Dombret H, Ottman OG, Rosti G, et al. Dasatinib (SPRYCEL) in patients (pts) with Philadelphia chromosome-positive acute lymphoblastic leukemia who are imatinib-resistant (im-r) or -intolerant (im-i): updated results from the CA180–015 START-L study. Blood 2006;108. Abstract 286.

61. Hochhaus A, Kim DW, Rousselot P, et al. Dasatinib (SPRYCEL®) 50mg or 70mg BID Versus 100mg or 140mg qd in patients with chronic myeloid leukemia in chronic phase (CML-CP) resistant or intolerant to imatinib: results of the CA180–034 study. Blood 2006;108. Abstract 166.

62. Kantarjian H, Ottmann O, Pasquini R, et al. Dasatinib (Sprycel®) 140 mg once daily (qd) vs 70 mg twice daily (bid) in patients (pts) with advanced phase chronic myeloid leukemia (ABP-CML) or Ph(+) ALL who are resistant or intolerant to imatinib (im): results of the CA180–035 study. Blood 2006;108. Abstract 746.

63. Cortes J, O'Brien S, Jones D, et al. Dasatinib in patients with previously untreated chronic myeloid leukemia in chronic phase. Blood 2006;108. Abstract 2161.

64. O'Hare T, Walters DK, Stoffregen EP, et al. In vitro activity of Bcr-Abl inhibitors AMN107 and BMS-354825 against clinically relevant imatinib-resistant Abl kinase domain mutants. Cancer Res 2005;65: 4500–5.

65. Weisberg E, Manley PW, Breitenstein W, et al. Characterization of AMN107, a selective inhibitor of native and mutant Bcr-Abl. Cancer Cell 2005;7:129–41.

66. Verstovsek S, Golemovic M, Kantarjian H, et al. AMN107, a novel aminopyrimidine inhibitor of p190 Bcr-Abl activation and of in vitro proliferation of Philadelphia-positive acute lymphoblastic leukemia cells. Cancer 2005;104:1230–6.

67. Jensen MR, Bruggen J, DiLea C, et al. AMN107: efficacy of the selective Bcr-Abl tyrosine kinase inhibitor in a murine model of chronic myelogenous leukemia. Proc Am Assoc Cancer Res 2006;47. Abstract 261.

68. Weisberg E, Manley P, Mestan J, et al. AMN107 (nilotinib): a novel and selective inhibitor of BCR-ABL. Br J Cancer 2006;94:1765–9.

69. Kantarjian H, Giles F, Wunderle L, et al. Nilotinib in imatinib-resistant CML and Philadelphia chromosome-positive ALL. N Engl J Med 2006;354:2542–51.

70. Le Coutre P, Bhalla K, Giles F, et al. A phase II study of nilotinib, a novel tyrosine kinase inhibitor administered to imatinib-resistant and -intolerant patients with chronic myelogenous leukemia (CML) in chronic phase (CP). Blood 2006;108. Abstract 165.

71. Kantarjian HM, Gattermann N, Hochhaus A, et al. A phase II study of nilotinib a novel tyrosine kinase inhibitor administered to imatinib-resistant or intolerant patients with chronic myelogenous leukemia (CML) in accelerated phase (AP). Blood 2006;108. Abstract 2169.

72. Ottmann O, Kantarjian H, Larson R, et al. A phase II study of nilotinib, a novel tyrosine kinase inhibitor administered to imatinib resistant or intolerant patients with chronic myelogenous leukemia (CML) in blast crisis (BC) or relapsed/refractory Ph+ acute lymphoblastic leukemia (ALL). Blood 2006;108. Abstract 1862.

73. Jabbour E, Cortes J, Giles F, et al. Preliminary activity of AMN107, a novel potent oral selective Bcr-Abl tyrosine kinase inhibitor, in newly diagnosed Philadelphia chromosome (Ph)-positive chronic phase chronic myelogenous leukaemia (CML-CP). Blood 2006;108. Abstract 2172.

74. Cortes J, Kantarjian HM, Baccarani M, et al. A phase 1/2 study of SKI-606, a dual Inhibitor of Src and Abl kinases, in adult patients with Philadelphia chromosome positive (Ph+) chronic myelogenous leukemia (CML) or acute lymphocytic leukemia (ALL) relapsed, refractory or intolerant of imatinib. Blood 2006;108. Abstract 168.

75. Craig AR, Kantarjian HM, Cortes JE, et al. Phase I study of INNO-406, a dual inhibitor of Abl and Lyn kinases, in adult patients with Philadelphia chromosome positive (Ph+) chronic myelogenous leukemia (CML) or acute lymphocytic leukemia (ALL) relapsed, refractory, or intolerant of imatinib. J Clin Oncol 2007; Abstract 7046.

76. Giles FJ, Cortes JE, Jones D, et al. MK-0457, a novel kinase inhibitor, is active in patients with chronic myeloid leukemia or acute lymphocytic leukemia with the T315I BCR-ABL mutation. Blood 2007;109: 500–2.

77. Cortes J, Albitar M, Thomas D, et al. Efficacy of the farnesyl transferase inhibitor R115777 in chronic myeloid leukemia and other hematologic malignancies. Blood 2003;101:1692–7.

78. Issa JP, Gharibyan V, Cortes J, et al. Phase II study of low-dose decitabine in patients with chronic myelogenous leukemia resistant to imatinib mesylate. J Clin Oncol 2005;23:3948–56.

79. Marin D, Kaeda JS, Andreasson C, et al. Phase I/II trial of adding semisynthetic homoharringtonine in chronic myeloid leukemia patients who have achieved partial or complete cytogenetic response on imatinib. Cancer 2005;103:1850–5.

80. Pinilla-Ibarz J, Cathcart K, Scheinberg DA. CML vaccines as a paradigm of the specific immunotherapy of cancer. Blood Rev 2000;14:111–20.

81. Quintas-Cardama A, Cortes J. Chronic myeloid leukemia: diagnosis and treatment. Mayo Clin Proc 2006;81:973–88.

82. Cathcart K, Pinilla-Ibarz J, Korontsvit T, et al. A multivalent bcr-abl fusion peptide vaccination trial in patients with chronic myeloid leukemia. Blood 2004;103:1037–42.

83. Bocchia M, Gentili S, Abruzzese E, et al. Effect of a p210 multipeptide vaccine associated with imatinib or interferon in patients with chronic myeloid leukaemia and persistent residual disease: a multicenter observational trial. Lancet 2005;365:657–62.

6 Targeted Therapy in Colorectal Cancer

Scott Kopetz, MD

CONTENTS

ABSTRACT

Despite U.S. Food and Drug Administration approval of three targeted therapeutics for colorectal cancer during the past several years, work remains in order to provide further meaningful advances. The tumor biology of colorectal cancer is well studied, with several distinct pathways leading to tumorigenesis: the chromosomal instability pathway, the mutator pathway, and the serrated adenoma pathway. EGFR and VEGF cytokines play a prominent role in colorectal cancer development and maintenance. Monoclonal antibodies targeting these pathways have provided benefit in the clinic. Despite active research, tyrosine kinase inhibitors have not yet found a place in the treatment of colorectal cancer. Further research is needed to bridge the gap between our growing knowledge of tumor biology and the development of agents that can provide clinical benefit. Combinations of therapeutic modalities, which include targeted therapy, may prove beneficial.

Key Words: Colorectal cancer, Targeted therapeutics, EGFR, VEGF, Monoclonal antibodies

1. INTRODUCTION

After years of treating patients with colon cancer therapies that had limited efficacy, recent advances have improved patient outcomes in both adjuvant and metastatic settings. Because of the increased use of endoscopic screening and polypectomy, mortality rates for colorectal cancer have fallen during the past two decades *(1)*. Six new agents have joined 5-fluorouracil (5-FU) as U.S. Food and Drug Administration (FDA)-approved therapies for metastatic colorectal cancer (Table 1) As a result, overall survival (OS) for metastatic colorectal has been extended from approximately 12 months with the use of 5-FU alone to more than 24 months with the use of modern chemotherapy regimens. Despite this incremental progress, much discovery is needed to increase survival.

From: *Current Clinical Oncology: Targeted Cancer Therapy*
Edited by: R. Kurzrock and M. Markman © Humana Press, Totowa, NJ

Table 1
Currently Approved Agents for Colorectal Cancer

Agent	Mechanism	Approval
5-Fluorouracil	Pyrimidine analogue	Adjuvant, metastatic
Irinotecan	Topoisomerase I inhibitor	Metastatic
Oxaliplatin	Alkylating agent	Adjuvant, metastatic
Capecitabine	Pyrimidine analogue	Adjuvant, metastatic
Bevacizumab	VEGF monoclonal antibody	Metastatic
Cetuximab	EGFR monoclonal antibody	Metastatic
Panitumumab	EGFR monoclonal antibody	Metastatic

1.1. Overview of Treatment

Most colorectal cancer patients present with localized disease (stage I and II) or regional lymph node involvement (stage III) (Table 2). Despite the high number of patients initially diagnosed with localized or regional disease, approximately 50% of patients with colorectal cancer present with or later develop metastatic disease. There are an estimated 75,000 patients in the United States being treated yearly for metastatic colorectal cancer. The lifetime risk of colorectal cancer has been estimated at 6%, although the rates are higher for patients with familial colorectal cancer syndromes or inflammatory bowel disease. The latter have a cumulative risk of colorectal cancer of 18% at 30 years (2).

Adjuvant therapy is routinely offered to patients diagnosed with stage III disease in an attempt to reduce their high rate of relapse. For almost 20 years, adjuvant chemotherapy with 5-FU has reduced the rate of relapse and improved OS (3). Recently, the combination of 5-FU, capecitabine, and oxaliplatin has improved the relapse rate, reducing the relative risk of recurrence by more than 50%, as reported in recent studies (4,5). Adjuvant chemotherapy for stage II colorectal cancer (limited to the colon or rectum without lymph node involvement) is controversial and may offer only limited benefit (6,7). Several high-risk features in stage II patients, such as lymphovascular involvement, poorly differentiated tumor, perforation, obstruction, and a small number of surgically recovered lymph nodes, are hallmarks of a subset of patients at high risk. Current guidelines do not advocate routine adjuvant therapy for patients with stage II disease (8).

Metastatic disease is commonly managed by combining various chemotherapy agents with 5-FU. Two common regimens combine 5-FU (given in a 2-day infusion) with oxaliplatin or irinotecan. These regimens, FOLFOX and FOLFIRI, respectively, are frequently also combined with a monoclonal antibody. Several studies showed that the selection of either

Table 2
Stage of Presentation and Survival of Colorectal Cancer

Stage at presentation[a]	Percent of patients	5-Year overall survival (%)
I or II (localized)	38	~90
III (regional)	38	~35
IV (metastatic)	19	~<10

[a]5% of patients were unstaged (144).

FOLFOX or FOLFIRI as the first regimen does not have an impact on treatment outcome *(9,10)*. Instead, it appears that the number of cytotoxic agents able to be administered to patients over the course of their therapy is the critical factor in determining OS. In two analyses, the proportion of patients treated with all three active cytoxic agents—5-FU (or capecitabine), oxaliplatin, irinotecan—was correlated with an improved OS rate *(11,12)*. As a result, current management focuses on administering regimens of one or two cytotoxic agents sequentially.

Other researchers recently questioned the previously established practice of continuous chemotherapy treatment for patients with metastatic disease. Several studies demonstrated that periods of less intense chemotherapy regimens followed by a return to traditional combination regimens does not significantly affect OS *(13,14)*. This research was initially prompted by the cumulative dose-limiting neurotoxicity of oxaliplatin but has been extended to irinotecan-containing regimens. Several recent studies have explored the impact of chemotherapy-free intervals, although this approach has not been widely adopted due to an apparently detrimental impact on OS *(15,16)*.

1.2. Familial Predispositions

It is estimated that 15% of colorectal cancer patients have an inherited disposition *(17)*. Of this group, two syndromes have been well described: hereditary nonpolyposis colorectal cancer (HNPCC) and familial adenomatous polyposis (FAP).

HNPCC is the most common form of familial colorectal cancer, accounting for 2% to 3% of all colorectal cancers *(18,19)*. It is characterized by an autosomal dominant pedigree and a deficiency in mismatch repair through germline mutation of one of the mismatch repair genes: *MSH2*, *MLH1*, and less commonly *MSH6*. Microsatellite instability is a common feature of HNPCC due to a deficient DNA repair mechanism, resulting in frameshift mutations in areas of basepair repeats, called microsatellites. Extracolonic tumors are common, including endometrial, ovarian, upper tract urothelial, small bowel, gastric, and hepatobiliary cancers. The lifetime risk for colorectal cancer approaches 80%, with a median onset at 44 years *(20)*. In contrast to sporadic colon cancer, most tumors occur in the transverse or right colon. Yearly colonoscopy is recommended beginning at the age of 20 to 25 for those with a family history of HNPCC *(21)*. Chemoprevention trials are exploring therapeutic options for this high-risk group, including cyclooxygenase-2 (COX-2) inhibitors.

Familial adenomatous polyposis is the second most common form of hereditary colorectal cancer, accounting for approximately 1% of patients *(22)*. FAP is caused by germline mutations in the adenomatous polyposis coli (*APC*) gene and is characterized by early onset of more than 100 polyps in the colon and rectum. In this setting, the rate of colorectal cancer approaches 100% by age 35. Risk-reducing surgery is recommended, including prophylactic total colectomy *(23)*. The extent of surgery requires discussions about the trade-off between preserving rectal function and the risk of recurrence in the remnant rectum. These patients are also at risk for developing extracolonic disease, including duodenal carcinomas, benign desmoid tumors, osteomas, and congenital hypertrophy of the retinal pigment epithelium. Attenuated forms of FAP exist that may be associated with alternate sites of mutation on the *APC* gene and a lower lifetime risk of colorectal cancer. The site of mutation on the *APC* gene appears to predict the subset of patients at higher risk for extracolonic manifestations *(24)*. An attenuated form of FAP exists, manifested by a lower number of polyps and increased prevalence of proximal colon tumors. Nevertheless, without prophylactic colectomy, FAP patients remain at high risk of colorectal cancer, with 80% developing carcinoma by age

70 *(25)*. Nonsteroidal antiinflammatory drugs (NSAIDs) have been shown to reduce adenoma development in the colon and duodenum *(26,27)*.

A third polyposis syndrome has recently been described. Patients in this group, representing 30% of the familial polyposis patients without APC mutations, carry a biallelic *MYH* gene mutation *(28)*. The inheritance pattern is autosomal recessive, with lifetime risks of colorectal cancer similar to individuals with attenuated FAP. Hamartomatous polyposis syndromes, including Peutz-Jeghers (autosomal dominant) and juvenile polyposis (autosomal dominant), confer a higher risk for colorectal and other gastrointestinal cancers *(29)*. A potential autosomal dominant familial syndrome has been isolated from a region on the long arm of chromosome 9 and is putatively related to the loss of a growth-suppressing micro-RNA or to another as yet unidentified gene *(30,31)*. Initial studies suggest that this mechanism may be relevant in 36% of familial kindreds that have not yet been classified. Further isolation of this region is ongoing.

2. MOLECULAR MECHANISMS

Colorectal cancer provides an ideal setting for developing targeted therapy. Some of the earliest work on understanding the biology of cancer was performed in colorectal cancer. Despite this large body of work, many of the complexities of colorectal cancer have yet to be elucidated. Emerging data on the profound heterogeneity of colorectal cancer clarify these difficulties.

Several distinct molecular mechanisms have been used to classify colorectal cancers. These classifiers include the presence or absence of particular mutations, cell surface receptors, genomic instability in microsatellites or at the chromosomal level, and extent of genomic methylation. These classifications have not yet been incorporated into clinical practice but are currently under investigation in a number of Phase III trials in adjuvant and metastatic settings.

2.1. Tumorigenesis Pathways

Mutations in three types of gene confer a tumorigeneic potential: oncogenes, tumor suppressor genes, and stability genes *(32)*. A direct growth advantage results from the mutation of oncogenes and tumor suppressor genes. Whereas oncogenes result from the activation of proto-oncogenes, tumor suppressor genes cause cancer when they are inactivated. Furthermore, whereas most oncogenes develop from mutations in normal genes (proto-oncogenes) during an individual's life (acquired mutations), tumor suppressor gene abnormalities can be inherited as well as acquired. The most common mutations in colorectal cancer include *APC*, *KRAS*, and *p53*. Fearon and Vogelstein described the classic multistep model of colorectal cancer development associated with the orderly occurrence of *APC*, *KRAS*, and *TP53* mutations *(17,33)*. Subsequent work has shown that these three classically described mutations are all present in only a small proportion of colon cancers (7%–11%) and, at least for *p53* and *KRAS*, likely represent separate pathways to tumorigenesis*(34,35)* (Fig. 1) This pathway to tumorigenesis is known as the chromosomal instability (CIN) pathway and best describes most sporadic colorectal cancers (Fig. 2) Mutations in CIN genes are manifested by the loss or gain of whole chromosomes or large portions of a chromosome during replication, resulting in more frequent loss of heterozygosity and aneuploidy.

In contrast, mutations in stability genes increase the potential for subsequent cellular mutations. This route to tumorigenesis has been termed the *mutator pathway* and is the

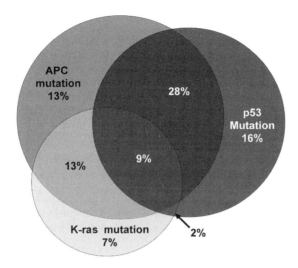

Fig. 1. Venn diagram of *APC*, *p53*, and K-*ras* mutations in colorectal cancer.

best model to describe approximately 15% of sporadic colorectal cancers and most HNPCC tumors *(36)*. Tumors derived from this pathway have high rates of microsatellite instability (MSI). This pathway is characterized by mutations or epigenetic silencing of mismatch repair genes. Several genes are particularly susceptible to MSI-induced mutations, including insulin-like growth factor receptor type 2 (*IGF-IIR*), transforming growth factor β receptor type 2 (*TGF-βIIR*), and the apoptosis-regulating gene *BAX (37)*. TGF-βIIR signals through SMAD proteins, leading to growth inhibition, apoptosis, and differentiation—functions that

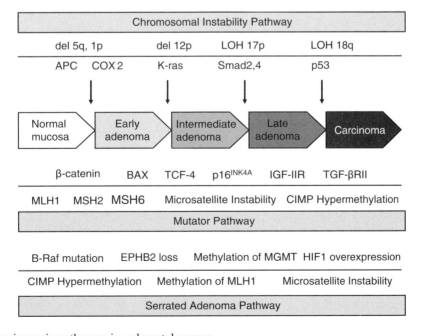

Fig. 2. Tumorigenesis pathways in colorectal cancer.

are lost with *TGF-βIIR* mutations *(38)*. In contrast, SMAD proteins are frequently mutated or lost by chromosomal instability in the CIN pathway, with a similar result *(39)*.

KRAS is a commonly mutated proto-oncogene in the CIN pathway. Mutation in the *K-Ras* coding gene *KRAS* results in constitutively activated signaling through the RAS/RAF/MAPK pathway, resulting in increased growth stimulation. *RAS* mutation is seen in late adenomas and carcinomas but is rarely present in adenomas < 1 cm in size *(40)*. Despite extensive study, there is no correlation between *RAS* mutations and sex, tumor site, or Duke's stage, but mutations may be slightly less common in poorly differentiated tumors *(41)*. In a collaborative database of more than 3000 patients, a particular mutation in codon 12 of *KRAS* was associated with a modestly worse time to relapse and OS, but in a separate study it was associated with a better response to chemoradiation *(42,43)*.

Although less common than mutations in *RAS*, *BRAF* is also mutated in colorectal cancer. In most of the patients with a *BRAF* mutation, hMLH1 is inactivated through methylation. As a result, *BRAF* mutations were more prevalent in tumors with high levels of MSI (18% vs. 1%),*(44)* but these mutations do not appear to be due solely to defects in mismatch repair *(45)*. This results in a third possible pathway to tumorigenesis, called the *serrated pathway*, described by epigenetic silencing of genes involved in DNA repair and cell cycle control. Histologically, these lesions develop from serrated and hyperplastic polyps *(46)*. CpG island methylation develops earlier in this pathway, with the MSI phenotype seen at a later time *(47,48)*.

APC is a tumor-suppressor gene that regulates β-catenin, which is critical to the regulation of apoptosis, cell cycle progression, and cell adhesion. The *APC* gene is located on the long arm of chromosome 5, and its function is frequently lost by chromosomal deletion or point mutation. Most of the mutations in *APC* are in the β-catenin-binding region. More than 300 mutations have been identified; and as a result, developing diagnostic tests has been technically difficult using standard techniques *(49)*. Some colorectal cancers with wild-type *APC* have β-catenin mutations rather than *APC* mutations, suggesting that inactivation of the *APC* tumor-suppressor pathway is a critical factor in most colorectal cancers.

P53 is a tumor suppressor whose gene, *TP53*, is located on the short arm of chromosome 17. A regulator of apoptosis and cell cycle progression, p53 is a target for inactivating point mutations and chromosomal loss of heterozygosity. Mutations in *TP53* result in compensatory overexpression of the gene product, which is readily detectable through immunohistochemistry *(50)*. *TP53* mutation rates are higher in the distal colon and rectal tumors and are associated with a worse prognosis after adjuvant therapy *(51)*. However, other research has provided mixed results, and the clinical significance of p53 mutation remains unclear *(52)*.

Src is another relevant tyrosine kinase in colorectal cancer. This nonreceptor tyrosine kinase is responsible for cytoskeletal arrangement, migration, and invasion. Src also recruits various signaling complexes and interacts with numerous receptors *(53,54)*. Src expression has been correlated with advanced clinical stage and a worse prognosis *(55)*.

The PI3K pathway is up-regulated in many colorectal cancers *(56)*. *PTEN*, a negative regulator of PI3K activity, is rarely mutated in colorectal cancer, in contrast to many other tumor types. Instead, activation of the pathway is through upstream signaling or through mutation of a gene encoding a subunit of PI3K *(57)*. Because the mammalian target of rapamycin, mTOR, is a downstream component of the PI3K pathway, it has been targeted for therapeutic intervention.

The recent quantification of mutations in the tyrosine kinome of colorectal cancer has resulted in a broader understanding of the complexity and extent of kinase mutations *(58)*.

This work demonstrated 69 mutated genes in a sample of 11 colorectal cell lines, with an average of 9 mutated genes per cell line. This variety of mutational combinations emphasizes the heterogeneity of colorectal cancer. Other genes that are mutated at high frequencies include metalloproteinase (MMP) genes and the EPH family of receptor tyrosine kinases.

2.2. Cytokine Mechanisms

Several cytokine receptors have been implicated in the development and maintenance of colorectal adenocarcinoma, including epidermal growth factor receptor (EGFR, also call ErbB-1 or HER1), vascular endothelial growth factor (VEGF), and insulin-like growth factor receptor (IGF-1R). These receptors have been targeted by several therapeutic agents that are either approved or are in the late stage of development.

2.2.1. EGFR

Present in normal colonic epithelium, the EGFR pathway is overexpressed in most colorectal cancer patients*(59,60)* and is associated with shorter survival and fewer responses to cytotoxic chemotherapy *(61,62)*. EGFR ligands include epidermal growth factor, transforming growth factor-α, amphiregulin, and epiregulin, among others. The receptor–ligand complex becomes activated through homodimerization or heterodimerization with other members of the HER family of receptors and subsequent autophosphorylation. Downstream signaling is through RAS/RAF/MAPK, PI3K/AKT, and Src, among others. The characteristic of the signaling generated by EGFR is dependent on both the particular ligand and the ErbB heterodimerization partner. EGFR signaling is relevant to colorectal carcinoma development and subsequent growth *(63)*.

Monoclonal antibodies inhibit EGFR by blocking ligand binding and increasing EGFR turnover through internalization and degradation *(64,67)*. Proliferation is reduced with the diminished activation of the RAS/RAF/MAPK pathway. The expression of angiogenic cytokines, such as VEGF and interleukin-8 (IL-8), and MMPs is reduced after treatment with an EGFR monoclonal antibody. The result is inhibited metastases and reduced microvessel density in *in vivo* models *(68,69)*. In addition, there are data suggesting that the induction of apoptosis may be augmented when a cytotoxic agent is combined with a monoclonal antibody, inhibiting the expression of EGFR *(70,72)*.

Although EGFR overexpression was initially believed to be a reasonable marker for EGFR pathway dependence, ligand expression and absence of an oncogenic KRAS mutation are seemingly more tightly coupled with a response to EGFR-targeting monoclonal antibodies *(73)*. Unlike non-small-cell lung cancer, EGFR activating mutations are rarely present in colorectal cancer, and their clinical significance is not known *(74,75)*. Other mechanisms under study include the impact of dimerization partners and receptor transactivation by alternate mechanisms.

2.2.2. VEGF

VEGF/VEGFR is a clearly established clinically relevant pathway in metastatic colorectal cancer. VEGF was simultaneously identified almost two decades ago as a potent stimulator of endothelial cell proliferation and vascular leakage *(76,77)*. Subsequent research identified several forms of VEGF ligand and receptors with different functions and expression patterns (Table 3) VEGF is overexpressed in colorectal cancer and is inversely correlated with prognosis *(78,80)*. Activation of the VEGF pathway leads to increased vascular proliferation, endothelial cell survival, and direct stimulation of tumor cell VEGFR *(81)*. It was

Table 3
Vascular Endothelial Growth Factor Ligands and Receptors

Parameter	Description
Ligand *(145)*	
VEGF-A	Ligand for VEGFR1 or VEGFR2
VEGF-B	Ligand for VEGFR1
VEGF-C	Ligand for VEGFR2 or VEGFR3
VEGF-D	Ligand for VEGFR2 or VEGFR3
VEGF-E	Ligand for VEGFR2
Receptor	
VEGFR1 (Flt-1)	Involved in endothelial cell migration and differentiation; also present on colon cancer cells and affects invasive phenotype *(146)*
VEGFR2 (Flk-1, KDR)	Predominant receptor for angiogenic and mitogenic stimuli in endothelial cells *(147)*
VEGFR3 (Flt-4)	Regulates lymphangiogenesis and lymphatic metastases *(148,149)*

historically thought that VEGF was expressed in the endothelial compartment, but recent data suggest that colon cancer cells express VEGFR-1, a mediator of cell migration and invasion *in vitro (82)*. It has also been postulated that VEGF blockade might improve pericyte coverage, thereby normalizing the vasculature and improving intratumoral delivery of chemotherapy *(83)*.

VEGF is expressed in most colorectal cancers and has been correlated with tumor stage and microvessel density *(79,84)*. Mutations in *TP53* and *KRAS* may be associated with higher VEGF expression *(84,85)*. Preclinical studies of VEGF inhibition with a murine monoclonal antibody to the VEGF ligand reduced the volume of the primary tumor and resulted in fewer liver metastases in a metastatic colon cancer model *(86)*.

2.2.3. IGFR

The insulin-like growth factor (IGF) pathway has been shown to play a role in the development and maintenance of colon cancer. A murine colon cancer model with a conditional IGF-1 knockout had diminished primary and hepatic tumor growth *(87)*. Plasma levels of IGF-1 have also been correlated with colorectal cancer risk *(88)*. Activation of the IGF-1 receptor (IGF-IR) results in growth and motility of colon cancer cells in in vitro and murine models. In contrast, the IGF-II receptor, which is commonly mutated in colorectal cancer, does not have an active kinase domain and appears to serve as a "sink" for IGF binding. The result may be an increased amount of IGF available to bind and activate IGF-IR. Downstream signaling includes the RAS/RAF/MAPK and PI3K/AKT pathways. In other tumor types, IGF-1R-targeted therapies have been ineffective in cells lines with constitutively activated AKT *(89)*.

3. MOLECULAR TARGETED THERAPIES

Molecular therapies targeting the VEGF and EGFR pathways have been approved for colorectal cancer over the last few years. Additional targeted therapies in advanced clinical trials in colorectal cancer include monoclonal antibodies to IGFR and tyrosine kinase inhibitors to mTOR (everolimus), enzastaurin, EGFR, VEGFR, and Src. COX-2 inhibitors have also been studied in colorectal cancer, with success limited to prevention studies.

3.1. VEGF

Bevacizumab is a humanized monoclonal antibody to VEGF. By binding circulating VEGF, VEGFR activation is significantly inhibited. Approval for this agent was based on the pivotal Phase III study of Hurwitz et al. Patients ($n = 813$) were randomized to one of three arms:(1) irinotecan/bolus 5-FU/leucovorin (IFL);(2) IFL/bevacizumab;(3) 5-FU/leucovorin (LV)/bevacizumab. After the safety of the bevacizumab- and irinotecan-containing arm was established, the 5-FU/LV/bevacizumab arm was discontinued. Results demonstrated clinically significant improvements in the radiographic response rate and progression-free survival (PFS) in the IFL/bevacizumab arm compared to the IFL alone arm. OS was also improved with the incorporation of bevacizumab (20.3 vs. 15.6 months) *(83)*. This initial significant benefit was not as obvious in a more recent trial of FOLFOX or XELOX (capecitabine combined with oxaliplatin) with or without bevacizumab *(90)*. Although the trial met its primary endpoint of improving PFS with the addition of bevacizumab, the incremental improvement with bevacizumab was less than expected, and there was no improvement in response rates (Fig. 3).

Bevacizumab also produced benefit in previously treated patients. In a trial of FOLFOX for patients refractory to irinotecan, adding bevacizumab improved response rates and OS. Two randomized trials ongoing at the time of bevacizumab approval were amended

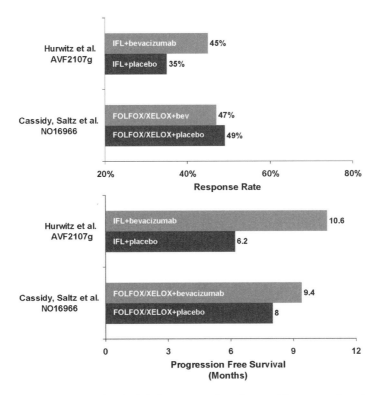

Fig. 3. Comparison of two randomized trials in untreated patients with metastatic colorectal cancer that evaluated bevacizumab benefit.

to include bevacizumab in both arms. These trials indirectly demonstrated the benefit of bevacizumab in previously untreated patients regardless of the chemotherapy combination utilized *(91,92)*.

Smaller studies demonstrated the benefit of bevacizumab when added to 5-FU-based chemoradiation for the neoadjuvant treatment of rectal cancer. Bevacizumab can decrease microvessel density and intratumoral pressure, and it subsequently improves pathologic complete response rates at the time of surgery *(93,94)*. The incorporation of this agent into the neoadjuvant treatment of rectal cancer is being explored in an ongoing Phase III study.

Side effects associated with bevacizumab include increased hypertension and epistaxis, and the less common but more severe toxicities of bowel perforation and arterial thromboembolic events. Subsequent studies confirmed that these rare toxicities are increased with bevacizumab utilization *(95,97)*. Elderly patients with preexisting arteriovascular disease are at the highest risk of developing a stroke or heart attack due to treatment with bevacizumab. Risk factors for bowel perforation include obstruction, acute diverticulitis, peritoneal carcinomatosis, and prior pelvic irradiation *(98)*. Having the primary tumor in place at the time of therapy has been reported to be a slight risk factor for perforation with bevacizumab in some studies *(98)* but not in others *(99,100)*. Epistaxis is a common occurrence and is associated with nasal septal ulceration that rarely leads to septal perforation *(101)*.

Several tyrosine kinase inhibitors of VEGFR have been developed, including vatalinib, sorafenib, semaxanib, sunitinib, and AZD2171 *(102)*. Vatalinib inhibits all VEGFR tyrosine kinases, and preclinical studies suggested a robust antiangiogenic response *(103)*. Vatalinib was tested in two large randomized Phase III trials in untreated and previously treated patients. Imaging correlates demonstrated a significant reduction in intratumoral blood flow, although the primary endpoints were not reached in either study *(104,105)*. Subgroup analysis pointed to a benefit for patients with elevated lactate dehydrogenase (LDH). Preclinical data suggest that LDH may be elevated in patients with increased tumor hypoxia, providing a scientific rationale for this subgroup benefit *(106)*. Additional studies are planned using a patient population enriched for elevated LDH.

In a randomized Phase III trial, semaxanib was studied in combination with 5-FU/LV in 737 patients; results showed no improvement in OS. Toxicity that included diarrhea, dehydration, vomiting, and sepsis was increased in the semaxanib-containing arm *(107)*. Sorafenib inhibits both VEGFRs and RAF kinase and is approved for treating advanced renal cell carcinoma. Phase II trials in combination with cetuximab and irinotecan are ongoing. Sunitinib, which inhibits VEGFRs and PDGFRβ, has also recently been approved for treating renal cell carcinoma. Preclinical data confirmed the expected antiangiogenic activity of the agent in colorectal cancer models *(108)*. A single-agent, Phase II study of sunitinib in previously treated patients failed to show significant clinical activity, although most of the patients had been previously treated with bevacizumab *(109)*. A Phase III, frontline study of FOLFIRI with or without sunitinib is ongoing.

AZD2171 is a pan-VEGFR tyrosine kinase inhibitor with additional selectivity for PDGFRβ that is administered as a once-daily oral dosing regimen. After early clinical responses were seen in the Phase I study,*(110)* the compound progressed through development and is currently undergoing evaluation in two Phase III trials in previously untreated patients with colorectal cancer.

3.2. EGFR

Cetuximab is a chimeric monoclonal antibody that binds to the extracellular domain of EGFR, resulting in inhibition of EGFR ligand binding, dimerization, and subsequent activation. Cetuximab was the first monoclonal antibody specifically targeting EGFR to be FDA approved for metastatic colorectal cancer. This approval was granted primarily on the basis of results of a trial in 329 patients with colorectal cancer refractory to irinotecan who were randomized to cetuximab or cetuximab and irinotecan *(59)*. Enrollment was limited to patients with EGFR expression as determined by immunohistochemistry. The result was a higher response rate (23% vs. 11%) and longer time to disease progression (4.1 vs. 1.5 months) with combination therapy. OS was not different between the groups, although this determination was potentially confounded by crossover.

The survival benefit of cetuximab was subsequently demonstrated in a randomized, international Phase III trial of cetuximab monotherapy versus best supportive care in 572 patients with refractory metastatic colorectal cancer. OS was increased from 4.6 months to 6.1 months. Acneiform rash, a common side effect of EGFR-targeted therapy, during or shortly after infusion of the monoclonal antibody *(111)*.

Several studies are ongoing to evaluate the role of cetuximab in untreated patients with metastatic disease, including a large intergroup trial in the United States comparing cetuximab, bevacizumab, or the combination of biologic agents with FOLFOX or FOLFIRI. A study of cetuximab in patients treated with one prior regimen failed to demonstrate improved OS. This study compared cetuximab plus irinotecan versus irinotecan alone in 1298 patients. The primary endpoint of OS was no different between the groups, although the irinotecan-alone arm was confounded by cetuximab after progression in almost 50% of the patients. PFS was higher with the combination regimen (4.0 vs. 2.6 months) *(112)*.

Small Phase II trials have been reported combining cetuximab with FOLFOX or FOLFIRI in untreated patients with high response rates. A Phase II trial of FOLFOX with cetuximab in untreated patients with metastatic disease had a response rate of 77% and a median PFS rate of 12.3 months *(113)*. This result is being pursued in a larger trial of previously untreated patients. A large Phase III trial of FOLFIRI with or without cetuximab has completed accrual, and preliminary results demonstrate improved PFS *(114)*.

Toxicities seen with cetuximab include acneiform rash, hypomagnesemia, and potentiation of irinotecan-induced diarrhea. Hypersensitivity reactions are seen in about 2% to 5% of patients, although there appears to be significant geographic variation in this rate for unclear reasons. The degree of rash has been strongly correlated with disease response rates and OS in a number of studies (Fig. 4) This reaction may reflect the underlying tumor biology or individual variations in the pharmacodynamics of the agent. In support of the later hypothesis, Van Cutsem et al. demonstrated an improved response rate in patients without a cetuximab-induced aceniform rash who were randomized to receive higher doses of cetuximab *(115)*.

Recent clinical data have suggested that *KRAS* mutations may select for a group of patients who do not respond to cetuximab *(73,116)*. The largest study reported to date evaluated 89 patients treated with cetuximab in combination with irinotecan or FOLFIRI. A *KRAS* mutation was present in 27% of the patients evaluated and resulted in a lower PFS and OS than in patients without the mutation (PFS of 10 weeks vs. 31 weeks; OS of 10 months vs. 14 months, respectively) (Table 4) The EGFR ligands amphiregulin and epiregulin may also predict response to therapy. Patients with low levels of epiregulin mRNA had a PFS of 57 days versus 104 days in patients with high levels; a similar correlation was seen with amphiregulin *(73)*.

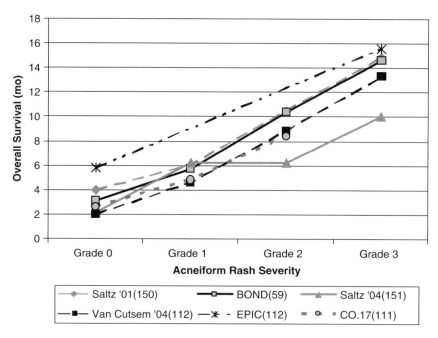

Fig. 4. Relation between cetuximab rash and overall survival.

Panitumumab, a second monoclonal antibody to EGFR, was approved by the FDA in 2006 for patients with refractory metastatic colorectal cancer. It is a fully human immunoglobulin G2 (IgG2) antibody that has the potential advantage of every-2-weeks dosing and fewer infusion reactions. FDA approval was based on improved PFS in a randomized study of panitumumab versus best supportive care in 463 colorectal cancer patients with metastatic refractory disease *(118)*. Because panitumumab and cetuximab have the same mechanism of action, several reports described substituting panitumumab for cetuximab in combination regimens. Pantimumab in combination with FOLFIRI was relatively safe but resulted in high rates of grade 3 and 4 diarrhea when combined with a regimen combining bolus 5-FU

Table 4
Summary of EGFR Response and KRAS Mutation Status

Setting	No. of patients	Definition of response	Response in KRAS mutation	Response in wild-type KRAS	References
Cetuximab with FOLFIRI or irinotecan	30	PR + SD	0% (0/13)	64% (11/17)	(116)
Cetuximab monotherapy	80	PR + SD	11% (3/29)	47% (24/51)	(73)
Cetuximab with FOLFIRI or irinotecan	89	PR	0% (0/24)	38% (25/40)	(117)

PR, partial response; SD, stable disease

and irinotecan *(119)*. Similarly, a randomized study of FOLFOX and bevacizumab with or without panitumamab was discontinued owing to high rates of diarrhea, dehydration, and infection in the panitumumab arm. A study of 900 patients comparing FOLFOX with or without panitumumab remains open for accrual. These findings demonstrate that further evaluation of panitumumab is required prior to its rapid incorporation into existing regimens.

The importance of the variations in the *EGFR* epitope is confirmed in preclinical studies of matuzumab, an investigational monoclonal EGFR antibody. Unlike cetuximab, matuzumab was not synergistic with irradiation or platinum-based chemotherapy in vitro. Cetuximab produced equal inhibition of EGFR phosphorylation but resulted in more profound inhibition of MAPK than matuzumab in one study, suggesting that EGFR antibodies are not necessarily interchangeable *(120)*.

Although its relevance has not clearly been demonstrated for colorectal cancer, antibody-dependent cell cytotoxicty (ADCC) has been hypothesized to play a role in the clinical efficacy of some monoclonal antibodies. Differences in the IgG subclasses of the two approved EGFR monoclonal antibodies may result in diverse clinical activity.

Tyrosine kinase inhibitors of EGFR, such as erlotinib and gefitinib, have been studied in metastatic colorectal cancer without success. As single agents, neither treatment demonstrated clinical benefit *(121–123)*. When EGFR tyrosine kinase inhibitors are combined with traditional cytotoxic chemotherapy regimens, clinical activity is evident but with unacceptable toxicity, primarily diarrhea and neutropenia *(124–127)*. After dose modification, a randomized Phase III study of FOLFOX (capecitabine substitution allowed) and bevacizumab, with or without erlotinib, was initiated and is still ongoing. EKB-569, an EGFR-specific, irreversible tyrosine kinase inhibitor combined with FOLFIRI in a Phase II trial did not show a clear benefit over historical results with FOLFIRI alone *(128)*.

3.3. Combination of VEGF and EGFR

Extensive preclinical work demonstrated that the VEGF and EGFR pathways are interrelated. EGFR activation results in VEGF up-regulation, and EGFR inhibition partially reduces VEGF levels *(129)*. Because complete blockade of VEGF is required for maximal tumor inhibition, the clinical impact of EGFR-mediated VEGF inhibition is unclear. VEGF has also been implicated in EGFR inhibitor resistance *(130,131)*. As a result of these interactions, it has been hypothesized that VEGF and EGFR inhibition may provide synergistic antitumor effects.

Cetuximab and bevacizumab were combined in a Phase II trial with a second arm also containing irinotecan. These results demonstrated an improved response rate and PFS from cetuximab and bevacizumab compared to historical results of cetuximab alone, although the different patient populations limit a cross-trial comparision (Table 5). A follow-up study is evaluating the benefit of cetuximab and bevacizumab therapy in patients who have previously progressed on bevacizumab-containing regimens. A large cooperative group trial in the United States is currently evaluating the benefit of cetuximab and bevacizumab in combination with cytotoxic chemotherapy in previously untreated patients with metastatic disease. All patients are treated with either FOLFOX or FOLFIRI and one of three arms: (1) bevacizumab; (2) cetuximab; (3) or bevacizumab/cetuximab.

Another approach under development targets both VEGFR and EGFR using tyrosine kinases with dual specificity. AEE788 is one such small-molecule inhibitor of both VEGFR and EGFR. In preclinical studies, AEE788 reduced colon cancer metastases in a murine

Table 5
Comparison of Response Rates for the BOND Trials

Trial and regimen	No. of patients in arm	Response rate (%)	Duration of disease control (months)
BOND (59)			
Cetuximab	111	11	1.5[a]
Cetuximab + irinotecan	218	23	4.1[a]
BOND-2 (152)			
Cetuximab + bevacizumab	40	20	5.6[b]
Cetuximab + bevacizumab + irinotecan	41	37	7.9[b]

[a]Median progression-free survival
[b]Median time to tumor progression

model (132). Phase I studies have been reported, with plans for further development in regard to colorectal cancer. Vandetanib is another tyrosine kinase inhibitor with activity against VEGFR, EGFR, and RET. In a colon cancer xenograft model with resistance to EGFR inhibitors, vandetanib as a single agent inhibited tumor growth (133). Whether the theoretical and preclinical benefit of dual inhibition extends to the clinical setting is yet to be established.

3.4. Other Agents in Late Development

To date, agents have been developed to target cytokine-driven pathways, and work is ongoing to target oncogenes and relevant intracellular kinases directly. Agents now in development for metastatic colorectal cancer target mTOR, protein kinase C (PKC), Src, and COX-2 (Table 6).

Rapamycin analogues such as everolimus (RAD-001) are undergoing clinical evaluation in patients with colorectal cancer. Because of the established dependence on the PI3K/AKT pathway in colorectal tumors with PI3CA mutations, a current Phase II trial of everolimus

Table 6
Agents in Late Development for Colorectal Cancer

Agent	Adjuvant	Untreated metastatic	Refractory metastatic
Bevacizumab	Phase III	Demonstrated (83)	Demonstrated (95)
Cetuximab	Phase III	Demonstrated (114)	Demonstrated (59)
Panitumumab		Phase III	Demonstrated (118)
Sunitinib		Phase III	
Semaxanib		Failed (107)	
Erlotinib		Phase III	Failed (121,124)
Gefitinib			Failed (122,123)
Valatinib		Failed (104,105)	
AZD2171		Phase III	
Enzastaurin		Phase III	
Everolimus		Phase III	
Celecoxib		Failed (92)	Phase III

is limited to patients with this mutation. This trial is the first in colorectal cancer to enrich the patient population for a mutation of interest while investigating a novel targeted agent.

Enzastaurin is a serine/threonine kinase inhibitor that inhibits PKC, resulting in a reduction in VEGF tumor secretion and suppression of colorectal cancer xenograft growth *(134)*. A Phase III study is underway that utilizes a novel trial design that combines enzastaurin with 5-FU and bevacizumab only after oxaliplatin is discontinued from the FOLFOX regimen. It is hoped that this "window" trial design will uncover the suspected disease-stabilizing characteristics of the agent.

Several Src inhibitors are undergoing testing in colorectal cancer. Preclinical work suggests that Src may interact with the EGFR pathway and synergize with oxaliplatin *(135,136)*. AZD0530, an oral Src kinase inhibitor, is being evaluated as a single agent in previously treated patients with metastatic colorectal cancer. Dasatinib, another oral Src kinase inhibitor approved for chronic myelogenous leukemia, is also being tested as a single agent as well as in combination with FOLFOX and cetuximab. Several other Src inhibitors are at earlier stages of development.

COX-2 has been implicated in the pathogenesis of colorectal cancer, and its use is correlated with colon cancer prognosis. Inhibition of COX-2 with celecoxib has been shown to reduce the number of recurrent polyps in large prevention trials *(137)*. The impact of COX-2 inhibition on metastatic disease was explored in a randomization of previously untreated patients with metastatic disease to either celecoxib or placebo. This trial, which enrolled 547 patients, did not find any impact of celecoxib on treatment efficacy or toxicity *(92)*. An ongoing separate Phase III trial is exploring the benefit of COX-2 inhibition in preventing capecitabine-induced hand-foot syndrome.

Several monoclonal antibodies to IGFR have been developed with both single-agent and combination studies in colorectal cancer currently ongoing. Murine studies have suggested benefit for IGFR monoclonal antibodies in combination with 5-FU and cetuximab *(89)*. Single-agent and combination studies are currently in Phase II testing.

Several other targets are of interest in colorectal cancer but are still in early development. Aurora kinase inhibitors, as mitotic regulators responsible for monitoring genomic stability, have demonstrated activity in colon cancer xenograft models *(138)*. Cyclin-dependent kinases such as flavopiridol have been tested without clear activity as a single agent in colorectal cancer, although combination studies are ongoing *(139)*.

4. FUTURE DIRECTIONS OF MOLECULAR THERAPEUTICS

The past several years have seen the introduction of three agents for targeted therapy of colorectal cancer. When combined with advances in cytotoxic chemotherapy, the result has been a doubling of the median OS for patients with metastatic colorectal cancer during the past decade. Although this is a promising start, continued development is needed to improve the outcome of patients with colorectal cancer.

4.1. Moving Beyond EGFR and VEGF

In a recent review of colorectal cancer trials, only 13% of ongoing trials incorporated an agent with a mechanism of action unique from currently approved colorectal cancer agents. Specifically, agents now in development favor therapeutic agents that target the EGFR and VEGF pathways. Although these EGFR- and VEGF-targeted agents may demonstrate interval improvement in efficacy or an improved side effect profile, a concerted effort to develop novel therapeutics is needed.

Despite many trials and positive preclinical work, small-molecule inhibitors have not yet found a place in the treatment of colorectal cancer. Instead of a limitation of a class of agents, the identified reasons for failure include difficulty with tolerance due to overlapping toxicities with cytotoxic chemotherapy, misjudgments in pharmacokinetics, and failure to identify a subgroup of patients most likely to respond to therapy.

4.2. Efficient Trial Design

Successful development of targeted therapy requires concurrent development of biomarkers of efficacy with prospective incorporation into clinical trials. This paradigm, as proposed by the FDA's Critical Path initiative *(140)*, has not yet been incorporated into the field addressing colorectal cancer. A recent review of colorectal trials demonstrated that only 3% of ongoing trials incorporated a novel tumor biomarker of efficacy into the trial design. Enrichment can improve the efficiency of drug development and provide a pathway to FDA approval *(141)*. Central to this new initiative is a required flexibility on the part of regulatory agencies to facilitate concurrent development of biomarker tests or combination therapy. Other recommendations of the FDA Critical Path initiative include the following: incorporation of novel Bayesian statistical methods, molecular imaging, and increased reliance on pharmacodynamic correlatives.

Novel trial designs, such as a randomized discontinuation trial, may be especially critical for evaluating the potential benefit of agents with an expectation for a best response of stable disease. With metastatic colorectal cancer, window trials investigate the potential benefit of a new agent after the development of cumulative toxicity or during planned combination chemotherapy holidays. Evaluating targeted therapy for neoadjuvant rectal cancer therapy allows incorporation of not otherwise practical pharmacodynamic endpoints and provides a rapid, quantifiable outcome based on pathologic response rates. The traditional model of adding novel agents to the current combination chemotherapy regimens is less feasible given increased patient toxicity and financial concerns. Instead, molecular-targeted therapy may allow sparing of cytotoxic agents while maintaining efficacy.

Molecular-targeted therapeutic agents have not yet been incorporated into the adjuvant setting. These trials require large sample sizes and significant financial resources. In addition, the involvement of healthier patients with a good prognosis alters the acceptable level of toxicity. Although several clinical trials are ongoing with bevacizumab in combination with FOLFOX, there remain concerns about the relevance of the low rates of bowel perforation or arteriothromboembolic events such as stroke or heart attack. Likewise, adjuvant patients, many of whom continue to work, may be less willing to accept the potentially severe acneiform rash associated with cetuximab treatment. In addition, long-term toxicities associated with many of these therapies have not yet been clearly identified given the poor prognosis of patients treated for metastatic disease. Despite these concerns, targeted therapies that are demonstrated to have activity in the metastatic setting will likely continue to undergo evaluation in the adjuvant setting.

4.3. Translating Our Understanding of Colorectal Biology to the Clinical Setting

Despite an increased understanding of the molecular biology of colorectal cancer, few therapeutic advances have been made other than targeted therapies directed against EGFR and VEGF. Distinct tumorigenesis pathways have been identified for colorectal cancer patients, potentially pinpointing differences in prognosis that may affect treatment choices and provide an opportunity to develop molecular therapeutics targeting these selective pathways.

The first Phase III study to incorporate this molecular prognostic information prospectively is currently ongoing. The ECGO 5202 trial is a randomized Phase III study comparing 5-FU/leucovorin/oxaliplatin versus 5-FU/leucovorin/oxaliplatin/bevacizumab in patients with stage II colon cancer at high risk for recurrence to determine prospectively the prognostic value of molecular markers. This trial of adjuvant therapy for stage II colon cancer patients stratifies patients with MSI and 18q loss of heterozygosity. Tumors without MSI or with 18q loss have a worse prognosis and are treated with chemotherapy, whereas patients with neither risk factor do not receive chemotherapy *(142,143)*.

We have recognized the heterogeneity of colorectal cancer for many years, yet our current treatment approaches have yet to incorporate this understanding. Of all the cancer subtypes, the biology of colon cancer has arguably been one of the most extensively studied. As a result, colon cancer clinical research should be poised to utilize molecularly targeted therapies rationally based on the biology of an individual patient's tumor. Only through such an approach can we double the survival rate of patients with metastatic colorectal cancer and advance the success of adjuvant chemotherapy.

4.4. Conclusions

The past several years have seen the development of monoclonal antibodies for treating colorectal cancer, with a substantial improvement in clinical outcomes. Both VEGF and EGFR have been validated as targets for drug development, and other targets are being evaluated. Further research is needed to bridge the gap between our growing knowledge of tumor biology and the development of agents that can provide clinical benefit.

5. REFERENCES

1. American Cancer Society. Cancer Facts and Figures. Atlanta: American Cancer Society; 2006.
2. Eaden JA, Abrams KR, Mayberry JF. The risk of colorectal cancer in ulcerative colitis: a meta-analysis. Gut 2001;48(4):526–35.
3. Moertel CG, Fleming TR, Macdonald JS, et al. Levamisole and fluorouracil for adjuvant therapy of resected colon carcinoma. N Engl J Med 1990;322(6):352–8.
4. Kuebler JP, Wieand HS, O'Connell MJ, et al. Oxaliplatin combined with weekly bolus fluorouracil and leucovorin as surgical adjuvant chemotherapy for stage II and III colon cancer: results from NSABP C-07. J Clin Oncol 2007;25(16):2198–204.
5. Andre T, Boni C, Mounedji-Boudiaf L, et al. Oxaliplatin, fluorouracil, and leucovorin as adjuvant treatment for colon cancer. N Engl J Med 2004;350(23):2343–51.
6. Figueredo A, Charette ML, Maroun J, et al. Adjuvant therapy for stage II colon cancer: a systematic review from the Cancer Care Ontario Program in Evidence-Based Care's Gastrointestinal Cancer Disease Site Group. J Clin Oncol 2004;22(16):3395–407.
7. Grothey A, Sargent DJ. FOLFOX for stage II colon cancer? A commentary on the recent FDA approval of oxaliplatin for adjuvant therapy of stage III colon cancer. J Clin Oncol 2005;23(15):3311–3.
8. Benson AB III, Schrag D, Somerfield MR, et al. American Society of Clinical Oncology recommendations on adjuvant chemotherapy for stage II colon cancer. J Clin Oncol 2004;22(16):3408–19.
9. Seymour MT. Fluorouracil, oxaliplatin and CPT-11 (irinotecan), use and sequencing (MRC FOCUS): a 2135-patient randomized trial in advanced colorectal cancer (ACRC). J Clin Oncol 2005;23(16S):3518.
10. Tournigand C, Andre T, Achille E, et al. FOLFIRI followed by FOLFOX6 or the reverse sequence in advanced colorectal cancer: a randomized GERCOR study. J Clin Oncol 2004;22(2):229–37.
11. Grothey A, Sargent D. Overall survival of patients with advanced colorectal cancer correlates with availability of fluorouracil, irinotecan, and oxaliplatin regardless of whether doublet or single-agent therapy is used first line. J Clin Oncol 2005;23(36):9441–2.

12. Grothey A, Sargent D, Goldberg RM, Schmoll HJ. Survival of patients with advanced colorectal cancer improves with the availability of fluorouracil-leucovorin, irinotecan, and oxaliplatin in the course of treatment. J Clin Oncol 2004;22(7):1209–14.

13. Tournigand C, Cervantes A, Figer A, et al. OPTIMOX1: A randomized study of FOLFOX4 or FOLFOX7 with oxaliplatin in a stop-and-go fashion in advanced colorectal cancer?a GERCOR study. J Clin Oncol 2006;24(3):394–400.

14. Gibson TB, Grothey A. Do all patients with metastatic colorectal cancer need chemotherapy until disease progression? Clin Colorectal Cancer 2006;6(3):196–201.

15. Maindrault-Goebel F, Lledo G, Chibaudel B, et al. OPTIMOX2, a large randomized phase II study of maintenance therapy or chemotherapy-free intervals (CFI) after FOLFOX in patients with metastatic colorectal cancer (MRC): a GERCOR study. J Clin Oncol 2006;24(18S):3504.

16. Labianca R, Floriani I, Cortesi E, et al. Alternating versus continuous "FOLFIRI" in advanced colorectal cancer (ACC): a randomized "GISCAD" trial. J Clin Oncol 2006;24(18S):3505.

17. Kinzler KW, Vogelstein B. Lessons from hereditary colorectal cancer. Cell 1996;87(2):159–70.

18. Lynch HT, Lynch JF. What the physician needs to know about Lynch syndrome: an update. Oncology (Williston Park) 2005;19(4):455–63; discussion 63–4, 66, 69.

19. Lynch HT, Lynch J. Lynch syndrome: genetics, natural history, genetic counseling, and prevention. J Clin Oncol 2000;18(suppl 1):19s-31.

20. Vasen HF, Wijnen JT, Menko FH, et al. Cancer risk in families with hereditary nonpolyposis colorectal cancer diagnosed by mutation analysis. Gastroenterology 1996;110(4):1020–7.

21. Lindor NM, Petersen GM, Hadley DW, et al. Recommendations for the care of individuals with an inherited predisposition to Lynch syndrome: a systematic review. JAMA 2006;296(12):1507–17.

22. Garber JE, Offit K. Hereditary cancer predisposition syndromes. J Clin Oncol 2005;23(2):276–92.

23. Guillem JG, Wood WC, Moley JF, et al. ASCO/SSO review of current role of risk-reducing surgery in common hereditary cancer syndromes. Ann Surg Oncol 2006;13(10):1296–321.

24. Bertario L, Russo A, Sala P, et al. Multiple approach to the exploration of genotype-phenotype correlations in familial adenomatous polyposis. J Clin Oncol 2003;21(9):1698–707.

25. Burt RW, Leppert MF, Slattery ML, et al. Genetic testing and phenotype in a large kindred with attenuated familial adenomatous polyposis. Gastroenterology 2004;127(2):444–51.

26. Giardiello FM, Yang VW, Hylind LM, et al. Primary chemoprevention of familial adenomatous polyposis with sulindac. N Engl J Med 2002;346(14):1054–9.

27. Phillips RKS, Wallace MH, Lynch PM, et al. A randomised, double blind, placebo controlled study of celecoxib, a selective cyclooxygenase 2 inhibitor, on duodenal polyposis in familial adenomatous polyposis. Gut 2002;50(6):857–60.

28. Sieber OM, Lipton L, Crabtree M, et al. Multiple colorectal adenomas, classic adenomatous polyposis, and germ-line mutations in MYH. N Engl J Med 2003;348(9):791–9.

29. Wirtzfeld DA, Petrelli NJ, Rodriguez-Bigas MA. Hamartomatous polyposis syndromes: molecular genetics, neoplastic risk, and surveillance recommendations. Ann Surg Oncol 2001;8(4):319–27.

30. Akao Y, Nakagawa Y, Naoe T. let-7 microRNA functions as a potential growth suppressor in human colon cancer cells. Biol Pharm Bull 2006;29(5):903–6.

31. Wiesner GL, Daley D, Lewis S, et al. A subset of familial colorectal neoplasia kindreds linked to chromosome 9q22.2–31.2. Proc Natl Acad Sci U S A 2003;100(22):12961–5.

32. Vogelstein B, Kinzler KW. Cancer genes and the pathways they control. Nat Med 2004;10(8):789–99.

33. Fearon ER, Vogelstein B. A genetic model for colorectal tumorigenesis. Cell 1990;61(5):759–67.

34. Smith G, Carey FA, Beattie J, et al. Mutations in APC, Kirsten-ras, and p53–alternative genetic pathways to colorectal cancer. Proc Natl Acad Sci U S A 2002;99(14):9433–8.

35. Samowitz WS, Slattery ML, Sweeney C, et al. APC mutations and other genetic and epigenetic changes in colon cancer. Mol Cancer Res 2007;5(2):165–70.

36. Loeb LA. Mutator phenotype may be required for multistage carcinogenesis. Cancer Res 1991;51(12): 3075–9.

37. Yamamoto H, Sawai H, Weber TK, et al. Somatic frameshift mutations in DNA mismatch repair and proapoptosis genes in hereditary nonpolyposis colorectal cancer. Cancer Res 1998;58(5):997–1003.

38. Markowitz SD, Roberts AB. Tumor suppressor activity of the TGF-beta pathway in human cancers. Cytokine Growth Factor Rev 1996;7(1):93–102.

39. Tang Y, Katuri V, Dillner A, et al. Disruption of transforming growth factor-beta signaling in ELF beta-spectrin-deficient mice. Science 2003;299(5606):574–7.

40. Vogelstein B, Fearon ER, Hamilton SR, et al. Genetic alterations during colorectal-tumor development. N Engl J Med 1988;319(9):525–32.

41. Andreyev HJ, Norman AR, Cunningham D, et al. Kirsten ras mutations in patients with colorectal cancer: the multicenter "RASCAL" study. J Natl Cancer Inst 1998;90(9):675–84.
42. Andreyev HJ, Norman AR, Cunningham D, et al. Kirsten ras mutations in patients with colorectal cancer: the 'RASCAL II' study. Br J Cancer 2001;85(5):692–6.
43. Luna-Perez P, Segura J, Alvarado I, et al. Specific c-K-ras gene mutations as a tumor-response marker in locally advanced rectal cancer treated with preoperative chemoradiotherapy. Ann Surg Oncol 2000;7(10):727–31.
44. Maestro M, Vidaurreta M, Sanz-Casla M, et al. Role of the BRAF mutations in the microsatellite instability genetic pathway in sporadic colorectal cancer. Ann Surg Oncol 2007;14(3):1229–36.
45. Wang L, Cunningham JM, Winters JL, et al. BRAF mutations in colon cancer are not likely attributable to defective DNA mismatch repair. Cancer Res 2003;63(17):5209–12.
46. Makinen MJ. Colorectal serrated adenocarcinoma. Histopathology 2007;50(1):131–50.
47. O'Brien MJ, Yang S, Mack C, et al. Comparison of microsatellite instability, CpG island methylation phenotype, BRAF and KRAS status in serrated polyps and traditional adenomas indicates separate pathways to distinct colorectal carcinoma end points. Am J Surg Pathol 2006;30(12):1491–501.
48. Kambara T, Simms LA, Whitehall VL, et al. BRAF mutation is associated with DNA methylation in serrated polyps and cancers of the colorectum. Gut 2004;53(8):1137–44.
49. Traverso G, Shuber A, Levin B, et al. Detection of APC mutations in fecal DNA from patients with colorectal tumors. N Engl J Med 2002;346(5):311–20.
50. Rodrigues NR, Rowan A, Smith ME, et al. p53 mutations in colorectal cancer. Proc Natl Acad Sci U S A 1990;87(19):7555–9.
51. Russo A, Bazan V, Iacopetta B, et al. The TP53 colorectal cancer international collaborative study on the prognostic and predictive significance of p53 mutation: influence of tumor site, type of mutation, and adjuvant treatment. J Clin Oncol 2005;23(30):7518–28.
52. Neal CP, Garcea G, Doucas H, et al. Molecular prognostic markers in resectable colorectal liver metastases: a systematic review. Eur J Cancer 2006;42(12):1728–43.
53. Summy JM, Gallick GE. Src family kinases in tumor progression and metastasis. Cancer Metast Rev 2003;22(4):337–58.
54. Summy JM, Gallick GE. Treatment for advanced tumors: SRC reclaims center stage. Clin Cancer Res 2006;12(5):1398–401.
55. Aligayer H, Boyd DD, Heiss MM, et al. Activation of Src kinase in primary colorectal carcinoma: an indicator of poor clinical prognosis. Cancer 2002;94(2):344–51.
56. Khaleghpour K, Li Y, Banville D, et al. Involvement of the PI 3-kinase signaling pathway in progression of colon adenocarcinoma. Carcinogenesis 2004;25(2):241–8.
57. Samuels Y, Wang Z, Bardelli A, et al. High frequency of mutations of the PIK3CA gene in human cancers. Science 2004;304(5670):554.
58. Sjoblom T, Jones S, Wood LD, et al. The consensus coding sequences of human breast and colorectal cancers. Science 2006;314(5797):268–74.
59. Cunningham D, Humblet Y, Siena S, et al. Cetuximab monotherapy and cetuximab plus irinotecan in irinotecan-refractory metastatic colorectal cancer. N Engl J Med 2004;351(4):337–45.
60. Díaz Rubio E, Tabernero J, Cutsem EV, et al. Cetuximab in combination with oxaliplatin/5-fluorouracil (5-FU)/folinic acid (FA) (FOLFOX-4) in the first-line treatment of patients with epidermal growth factor receptor (EGFR)-expressing metastatic colorectal cancer: an international phase II study. J Clin Oncol 2005;23(16S):3535.
61. Tabernero J, Salazar R, Casado E, et al. Targeted therapy in advanced colon cancer: the role of new therapies. Ann Oncol 2004;15(suppl 4):iv55–62.
62. Mendelsohn J, Baselga J. The EGF receptor family as targets for cancer therapy. Oncogene 2000; 19(56):6550–65.
63. Mendelsohn J, Baselga J. Status of epidermal growth factor receptor antagonists in the biology and treatment of cancer. J Clin Oncol 2003;21(14):2787–99.
64. Hadari Y, Doody J, Wang Y. The IgG1 monoclonal antibody cetuximab induces degradation of the epidermal growth factor receptor. In: ASCO Gastrointestinal Cancers Symposium 2004. San Francisco, 2004. Abstract 234.
65. Prewett M, Rockwell P, Rockwell RF, et al. The biologic effects of C225, a chimeric monoclonal antibody to the EGFR, on human prostate carcinoma. J Immunother Emphasis Tumor Immunol 1996; 19(6):419–27.
66. Prewett M, Rothman M, Waksal H, et al. Mouse-human chimeric anti-epidermal growth factor receptor antibody C225 inhibits the growth of human renal cell carcinoma xenografts in nude mice. Clin Cancer Res 1998;4(12):2957–66.

67. Goldstein NI, Prewett M, Zuklys K, et al. Biological efficacy of a chimeric antibody to the epidermal growth factor receptor in a human tumor xenograft model. Clin Cancer Res 1995;1(11):1311–8.

68. O-Charoenrat P, Rhys-Evans P, Modjtahedi H, et al. Overexpression of epidermal growth factor receptor in human head and neck squamous carcinoma cell lines correlates with matrix metalloproteinase-9 expression and in vitro invasion. Int J Cancer 2000;86(3):307–17.

69. Perrotte P, Matsumoto T, Inoue K, et al. Anti-epidermal growth factor receptor antibody C225 inhibits angiogenesis in human transitional cell carcinoma growing orthotopically in nude mice. Clin Cancer Res 1999;5(2):257–65.

70. Bruns CJ, Harbison MT, Davis DW, et al. Epidermal growth factor receptor blockade with C225 plus gemcitabine results in regression of human pancreatic carcinoma growing orthotopically in nude mice by antiangiogenic mechanisms. Clin Cancer Res 2000;6(5):1936–48.

71. Inoue K, Slaton JW, Perrotte P, et al. Paclitaxel enhances the effects of the anti-epidermal growth factor receptor monoclonal antibody ImClone C225 in mice with metastatic human bladder transitional cell carcinoma. Clin Cancer Res 2000;6(12):4874–84.

72. Ciardiello F, Bianco R, Damiano V, et al. Antitumor activity of sequential treatment with topotecan and anti-epidermal growth factor receptor monoclonal antibody C225. Clin Cancer Res 1999;5(4):909–16.

73. Ford SK, Perkins N-A, Huang X, et al. Preclinical discovery and clinical validation of predictive markers of response to cetuximab (ErbituxTM) in metastatic colorectal cancer. AACR Meet Abstr 2006; 2006(1):950-a.

74. Lynch TJ, Bell DW, Sordella R, et al. Activating mutations in the epidermal growth factor receptor underlying responsiveness of non-small-cell lung cancer to gefitinib. N Engl J Med 2004;350(21):2129–39.

75. Lenz HJ, Van Cutsem E, Khambata-Ford S, et al. Multicenter phase II and translational study of cetuximab in metastatic colorectal carcinoma refractory to irinotecan, oxaliplatin, and fluoropyrimidines. J Clin Oncol 2006;24(30):4914–21.

76. Connolly DT, Olander JV, Heuvelman D, et al. Human vascular permeability factor: isolation from U937 cells. J Biol Chem 1989;264(33):20017–24.

77. Ferrara N, Henzel WJ. Pituitary follicular cells secrete a novel heparin-binding growth factor specific for vascular endothelial cells. Biochem Biophys Res Commun 1989;161(2):851–8.

78. Ferrara N, Davis-Smyth T. The biology of vascular endothelial growth factor. Endocr Rev 1997;18(1):4–25.

79. Frank RE, Saclarides TJ, Leurgans S, et al. Tumor angiogenesis as a predictor of recurrence and survival in patients with node-negative colon cancer. Ann Surg 1995;222(6):695–9.

80. Choi HJ, Hyun MS, Jung GJ, et al. Tumor angiogenesis as a prognostic predictor in colorectal carcinoma with special reference to mode of metastasis and recurrence. Oncology 1998;55(6):575–81.

81. Ellis LM. Angiogenesis and its role in colorectal tumor and metastasis formation. Semin Oncol 2004;31(suppl 17):3–9.

82. Fan F, Wey JS, McCarty MF, et al. Expression and function of vascular endothelial growth factor receptor-1 on human colorectal cancer cells. Oncogene 2005;24(16):2647–53.

83. Hurwitz H, Fehrenbacher L, Novotny W, et al. Bevacizumab plus irinotecan, fluorouracil, and leucovorin for metastatic colorectal cancer. N Engl J Med 2004;350(23):2335–42.

84. Konishi N, Miki C, Yoshida T, et al. Interleukin-1 receptor antagonist inhibits the expression of vascular endothelial growth factor in colorectal carcinoma. Oncology 2005;68(2–3):138–45.

85. Zhang X, Gaspard JP, Chung DC. Regulation of vascular endothelial growth factor by the Wnt and K-ras pathways in colonic neoplasia. Cancer Res 2001;61(16):6050–4.

86. Warren RS, Yuan H, Matli MR, et al. Regulation by vascular endothelial growth factor of human colon cancer tumorigenesis in a mouse model of experimental liver metastasis. J Clin Invest 1995;95(4):1789–97.

87. Wu Y, Yakar S, Zhao L, et al. Circulating insulin-like growth factor-I levels regulate colon cancer growth and metastasis. Cancer Res 2002;62(4):1030–5.

88. Ma J, Pollak MN, Giovannucci E, et al. Prospective study of colorectal cancer risk in men and plasma levels of insulin-like growth factor (IGF)-I and IGF-binding protein-3. J Natl Cancer Inst 1999;91(7):620–5.

89. Sachdev D, Yee D. Disrupting insulin-like growth factor signaling as a potential cancer therapy. Mol Cancer Ther 2007;6(1):1–12.

90. Saltz LB, Clarke S, Diaz-Rubio E, et al. Bevacizumab (Bev) in combination with XELOX or FOLFOX4: efficacy results from XELOX-1/NO16966, a randomized phase III trial in the first-line treatment of metastatic colorectal cancer (MCRC). In: ASCO Gastrointestinal Cancers Symposium 2007, Orlando, FL, 2007. Abstract 238.

91. Hochster H, Hart LL, Ramanathan RK, et al. Safety and efficacy of oxaliplatin/fluoropyrimidine regimens with or without bevacizumab as first-line treatment of metastatic colorectal cancer (mCRC): final analysis of the TREE study. J Clin Oncol 2006;24(18S):3510.

92. Fuchs C, Marshall J, Mitchell E, et al. A randomized trial of first-line irinotecan/fluoropymidine combinations with or without celecoxib in metastatic colorectal cancer (BICC-C). J Clin Oncol 2006;24(18S):3506.
93. Willett CG, Boucher Y, di Tomaso E, et al. Direct evidence that the VEGF-specific antibody bevacizumab has antivascular effects in human rectal cancer. Nat Med 2004;10(2):145–7.
94. Willett CG, Duda DG, Boucher Y, et al. Phase I/II study of neoadjuvant bevacizumab with radiation therapy and 5-fluorouracil in patients with rectal cancer: initial results. In: ASCO Annual Meeting, Chicago, 2007. Abstract 4041.
95. Giantonio B, Catalano PJ, Meropol NJ, et al. High-dose bevacizumab improves survival when combined with FOLFOX4 in previously treated advanced colorectal cancer: results from the Eastern Cooperative Oncology Group (ECOG) study E3200. J Clin Oncol 2005;23(16S). Abstract 2.
96. Hochster HS, Welles L, Hart L, et al. Safety and efficacy of bevacizumab (Bev) when added to oxali-platin/fluoropyrimidine (O/F) regimens as first-line treatment of metastatic colorectal cancer (mCRC): TREE 1 & 2 Studies. J Clin Oncol 2005;23(16S). Abstract 3515.
97. Kabbinavar F, Hurwitz HI, Fehrenbacher L, et al. Phase II, randomized trial comparing bevacizumab plus fluorouracil (FU)/leucovorin (LV) with FU/LV alone in patients with metastatic colorectal cancer. J Clin Oncol 2003;21(1):60–5.
98. Sugrue M, Kozloff M, Hainsworth J, et al. Risk factors for gastrointestinal perforations in patients with metastatic colorectal cancer receiving bevacizumab plus chemotherapy. J Clin Oncol 2006;24(18S):3535.
99. Kretzschmar A, Cunningham D, Berry S, et al. Incidence of gastrointestinal perforations and bleeding in patients starting bevacizumab treatment in first-line mCRC without primary tumour resection: preliminary results from the first BEATrial. In: ASCO Gastrointestinal Cancers Symposium 2006. Abstract 248.
100. Kopetz S, Dang J, Overman M, et al. Bevacizumab toxicity and efficacy are unaffected by regimen or resection status: a single institution retrospective study. In: ASCO Gastrointestinal Cancers Symposium 2006. Abstract 243.
101. Traina TA, Norton L, Drucker K, et al. Nasal septum perforation in a bevacizumab-treated patient with metastatic breast cancer. Oncologist 2006;11(10):1070–1.
102. Morabito A, De Maio E, Di Maio M, et al. Tyrosine kinase inhibitors of vascular endothelial growth factor receptors in clinical trials: current status and future directions. Oncologist 2006;11(7):753–64.
103. Drevs J, Muller-Driver R, Wittig C, et al. PTK787/ZK 222584, a specific vascular endothelial growth factor-receptor tyrosine kinase inhibitor, affects the anatomy of the tumor vascular bed and the functional vascular properties as detected by dynamic enhanced magnetic resonance imaging. Cancer Res 2002;62(14):4015–22.
104. Hecht J, Trarbach T, Jaeger E. A randomized, double-blind, placebo-controlled phase III study in patients with metastatic adenocarcinoma of the colon or rectum receiving first-line chemotherapy with oxaliplatin/5-fluorouracil/leucovorin and PTK787/ZK 222584 or placebo. (CONFIRM-1). J Clin Oncol 2005;23(16S). Abstract LBA3a.
105. Koehne C, Bajetta E, Lin E. Results of an interim analysis of a multinational randomized, double-blind, phase III study in patients with previously treated metastatic colorectal cancer receiving FOLFOX4 and PTK787/ZK 222584 or placebo (CONFIRM 2). J Clin Oncolo 2006;24(16S). Abstract 148.
106. Harris AL. Hypoxia—a key regulatory factor in tumour growth. Nat Rev Cancer 2002;2(1):38–47.
107. Longo R, Sarmiento R, Fanelli M, et al. Anti-angiogenic therapy: rationale, challenges and clinical studies. Angiogenesis 2002;5(4):237–56.
108. Marzola P, Degrassi A, Calderan L, et al. Early antiangiogenic activity of SU11248 evaluated in vivo by dynamic contrast-enhanced magnetic resonance imaging in an experimental model of colon carcinoma. Clin Cancer Res 2005;11(16):5827–32.
109. Lenz HJ, Marshall JL, Rosen LS, et al. Phase II trial of SU11248 in patients with metastatic colorectal cancer after failure of standard chemotherapy. J Clin Oncol 2006;24(16S). Abstract 241.
110. Morris C, Jurgensmeier J, Robertson J, et al. AZD2171, an oral, highly potent, and reversible inhibitor of VEGFR signaling with potential for treatment of advanced colorectal cancer. In: GI ASCO, 2006. Abstract 242.
111. Jonker D, Karapetis CS, Moore MJ, et al. Randomized phase III trial of cetuximab monotherapy plus best supportive care (BSC) versus BSC alone in patients with pretreated metastatic epidermal growth factor receptor [EGFR]-positive colorectal carcinoma: a trial of the National Cancer Institute of Canada Clinical Trials Group (NCIC CTG) and the Australasian Gastro-Intestinal Trials Group (AGITG). In: AACR Meeting Abstracts, 2007, p. 3536-a.
112. Sobrero A, Fehrenbacher L, Rivera F, et al. Randomized phase III trial of cetuximab plus irinotecan alone for metastatic colorectal cancer (mCRC) in 1298 patients who have failed prior oxaliplatin-based therapy: the EPIC trial. In: AACR Meeting Abstracts, 2007, p. 3536-a.
113. Andre T, Tabernero J, Van Cutsem E, et al. Phase II study with cetuximab plus FOLFOX-4 in first-line setting for epidermal growth factor receptor (EGFR)-expressing metastatic colorectal cancer (mCRC): final results. In: ASCO Gastrointestinal Cancers Symposium, 2007. Abstract 334.

114. Van Cutsem E, Nowacki M, Lang I, et al. Randomized phase III study of irinotecan and 5-FU/FA with or without cetuximab in the first-line treatment of patients with metastatic colorectal cancer (mCRC): the CRYSTAL trial. In: ASCO Annual Meeting Abstracts, 2007. Abstract 4000.

115. Van Cutsem E, Humblet Y, Gelderblom H, et al. Cetuximab dose-escalation study in patients with metastatic colorectal cancer (mCRC) with no or slight skin reactions on cetuximab standard dose treatment (EVEREST): pharmacokinetic and efficacy data of a randomized study. In: ASCO Gastrointestinal Cancers Symposium 2007, Orlando, FL, 2007. Abstract 237.

116. Lievre A, Bachet JB, Le Corre D, et al. KRAS mutation status is predictive of response to cetuximab therapy in colorectal cancer. Cancer Res 2006;66(8):3992–5.

117. Lievre A, Bachet JB, Ychou M, et al. KRAS mutations in colorectal cancer is a predictive factor of response and progression free survival in patients treated with Cetuximab. In: AACR Meeting Abstracts, 2007, 5671-a.

118. Van Cutsem E, Peeters M, Siena S, et al. Open-label phase III trial of panitumumab plus best supportive care compared with best supportive care alone in patients with chemotherapy?refractory metastatic colorectal cancer. J Clin Oncol 2007;25(13):1658–64.

119. Hecht J, Posey J, Techekmedyian S. Panitumumab in combination with 5-fluorouracil, leucovorin, and irinotecan (IFL) or FOLFIRI for first-line treatment of metastatic colorectal cancer (mCRC). In: ASCO Gastrointestinal Cancers Symposium, San Francisco, 2006. Abstract 327.

120. Meira D, Nobrega N, Monoro J. Differences in activity between matuzumab and cetuximab in A431 cells may rely on MAPK cascade inhibition. In: AACR Annual Conference, Los Angeles, 2007. Abstract 336.

121. Townsley CA, Major P, Siu LL, et al. Phase II study of erlotinib (OSI-774) in patients with metastatic colorectal cancer. Br J Cancer 2006;94(8):1136–43.

122. Rothenberg ML, LaFleur B, Levy DE, et al. Randomized phase II trial of the clinical and biological effects of two dose levels of gefitinib in patients with recurrent colorectal adenocarcinoma. J Clin Oncol 2005;23(36):9265–74.

123. Mackenzie MJ, Hirte HW, Glenwood G, et al. A phase II trial of ZD1839 (Iressa) 750 mg per day, an oral epidermal growth factor receptor-tyrosine kinase inhibitor, in patients with metastatic colorectal cancer. Invest New Drugs 2005;23(2):165–70.

124. Meyerhardt JA, Zhu AX, Enzinger PC, et al. Phase II study of capecitabine, oxaliplatin, and erlotinib in previously treated patients with metastastic colorectal cancer. J Clin Oncol 2006;24(12):1892–7.

125. Veronese ML, Sun W, Giantonio B, et al. A phase II trial of gefitinib with 5-fluorouracil, leucovorin, and irinotecan in patients with colorectal cancer. Br J Cancer 2005;92(10):1846–9.

126. Messersmith WA, Laheru DA, Senzer NN, et al. Phase I trial of irinotecan, infusional 5-fluorouracil, and leucovorin (FOLFIRI) with erlotinib (OSI-774): early termination due to increased toxicities. Clin Cancer Res 2004;10(19):6522–7.

127. Kuo T, Cho CD, Halsey J, et al. Phase II study of gefitinib, fluorouracil, leucovorin, and oxaliplatin therapy in previously treated patients with metastatic colorectal cancer. J Clin Oncol 2005;23(24):5613–9.

128. Salazar R, Koehne C, Cortes-Funes H. Preliminary report of a phase 1/2 open-label study of EKB-569 in combination with 5-fluorouracil, leucovorin, and irinotecan in patients with advanced colorectal cancer. In: AACR Molecular Targets and Cancer Therapeutics, Boston, 2003. Abstract 125.

129. Ellis LM. Epidermal growth factor receptor in tumor angiogenesis. Hematol Oncol Clin North Am 2004;18(5):1007–21, viii.

130. Viloria-Petit A, Crombet T, Jothy S, et al. Acquired resistance to the antitumor effect of epidermal growth factor receptor-blocking antibodies in vivo: a role for altered tumor angiogenesis. Cancer Res 2001;61(13):5090–101.

131. Tabernero J. The role of VEGF and EGFR inhibition: implications for combining anti-VEGF and anti-EGFR agents. Mol Cancer Res 2007;5(3):203–20.

132. Yokoi K, Thaker PH, Yazici S, et al. Dual inhibition of epidermal growth factor receptor and vascular endothelial growth factor receptor phosphorylation by AEE788 reduces growth and metastasis of human colon carcinoma in an orthotopic nude mouse model. Cancer Res 2005;65(9):3716–25.

133. Ciardiello F, Bianco R, Caputo R, et al. Antitumor activity of ZD6474, a vascular endothelial growth factor receptor tyrosine kinase inhibitor, in human cancer cells with acquired resistance to antiepidermal growth factor receptor therapy. Clin Cancer Res 2004;10(2):784–93.

134. Keyes K, Cox K, Treadway P, et al. An in vitro tumor model: analysis of angiogenic factor expression after chemotherapy. Cancer Res 2002;62(19):5597–602.

135. Lesslie DP III, Parikh NU, Shah A, et al. Combined activity of dasatinib (BMS-354825) and oxaliplatin in an orthotopic model of metastatic colorectal carcinoma. In: AACR Meeting Abstracts, 2006, p. ; 1114-c.

136. Kopetz S, Wu J, Davies M, et al. Synergistic activity of Src and EGFR inhibitors in colon cancer. In: AACR Meeting Abstracts, 2007.

137. Nelson NJ. Celecoxib shown effective in preventing colon polyps. J Natl Cancer Inst 2006;98(10):665–7.

138. Harrington EA, Bebbington D, Moore J, et al. VX-680, a potent and selective small-molecule inhibitor of the Aurora kinases, suppresses tumor growth in vivo. Nat Med 2004;10(3):262–7.
139. Aklilu M, Kindler HL, Donehower RC, et al. Phase II study of flavopiridol in patients with advanced colorectal cancer. Ann Oncol 2003;14(8):1270–3.
140. Food and Drug Administration: Challenge and Opportunity on the Critical Path to New Medical Products. Washington, DC: US Department of Health and Human Services; 2004. http://www.fda.gov/oc/initiatives/criticalpath/whitepaper.pdf/.
141. Temple RJ. Enrichment designs: efficiency in development of cancer treatments. J Clin Oncol 2005;23(22):4838–9.
142. Jen J, Kim H, Piantadosi S, et al. Allelic loss of chromosome 18q and prognosis in colorectal cancer. N Engl J Med 1994;331(4):213–21.
143. Halling KC, French AJ, McDonnell SK, et al. Microsatellite instability and 8p allelic imbalance in stage B2 and C colorectal cancers. J Natl Cancer Inst 1999;91(15):1295–303.
144. Ries L, Eisner M, Kosary C, et al (eds). SEER Cancer Statistics Review, 1975–2000. http://seer.cancer.gov/csr/1975_2000/ed. Bethesda, MD: National Cancer Institute; 2003.
145. Hicklin DJ, Ellis LM. Role of the vascular endothelial growth factor pathway in tumor growth and angiogenesis. J Clin Oncol 2005;23(5):1011–27.
146. Zeng H, Dvorak HF, Mukhopadhyay D. Vascular permeability factor (VPF)/vascular endothelial growth factor (VEGF) peceptor-1 down-modulates VPF/VEGF receptor-2-mediated endothelial cell proliferation, but not migration, through phosphatidylinositol 3-kinase-dependent pathways. J Biol Chem 2001;276(29):26969–79.
147. Millauer B, Wizigmann-Voos S, Schnurch H, et al. High affinity VEGF binding and developmental expression suggest Flk-1 as a major regulator of vasculogenesis and angiogenesis. Cell 1993;72(6):835–46.
148. Stacker SA, Caesar C, Baldwin ME, et al. VEGF-D promotes the metastatic spread of tumor cells via the lymphatics. Nat Med 2001;7(2):186–91.
149. Mandriota SJ, Jussila L, Jeltsch M, et al. Vascular endothelial growth factor-C-mediated lymphangiogenesis promotes tumour metastasis. EMBO J 2001;20(4):672–82.
150. Saltz LB, Rubin M, Hochster HS, et al. Cetuximab (IMC-C225) plus irinotecan (CPT-11) is active in CPT-11-refractory colorectal cancer (CRC) that expresses epidermal growth factor receptor (EGFR). In: ASCO Annual Meeting, 2001. Abstract 7.
151. Saltz LB, Meropol NJ, Loehrer PJ Sr, et al. Phase II trial of cetuximab in patients with refractory colorectal cancer that expresses the epidermal growth factor receptor. J Clin Oncol 2004;22(7):1201–8.
152. Saltz LB. Randomized phase II trial of cetuximab/bevacizumab/irinotecan versus cetuximab/bevacizumab in irinotecan-refractory colorectal cancer. J Clin Oncol 2005;23(16S). Abstract 248.

7

Targeted Therapy in Non-Small Cell Lung Cancer

David J. Stewart, MD, FRCPC

CONTENTS

SUMMARY

Despite advances in standard therapies and chemotherapeutic regimens, survival remains poor for patients with lung cancer, the leading cause of cancer death in the world. Consequently, there is substantial interest in identifying potentially exploitable new targets in lung cancer. Over the past 5 years, targeted therapies have become firmly established as therapeutic options in non-small-cell lung cancer. The epidermal growth factor receptor inhibitors and vascular endothelial growth factor receptor inhibitors have proven activity and have rapidly gained widespread use. It is anticipated that the usefulness of additional classes of agents will be established in the near future. Of particular interest and importance are agents that are effective against tumor cells resistant to chemotherapy. Several new classes of agents are currently under investigation, including histone deacetylase inhibitors, DNA-methyltransferase inhibitors, proapoptotic agents, agents that antagonize antiapoptosis molecules, heat shock protein inhibitors, and hypoxia-inducible factor-1α antagonists, among others. Further development of these approaches is awaited with interest.

Key Words: Non-small-cell lung cancer, EGFR, Erlotinib, Gefitinib, VEGFR

1. INTRODUCTION

Lung cancer (the leading cause of cancer death in the world) is responsible for 33% of cancer deaths in American men, 25% of cancer deaths in American women, and 5% of U.S.

From: *Current Clinical Oncology: Targeted Cancer Therapy*
Edited by: R. Kurzrock and M. Markman © Humana Press, Totowa, NJ

deaths from all causes *(1)*. Non-small-cell lung cancer (NSCLC) accounts for 85% of all lung cancer cases *(1)*. Only 15% of lung cancer patients survive 5 years *(1)*.

Adjuvant/neoadjuvant chemotherapy modestly improves survival in patients with operable NSCLC *(2,3)*. However, fewer than 40% of patients have operable disease at diagnosis *(4)*, and most patients who undergo surgery ultimately relapse and die despite adjuvant therapy *(5)*. With advanced NSCLC, 20% to 40% of patients respond to chemotherapy, and approximately 70% have "disease control" (response or stable disease) *(4)*. Chemotherapy improves the average life expectancy by a few months *(4)*. For patients with tumor progression after frontline chemotherapy, second-line chemotherapy with docetaxel is superior to best supportive care (BSC) *(6)*, and pemetrexed is also useful *(7)*.

In NSCLC, dose–response curves flatten at higher chemotherapy doses *(8)*, suggesting that something required for efficacy is saturated at higher drug doses *(9)*. Our current thinking *(8)* is that noncycling quiescent cells, which are generally resistant to chemotherapy, may survive the first cycle of chemotherapy. Available evidence indicates that after initial chemotherapy exposure, surviving cells rapidly undergo epigenetic changes that render them resistant to subsequent therapy. Some cells may up-regulate the expression of resistance factors after chemotherapy exposure, and this might permit rapid tumor regrowth between chemotherapy cycles *(8)*, whereas others might rapidly down-regulate membrane transporters *(10,11)* and become more resistant through reversible quiescence. Overall, the broad cross-resistance between chemotherapy regimens and the absence of benefit from higher doses suggest that a common set of factors is limiting the efficacy of chemotherapy, and that saturation or down-regulation of expression of some factor required for drug efficacy may be playing an important role in therapy failure *(8)*.

2. PUTATIVE TARGETS AND AGENTS IN NSCLC: ErbB FAMILY MEMBERS

Most chemotherapy agents target primarily DNA or DNA synthesis mechanisms, topoisomerases, or tubulin. There is substantial interest in identifying other potentially exploitable new targets. Of particular interest for new targeted therapies are growth factor receptors and their ligands, signaling pathways, the proteosome, and angiogenesis. Here we discuss the experience to date with new targeted therapies for NSCLC.

2.1. Epidermal Growth Factor Receptor

With respect to targeted therapies in NSCLC, most is known about agents that may inhibit epidermal growth factor receptors (EGFRs; erbB1). We review the efficacy and toxicity of these agents and discuss factors that have an impact on efficacy.

2.1.1. EGFR EXPRESSION BY IMMUNOHISTOCHEMISTRY

In NSCLC, as many as 70% of tumors express EGFR by IHC *(12,13)*. EGFR expression is more common in squamous cell carcinoma of the lung than in adenocarcinoma *(12,14)*, in nonmucinous variants of bronchioloalveolar carcinoma (BAC) than in mucinous variants *(15)*, and in cavitating than in noncavitating tumors *(12)*. In a meta-analysis, EGFR overexpression was noted in 58% of lung squamous cell carcinomas, 39% of adenocarcinomas, and 38% of large-cell carcinomas; it did not correlate significantly with survival *(16)*. In adenocarcinomas, EGFR expression may be higher in smokers than in nonsmokers *(17)*. EGFR expression may be substantially higher in tumors with EGFR gene amplification than in others *(18)*, but this has not been noted in all studies *(19)*.

2.1.2. EGFR Tyrosine Kinase Inhibitors

Gefitinib and erlotinib are oral small molecules that inhibit EGFR tyrosine kinase (TK) by competing with ATP for access to TK's intracellular ATP binding pocket *(20)*. Gefitinib-sensitive lines undergo G_1 arrest following gefitinib exposure and inactivation of downstream signaling proteins, whereas resistant lines have no change in these proteins *(21)*. After oral administration of EGFR TKI inhibitors (TKIs), high tumor concentrations are achieved. In patients who received gefitinib 250 mg orally daily for 28 days prior to resection of stage I to III NSCLC, the concentration of gefitinib found in tumors (0.5–135 µM) was substantially higher than plasma concentrations (0.07–1.2 µM) *(22)*, suggesting that drug uptake into the tumor is not a major issue with respect to efficacy.

2.1.3. Gefitinib in Previously Treated NSCLC Patients

In NSCLC patients who had previously been treated with chemotherapy, gefitinib resulted in partial remissions in 1% to 19% of patients and stable disease in 26% to 46% of patients, with a median time to progression (TTP) or progression-free survival (PFS) of 2.5 to 3.3 months, a median overall survival (OS) time of 4.1 to 8.0 months, and a 1-year survival rate of 24% to 29% *(20,23–30)*. Efficacy was somewhat greater in a study done in China, where the response rate was 33.5%, with a median PFS of 5.5 months and a median OS of 11.5 months *(31)*. In a randomized trial of second-line gefitinib versus docetaxel, outcomes were similar with the two therapies, with symptom improvement in 37% versus 26%, quality of life improvement in 34% versus 26%, responses in 13% versus 14%, median OS time of 7.5 versus 7.1 months, and better tolerance of the gefitinib *(28)*.

With gefitinib, the dose–response curve appears to be relatively flat. In the IDEAL1 and IDEAL2 trials in which previously treated NSCLC patients were randomized between 250 mg and 500 mg daily of gefitinib, response rates, PFS, median OS, and 1-year survival rates were similar for the two doses, whereas toxicity was greater at the higher dose *(29,32)*. Cancer-related symptoms improved in 37% to 43% of treated patients *(29,32)*.

In a randomized trial of gefitinib 250 mg/day versus placebo in 1692 previously treated NSCLC patients, gefitinib was either significantly superior to placebo or there was a trend toward gefitinib being superior for of the median survival (MS) (5.6 vs. 5.1 months, hazard ratio 0.89, $p = 0.087$), TTP (3.0 vs. 2.6 months, $p = 0.0006$), and response rate (8.0% vs. 1.3%) *(30)*. In patients with adenocarcinoma, MS was 6.3 months with gefitinib versus 5.4 months with placebo ($p = 0.089$) *(30)*. In a Cox multivariate survival analysis, gefitinib was superior to placebo in the overall group ($p = 0.03$) and in adenocarcinoma patients ($p = 0.033$) *(30)*.

2.1.4. Erlotinib in Previously Treated NSCLC Patients

In 57 previously treated North American patients with EGFR-expressing NSCLC, the response rate to erlotinib 150 mg orally was 12.3% *(33)*. Responses were seen regardless of the number of prior chemotherapy regimens *(33)*. The median survival was 8.4 months, and the 1-year survival rate was 40% *(33)*. In a randomized trial of erlotinib versus BSC in second- or third-line treatment of NSCLC involving 731 patients, the response rate for erlotinib was 8.9%, and erlotinib was superior to placebo with respect to PFS (2.2 vs. 1.8 months, $p < 0.001$) and OS (6.7 vs. 4.7 months, $p < 0.001$) *(34)*. Overall, efficacy in NSCLC appears to be similar for erlotinib and gefitinib.

Erlotinib has a half-life of approximately 36 hours and is generally given on a daily basis *(35)*. Although some preclinical studies have suggested that prolonged continuous exposure to EGFR TKIs is important for optimal tumor control, others suggested that intermittent high-dose administration inhibits additional sites downstream of EGFR, with greater antitumor activity *(36)*. In Phase I/II trials of weekly administration of high-dose erlotinib, the response rate of 5%, MS of 9.5 months, and toxicity profile appeared similar to that with daily administration *(36)*.

2.1.5. GEFITINIB AND ERLOTINIB IN CHEMONAIVE PATIENTS

Both gefitinib 250 mg daily and erlotinib 150 mg daily have been tested in chemonaive NSCLC patients. In 58 European patients treated with frontline gefitinib, the response rate was 5%, whereas 40% had stable disease; the median PFS was 1.6 months; and the MS was 6.7 months *(37)*. The efficacy of gefitinib appeared to be greater in chemonaive East Asian patients than in the European trial, with response rates of 27% to 69%, MS of 13.9 to 14.1 months, and estimated 1-year survival rates of 55% to 73% *(38–40)*. In chemonaive European and North American patients, erlotinib conferred response rates of 10% to 23%, with tumor control rates (response plus stable disease) of 51% to 53%, median TTP of 2.8 to 3.5 months, and median OS of 11 to 13 months *(41,42)*. Patients subsequently treated with chemotherapy after erlotinib experienced a response rate to chemotherapy of 6%, suggesting that there may be some degree of cross-resistance *(42)*.

2.1.6. EGFR TKIs ADDED TO FRONTLINE CHEMOTHERAPY AND CHEMORADIOTHERAPY

When gefitinib was administered to patients who had completed chemoradiotherapy for stage III NSCLC, it did not add any benefit. Survival was significantly shorter in the gefitinib arm than in the placebo arm *(43)*. Similarly, neither gefitinib *(44,45)* nor erlotinib *(46,47)* significantly prolonged PFS or OS for most NSCLC patients when added to frontline chemotherapy for advanced disease, despite substantially augmenting the efficacy of chemotherapy when added to it in preclinical systems. However, longer survival and PFS was seen with the addition of erlotinib to chemotherapy in the subset of patients who had never smoked *(46,47)*. In addition, for patients with adenocarcinomas who underwent ≥ 90 days of chemotherapy, there was significant prolongation of survival for gefitinib plus chemotherapy compared to chemotherapy alone, suggesting a possible maintenance effect of gefitinib *(44)*.

Reasons for the negative results when EGFR TKIs are added to frontline chemotherapy in NSCLC are unclear, although it has been suggested that the EGFR TKIs may alter cell cycle distribution of tumor cells such that they are in a phase of the cell cycle that is less sensitive to chemotherapy *(48)*. As an alternative explanation, it is possible that all the tumor cells that can be killed by therapy are already being killed by the two chemotherapy agents. Generally, there are no or few situations in NSCLC in which addition of a third agent targeting the tumor cell has improved outcome over dual-agent chemotherapy *(8)*. The factors that lead to flattening of dose–response curves in NSCLC and that limit the efficacy of three-drug chemotherapy regimens and of alternating chemotherapy approaches may also limit the ability of EGFR TKIs and other targeted agents to improve the efficacy of frontline therapy. We have proposed that something required for therapy efficacy is being saturated *(8)*. It remains unclear whether addition of an EGFR to a single chemotherapy agent would also fail to add to the treatment efficacy.

2.1.7. EGFR TKIs for NSCLC Brain Metastases

Several publications have documented the efficacy of EGFR TKIs against NSCLC brain metastases *(38,49–52)*. Among 10 chemonaive Korean never smokers with lung adeno-carcinomas treated with gefitinib for brain metastases, 7 had responses in both brain and extracranial sites, 1 had extracranial response and brain stability, and 2 had progression in both brain and extracranial sites *(38)*. In a study from Taiwan involving 57 patients with measurable brain metastases, 33.3% responded and the disease control rate was 63.2%, with PFS of 5.0 months and a median OS of 9.9 months *(51)*. Of 21 patients with simultaneously assessable extracranial and brain lesions, 17 (81%) had comparable responses in both sites, and survival was analogous to versus without brain metastases *(51)*. In another study of 41 patients from Italy with measurable brain metastases, 10% responded to gefitinib and 17% had stable disease, with a median PFS of 3 months *(52)*. Hence, overall the efficacy of gefitinib against NSCLC brain metastases appears to be similar to its efficacy against extracranial disease.

We previously documented that most chemotherapy agents tested achieve high concentrations in human brain tumors irrespective of concentrations achieved in the normal central nervous system and have advocated using agents that are active against a tumor regardless of whether they reach high concentrations in the normal nervous system *(53)*. This documentation of activity of gefitinib in brain metastases is in keeping with our thinking. Although there is less information on the efficacy of erlotinib in brain metastases, we would not anticipate substantial differences between erlotinib and gefitinib.

2.1.8. Agents That Act Against EGFR Plus Other erbB Targets

CI-1033 is a pan-erbB inhibitor that binds irreversibly in the EGFR ATP receptor pocket *(54)*. In a Phase I trial that included 18 patients with NSCLC, there were no responses, but there was evidence of down-regulation of EGFR, HER2, and Ki-67 in tumor tissues *(54)*. When combined with frontline paclitaxel and carboplatin, 26% of patients responded, 28% had stable disease, MS was 12.4 months, and PFS was 5.1 months *(55)*. Hence, its addition to chemotherapy did not appear to augment efficacy substantially.

In single-agent studies of the EGFR and erbB2 TKI lapatinib as first- or second-line therapy for patients with BAC or with no history of smoking, the response rate was only 2%, but 20% of patients had stable disease for $\geq$ 24 weeks *(56)*.

2.1.9. Clinical Prognostic and Predictive Factors in EGFR TKI Clinical Trials

Factors correlating with response or disease control with gefitinib and erlotinib (Table 1) include East Asian race *(23,30,34,57,58)*, adenocarcinoma *(26,30,34,37,59,60)* or BAC *(15)* histology (particularly nonmucinous, in contrast to mucinous, variants of BAC *(15)*), tumors with high TTF-1 expression *(15)*, female sex *(15,30,34,37,40,59,60)*, history of never having smoked *(15,23,26,30,34,37,59,60)*, good performance status *(60)*, no prior chemotherapy *(61)*, and development of skin rash *(51)* or diarrhea *(23)* with EGFR TKI therapy. Efficacy of prior chemotherapy *(34)*, type of prior chemotherapy (platinum vs. not) *(34)*, time since last chemotherapy *(26)*, number of prior chemotherapy regimens *(26,34)*, and patient age *(34)* were not associated with EGFR TKI response rates; and in occasional studies, a correlation of efficacy was not seen with sex *(26)*, tumor type *(40)*, smoking history *(40)*, and performance status *(34,0)*.

Table 1
Clinical Factors Possibly or Definitely Associated with
Improved Outcome on EGFR TKIs

East Asian race
Histology
    Adenocarcinoma
    BAC (particularly nonmucinous)
    High TTF-1 expression
Female sex
History of never having smoked
Good performance status
Less weight loss
No prior chemotherapy
Time from diagnosis
EGFR TKI toxicity
    Skin rash
    Diarrhea

BAC, bronchioloalveolar carcinoma; EGFR, epidermal growth factor receptor; TKI, thymidine kinase inhibitor

In univariate analyses, factors correlating with survival have been similar for gefitinib and erlotinib and have included Asian race *(58)*, female sex *(25,60,61)*, history of never having smoked *(42,60–62)*, good performance status *(25,27,33,60,61,63)*, adenocarcinoma histology *(25,60)*, development of a rash with EGFR TKI therapy *(27,33,42,46,51,61)* and rash severity *(33)*, history of less initial weight loss *(42)*, no prior chemotherapy *(63)*, and time from diagnosis to initiation of therapy with the EGFR TKI *(33)*. As with response, the correlation of these clinical factors with survival did not hold in all instances. In two trials, there was a trend toward an association between female sex and better survival, but statistical significance was not reached *(26,42)*; whereas in others, tumor histology *(27,42)*, performance status *(42)*, sex *(27)*, and development of diarrhea *(27)* did not correlate with survival.

In multivariate analyses, prognostic factors that have emerged as being independent significant predictors of survival in various trials of EGFR TKIs have included female sex *(25)*, good performance status *(25,63,64)*, adenocarcinoma histology *(25)*, history of no prior chemotherapy *(63)*, Asian race *(64)*, never having smoked *(64)*, less than 5% weight loss *(64)*, no prior cisplatin *(64)*, and a greater than a 12-month interval from time of diagnosis to enrollment in the trial *(64)*.

With respect to the greater efficacy of EGFR TKIs in nonsmokers compared to smokers, erlotinib clearance was 24% faster in current smokers than in former smokers or never smokers *(35)*, suggesting that part of the effect of smoking on outcome could be mediated by pharmacologic factors. Similarly, with respect to the link between the development of rash and EGFR TKI efficacy, pharmacology studies suggest that rash may increase with increasing erlotinib exposure, but there was no apparent relation between pharmacology and diarrhea *(35)*. Overall, these observations suggest that some factors that affect EGFR TKI efficacy may do so by altering drug pharmacology. However, the flat dose–response curves demonstrated in randomized trials for gefitinib *(29,32)* raise questions as to the importance of this altered metabolism in drug efficacy.

In addition to the above prognostic factors associated with duration of patient survival on EGFR TKIs, various *predictive factors* have been described that discern which patients will (versus will not) benefit from an EGFR TKI. In a randomized study comparing erlotinib to BSC in previously treated patients, the favorable impact of erlotinib on survival was greater in never smokers than in smokers, but there did nevertheless appear to be a beneficial effect in smokers as well *(62)*. In this trial, most groups assessed appeared to derive a survival benefit from the addition of erlotinib; and in the univariate analysis it attained statistical significance ($p < 0.05$) for the following factors: patients both older and younger than 60; male sex; adenocarcinomas and other tumor types; ECOG performance status 0 to 1; patients with a response to prior therapy; patients with one, two, or three prior regimens; patients with prior platinum-based therapy; never smokers; and race other than Asian. It approached significance ($p < 0.15$) for the following factors: female sex, ECOG performance status 2, current or ever smokers, and Asians *(34)*. Even male ever-smokers appeared to benefit from erlotinib *(62)*.

In the ISEL trial of gefitinib versus placebo, Asian patients had a significant improvement in OS, TTP, and objective response rates, whereas non-Asian patients did not have a significant improvement in survival parameters *(58)*. The other factor predicting a significant positive impact on survival with gefitinib in this trial was a history of never having smoked *(30)*.

Overall, it appears that patients with a broad range of characteristics may benefit from EGFR TKIs. Although some groups appear to benefit more than others, most groups appear to derive at least some benefit.

2.1.10. MOLECULAR FACTORS LINKED TO EGFR TKI EFFICACY OR RESISTANCE

Several molecular factors have been linked with efficacy of (Table 2) or resistance to (Table 3) EGFR TKIs.

2.1.10.1. EGFR Mutations and Their Impact on Efficacy of EGFR TKIs. Somatic mutations in the EGFR tyrosine kinase domain have been described in NSCLC and were

Table 2
Molecular Factors Possibly or Definitely Associated with Improved Outcome on EGFR TKIs

EGFR mutations
    Exon 19 deletions
    Exon 21 L858R point mutations
    Others?
High *EGFR* gene copy number
    EGFR amplification
    Chromosome 7 polysomy
EGFR protein expression?
p-AKT
    Low if *EGFR* wild-type
    High if *EGFR* mutation
PTEN expression
TP53 mutation
High *erbB2* gene copy number?
High *erbB3* gene copy number?
E-cadherin-positive

Table 3
Molecular Factors Associated with Possible or Probable
Resistance to EGFR Tyrosine Kinase Inhibitors

EGFR T790M mutations
erbB2 mutation?
KRAS mutation
p-ERK?
Epithelial to mesenchymal transition
Mesenchymal phenotype
Epithelial membrane protein-1
MET amplification

significantly associated with tumor EGFR overexpression in some series *(65)* and with mutations found in circulating DNA in the serum *(66)*. EGFR mutations have also been found in normal bronchial epithelium adjacent to tumors bearing the mutation, suggesting that such mutations may be an early event in the development of some NSCLCs *(67)*.

EGFR mutations are found in tumors from approximately 7% to 12% of North American or European NSCLC patients *(13,18,19,68–70)* (and have been seen in as many as 24% of a selected group of patients *(71)*), whereas they are seen in 19% to 59% of NSCLC cases in East Asians *(19,39,65,72–75)*. An additional 5% of North American patients may display novel gene variations consistent with germline polymorphisms *(69)*. Patients with EGFR mutations have a significantly better postoperative prognosis than patients with wild-type EGFR *(65)*.

Overall, there is a striking overlap between factors that predict efficacy of EGFR TKIs in NSCLC (as discussed above) and factors that are associated with EGFR mutations (Table 4). In one series *(19)*, EGFR mutations were found in 17% of lung adenocarcinomas versus 5% in other histologies, in 19% of women versus 9% of males, in 26% of nonsmokers versus 8% of smokers, and in 19% of Asians versus 11% of non-Asians. Overall, EGFR mutations appear to be more common in adenocarcinomas than in other histologies *(19, 59,73,76)*, in nonmucinous than in mucinous BACs *(15)*, in papillary tumors and tumors with BAC features than in other adenocarcinomas *(65)*, in women than in men *(19,59,66, 70,73,76,77)*, in nonsmokers than in smokers *(19,59,65,66,70,71,73,76,77)*, in Asians than in Caucasians *(19,71,77)*, in younger patients than in older patients *(19)*, in stage I tumors

Table 4
Clinical Factors Associated with *EGFR* Gene
Mutations

East Asian race
Histology
    Adenocarcinomas
    BAC features
    Nonmucinous BACs
    Papillary
Female sex
Nonsmokers
Age < 65 years
Stage I

versus later-stage tumors *(70)*, and in patients with an absence of emphysema or fibrosis on computed tomography (CT) *(65)*, but they are not restricted to these groups *(69,72,78,79)*. A significant association of mutations with female sex *(71)* and with adenocarcinoma or BAC *(71)* has not been noted in all series, and squamous cell carcinomas with EGFR mutations have been described *(71)*. In a multivariate analysis of Chinese NSCLC patients, adenocarcinoma and nonsmoker status were independent predictors of EGFR mutations *(73)*. Although the incidence of EGFR mutations is higher in Asians than in Caucasians, factors associated with increased probability of mutations appears to be similar in the two groups.

With respect to smoking, the probability of having an EGFR mutation is inversely proportional to prior tobacco exposure *(71,78)*. Mutations were found in 54% of never smokers *(71)*, 43% of ex-smokers *(71)*, and in 3% of current smokers *(71)*. The higher rate of EGFR mutations in females than in males may be related to the fact that most of the never smokers with NSCLC are female *(77)*.

Generally, exon 19 deletions in the tyrosine kinase ATP binding domain are the most common EGFR mutations seen, followed by exon 21 L858R point mutations *(13,15,59, 65,66,71,74,80)*. Other EGFR mutations that have been described in a small proportion of NSCLCs include exon 18 G719A, G179S, and G719C missense mutations; exon 19 A743S mutations; and exon 21 L861Q mutations *(13,74)*. In NSCLCs, it is uncommon to find EGFR mutations other than in exons encoding the kinase domain, although the EGFRvIII mutation is seen occasionally, particularly in squamous cell carcinoma *(77)*.

Tumor cells with EGFR mutations are more sensitive to gefitinib than are cells with wild-type EGFR *(21,77,81)*, particularly if the mutations consist of L858R point mutations on exon 21, G719S mutations on exon 18, or E746-A750 deletions on exon 19 *(77,81)*. On the other hand, S7681 and E709G mutations may actually confer resistance to gefitinib *(81)*, as may an exon 19 point mutation (D761Y), an exon 20 point mutation (T790M), and an exon 20 insertion (D770_N771insNPG) *(77)*.

NSCLC patients with tumors bearing EGFR mutations are more likely to respond to EGFR TKIs than patients with tumors bearing wild-type EGFR *(13,15,19,64,68,73,75–77)*; and in patients with mutations, responses can be rapid, dramatic, and prolonged. In previously treated patients, a response to gefitinib and erlotinib was seen in 16% to 83% with EGFR mutations versus 3% to18% with wild-type EGFR *(13,19,59,64,73,75,77)*. Similarly, in chemonaive patients, the EGFR TKI response rates of 75% to 100% reported in patients with EGFR mutations *(39,72,74)* are substantially higher than response rates in chemonaive patients with EGFR wild-type *(42,74)*. In multivariate analyses involving previously treated patients, EGFR mutation, adenocarcinoma, and a history of being a nonsmoker were independent predictors of response to gefitinib in one trial *(73)*, whereas EGFR mutational status, chromosome 7 polysomy, and never smoking predicted response to gefitinib were independent predictors in another trial *(82)*.

In randomized frontline trials of chemotherapy combined with placebo versus chemotherapy combined with an EGFR TKI, there was a trend toward higher response rates in the chemotherapy-EGFR TKI group for patients with EGFR mutations than for patients with EGFR wild-type *(19,83)*, and patients with mutations had a higher response rate with chemotherapy plus EGFR TKI than they did with chemotherapy plus placebo *(19)*.

Although there is a consensus that EGFR mutations increase the probability of response to EGFR TKIs, there is less certainty about the impact of mutations on survival. In previously treated and chemonaive patients receiving EGFR TKIs, patients with EGFR mutations had median OSs of 13 to 31 months *(71,74,77)* (with no apparent difference between gefitinib and erlotinib *(71)*), whereas in patients with EGFR wild-type, MS times were 5 to 14 months *(74,77)*. In some studies EGFR mutation was significantly associated with better PFS or TTP *(19,42,74–76)* and OS *(42,74–76,82)*, or the association with survival approached significance *(73)*, whereas in other trials mutation status did not significantly affect survival despite being associated with an improved response rate *(19,59,64,68)*. In patients with EGFR mutations, smoking history may be an independent predictor of survival, with never smokers surviving longer than those who have a $\geq$ 8 pack-year history *(71)*.

Although some studies have suggested that patients with EGFR mutations live longer than patients without EGFR mutations when treated with EGFR TKIs, both the mutant group and the wild-type group may derive benefit from EGFR TKIs. In a randomized trial of erlotinib versus placebo, the hazard ratio for survival was 0.73 in the EGFR wild-type group ($p = 0.13$) versus 0.77 in the EGFR mutation group ($p = 0.45$), suggesting that impact of erlotinib on survival was similar to with versus without EGFR mutation *(64)*.

EGFR-mutant patients treated with chemotherapy alone had a longer OS than EGFR wild-type patients treated with chemotherapy alone *(19,83)*. PFS was also longer for the mutant group *(19)*, suggesting that the presence of an EGFR mutation may alter either the tumor growth rate or the sensitivity to chemotherapy. On the other hand, although the differences were not statistically significant, in patients receiving adjuvant chemotherapy following resection of NSCLCs the median TTP and OS in patients with EGFR mutations were 13.2 and 40 months, respectively, whereas they were 22.9 and 43.2 months, respectively, in patients without EGFR mutations *(70)*. Furthermore, for reasons that are unclear, EGFR-mutant patients who were treated with chemotherapy plus an EGFR TKI did not have a longer survival than EGFR wild-type patients treated with chemotherapy plus an EGFR TKI *(83)*, although there was a trend toward a longer TTP in the mutant-type patients compared to the wild-type patients treated with chemotherapy plus an EGFR TKI *(83)*. EGFR-mutant patients treated with chemotherapy plus an EGFR TKI did not have better survival than EGFR-mutant patients treated with chemotherapy alone *(19,83)*.

Among patients with EGFR mutations, those with exon 19 deletions may be more sensitive to EGFR TKIs than patients with other types of mutation *(42,66,71,73,81,84)*, and exon 19 deletions are more common in patients having clinical characteristics associated with sensitivity to EGFR TKIs than are other types of EGFR mutation *(84)*. In patients treated with erlotinib or gefitinib, those with exon 19 deletions had a TTP of 12 months versus 5 months for those with L858R mutations and had an MS of 34 versus 8 months ($p = 0.01$) *(71)*. Response to gefitinib was seen in all of 16 patients with exon 19 deletions versus 8 of 13 patients with L858R mutations and other mutations *(59)*. Furthermore, among those with EGFR mutations, response to chemotherapy was seen only in those with exon 19 deletions *(85)*, suggesting that the EGFR mutation type could affect not only sensitivity to EGFR TKIs but also sensitivity to chemotherapy.

Overall, EGFR-activating mutations are associated with increased response rates to EGFR TKIs and may also be associated with improved survival with EGFR TKI therapy. Clinical characteristics associated with increased benefit from EGFR TKIs are also associated with increased an incidence of EGFR mutation. EGFR exon 19 deletions appear to confer the greatest degree of sensitivity to EGFR TKIs.

2.1.10.2. Increase in EGFR Copy Number Through Gene Amplification or Polysomy and Efficacy of EGFR TKIs. An increase in the gene copy number ("high gene copy number") can occur through either gene amplification (extra copies of the gene on a chromosome) or polysomy (extra copies of the chromosome). When gene amplification is seen, it is frequently wild-type EGFR that is amplified *(19)*, although high EGFR copy number with amplification of a mutant allele has also been reported *(74)*. EGFR polysomy or trisomy was more frequent with EGFR mutation than with EGFR wild-type *(86)*, and in one study all patients with EGFR mutation also had had EGFR polysomy or trisomy *(86)*.

In another study, high polysomy (defined as four or more gene copies in 40% of cells) was seen in 17% of patients; gene amplification (gene/chromosome ratio $\geq$ 2, or $\geq$ 15 gene copies per cell in $\geq$ 10% of cells) was seen in 14%; low polysomy ($\geq$ 4 gene copies in 10%–39% of cells) was seen in 27%; low trisomy (3 gene copies in 10%–39% of cells) was seen in 24% of patients; high trisomy (3 gene copies in $\geq$ 40% of cells) was seen in 2%; and disomy ($\leq$ 2 gene copies in > 90% of cells) was seen in 16% *(13)*. In other studies, high EGFR gene copy number was reported in 15% to 54% of NSCLC patients *(15,68,74,86,87)*. Tumors with EGFR polysomy or trisomy also had HER2 polysomy or trisomy in a high proportion of cases *(86)*. EGFR amplification might also be somewhat associated with increased EGFR protein expression as assessed by immunohistochemistry *(14)*.

Despite the fact that EGFR mutations may be associated with trisomy and polysomy, the factors that predict an increased incidence of mutations do not predict well for high gene copy number *(76)*. For example, whereas EGFR mutations are more common in Asians than Caucasians, the opposite may be true for EGFR gene amplification or increased copy number*(19,57)*; and the gene copy number or amplification (unlike mutation) was not significantly associated with sex *(19,76)*, pathologic subtype *(19,76)*, or smoking status *(19,76)*. Poorly differentiated tumors were more likely to have a high EGFR copy number than were well-differentiated tumors *(14)*. As with EGFR mutations, in patients with BAC variants EGFR high polysomy or amplification was seen significantly more often in patients with nonmucinous variants than in those with mucinous variants *(15)*.

In NSCLC cell lines, gefitinib sensitivity correlated with EGFR gene copy number (in addition to correlating with EGFR mutations) *(21)*. Clinically, the efficacy of EGFR TKIs may correlate with increased EGFR gene copy number, EGFR gene amplification, or polysomy for chromosome 7 (the chromosome on which the EGFR gene is located) *(19,64,74,75,82,86,88,89)*. Some studies have suggested that EGFR gene copy number may be a better predictor of response to EGFR TKIs than EGFR mutation *(86)*, and patients with both an EGFR mutation and a high gene copy number may be particularly likely to respond *(68)*. Patients with high gene copy number, revealed by fluorescence in situ hybridization (FISH), were more sensitive to EGFR TKIs than to chemotherapy, whereas EGFR FISH-negative patients were more sensitive to chemotherapy *(85)*. In previously treated patients, EGFR TKIs gave response rates of 20% to 32% in those with high gene copy numbers versus 2% to 15% in patients with low gene copy numbers *(19,64,75)*. The response to EGFR TKIs was noted in 60% of patients who had either a EGFR mutation or amplification versus 10% of patients who had neither amplification nor mutation *(19)*. In chemonaive Japanese patients, EGFR TKIs conferred a response rate of 72% in patients with a high EGFR gene copy number versus 38% in patients with a low gene copy number *(74)*. However, the gene copy number did not correlate with EGFR TKI efficacy in all trials *(68,90)*.

In some therapeutic trials of EGFR TKIs, high EGFR gene copy number was associated with longer TTP*(74)* or survival *(13,64,82)*, or a trend toward longer survival *(75)*, but this association was not seen in some other trials *(68,90)*. In randomized studies of gefitinib or erlotinib versus placebo in previously treated patients with NSCLC, a greater beneficial effect of gefitinib and erlotinib on survival was seen for patients with high a EGFR copy number than for patients with a low copy number *(13,64)*. In the erlotinib trial, EGFR amplification was prognostic for poorer survival overall ($p = 0.005$) but was predictive for a differential survival benefit with erlotinib *(91)*.

Despite the apparent association of EGFR gene copy number with response to EGFR TKIs, in randomized trials of chemotherapy plus EGFR TKI versus placebo, patients with a high gene copy number were no more likely to respond to chemotherapy plus EGFR TKI than they were to chemotherapy plus placebo*(19,87)*; and for patients in the chemotherapy plus EGFR TKI arm, response rates were comparable in the high gene copy number and low gene copy number patient groups *(19)*. Adding EGFR TKI to chemotherapy also did not augment survival in patients with a high EGFR gene copy *(87)*, whereas in one trial patients with EGFR high gene copy number treated with chemotherapy alone had a trend toward a longer survival compared to patients with a low gene copy number *(19)*.

Overall, as with EGFR gene mutations, patients with a high EGFR gene copy number appear to have higher response rates with EGFR TKIs than do patients with a low EGFR gene copy number; moreover, some studies also suggest more of a survival benefit from EGFR TKIs in the high gene copy number group than in the low gene copy number group. Patients who have either an EGFR mutation or a high gene copy number may derive more benefit from EGFR TKIs than patients who have neither. However, as with EGFR mutations, the addition of EGFR TKIs to chemotherapy does not appear to have substantial benefit in even the high gene copy group, and a high gene copy number may be associated with longer survival in patients treated with chemotherapy alone compared to those with a low gene copy number.

2.1.10.3. Impact of EGFR Protein Expression on Efficacy of EGFR TKIs seen by Immunohistochemistry. In some cell lines, there was no association between constitutive expression of EGFR and sensitivity to gefitinib *(92)*. In others, EGFR protein expression was necessary but not sufficient for gefitinib sensitivity *(21)*, whereas in still other cell lines, correlation between EGFR protein expression and sensitivity to EGFR TKIs was strongly positive *(20)*.

Clinically, EGFR protein expression may correlate with EGFR TKI benefit. In a randomized study of gefitinib versus placebo in previously treated patients with NSCLC, a beneficial effect of gefitinib on survival was seen in patients with positive EGFR protein expression by immunohistochemistry (IHC) [hazard ratio (HR) = 0.77] but not those who were EGFR negative (HR = 1.57) ($p = 0.049$) *(13)*. Similarly, in a randomized trial of erlotinib versus placebo as second- or third-line therapy, responses were noted in 11.3% of patients with EGFR-positive tumors, 3.8% in EGFR-negative tumors, and 9.5% in tumors with unknown EGFR status ($p = 0.10$) *(34)*. Erlotinib had a significantly beneficial impact on survival ($p < 0.05$) in EGFR-positive patients and in those whose EGFR status was not known but not in EGFR-negative patients, for whom the hazard ratio was 0.9 ($p = 0.70$) *(34)*. In multivariate analysis in this trial, adenocarcinoma ($p = 0.01$), never smoking ($p < 0.001$), and expression of EGFR ($p = 0.03$) were associated with response *(64)*, whereas EGFR expression did not influence survival with erlotinib in the multivariate analysis *(64)*. EGFR expression also was not a significant independent predictor of survival in a multivariate analysis of another erlotinib trial *(33)*, although there was a trend toward a greater benefit for erlotinib in the EGFR-positive group than in the EGFR-negative group in other studies *(62,93)*. In a randomized trial of erlotinib versus placebo, patients receiving placebo had slightly worse survival if their tumors expressed EGFR than if they did not *(93)*.

2.1.10.4. Impact of *KRAS* Mutations on Efficacy of EGFR TKIs. *KRAS* mutations occur in 8% to 23% of patients with NSCLC(*13,15,18,68,70,75,83*) and generally not in tumors that have EGFR mutations. If the tumor exhibits one mutation, it generally does not exhibit the other (*18,42,70,78,84*), and patient population characteristics differ with respect to the two mutation types (*78*). *KRAS* mutations are generally seen in smokers (*18,42*), unlike EGFR mutations. This suggests that smoking-related carcinogenesis may lead to lung cancer development through *KRAS* mutations and other pathways, whereas EGFR tyrosine kinase mutation is not usually caused by smoking and may drive tumor development in patients who have never smoked.

Tumors with *KRAS* mutations are generally resistant to EGFR TKIs (*15,41,42,75,89*). In patients with previously treated NSCLCs who received gefitinib or erlotinib, *KRAS* mutations correlated with progressive disease and with a shorter median TTP but did not correlate with survival (*68*). Patients with *KRAS* mutation with or without an increase in *KRAS* gene copy number had a greater than 96% probability of tumor progression (*68*). Patients with tumor *KRAS* mutations who had erlotinib added to their frontline chemotherapy in the TRIBUTE trial had a worse TTP and OS than patients treated with chemotherapy plus placebo (*83*). Hence, as a rule, patients with *KRAS* mutations generally do not derive benefit from EGFR TKIs.

2.1.10.5. Impact of p-AKT, PTEN Loss, p-ERK, and p53 on Efficacy of EGFR TKIs. Approximately 28% to 41% of NSCLCs are p-AKT-positive (*13,75*), and 32% have reduced PTEN expression (*75*). In Korean patients with wild-type EGFR who were treated with gefitinib, the presence of either a *KRAS* mutation or strong p-AKT expression was associated with significantly reduced response rates and significant shortening of PFS (*75*). No patient exhibited both *KRAS* mutation and p-AKT overexpression (*75*). On the other hand, in patients with EGFR mutations, p-AKT overexpression was associated with prolonged TTP (*80*). In still other studies, there was no apparent association between PTEN expression and gefitinib efficacy, despite the role of PTEN in suppressing activation of AKT (*13,19,75,94*).

In yet another study, expression of both p-AKT and PTEN correlated with improved survival after gefitinib treatment (*82*). In the latter study, there was a significant difference in OS between patients with chromosome 7 polysomy versus the groups with both chromosome 7 polysomy and p-AKT overexpression ($p = 0.002$) and both chromosome 7 polysomy and PTEN expression ($p = 0.04$). In the multivariate analysis, chromosome 7 polysomy and PTEN expression were both significantly associated with prolongation of OS ($p = 0.004$ and $p = 0.017$, respectively) (*82*).

Overall, the data suggest that the impact of p-AKT on EGFR TKI efficacy may be opposite for patients with versus without EGFR mutations or high EGFR gene copy number, with it being an adverse factor when associated with EGFR wild-type and low copy number versus a beneficial factor if associated with EGFR mutation or high copy number.

In one study in which 64% of tumors were p-ERK-positive, patients with p-ERK expression had a borderline reduction in the response rate to gefitinib (16% vs. 36%, $p = 0.057$) (*75*). *TP53* mutations have been reported in 33% of patients who responded to gefitinib versus 14% of nonresponders (*19*).

2.1.10.6. Impact of erbB2 and erbB3 Expression on Efficacy of EGFR TKIs. ErbB2 protein expression as determined by IHC is positive in tumor samples from 7% to 50% of NSLCC patients (*12,95,96*). Many NSCLC cell lines overexpress erbB2 (*96*), but strong overexpression (3+ IHC staining) is relatively uncommon (*97*). ErbB2 expression is associated with a poor prognosis (*96*). Whereas *erbB2* (*HER2/neu*) gene mutations are uncommon in NSCLC *(95)*, approximately 2% to 23% of patients with NSCLC have high *erbB2* gene copy number (high polysomy or gene amplification) *(95,97,98)*. The *erbB2* gene copy number did not correlate significantly with *EGFR* mutation or with *EGFR* gene copy number in one study *(76)*, whereas in another study if there was *EGFR* polysomy or trisomy there was also *erbB2* polysomy or trisomy in a high proportion of cases *(86)*.

EGFR and other erbB family members may undergo heterodimerization with erbB2 *(98)*. There is no consensus on how erbB2 affects EGFR TKI activity. In some cell lines *(81)* overexpression of erbB2 or erbB3 confers sensitivity to gefitinib *(81)*; and in gene expression arrays in NSCLC cell lines, sensitivity to gefitinib was associated with expression of several genes involved in the erbB signaling pathway or in pathways that interrelate with the erbB signaling pathway *(99)*. In keeping with this, some clinical studies have suggested that increased *erbB2* gene copy number might be associated with improved outcome in patients treated with gefitinib *(81,86,95)*, with a higher response rate (34.8% in erbB2 FISH-positive versus 6.4% in FISH-negative patients, $p = 0.001$), disease control rate (56.5% vs. 33.3%, $p = 0.04$), TTP (9.05 vs. 2.7 months, $p = 0.02$), and a trend toward longer OS (20.8 vs. 8.4 months, $p = 0.056$). Patients who are both erbB2-positive and also have increased EGFR protein expression or *EGFR* gene gain or mutation have significantly better response rates, disease control rates, TTP, and OS than patients who are negative for both *(95)*.

However, some preclinical studies have noted no impact of erbB2 on gefitinib sensitivity *(92)*. Still others have noted either no effect on EGFR TKI efficacy of *erbB2* or *erbB3* positivity in FISH analysis *(81)*, or else disease control rates with gefitinib were slightly lower in patients whose tumors overexpressed erbB2 than in those who did not overexpress it *(24)*. In addition, some clinical studies have suggested that *erbB2* mutations render cells resistant to EGFR TKIs *(89)*.

ErbB3 high polysomy or gene amplification was reported in 27% of NSCLC patients and was significantly associated with female sex and a history of having never smoked *(100)*. Patients with *erbB3*-positive tumors (26.8%) had a significantly longer TTP on gefitinib than did *erbB3*-negative tumors (3.7 vs. 2.7 months, $p = 0.04$) but did not have improved response rates or OS *(100)*.

Overall, the impact of erbB2 and erbB3 on EGFR TKI efficacy remains unclear. In patients undergoing frontline chemotherapy for advanced NSCLC, the response rate was not associated with EGFR, erbB2, or p-AKT status *(85)*.

2.1.10.7. Impact of E-cadherin and Epithelial-to-Mesenchymal Transition on EGFR TKI Efficacy. E-cadherin expression is substantially reduced or absent in approximately 10% of NSCLC tumor samples. Loss of E-cadherin expression is associated with dedifferentiation in squamous cell lung cancers, with local invasion and nodal metastases; and it is an independent prognostic factor associated with shortened survival of patients with NSCLC *(101)*. Tumor cells that are E-cadherin-positive appear to be more sensitive to EGFR TKIs than E-cadherin-negative tumor cells *(102)*; and epithelial-to-mesenchymal transition *(102)* or a mesenchymal phenotype *(81)* is associated with EGFR TKI resistance in NSCLC cell lines and xenografts.

In a randomized trial of erlotinib versus placebo combined with frontline chemotherapy, there was a trend toward longer survival among patients treated with chemotherapy plus erlotinib versus chemotherapy plusplacebo if their tumors stained positively for E-cadherin *(102)*. In contrast, there was a trend toward shorter survival in the group receiving erlotinib with chemotherapy if their tumors stained negatively for E-cadherin *(102)*. E-cadherin positivity was associated with a trend toward longer survival regardless of whether erlotinib was included in the treatment, suggesting that E-cadherin staining is a prognostic marker *(102)*. On the other hand, another epithelial marker, epithelial membrane protein-1 (EMP-1), is associated with resistance to gefitinib in lung adenocarcinoma xenografts and in clinical NSCLC tumor samples *(103)*.

2.1.11. ACQUIRED RESISTANCE TO EGFR TKIs

Some patients who initially responded to an EGFR TKI and then progressed were found to have a new T790M mutation in the EGFR TK ATP binding pocket domain *(79,104,105)*, a mutation that has also been reported in patients with disease resistant to erlotinib from the initiation of therapy *(41)*. The T790M mutation may develop primarily in cells that have a prior EGFR activating mutation *(104)*. This T790M mutation alters the ATP binding pocket such that erlotinib and gefitinib no longer fit in it and can no longer inhibit the TK *(79)*. However, irreversible inhibitors of EGFR TK are effective against tumor cells with these T790M mutations in preclinical systems and are now being tested clinically *(79)*.

Occasional cells with the T790M mutation have been found in tumors that have not been exposed to EGFR TKIs *(106)*, and tumors with T790M mutations present at baseline are less likely to respond to EGFR TKIs than tumors without such mutations *(106)*. This suggests that such tumor cells may in some cases exist at the time of initiation of therapy with EGFR TKIs and that over time they would be selected for, and would outgrow, the original tumor cell population.

Development of *MET* amplification in a gefitinib-sensitive NSCLC cell line was associated with onset of resistance to gefitinib, and inhibition of MET signaling restored sensitivity *(107)*. Evidence suggested that *MET* amplification caused gefitinib resistance by driving erbB3-dependent activation of PI3K *(107)*. In addition, *MET* amplification was found in 4 of 18 NSCLC clinical tumor specimens from patients who had developed EGFR TKI resistance *(107)*.

Overall, there is interest in exploring both irreversible EGFR TKIs and MET inhibitors as therapeutic options to overcome resistance to EGFR TKIs.

2.1.12. TOXICITY OF EGFR TKIs

Acneiform rash (in 50%–75% of patients) and diarrhea (in 20%–60%) are the most common side effects seen with EGFR TKIs *(30,33,34,37,39,40)*. Toxicity is usually grade 1 to 2. Severe toxicity is relatively uncommon. Fatigue, ocular toxicity (dry eyes or abnormal eyelash growth), alopecia, infection, and reversible hepatic dysfunction are seen occasionally *(34,39)*. Life-threatening or fatal interstitial lung disease is seen in about 1% of North American and European patients *(30)*, with a higher incidence in Asian patients *(39,60)*. In Japanese patients, 3.5% developed lung toxicity and 1.6% died *(60)*. Risk factors for development of lung toxicity included male sex, history of smoking, and presence of interstitial pneumonia *(60)*. EGFR mutation in the tumor is not associated with worsening toxicity of EGFR TKIs *(108)*.

2.1.13. ANTI-EGFR ANTIBODIES

In a Phase II study in previously treated NSCLC patients (who had tumors with the most expressed EGFR), the humanized anti-EGFR monoclonal antibody C225 (Cetuximab) resulted in a response rate of 4.5%, with stable disease in 30%, median TTP of 2.3 months, and MS of 8.9 months *(109)*. When cetuximab was added to frontline chemotherapy, the response and survival parameters were comparable to those expected with chemotherapy alone: response rates of 26% to 34%, median PFS or TTP of 4 to 5 months, and MS of 10 to 11 months *(110–112)*. When added to second-line docetaxel, efficacy appeared to be somewhat greater than would be expected with docetaxel alone, with a response rate of 28% and median TTP of 3 months *(113)*. Studies are underway combining cetuximab with chemotherapy plus bevacizumab as frontline therapy for advanced NSCLC and combining it with chemoradiotherapy for stage III disease.

In preclinical studies, the anti-EGFR monoclonal antibody B4G7 stimulated tumor cell growth. It led to heterodimerization with erbB2 and erbB3 and to phosphorylation of erbB3. The erbB3 phosphorylation and the stimulation of growth were blocked by a specific inhibitor of erbB2 *(114)*.

2.2. Anti-erbB2 Antibodies

As noted previously, approximately 2% to 23% of patients with NSCLC have a high erbB2 gene copy number *(95,97,98)*, and erbB2 protein expression (seen by IHC) is positive in tumor samples from 7% to 50% of NSLCC patients *(12,95,96)*. However, high overexpression (3+ staining on IHC) is uncommon *(97)*. Antibodies directed against erbB2 inhibit the dimerization of erbB2 with EGFR, erbB3, or erbB4 and have demonstrated activity against NSCLC xenografts in preclinical studies *(97)*. It has been postulated that the disruption of heterodimerization of erbB2 with other erbB members could prove therapeutically useful even in the absence of erbB2 overexpression *(98)*. In a Phase II trial of the anti-erbB2 antibody trastuzumab combined with paclitaxel plus carboplatin in NSCLC patients with tumors that stained ≥ 1+ for erbB2 on IHC, 24.5% responded, the median PFS was 3.3 months, the median OS was 10.1 months, and 1-year survival was 42% *(96)*. Although overall efficacy was similar to that expected with chemotherapy alone, the outcome may have been somewhat improved by the addition of trastuzumab in the 9% of patients whose tumors stained 3+ for erbB2 compared to expectations from historical controls *(96)*. However, in a Phase II trial of the humanized anti-erbB2 antibody pertuzumab, 0 of 33 NSCLC patients responded *(97)*.

3. PUTATIVE TARGETS AND AGENTS IN NSCLC: VASCULAR ENDOTHELIAL GROWTH FACTOR AND ITS RECEPTOR

3.1. Bevacizumab

High preoperative serum VEGF levels are associated with a poor prognosis in patients with stage I/II NSCLC *(115)*. The monoclonal antibody bevacizumab antagonizes tumor angiogenesis by binding and inactivating VEGF. In a randomized Phase II trial comparing the combination of two different doses of bevacizumab with carboplatin and paclitaxel to chemotherapy alone in the frontline therapy of advanced NSCLC, administration of bevacizumab was associated with an increased response rate and prolonged PFS and OS *(116)*. In addition, 19 patients who progressed on chemotherapy alone were crossed over to single-agent bevacizumab, and 5 of them experienced stable disease *(116)*. On bevacizumab, there was an increased risk of life-threatening or fatal hemoptysis in patients with squamous cell carcinoma of the lung, tumors located near large blood vessels, or tumor necrosis or cavitation *(116)*. In a subsequent Phase III randomized trial of chemotherapy alone versus chemotherapy plus bevacizumab, the addition of bevacizumab was associated with a significant increase in response rate (35% with bevacizumab versus 15% without it) and prolongation of PFS (6.2 vs. 4.5 months) and OS (12.3 vs. 10.3 months) *(117)*. Benefit of adding bevacizumab to chemotherapy appeared to be more pronounced for men than for women (117). Despite patients with squamous cell carcinoma being excluded from this Phase III trial, the risk of significant bleeding and fatal pulmonary hemorrhage was higher in the bevacizumab arm than in the control arm (117). Studies are currently underway to assess whether delivering low-dose radiation to squamous cell carcinomas prior to initiation of bevacizumab can reduce the risk of major hemoptysis.

Preclinical data indicate that VEGF signaling may be up-regulated by EGFR expression, and VEGF up-regulation may increase resistance to EGFR inhibitors (118). Preclinical data also suggest that VEGF inhibitors and EGFR inhibitors may have additive or supra-additive effects (118,119). When the combination of bevacizumab and erlotinib was tested in previously treated patients with advanced NSCLC, the response rate of 20%, stable disease rate of 65%, PFS of 6.2 months, and median OS of 12.6 months were higher than would be expected with erlotinib alone (119).

3.2. VEGF Trap (AVE0005)

Studies in advanced NSCLC have recently been initiated with VEGF Trap (AVE0005), a recombinant molecule consisting of the human VEGFR extracellular domains fused with the F_c portion of human IgG1 (120). Like bevacizumab, VEGF Trap binds and inactivates VEGF, but it has a greater affinity for VEGF than does bevacizumab. Among the first 33 patients evaluated, 2 responded, indicating at least a modest level of activity (120).

3.3. ZD6474 (Vandetanib)

ZD6474 is a small molecule that inhibits VEGFR TK and at higher concentrations also inhibits EGFR tyrosine kinase and RET (121). In a Phase I study of ZD6474, four of nine patients with refractory NSCLC achieved partial responses (122). In a randomized trial comparing ZD6474 to gefitinib in patients with previously treated NSCLC, PFS was 11.0 weeks in the ZD6474 arm versus 8.1 weeks in the gefitinib arm ($p = 0.025$), and disease control was seen in 45% of ZD6474 patients versus 34% of gefitinib patients (123). A higher proportion of patients achieved stable disease when crossed over from gefitinib to ZD6474 than with crossover from ZD6474 to gefitinib (123).

In randomized studies comparing chemotherapy alone to chemotherapy combined with two dose levels of ZD6474 as second-line therapy for NSCLC, there was a trend toward improved PFS in the ZD6474 100 mg/day arm (19 weeks with ZD6474 100 mg/day versus 12 weeks for docetaxel alone, $p = 0.07$) (124). The PFS in the group receiving ZD6474 300 mg/day with docetaxel was 17 weeks (124). Additional studies are needed to assess the impact on OS.

More recently, in a randomized Phase II study of carboplatin plus paclitaxel versus carboplatin plus paclitaxel plus ZD6474 versus ZD6474 alone as frontline therapy for advanced NSCLC, the ZD6474 alone arm was inferior to the two arms that included chemotherapy (125). There was a trend to longer PFS in the group receiving ZD6474 with chemotherapy compared to the chemotherapy-alone arm ($p = 0.098$) (125). Response rates were 32%, 25%, and 7%, respectively, for ZD6474 plus chemotherapy versus chemotherapy alone versus ZD6474 alone (125). Subgroup analysis suggested that women in particular may benefit from the addition of ZD6474 to chemotherapy (125), unlike the addition of bevacizumab to chemotherapy with a male predilection (117). High baseline serum E-selectin and IL-2R were adverse prognostic factors for PFS (121). Low levels of serum HGF and

IL-2R were associated with prolonged PFS in the group receiving ZD6474 alone but not in the chemotherapy-alone or chemotherapy plus ZD6474 arms *(121)*.

3.4. Sorafenib (BAY 43-9006)

Sorafenib (BAY 43-9006) inhibits VEGFR 1-3, PDGFRα and PDGFRβ, c-Kit, FLT3, RET, and the RAF/MAPK pathway; it is effective in NSCLCs in preclinical systems and is additive with gefitinib *(126)*. Only a small proportion of NSCLCs (0%–3%) harbor B-*raf* mutations *(13,127)*, but cells that do possess B-*raf* mutations may have increased sensitivity to gefitinib *(128)*. In a Phase II trial of sorafenib in patients with refractory NSCLC, no partial responses were seen, but 63% had stable disease with 48% overall having minor responses *(129)*. Four patients with stable disease developed tumor cavitation, including one who died of hemoptysis. The median PFS was 11.9 weeks *(130)*. In a Phase I trial of sorafenib plus gefitinib in patients with refractory NSCLC, the combination was well tolerated *(126)*. Additional studies are needed to assess efficacy, and further combination trials are underway.

3.5. Sunitinib

Sunitinib inhibits PDGFR, KIT, FMS-like tyrosine kinase 3, and VEGFR *(131)*. In a Phase II trial of sunitinib in refractory NSCLC, the response rate in 63 evaluable patients was 9.5%, and 43% of patients had stable disease *(132)*. The median PFS was 11.3 weeks, and the median OS was 23.9 weeks *(132)*. Fatal pulmonary hemorrhage occurred in two patients with squamous cell carcinomas, and a fatal cerebral hemorrhage occurred in one patient *(132)*. The agent is currently being explored further in combination with other agents.

3.6. Axitanib (AG-013736)

Axitanib (AG-013736) is a potent small-molecule inhibitor of VEGFR-1, -2, and -3 that at higher concentrations also inhibits PDGFRβ and KIT *(133)*. In preliminary studies in patients with advanced NSCLC (some of whom were treatment-naive), the response rate was 9.4%, with an MS of 12.8 months and a median PFS of 5.8 months *(133)*.

3.7. Nitroglycerin

Preoperative treatment with nitroglycerin has been reported to decrease expression of HIF-1α and VEGF in resected NSCLC tumor specimens *(134)*. It has also been associated with reduced plasma VEGF levels *(132)* and possibly increased chemotherapy efficacy *(134,135)*.

4. NSCLC AND OTHER ANTIANGIOGENIC AGENTS

Overall, the positive studies with bevacizumab provide solid evidence that antiangiogenic therapy is useful in NSCLCs. Although it is too early to assess fully the impact of orally available anti-VEGFR on small molecules in NSCLC, the preliminary data are encouraging.

4.1. CXCL8 (Interleukin-8) and CXCR2 Antagonists

When one angiogenic target is inhibited, there may be up-regulation of other angiogenic signaling cascades *(136)*, and there has been interest in CXCR2 as a possible mediator of resistance to anti-VEGF therapy. CXC chemokines are heparin-binding proteins *(137,138)*;

and family members that possess three amino acid residues, referred to as the "ELR" motif, at the NH_2-terminus are as potent as basic fibroblastic growth factor (bFGF) and VEGF with respect to their angiogenic effect *(139)*. The ERL-positive CXC chemokine CXCL8 (or interleukin-8, IL-8) is an autocrine growth factor for some cancer cells; it recruits neutrophils, macrophages, and endothelial cells to tumors that might support and stimulate tumor growth *(140–145)* and that might mediate aberrant angiogenesis *(146,147)*. CXCL8 is readily demonstrated in human NSCLC specimens *(148–150)*.

Receptors for CXCL8 include CXCR1, CXCR2, and Duffy antigen receptor; and binding of CXCL8 to CXCR2 promotes several aspects of angiogenesis *(138,151,152)*. Hypoxia and acidosis up-regulate CXCL8 expression through up-regulation of NFkB *(153,154)*, and EGFR-mediated signaling also stimulates CXCL8 production *(155)*. *KRAS*-induced tumor angiogenesis may be at least partially mediated through CXCR2*(156)*; and in *KRAS*-mutant mice that spontaneously develop lung cancer, CXCR2 neutralization blocks lung tumorigenesis *(157)* and induces endothelial cell apoptosis *(157,158)*. For these reasons, there is interest in exploring anti-CXCR2 strategies clinically.

4.2. Matrix Metalloproteinase Inhibitors

Matrix metalloproteinases (MMPs) secreted by endothelial cells may play a role in the invasion of endothelial cells into tissues during angiogenesis, and high preoperative MMP-9 serum levels were associated with poor prognosis in patients with stage I/II NSCLC *(115)*. In human NSCLC xenografts, the MMP inhibitor (MMPI) AG3340 inhibited angiogenesis and tumor growth, induced tumor necrosis, and potentiated chemotherapy *(159)*. However, in clinical trials in advanced NSCLC, MMPIs did not add substantially to chemotherapy. In randomized Phase II and III trials, addition of the MMPI BMS-275291 to frontline chemotherapy with paclitaxel and carboplatin did not improve the response rate *(160, 161)*, PFS, or OS *(161)*. Similarly, the MMPI prinomastat added to chemotherapy did not significantly improve response rates, PFS, or OS in advanced NSCLC compared to chemotherapy alone *(162)*, and it approximately doubled the hazard ratio for the development of venous thromboembolism *(163)*. The MMPI marimastat administered to patients with small-cell lung cancer after response to frontline chemotherapy also failed to improve outcome *(164)*.

4.3. Interferons

Interferons are potent inhibitors of angiogenesis in preclinical systems *(165)* and have been tested extensively in NSCLC clinical trials. However, addition of interferon-α (IFNα) alone to irradiation or chemotherapy *(166–173)* or the addition of IFNα plus retinoids *(174–178)* to chemotherapy in small Phase I-II trials did not appear to improve efficacy. In some randomized trials involving addition of IFNα to frontline chemotherapy for NSCLC, there appeared to be some favorable impact on response rates *(179,180)* or PFS *(179)* but no improvement in survival *(180)*.

Single-agent IFNβ induced no response in advanced NSCLC *(181)*. Phase II studies of IFNβ added to radiotherapy for locally advanced NSCLC induced quite high response rates and MS times *(182–184)*; but in a randomized trial, there was no significant improvement in MS (9.5 months for radiotherapy alone versus 10.3 months for radiotherapy plus IFNβ) or in the 1-year survival (44% vs. 42%) *(185)*. In Phase II trials, there was also little indication that IFNβ increased the efficacy of systemic regimens *(186,187)*. In a randomized trial, addition to chemotherapy of IFNγ or IFNγ plus IFNα also did not improve outcome *(188)*.

Overall, there is little indication that interferons are therapeutically useful in NSCLC.

5. OTHER INHIBITORS TO GROWTH IN NSCLCs

5.1. Src Inhibitors

Immunohistochemical assessments of NSCLC biopsy samples revealed activated Src in 33% of samples analyzed *(189)*, particularly in adenocarcinomas *(190)*. The ATP-competitive small-molecule TKI dasatinib (BMS-354825) inhibits Src; and in NSCLC cell lines it inhibited migration and invasion, altered cell morphology, blocked G_1 to S transition, and induced cell cycle arrest and apoptosis *(191)*. Src is both an upstream activator and downstream mediator of EGFR, and Src inhibition in NSCLC cell lines reduced phosphorylation of EGFR, erbB3, and erbB3; caused apoptosis in EGFR-dependent cell lines; and markedly potentiated gefitinib-induced apoptosis *(189)*. Clinical trials of Src inhibitors alone and Src inhibitors combined with erlotinib are currently underway in patients with NSCLC.

5.2. KRAS Inhibitors

KRAS mutations are found in about 8% to 23% of NSCLC tumor samples *(13,15,18,68, 70,75,83)* and are more common in adenocarcinomas than other tumor types, in smokers than in nonsmokers, in males than in females, and in poorly differentiated than in well-differentiated tumors *(78)*. As noted previously, *KRAS* mutations and *EGFR* mutations are generally mutually exclusive *(78)*. Regression analysis suggests that smoking history is the major determinant of *KRAS* versus *EGFR* mutation, and sex is a confounding variable *(78)*.

There was a trend toward worsened survival in NSCLC patients treated with postoperative adjuvant chemotherapy plus radiotherapy if their tumors harbored the *KRAS* mutation compared to patients with wild-type *KRAS* in one study *(192)*; and in another trial, patients treated with neoadjuvant chemotherapy prior to resection of early-stage NSCLC had shorter MS times and an increased risk of developing distant metastases if they had a *KRAS* mutation *(193)*.

Farnesyltransferase inhibitors interfere with membrane localization of KRAS by reducing farnesylation. When tested as a single agent in patients with advanced chemonaive NSCLC, the farnesyltransferase inhibitor R115777 did not result in objective responses in any of 44 patients, although 16% of patients did have disease stabilization for more than 6 months, and the MS time was 7.7 months, with the TTP 2.7 months *(194)*. The farnesyltransferase inhibitor L-778123 was also inactive in NSCLC *(195)*. Overall, despite the importance of *KRAS* mutations in NSCLC, K-ras inhibition by farnesyltransferase inhibition does not appear to be therapeutically effective.

5.3. Insulin-like Growth Factor and Its Receptor and the Receptor Inhibitors

In IHC assessments of human NSCLC tumor samples, 39% were positive for insulin-like growth factor-1 receptor (IGF-1R) *(94)*. The IGF pathway involves the ligands IGF-1 and IGF-2, six binding proteins (IGFBP-1–6), and two cell surface receptors (IGF-1R, IGF-2R) *(196)*. Lung cancers may display autocrine production and high levels of IGF-1 and overexpression of IGF-1R *(196)*. IGF-mediated signaling may potentiate lung cancer cell proliferation, survival, and metastasis *(196)*. Growth hormone regulates normal tissue production of IGF, but inhibition of growth hormone receptors by somatostatin has not proven helpful, possibly because tumor cell production of IGF may not be under growth hormone control *(196)*.

In preclinical systems, IGF-1R kinase inhibitors were effective against both NSCLC and small-cell lung cancer models, and anti-IGF-1R monoclonal antibodies have single-agent activity in NSCLC models and also potentiate chemotherapy *(196)*. Human trials of anti-IGF-1R antibodies are underway *(196)*. In a preliminary analysis of the addition of the anti-IGF-1R antibody CP-751871 to frontline NSCLC chemotherapy, the overall response rate after addition of the antibody was 46% versus 32% with chemotherapy alone *(197)*. The response rate of 52% with the combination was higher in nonadenocarcinomas than that in adenocarcinomas *(197)*. Among four patients who were switched to antibody after progression on chemotherapy, one experienced a response to antibody *(197)*.

Preclinical studies had suggested that the IGF-1R pathway is involved in resistance to EGFR targeting agents in NSCLC. Gefitinib *(198)* and erlotinib *(199)* (but not cetuximab) induced heterodimerization of EGFR:IGF-1R in cell lines with high IGF-1R expression, with activation of IGF-1R, activation of its downstream signaling mediators, increased survivin expression *(198,199)*, and stimulation of mTOR-mediated synthesis of EGFR *(199)*. Inhibition or reduction of IGF-1R *(198,199)*, survivin *(198,199)*, or mTOR activity *(199)* increased gefitinib-induced *(198)* and erlotinib-induced *(199)* apoptosis and reversed EGFR TKI resistance, whereas augmentation of survivin protected cells with low IGF-1R from gefitinib-induced apoptosis *(198)*. Human NSCLC tumors that overexpressed EGFR also generally had high IGF-1R expression *(198)*.

However, in clinical trials of gefitinib, IGF-1R expression did not correlate with gefitinib efficacy *(194)*, and patients whose tumors expressed IGF-1R had significantly longer survival times than those with IGF-1R-negative tumors in both univariate and multivariate analyses *(194)*. Similarly, in multivariate assessment of NSCLC patients treated with chemotherapy, high pretreatment plasma levels of IGF-1 and IGFBP-3 were independent factors for longer PFS ($p < 0.0001$ and $p = 0.001$, respectively), and high IGF-1, IGF-2, and IGFBP-3 levels were independently predictive for OS ($p = 0.004$, $p = 0.001$, and $p = 0.043$, respectively) *(200)*.

Trials of anti-IGF-1R antibody with chemotherapy are ongoing, and further trials are planned combining them with both chemotherapy and EGFR inhibitors. Clinical trials of oral small-molecule IGF-1R inhibitors are also starting.

5.4. mTOR Inhibitors

The mTOR inhibitor RAD001 (everolimus) gave a response rate of 5.3%, a stable disease rate of 45%, and median PFS of 11.3 weeks in NSCLC patients who had previously received chemotherapy, with a somewhat lower response rate and PFS in those who had previously failed both chemotherapy and treatment with an EGFR TKI *(201)*. Preclinical data suggest that inhibition of the PI3K/AKT/mTOR pathway reverses resistance to EGFR TKIs *(202)*. When RAD001 was combined with gefitinib in current or former smokers, responses were seen in 4 of 23 patients, including one with a *KRAS* mutation *(202)*. Enrollment on this trial continues, and a trial of RAD001 with erlotinib is also underway.

5.5. Protein Kinase C Inhibitors

Tamoxifen and toremifene may potentiate the effect of cisplatin by inhibiting protein kinase C (PKC) *(203)*. In a Phase II trial of high-dose toremifene added to cisplatin in the treatment of advanced NSCLC, toremifene blood levels matched those required in vitro for cisplatin potentiation *(203)*. The new agent enzastaurin inhibited PKC, the PI3K/AKT pathway, and proliferation and angiogenesis in preclinical systems; and it induced tumor cell apoptosis *(204)*. In a Phase II trial in previously treated patients with NSCLC, no patients responded, but 35% had stable disease, 14% of patients were progression-free at 6 months, the median PFS was 1.9 months, the median OS was 9.9 months, and 1-year survival was 46% *(204)*. Of interest, one patient who entered the trial experienced improvement of biopsy-proven nodal disease on positron emission tomography/computed tomography (PET/CT) scans, had progression of disease after 9 months on therapy, discontinued treatment with enzastaurin, and then had resolution of all enlarged nodes with no further therapy. She has been off treatment now for 14 months with no evidence of tumor regrowth (D.J. Stewart, unpublished data). The high proportion of patients stable for = 6 months with this agent suggests that further studies are warranted.

5.6. Proteosome Inhibitors

The proteosome is responsible for breaking down ubiquinated proteins and is important in the maintenance of protein homeostasis. Proteosome inhibition leads to cell cycle disruption, inhibition of transcription factors, inhibition of angiogenesis, reduced tumor cell proliferation, and increased apoptosis *(205)*. In a randomized Phase II trial in previously treated patients with advanced NSCLC, the proteosome inhibitor bortezomib (Velcade) resulted in an 8% response rate and a 29% disease control rate, with a median TTP of 1.5 months, MS of 7.4 months, and 1-year survival rate of 39% *(205)*. The disease control rate was higher at 54%, and the TTP was longer at 4.0 months in the comparator arm involving bortezomib plus docetaxel; but the response rates, MS times, and 1-year survival rates were comparable in the two arms. The efficacy of the two-drug combination did not appear to be much different from that expected with single-agent docetaxel, but it remains uncertain whether bortezomib adds benefit when combined with docetaxel *(205)*.

5.7. Retinoid X Receptor β Targeting

Expression of retinoid X receptor β (RXR β) is decreased in NSCLC compared to normal tissues, and higher RXR β expression is associated with improved survival. Bexarotene binding to RXR β induces heterodimerization and activation of proapoptotic genes *(206)*. In a Phase II trial of bexarotene in heavily pretreated NSCLC patients, MS was 5 months with a 1-year survival rate of 23% *(206)*. Survival was longer in patients with toxicity consisting of hypertriglyceridemia and rash than in others *(206)*.

In vitro, bexarotene enhances the growth suppression induced by erlotinib, and it repressed cyclin D1 expression *(207)*. Clinically, the combination of bexarotene and erlotinib was tolerable, and responses were seen in groups not usually responding to erlotinib alone, including men and smokers *(207)*. When bexarotene was combined with carboplatin and gemcitabine in previously untreated NSCLC patients, efficacy was comparable to that expected with chemotherapy alone *(208)*, and the MS was somewhat better than expected (14 months) when bexarotene was combined with cisplatin plus vinorelbine *(209)*. However, in randomized trials, bexarotene did not improve outcome when added to frontline NSCLC chemotherapy *(210)*. Some studies combining bexarotene with erlotinib continue.

5.8. Cyclooxygenase-2 Inhibitors

Cyclooxygenase-2 (COX-2) is overexpressed in 70% to 90% of NSCLCs *(211)*. The COX-2 inhibitor celecoxib reduced urinary prostaglandin metabolites but did not appear to increase the efficacy of docetaxel in a Phase II trial in previously treated NSCLC patients (response rate 11%, MS 6 months) *(211)*, although efficacy of the paclitaxel-celecoxib combination in a similar patient population did appear to be somewhat superior to what would have been expected with taxane alone (24% response rate, 41% stable disease, median TTP 5 months, MS 11 months) *(212)*. In addition, when celecoxib was added to radiotherapy for locally advanced NSCLC, the observed PFS rates of 66% at 1 year and 42% at 2 years were thought to be sufficiently promising to warrant further study *(213)*. When added to neoadjuvant paclitaxel plus carboplatin in patients with operable NSCLC, the addition of celecoxib abrogated the marked rise in tumor prostaglandin levels expected with chemotherapy alone, and a complete response rate of 17% and overall response rate of 65% were thought to be better than what would be expected with chemotherapy alone *(214)*.

The addition of celecoxib to gefitinib gave a response rate of 7% in patients with platinum-refractory NSCLC and hence did not appear to increase efficacy compared to what would be expected with gefitinib alone *(215)*. It remains uncertain whether COX-2 inhibitors have useful activity in NSCLC.

5.9. SGN-15

The Lewis Y antigen is expressed by most NSCLC tumors. SGN-15 is an antibody–drug conjugate with a chimeric murine monoclonal antibody against the Lewis Y antigen conjugated to doxorubicin. SGN-15 was administered with docetaxel as second-line or third-line therapy to patients with advanced NSCLC in a randomized Phase II trial. Survival was modestly longer in the arm that included SGN-15 than in the arm with docetaxel alone, and further studies are ongoing *(216)*.

6. CONCLUSION

Targeted therapies are now firmly established as therapeutic options for NSCLC. The EGFR inhibitors and VEGFR inhibitors have proven activity and are now in widespread use. It is anticipated that the usefulness of additional classes of agents will be established in the near future. Of particular interest and importance are agents effective against tumor cells that are resistant to chemotherapy, whether the resistance arises because of overexpression of resistance factors or it is, instead, due to down-regulation of transport and onset of reversible quiescence. Several new classes of agents are currently under investigation, including histone deacetylase inhibitors, DNA-methyltransferase inhibitors, proapoptotic agents, agents that antagonize antiapoptosis molecules, heat shock protein inhibitors, HIF-1α antagonists, and others. Further development of these approaches is awaited with interest.

REFERENCES

1. Thompson E. Latest advances and research in lung cancer. Drug News Perspect 2005;18(6):405–11.
2. Pignon J, Tribodet H, Scagliotti G, et al. Lung Adjuvant Clinical Evaluation (LACE): a pooled analysis of five randomized clinical trials including 4,584 patients. J Clin Oncol 2006;24(18s):366s.
3. Berghmans T, Paesmans M, Meert AP, et al. Survival improvement in resectable non-small cell lung cancer with (neo)adjuvant chemotherapy: results of a meta-analysis of the literature. Lung Cancer 2005;49(1):13–23.
4. Spiro SG, Silvestri GA. The treatment of advanced non-small cell lung cancer. Curr Opin Pulm Med 2005;11(4):287–91.
5. Cappuzzo F, Bartolini S, Calandri C,et al. Induction therapy for early-stage non-small-cell lung cancer. Oncology (Williston Park) 2004;18(suppl 5):32–7.

6. Shepherd FA, Fossella FV, Lynch T, et al. Docetaxel (Taxotere) shows survival and quality-of-life benefits in the second-line treatment of non-small cell lung cancer: a review of two phase III trials. Semin Oncol 2001;28(suppl 2):4–9.

7. Hanna N, Shepherd FA, Fossella FV, et al. Randomized phase III trial of pemetrexed versus docetaxel in patients with non-small-cell lung cancer previously treated with chemotherapy. J Clin Oncol 2004;22(9):1589–97.

8. Stewart DJ, Chiritescu G, Dahrouge S, et al. Chemotherapy dose-response relationships in non-small cell lung cancer and implied resistance mechanisms. Cancer Treat Rev 2007;33(2):101–37.

9. Stewart DJ, Raaphorst GP, Yau J, et al. Active vs. passive resistance, dose-response relationships, high dose chemotherapy, and resistance modulation: a hypothesis. Invest New Drugs 1996;14(2):115–30.

10. Liang XJ, Shen DW, Gottesman MM. A pleiotropic defect reducing drug accumulation in cisplatin-resistant cells. J Inorg Biochem 2004;98(10):1599–606.

11. Shen DW, Su A, Liang XJ, et al. Reduced expression of small GTPases and hypermethylation of the folate binding protein gene in cisplatin-resistant cells. Br J Cancer 2004;91(2):270–6.

12. Onn A, Choe DH, Herbst RS, et al. Tumor cavitation in stage I non-small cell lung cancer: epidermal growth factor receptor expression and prediction of poor outcome. Radiology 2005;237(1):342–7.

13. Hirsch FR, Varella-Garcia M, Bunn PA Jr, et al. Molecular predictors of outcome with gefitinib in a phase III placebo-controlled study in advanced non-small-cell lung cancer. J Clin Oncol 2006;24(31):5034–42.

14. Dacic S, Flanagan M, Cieply K, et al. Significance of EGFR protein expression and gene amplification in non-small cell lung carcinoma. Am J Clin Pathol 2006;125(6):860–5.

15. Wislez M, Antoine M, Poulot V, et al. IFCT0401-bio trial: predictive biological markers for disease control of patients with non-resectable, adenocarcinoma with bronchioloalvelolar features treated with gefitinib. J Clin Oncol 2007;25(suppl). Abstract 7653.

16. Nakamura H, Kawasaki N, Taguchi M, et al. Survival impact of epidermal growth factor receptor overexpression in patients with non-small cell lung cancer: a meta-analysis. Thorax 2006;61(2):140–5.

17. Dutu T, Michiels S, Fouret P, et al. Differential expression of biomarkers in lung adenocarcinoma: a comparative study between smokers and never-smokers. Ann Oncol 2005;16(12):1906–14.

18. Laack E, Schneider C, Gutjahr T, et al. Association between different potential predictive markers from TRUST, a trial of erlotinib in non-small cell lung cancer. J Clin Oncol 2007;25(suppl). Abstract 7651.

19. Bell DW, Lynch TJ, Haserlat SM, et al. Epidermal growth factor receptor mutations and gene amplification in non-small-cell lung cancer: molecular analysis of the IDEAL/INTACT gefitinib trials. J Clin Oncol 2005;23(31):8081–92.

20. Dassonville O, Bozec A, Fischel JL, et al. EGFR targeting therapies: monoclonal antibodies versus tyrosine kinase inhibitors: similarities and differences. Crit Rev Oncol Hematol 2007;62(1):53–61.

21. Helfrich BA, Raben D, Varella-Garcia M, et al. Antitumor activity of the epidermal growth factor receptor (EGFR) tyrosine kinase inhibitor gefitinib (ZD1839, Iressa) in non-small cell lung cancer cell lines correlates with gene copy number and EGFR mutations but not EGFR protein levels. Clin Cancer Res 2006;12(23):7117–25.

22. Haura E, Sommers E, Becker A, et al. Pilot phase II study of preoperative gefitinib in early stage non-small cell lung cancer with assessment of intratumor gefitinib levels and tumor target modulation. J Clin Oncol 2007;25 (suppl). Abstract 7603.

23. Thomas SK, Fossella FV, Liu D, et al. Asian ethnicity as a predictor of response in patients with non-small-cell lung cancer treated with gefitinib on an expanded access program. Clin Lung Cancer 2006;7(5):326–31.

24. Cappuzzo F, Gregorc V, Rossi E, et al. Gefitinib in pretreated non-small-cell lung cancer (NSCLC): analysis of efficacy and correlation with HER2 and epidermal growth factor receptor expression in locally advanced or metastatic NSCLC. J Clin Oncol 2003;21(14):2658–63.

25. Janne PA, Gurubhagavatula S, Yeap BY, et al. Outcomes of patients with advanced non-small cell lung cancer treated with gefitinib (ZD1839, "Iressa") on an expanded access study. Lung Cancer 2004;44(2):221–30.

26. Haringhuizen A, van Tinteren H, Vaessen HF, et al. Gefitinib as a last treatment option for non-small-cell lung cancer: durable disease control in a subset of patients. Ann Oncol 2004;15(5):786–92.

27. Mohamed MK, Ramalingam S, Lin Y, et al. Skin rash and good performance status predict improved survival with gefitinib in patients with advanced non-small cell lung cancer. Ann Oncol 2005;16(5):780–5.

28. Cufer T, Vrdoljak E, Gaafar R, et al. Phase II, open-label, randomized study (SIGN) of single-agent gefitinib (IRESSA) or docetaxel as second-line therapy in patients with advanced (stage IIIb or IV) non-small-cell lung cancer. Anticancer Drugs 2006;17(4):401–9.

29. Fukuoka M, Yano S, Giaccone G, et al. Multi-institutional randomized phase II trial of gefitinib for previously treated patients with advanced non-small-cell lung cancer (The IDEAL 1 Trial) [corrected]. J Clin Oncol 2003;21(12):2237–46.

30. Thatcher N, Chang A, Parikh P, et al. Gefitinib plus best supportive care in previously treated patients with refractory advanced non-small-cell lung cancer: results from a randomised, placebo-controlled, multicentre study (Iressa Survival Evaluation in Lung Cancer). Lancet 2005;366(9496):1527–37.

31. Mu XL, Li LY, Zhang XT, et al. Evaluation of safety and efficacy of gefitinib ('iressa', zd1839) as monotherapy in a series of Chinese patients with advanced non-small-cell lung cancer: experience from a compassionate-use programme. BMC Cancer 2004;4:51.

32. Kris MG, Natale RB, Herbst RS, et al. Efficacy of gefitinib, an inhibitor of the epidermal growth factor receptor tyrosine kinase, in symptomatic patients with non-small cell lung cancer: a randomized trial. JAMA 2003;290(16):2149–58.

33. Perez-Soler R, Chachoua A, Hammond LA, et al. Determinants of tumor response and survival with erlotinib in patients with non-small-cell lung cancer. J Clin Oncol 2004;22(16):3238–47.

34. Shepherd FA, Rodrigues Pereira J, Ciuleanu T, et al. Erlotinib in previously treated non-small-cell lung cancer. N Engl J Med 2005;353(2):123–32.

35. Lu JF, Eppler SM, Wolf J, et al. Clinical pharmacokinetics of erlotinib in patients with solid tumors and exposure-safety relationship in patients with non-small cell lung cancer. Clin Pharmacol Ther 2006;80(2):136–45.

36. Milton DT, Azzoli CG, Heelan RT, et al. A phase I/II study of weekly high-dose erlotinib in previously treated patients with nonsmall cell lung cancer. Cancer 2006;107(5):1034–41.

37. Reck M, Buchholz E, Romer KS, et al. Gefitinib monotherapy in chemotherapy-naive patients with inoperable stage III/IV non-small-cell lung cancer. Clin Lung Cancer 2006;7(6):406–11.

38. Lee DH, Han JY, Lee HG, et al. Gefitinib as a first-line therapy of advanced or metastatic adenocarcinoma of the lung in never-smokers. Clin Cancer Res 2005;11(8):3032–7.

39. Niho S, Kubota K, Goto K, et al. First-line single agent treatment with gefitinib in patients with advanced non-small-cell lung cancer: a phase II study. J Clin Oncol 2006;24(1):64–9.

40. Suzuki R, Hasegawa Y, Baba K, et al. A phase II study of single-agent gefitinib as first-line therapy in patients with stage IV non-small-cell lung cancer. Br J Cancer 2006;94(11):1599–603.

41. Giaccone G, Gallegos Ruiz M, et al. Erlotinib for frontline treatment of advanced non-small cell lung cancer: a phase II study. Clin Cancer Res 2006;12(20 Pt 1):6049–55.

42. Jackman DM, Yeap BY, Lindeman NI, et al. Phase II clinical trial of chemotherapy-naive patients > or = 70 years of age treated with erlotinib for advanced non-small-cell lung cancer. J Clin Oncol 2007;25(7):760–6.

43. Kelly K, Chansky K, Gaspar LE, et al. Updated analysis of SWOG 0023: a randomized phase III trial of gefitinib vs placebo maintenance after defintive chemoradiation followed by docetaxel in patients with locally advanced stage III non-small cell lung cancer. J Clin Oncol 2007;25(suppl). Abstract 7513.

44. Herbst RS, Giaccone G, Schiller JH, et al. Gefitinib in combination with paclitaxel and carboplatin in advanced non-small-cell lung cancer: a phase III trial—INTACT 2. J Clin Oncol 2004;22(5):785–94.

45. Giaccone G, Herbst RS, Manegold C, et al. Gefitinib in combination with gemcitabine and cisplatin in advanced non-small-cell lung cancer: a phase III trial—INTACT 1. J Clin Oncol 2004;22(5):777–84.

46. Gatzemeier U, Pluzanska A, Szczesna A, et al. Phase III study of erlotinib in combination with cisplatin and gemcitabine in advanced non-small-cell lung cancer: the Tarceva Lung Cancer Investigation Trial. J Clin Oncol 2007;25(12):1545–52.

47. Herbst RS, Prager D, Hermann R, et al. TRIBUTE: a phase III trial of erlotinib hydrochloride (OSI-774) combined with carboplatin and paclitaxel chemotherapy in advanced non-small-cell lung cancer. J Clin Oncol 2005;23(25):5892–9.

48. Davies AM, Ho C, Lara PN Jr, et al. Pharmacodynamic separation of epidermal growth factor receptor tyrosine kinase inhibitors and chemotherapy in non-small-cell lung cancer. Clin Lung Cancer 2006;7(6):385–8.

49. Cappuzzo F, Ardizzoni A, Soto-Parra H, et al. Epidermal growth factor receptor targeted therapy by ZD 1839 (Iressa) in patients with brain metastases from non-small cell lung cancer (NSCLC). Lung Cancer 2003;41(2):227–31.

50. Hotta K, Kiura K, Ueoka H, et al. Effect of gefitinib ('Iressa', ZD1839) on brain metastases in patients with advanced non-small-cell lung cancer. Lung Cancer 2004;46(2):255–61.

51. Chiu CH, Tsai CM, Chen YM, et al. Gefitinib is active in patients with brain metastases from non-small cell lung cancer and response is related to skin toxicity. Lung Cancer 2005;47(1):129–38.

52. Ceresoli GL, Cappuzzo F, Gregorc V, et al. Gefitinib in patients with brain metastases from non-small-cell lung cancer: a prospective trial. Ann Oncol 2004;15(7):1042–7.

53. Stewart DJ. A critique of the role of the blood-brain barrier in the chemotherapy of human brain tumors. J Neurooncol 1994;20(2):121–39.

54. Zinner RG, Nemunaitis J, Eiseman I, et al. Phase I clinical and pharmacodynamic evaluation of oral CI-1033 in patients with refractory cancer. Clin Cancer Res 2007;13(10):3006–14.

55. Chiappori AA, Ellis PM, Hamm JT, et al. A phase I evaluation of oral CI-1033 in combination with paclitaxel and carboplatin as first-line chemotherapy in patients with advanced non-small cell lung cancer. J Thorac Oncol 2006;1(9):1010–9.

56. Smylie M, Blumenschein G, Dowlati A, et al. A phase II multicenter trial comparing two schedules of lapatinib as first or second line monotherapy in subjects with advanced or metasatic non-small lung cancer with either bronchioloalveolar carcinoma or no smoking history. J Clin Oncol 2007;25(suppl). Abstract 7611.

57. Calvo E, Baselga J. Ethnic differences in response to epidermal growth factor receptor tyrosine kinase inhibitors. J Clin Oncol 2006;24(14):2158–63.

58. Chang A, Parikh P, Thongprasert S, et al. Gefitinib (IRESSA) in patients of Asian origin with refractory advanced non-small cell lung cancer: subset analysis from the ISEL study. J Thorac Oncol 2006;1(8):847–55.

59. Mitsudomi T, Kosaka T, Endoh H, et al. Mutations of the epidermal growth factor receptor gene predict prolonged survival after gefitinib treatment in patients with non-small-cell lung cancer with postoperative recurrence. J Clin Oncol 2005;23(11):2513–20.

60. Ando M, Okamoto I, Yamamoto N, et al. Predictive factors for interstitial lung disease, antitumor response, and survival in non-small-cell lung cancer patients treated with gefitinib. J Clin Oncol 2006;24(16):2549–56.

61. West HL, Franklin WA, McCoy J, et al. Gefitinib therapy in advanced bronchioloalveolar carcinoma: Southwest Oncology Group study S0126. J Clin Oncol 2006;24(12):1807–13.

62. Clark GM, Zborowski DM, Santabarbara P, et al. Smoking history and epidermal growth factor receptor expression as predictors of survival benefit from erlotinib for patients with non-small-cell lung cancer in the National Cancer Institute of Canada Clinical Trials Group study BR.21. Clin Lung Cancer 2006;7(6): 389–94.

63. Lee DH, Han JY, Yu SY, et al. The role of gefitinib treatment for Korean never-smokers with advanced or metastatic adenocarcinoma of the lung: a prospective study. J Thorac Oncol 2006;1(9):965–71.

64. Tsao MS, Sakurada A, Cutz JC, et al. Erlotinib in lung cancer: molecular and clinical predictors of outcome. N Engl J Med 2005;353(2):133–44.

65. Ohtsuka K, Ohnishi H, Furuyashiki G, et al. Clinico-pathological and biological significance of tyrosine kinase domain gene mutations and overexpression of epidermal growth factor receptor for lung adenocarcinoma. J Thorac Oncol 2006;1(8):787–95.

66. Moran T, Paz-Ares L, Isla D, et al. High correspondence between EGFR mutations in tissue and in circulating DNA from non-small cell lung cancer patients with poor performance status. J Clin Oncol 2007;25(suppl). Abstract 7505.

67. Tang X, Shigematsu H, Bekele BN, et al. EGFR tyrosine kinase domain mutations are detected in histologically normal respiratory epithelium in lung cancer patients. Cancer Res 2005;65(17):7568–72.

68. Massarelli E, Varella-Garcia M, Tang X, et al. KRAS mutation is an important predictor of resistance to therapy with epidermal growth factor receptor tyrosine kinase inhibitors in non-small-cell lung cancer. Clin Cancer Res 2007;13(10):2890–6.

69. Yang SH, Mechanic LE, Yang P, et al. Mutations in the tyrosine kinase domain of the epidermal growth factor receptor in non-small cell lung cancer. Clin Cancer Res 2005;11(6):2106–10.

70. Murray S, Timotheadou E, Linardou H, et al. Mutations of the epidermal growth factor receptor tyrosine kinase domain and associations with clinicopathological features in non-small cell lung cancer patients. Lung Cancer 2006;52(2):225–33.

71. Riely GJ, Pao W, Pham D, et al. Clinical course of patients with non-small cell lung cancer and epidermal growth factor receptor exon 19 and exon 21 mutations treated with gefitinib or erlotinib. Clin Cancer Res 2006;12(Pt 1):839–44.

72. Inoue A, Suzuki T, Fukuhara T, et al. Prospective phase II study of gefitinib for chemotherapy-naive patients with advanced non-small-cell lung cancer with epidermal growth factor receptor gene mutations. J Clin Oncol 2006;24(21):3340–6.

73. Wu YL, Zhong WZ, Li LY, et al. Epidermal growth factor receptor mutations and their correlation with gefitinib therapy in patients with non-small cell lung cancer: a meta-analysis based on updated individual patient data from six medical centers in mainland China. J Thorac Oncol 2007;2(5):430–9.

74. Takano T, Ohe Y, Sakamoto H, et al. Epidermal growth factor receptor gene mutations and increased copy numbers predict gefitinib sensitivity in patients with recurrent non-small-cell lung cancer. J Clin Oncol 2005;23(28):6829–37.

75. Han SW, Kim TY, Jeon YK, et al. Optimization of patient selection for gefitinib in non-small cell lung cancer by combined analysis of epidermal growth factor receptor mutation, K-ras mutation, and Akt phosphorylation. Clin Cancer Res 2006;12(8):2538–44.

76. Endo K, Sasaki H, Yano M, et al. Evaluation of the epidermal growth factor receptor gene mutation and copy number in non-small cell lung cancer with gefitinib therapy. Oncol Rep 2006;16(3):533–41.

77. Riely GJ, Politi KA, Miller VA, Pao W. Update on epidermal growth factor receptor mutations in non-small cell lung cancer. Clin Cancer Res 2006;12(24):7232–41.
78. Tam IY, Chung LP, Suen WS, et al. Distinct epidermal growth factor receptor and KRAS mutation patterns in non-small cell lung cancer patients with different tobacco exposure and clinicopathologic features. Clin Cancer Res 2006;12(5):1647–53.
79. Haber DA, Bell DW, Sordella R, et al. Molecular targeted therapy of lung cancer: EGFR mutations and response to EGFR inhibitors. Cold Spring Harb Symp Quant Biol 2005;70:419–26.
80. Han SW, Kim TY, Hwang PG, et al. Predictive and prognostic impact of epidermal growth factor receptor mutation in non-small-cell lung cancer patients treated with gefitinib. J Clin Oncol 2005;23(11):2493–501.
81. Rosell R, Taron M, Reguart N, et al. Epidermal growth factor receptor activation: how exon 19 and 21 mutations changed our understanding of the pathway. Clin Cancer Res 2006;12(24):7222–31.
82. Buckingham LE, Coon JS, Morrison LE, et al. The prognostic value of chromosome 7 polysomy in non-small cell lung cancer patients treated with gefitinib. J Thorac Oncol 2007;2(5):414–22.
83. Eberhard DA, Johnson BE, Amler LC, et al. Mutations in the epidermal growth factor receptor and in KRAS are predictive and prognostic indicators in patients with non-small-cell lung cancer treated with chemotherapy alone and in combination with erlotinib. J Clin Oncol 2005;23(25):5900–9.
84. Van Zandwijk N, Mathy A, Boerrigter L, et al. EGFR and KRAS mutations as criteria for treatment with tyrosine kinase inhibitors: retro- and prospective observations in non-small-cell lung cancer. Ann Oncol 2007;18(1):99–103.
85. Cappuzzo F, Ligorio C, Toschi L, et al. EGFR and HER2 gene copy number and response to first-line chemotherapy in patients with advanced non-small cell lung cancer (NSCLC). J Thorac Oncol 2007;2(5):423–9.
86. Daniele L, Macri L, Schena M, et al. Predicting gefitinib responsiveness in lung cancer by fluorescence in situ hybridization/chromogenic in situ hybridization analysis of EGFR and HER2 in biopsy and cytology specimens. Mol Cancer Ther 2007;6(4):1223–9.
87. Hirsch FR, Varella-Garcia M, Bunn PA, et al. Fluorescence in situ hybridization (FISH) subgroup analysis of TRIBUTE, a phase III trial of erlotinib plus carboplatin and paclitaxel in NSCLC. J Clin Oncol 2007;25(suppl). Abstract 7570.
88. Amler LC, Goddard AD, Hillan KJ. Predicting clinical benefit in non-small-cell lung cancer patients treated with epidermal growth factor tyrosine kinase inhibitors. Cold Spring Harb Symp Quant Biol 2005;70:483–8.
89. Cappuzzo F. Predictive factors for response and for resistance to tyrosine kinase inhibitor therapy in lung cancer. J Thorac Oncol 2007;2(suppl):S12–4.
90. Dziadziuszko R, Witta SE, Cappuzzo F, et al. Epidermal growth factor receptor messenger RNA expression, gene dosage, and gefitinib sensitivity in non-small cell lung cancer. Clin Cancer Res 2006;12(10):3078–84.
91. Shepherd F, Ding K, Sakurada A, et al. Updated molecular analysis of exons 19 and 21 of the epidermal growth factor gene and codons 12 and 13 of the KRAS gene in non-small cell lung cancer patients treated with erlotinib in National Cancer Institute of Canada. J Clin Oncol 2007;25(suppl). Abstract 7571.
92. Van Schaeybroeck S, Kyula J, Kelly DM, et al. Chemotherapy-induced epidermal growth factor receptor activation determines response to combined gefitinib/chemotherapy treatment in non-small cell lung cancer cells. Mol Cancer Ther 2006;5(5):1154–65.
93. Clark GM, Zborowski DM, Culbertson JL, et al. Clinical utility of epidermal growth factor receptor expression for selecting patients with advanced non-small cell lung cancer for treatment with erlotinib. J Thorac Oncol 2006;1(8):837–46.
94. Cappuzzo F, Toschi L, Tallini G, et al. Insulin-like growth factor receptor 1 (IGFR-1) is significantly associated with longer survival in non-small-cell lung cancer patients treated with gefitinib. Ann Oncol 2006;17(7):1120–7.
95. Cappuzzo F, Varella-Garcia M, Shigematsu H, et al. Increased HER2 gene copy number is associated with response to gefitinib therapy in epidermal growth factor receptor-positive non-small-cell lung cancer patients. J Clin Oncol 2005;23(22):5007–18.
96. Langer CJ, Stephenson P, Thor A, et al. Trastuzumab in the treatment of advanced non-small-cell lung cancer: is there a role? Focus on Eastern Cooperative Oncology Group study 2598. J Clin Oncol 2004;22(7):1180–7.
97. Johnson BE, Janne PA. Rationale for a phase II trial of pertuzumab, a HER-2 dimerization inhibitor, in patients with non-small cell lung cancer. Clin Cancer Res 2006;12(14 Pt 2):4436s-40s.
98. Swanton C, Futreal A, Eisen T. Her2-targeted therapies in non-small cell lung cancer. Clin Cancer Res 2006;12(14 Pt 2):4377s-83s.
99. Coldren CD, Helfrich BA, Witta SE, et al. Baseline gene expression predicts sensitivity to gefitinib in non-small cell lung cancer cell lines. Mol Cancer Res 2006;4(8):521–8.
100. Cappuzzo F, Toschi L, Domenichini I, et al. HER3 genomic gain and sensitivity to gefitinib in advanced non-small-cell lung cancer patients. Br J Cancer 2005;93(12):1334–40.

101. Bremnes RM, Veve R, Gabrielson E, et al. High-throughput tissue microarray analysis used to evaluate biology and prognostic significance of the E-cadherin pathway in non-small-cell lung cancer. J Clin Oncol 2002;20(10):2417–28.

102. Yauch RL, Januario T, Eberhard DA, et al. Epithelial versus mesenchymal phenotype determines in vitro sensitivity and predicts clinical activity of erlotinib in lung cancer patients. Clin Cancer Res 2005; 11(24 Pt 1):8686–98.

103. Jain A, Tindell CA, Laux I, et al. Epithelial membrane protein-1 is a biomarker of gefitinib resistance. Proc Natl Acad Sci U S A 2005;102(33):11858–63.

104. Kosaka T, Yatabe Y, Endoh H, et al. Analysis of epidermal growth factor receptor gene mutation in patients with non-small cell lung cancer and acquired resistance to gefitinib. Clin Cancer Res 2006; 12(19):5764–9.

105. Balak MN, Gong Y, Riely GJ, et al. Novel D761Y and common secondary T790M mutations in epidermal growth factor receptor-mutant lung adenocarcinomas with acquired resistance to kinase inhibitors. Clin Cancer Res 2006;12(21):6494–501.

106. Inukai M, Toyooka S, Ito S, et al. Presence of epidermal growth factor receptor gene T790M mutation as a minor clone in non-small cell lung cancer. Cancer Res 2006;66(16):7854–8.

107. Engelman JA, Zejnullahu K, Mitsudomi T, et al. MET amplification leads to gefitinib resistance in lung cancer by activating ERBB3 signaling. Science 2007;316(5827):1039–43.

108. Fujiwara Y, Kiura K, Toyooka S, et al. Relationship between epidermal growth factor receptor gene mutations and the severity of adverse events by gefitinib in patients with advanced non-small cell lung cancer. Lung Cancer 2006;52(1):99–103.

109. Hanna N, Lilenbaum R, Ansari R, et al. Phase II trial of cetuximab in patients with previously treated non-small-cell lung cancer. J Clin Oncol 2006;24(33):5253–8.

110. Thienelt CD, Bunn PA Jr, Hanna N, et al. Multicenter phase I/II study of cetuximab with paclitaxel and carboplatin in untreated patients with stage IV non-small-cell lung cancer. J Clin Oncol 2005;23(34):8786–93.

111. Bareschino MA, Morgillo F, Ciardiello F. Combination of standard chemotherapy and targeted agents. J Thorac Oncol 2007;2(suppl):S19–23.

112. Herbst RS, Chansky K, Kelly K, et al. A phase II randomized selection trial evaluating concurrent chemotherapy plus cetuximab or chemotherapy followed by cetuximab in patients with advanced NSCLC: final report of SWOG 0342. J Clin Oncol 2007;25(suppl). Abstract 7545.

113. Kim ES, Mauer A, Tran HT, et al. A phase II study of cetuximab, an epidermal growth factor receptor blocking antibody, in combination with docetaxel in chemotherapy refractory/resistant patients with advanced non-small cell lung cancer: final report. Proc Am Soc Clin Oncol 2003;22. Abstract 2581.

114. Maegawa M, Takeuchi K, Funakoshi E, et al. Growth stimulation of non-small cell lung cancer cell lines by antibody against epidermal growth factor receptor promoting formation of ErbB2/ErbB3 heterodimers. Mol Cancer Res 2007;5(4):393–401.

115. Laack E, Kohler A, Kugler C, et al. Pretreatment serum levels of matrix metalloproteinase-9 and vascular endothelial growth factor in non-small-cell lung cancer. Ann Oncol 2002;13(10):1550–7.

116. Johnson DH, Fehrenbacher L, Novotny WF, et al. Randomized phase II trial comparing bevacizumab plus carboplatin and paclitaxel with carboplatin and paclitaxel alone in previously untreated locally advanced or metastatic non-small-cell lung cancer. J Clin Oncol 2004;22(11):2184–91.

117. Sandler A, Gray R, Perry MC, et al. Paclitaxel-carboplatin alone or with bevacizumab for non-small-cell lung cancer. N Engl J Med 2006;355(24):2542–50.

118. Tabernero J. The role of VEGF and EGFR inhibition: implications for combining anti-VEGF and anti-EGFR agents. Mol Cancer Res 2007;5(3):203–20.

119. Herbst RS, Johnson DH, Mininberg E, et al. Phase I/II trial evaluating the anti-vascular endothelial growth factor monoclonal antibody bevacizumab in combination with the HER-1/epidermal growth factor receptor tyrosine kinase inhibitor erlotinib for patients with recurrent non-small-cell lung cancer. J Clin Oncol 2005;23(11):2544–55.

120. Massarelli E, Miller V, Leighl N, et al. Phase II study of the efficacy of intravenous AVE0005 (VEGF trap) given every 2 weeks in patients with platinum- and erlotinib-resistant adenocarcinoma of the lung. J Clin Oncol 2007;25(suppl). Abstract 7627.

121. Hanrahan EO, Lin HY, Du D, et al. Correlative analyses of plasma cytokine/angiogenic factor profile, sex and outcome in a randomized, three-arm, phase II trial of first-line vanbdetanib and/or carboplatin plus paclitaxel for advanced non-small cell lung cancer. J Clin Oncol 2007;25(suppl). Abstract 7593.

122. Herbst RS, Onn A, Sandler A. Angiogenesis and lung cancer: prognostic and therapeutic implications. J Clin Oncol 2005;23(14):3243–56.

123. Natale R, Bodkin D, Govindan R, et al. ZD6474 versus gefitinib in patients with advanced NSCLC: final results from a two-part, double-blind, randomized phase II trial. J Clin Oncol 2006;24(suppl). Abstract 7000.

124. Heymach JV, Johnson BE, Prager D, et al. A phase II trial of ZD6474 plus docetaxel in patients with previously treated NSCLC: follow-up results. J Clin Oncol 2006;24(suppl). Abstract 7016.

125. Heymach JV, Paz-Ares L, De Braud F, et al. Randomized phase II study of vandetanib alone or in combination with carboplatin and paclitaxel as first-line treatment for advanced non-small cell lung cancer. J Clin Oncol 2007;25(suppl). Abstract 7544.

126. Adjei AA, Molina JR, Mandrekar SJ, et al. Phase I trial of sorafenib in combination with gefitinib in patients with refractory or recurrent non-small cell lung cancer. Clin Cancer Res 2007;13(9):2684–91.

127. Brose MS, Volpe P, Feldman M, et al. BRAF and RAS mutations in human lung cancer and melanoma. Cancer Res 2002;62(23):6997–7000.

128. Toyooka S, Uchida A, Shigematsu H, et al. The effect of gefitinib on B-RAF mutant non-small cell lung cancer and transfectants. J Thorac Oncol 2007;2(4):321–4.

129. Blumenschein G, Heymach JV. Angiogenesis inhibitors for lung cancer: clinical developments and future directions. J Thorac Oncol 2006;1(7):744–8.

130. Blumenschein GR, Gatzenmeier U, Fossella F, et al. A phase II multicenter uncontrolled trial of single agent sorafenib (BAY 43–9006) in patients with relapsed or refractory advanced non-small cell lung carcinoma. In: Proceedings of the AACR-NCI-EORTC International Conference "Molecular Targets and Cancer Therapeutics," 2005, p. 46.

131. Gridelli C, Maione P, Del Gaizo F, et al. Sorafenib and sunitinib in the treatment of advanced non-small cell lung cancer. Oncologist 2007;12(2):191–200.

132. Socinski M, Novello S, Sanchez J. Efficacy and safety of sunitinib in previously treated, advanced non-small cell lung cancer: preliminary results of a multicenter phase II trial. J Clin Oncol 2006;24(suppl). Abstract 7001.

133. Schiller JH, Larson T, Ou S, et al. Efficacy and safety of axitinib (AG-013736) in patients with advanced non-small cell lung cancer: a phase II trial. J Clin Oncol 2007;25(suppl). Abstract 7507.

134. Yasuda H, Nakayama K, Watanabe M, et al. Nitroglycerin treatment may enhance chemosensitivity to docetaxel and carboplatin in patients with lung adenocarcinoma. Clin Cancer Res 2006;12(22):6748–57.

135. Yasuda H, Yamaya M, Nakayama K, et al. Randomized phase II trial comparing nitroglycerin plus vinorelbine and cisplatin with vinorelbine and cisplatin alone in previously untreated stage IIIB/IV non-small-cell lung cancer. J Clin Oncol 2006;24(4):688–94.

136. Horn L, Sandler A. Chemotherapy and antiangiogenic agents in non-small-cell lung cancer. Clin Lung Cancer 2007;8(suppl 2):S68–73.

137. Strieter RM, Burdick MD, Gomperts BN, et al. CXC chemokines in angiogenesis. Cytokine Growth Factor Rev 2005;16(6):593–609.

138. Strieter RM, Burdick MD, Mestas J, et al. Cancer CXC chemokine networks and tumour angiogenesis. Eur J Cancer 2006;42(6):768–78.

139. Belperio JA, Keane MP, Arenberg DA, et al. CXC chemokines in angiogenesis. J Leukoc Biol 2000;68(1):1–8.

140. Rampart M, Van Damme J, Zonnekeyn L, et al. Granulocyte chemotactic protein/interleukin-8 induces plasma leakage and neutrophil accumulation in rabbit skin. Am J Pathol 1989;135(1):21–5.

141. Murphy C, McGurk M, Pettigrew J, et al. Nonapical and cytoplasmic expression of interleukin-8, CXCR1, and CXCR2 correlates with cell proliferation and microvessel density in prostate cancer. Clin Cancer Res 2005;11(11):4117–27.

142. Schadendorf D, Moller A, Algermissen B, et al. IL-8 produced by human malignant melanoma cells in vitro is an essential autocrine growth factor. J Immunol 1993;151(5):2667–75.

143. Zhu YM, Webster SJ, Flower D, et al. Interleukin-8/CXCL8 is a growth factor for human lung cancer cells. Br J Cancer 2004;91(11):1970–6.

144. Strieter RM, Kasahara K, Allen RM, et al. Cytokine-induced neutrophil-derived interleukin-8. Am J Pathol 1992;141(2):397–407.

145. Strieter RM, Polverini PJ, Kunkel SL, et al. The functional role of the ELR motif in CXC chemokine-mediated angiogenesis. J Biol Chem 1995;270(45):27348–57.

146. Keane MP, Burdick MD, Xue YY, et al. The chemokine receptor, CXCR2, mediates the tumorigenic effects of ELR+ CXC chemokines. Chest 2004;125(suppl):133S.

147. Keane MP, Belperio JA, Xue YY, et al. Depletion of CXCR2 inhibits tumor growth and angiogenesis in a murine model of lung cancer. J Immunol 2004;172(5):2853–60.

148. Wislez M, Rabbe N, Marchal J, et al. Hepatocyte growth factor production by neutrophils infiltrating bronchioloalveolar subtype pulmonary adenocarcinoma: role in tumor progression and death. Cancer Res 2003;63(6):1405–12.

149. Dazzi C, Cariello A, Maioli P, et al. Prognostic and predictive value of intratumoral microvessels density in operable non-small-cell lung cancer. Lung Cancer 1999;24(2):81–8.

150. Yuan A, Yang PC, Yu CJ, et al. Interleukin-8 messenger ribonucleic acid expression correlates with tumor progression, tumor angiogenesis, patient survival, and timing of relapse in non-small-cell lung cancer. Am J Respir Crit Care Med 2000;162(5):1957–63.

151. Addison CL, Daniel TO, Burdick MD, et al. The CXC chemokine receptor 2, CXCR2, is the putative receptor for ELR+ CXC chemokine-induced angiogenic activity. J Immunol 2000;165(9):5269–77.

152. Strieter RM, Belperio JA, Burdick MD, et al. CXC chemokines: angiogenesis, immunoangiostasis, and metastases in lung cancer. Ann N Y Acad Sci 2004;1028:351–60.

153. Shi Q, Abbruzzese JL, Huang S, et al. Constitutive and inducible interleukin 8 expression by hypoxia and acidosis renders human pancreatic cancer cells more tumorigenic and metastatic. Clin Cancer Res 1999;5(11):3711–21.

154. Shi Q, Le X, Abbruzzese JL, et al. Cooperation between transcription factor AP-1 and NF-kappaB in the induction of interleukin-8 in human pancreatic adenocarcinoma cells by hypoxia. J Interferon Cytokine Res 1999;19(12):1363–71.

155. Bruns CJ, Solorzano CC, Harbison MT, et al. Blockade of the epidermal growth factor receptor signaling by a novel tyrosine kinase inhibitor leads to apoptosis of endothelial cells and therapy of human pancreatic carcinoma. Cancer Res 2000;60(11):2926–35.

156. Sparmann A, Bar-Sagi D. Ras-induced interleukin-8 expression plays a critical role in tumor growth and angiogenesis. Cancer Cell 2004;6(5):447–58.

157. Wislez M, Fujimoto N, Izzo JG, et al. High expression of ligands for chemokine receptor CXCR2 in alveolar epithelial neoplasia induced by oncogenic kras. Cancer Res 2006;66(8):4198–207.

158. Wislez M, Spencer ML, Izzo JG, et al. Inhibition of mammalian target of rapamycin reverses alveolar epithelial neoplasia induced by oncogenic K-ras. Cancer Res 2005;65(8):3226–35.

159. Shalinsky DR, Brekken J, Zou H, et al. Marked antiangiogenic and antitumor efficacy of AG3340 in chemoresistant human non-small cell lung cancer tumors: single agent and combination chemotherapy studies. Clin Cancer Res 1999;5(7):1905–17.

160. Douillard JY, Peschel C, Shepherd F, et al. Randomized phase II feasibility study of combining the matrix metalloproteinase inhibitor BMS-275291 with paclitaxel plus carboplatin in advanced non-small cell lung cancer. Lung Cancer 2004;46(3):361–8.

161. Leighl NB, Paz-Ares L, Douillard JY, et al. Randomized phase III study of matrix metalloproteinase inhibitor BMS-275291 in combination with paclitaxel and carboplatin in advanced non-small-cell lung cancer: National Cancer Institute of Canada-Clinical Trials Group Study BR.18. J Clin Oncol 2005;23(12):2831–9.

162. Bissett D, O'Byrne KJ, von Pawel J, et al. Phase III study of matrix metalloproteinase inhibitor prinomastat in non-small-cell lung cancer. J Clin Oncol 2005;23(4):842–9.

163. Behrendt CE, Ruiz RB. Venous thromboembolism among patients with advanced lung cancer randomized to prinomastat or placebo, plus chemotherapy. Thromb Haemost 2003;90(4):734–7.

164. Shepherd FA, Giaccone G, Seymour L, et al. Prospective, randomized, double-blind, placebo-controlled trial of marimastat after response to first-line chemotherapy in patients with small-cell lung cancer: a trial of the National Cancer Institute of Canada-Clinical Trials Group and the European Organization for Research and Treatment of Cancer. J Clin Oncol 2002;20(22):4434–9.

165. Majewski S, Marczak M, Mlynarczyk B, et al. Imiquimod is a strong inhibitor of tumor cell-induced angiogenesis. Int J Dermatol 2005;44(1):14–9.

166. Maasilta P, Holsti LR, Halme M, et al. Natural alpha-interferon in combination with hyperfractionated radiotherapy in the treatment of non-small cell lung cancer. Int J Radiat Oncol Biol Phys 1992;23(4):863–8.

167. Kataja V, Yap A. Combination of cisplatin and interferon-alpha 2a (Roferon-A) in patients with non-small cell lung cancer (NSCLC): an open phase II multicentre study. Eur J Cancer 1995;31A(1):35–40.

168. Chao TY, Hwang WS, Yang MJ, et al. Combination chemoimmunotherapy with interferon-alpha and cisplatin in patients with advanced non-small cell lung cancer. Zhonghua Yi Xue Za Zhi (Taipei) 1995;56(4):232–8.

169. Mandanas R, Einhorn LH, Wheeler B, et al. Carboplatin (CBDCA) plus alpha interferon in metastatic non-small cell lung cancer: a Hoosier Oncology Group phase II trial. Am J Clin Oncol 1993;16(6):519–21.

170. Fuxius S, Mross K, Mansouri K, et al. Gemcitabine and interferon-alpha 2b in solid tumors: a phase I study in patients with advanced or metastatic non-small cell lung, ovarian, pancreatic or renal cancer. Anticancer Drugs 2002;13(9):899–905.

171. Quan WD, Jr., Casal R, Rosenfeld M, et al. Alpha interferon-2b, leucovorin, and 5-fluorouracil (ALF) in non-small cell lung cancer. Cancer Biother Radiopharm 1996;11(4):229–34.

172. Ardizzoni A, Rosso R, Salvati F, et al. Combination chemotherapy and interferon alpha 2b in the treatment of advanced non-small-cell lung cancer: the Italian Lung Cancer Task Force (FONICAP). Am J Clin Oncol 1991;14(2):120–3.

173. Silva RR, Bascioni R, Rossini S, et al. A phase II study of mitomycin C, vindesine and cisplatin combined with alpha interferon in advanced non-small cell lung cancer. Tumori 1996;82(1):68–71.

174. Athanasiadis I, Kies MS, Miller M, et al. Phase II study of all-trans-retinoic acid and alpha-interferon in patients with advanced non-small cell lung cancer. Clin Cancer Res 1995;1(9):973–9.

175. Goncalves A, Camerlo J, Bun H, et al. Phase II study of a combination of cisplatin, all-trans-retinoic acid and interferon-alpha in squamous cell carcinoma: clinical results and pharmacokinetics. Anticancer Res 2001;21(2B):1431–7.

176. Roth AD, Abele R, Alberto P. 13-Cis-retinoic acid plus interferon-alpha: a phase II clinical study in squamous cell carcinoma of the lung and the head and neck. Oncology 1994;51(1):84–6.

177. Roth AD, Morant R, Alberto P. High dose etretinate and interferon-alpha—a phase I study in squamous cell carcinomas and transitional cell carcinomas. Acta Oncol 1999;38(5):613–7.

178. Rinaldi DA, Lippman SM, Burris HA 3rd, et al. Phase II study of 13-cis-retinoic acid and interferon-alpha 2a in patients with advanced squamous cell lung cancer. Anticancer Drugs 1993;4(1):33–6.

179. Salvati F, Rasi G, Portalone L, et al. Combined treatment with thymosin-alpha1 and low-dose interferon-alpha after ifosfamide in non-small cell lung cancer: a phase-II controlled trial. Anticancer Res 1996;16(2):1001–4.

180. Ardizzoni A, Salvati F, Rosso R, et al. Combination of chemotherapy and recombinant alpha-interferon in advanced non-small cell lung cancer: multicentric randomized FONICAP trial report; the Italian Lung Cancer Task Force. Cancer 1993;72(10):2929–35.

181. Wheeler RH, Herndon JE, Clamon GH, et al. A phase II study of recombinant beta-interferon at maximum tolerated dose in patients with advanced non-small cell lung cancer: a cancer and leukemia group B study. J Immunother Emphasis Tumor Immunol 1994;15(3):212–6.

182. McDonald S, Chang AY, Rubin P, et al. Combined Betaseron R (recombinant human interferon beta) and radiation for inoperable non-small cell lung cancer. Int J Radiat Oncol Biol Phys 1993;27(3):613–9.

183. Byhardt RW, Vaickus L, Witt PL, et al. Recombinant human interferon-beta (rHuIFN-beta) and radiation therapy for inoperable non-small cell lung cancer. J Interferon Cytokine Res 1996;16(11):891–902.

184. Bunn PA Jr. Early-stage non-small-cell lung cancer: current perspectives in combined-modality therapy. Clin Lung Cancer 2004;6(2):85–98.

185. Bradley JD, Scott CB, Paris KJ, et al. A phase III comparison of radiation therapy with or without recombinant beta-interferon for poor-risk patients with locally advanced non-small-cell lung cancer (RTOG 93–04). Int J Radiat Oncol Biol Phys 2002;52(5):1173–9.

186. Tester WJ, Kim KM, Krigel RL, et al. A randomized phase II study of interleukin-2 with and without beta-interferon for patients with advanced non-small cell lung cancer: an Eastern Cooperative Oncology Group study (PZ586). Lung Cancer 1999;25(3):199–206.

187. Recchia F, Sica G, De Filippis S, et al. Combined chemotherapy and differentiation therapy in the treatment of advanced non-small-cell lung cancer. Anticancer Res 1997;17(5B):3761–5.

188. Halme M, Maasilta PK, Pyrhonen SO, et al. Interferons combined with chemotherapy in the treatment of stage III-IV non-small cell lung cancer—a randomised study. Eur J Cancer 1994;30A(1):11–5.

189. Zhang J, Kalyankrishna S, Wislez M, et al. SRC-family kinases are activated in non-small cell lung cancer and promote the survival of epidermal growth factor receptor-dependent cell lines. Am J Pathol 2007;170(1):366–76.

190. Masaki T, Igarashi K, Tokuda M, et al. pp60c-src activation in lung adenocarcinoma. Eur J Cancer 2003;39(10):1447–55.

191. Johnson FM, Saigal B, Talpaz M, et al. Dasatinib (BMS-354825) tyrosine kinase inhibitor suppresses invasion and induces cell cycle arrest and apoptosis of head and neck squamous cell carcinoma and non-small cell lung cancer cells. Clin Cancer Res 2005;11(19 Pt 1):6924–32.

192. Schiller JH, Adak S, Feins RH, et al. Lack of prognostic significance of p53 and K-ras mutations in primary resected non-small-cell lung cancer on E4592: a laboratory ancillary study on an Eastern Cooperative Oncology Group prospective randomized trial of postoperative adjuvant therapy. J Clin Oncol 2001;19(2):448–57.

193. Rosell R, Font A, Pifarre A, et al. The role of induction (neoadjuvant) chemotherapy in stage IIIA NSCLC. Chest 1996;109(suppl):102S-6S.

194. Adjei AA, Mauer A, Bruzek L, et al. Phase II study of the farnesyl transferase inhibitor R115777 in patients with advanced non-small-cell lung cancer. J Clin Oncol 2003;21(9):1760–6.

195. Evans T, Fidias P, Skarin A, et al. A phase II study of the efficacy and tolerability of the farnesyl transferase inhibitor L-778,123 as first-line therapy in patients with advanced non-small cell lung cancer. Proc Am Soc Clin Oncol 2002;21. Abstract 1861.

196. Velcheti V, Govindan R. Insulin-like growth factor and lung cancer. J Thorac Oncol 2006;1(7):607–10.

197. Karp D, Paz-Ares L, Blakely L, et al. Efficacy of the anti-insulin like growth factor 1 receptor (IGF-1R) antibody CP-751871 in combination with paclitaxel and carboplatin as first-line treatment for advanced non-small cell lung cancer. J Clin Oncol 2007;25(suppl). Abstract 7506.

198. Morgillo F, Kim WY, Kim ES, et al. Implication of the insulin-like growth factor-IR pathway in the resistance of non-small cell lung cancer cells to treatment with gefitinib. Clin Cancer Res 2007;13(9):2795–803.

199. Morgillo F, Woo JK, Kim ES, et al. Heterodimerization of insulin-like growth factor receptor/epidermal growth factor receptor and induction of survivin expression counteract the antitumor action of erlotinib. Cancer Res 2006;66(20):10100–11.

200. Han JY, Choi BG, Choi JY, et al. The prognostic significance of pretreatment plasma levels of insulin-like growth factor (IGF)-1, IGF-2, and IGF binding protein-3 in patients with advanced non-small cell lung cancer. Lung Cancer 2006;54(2):227–34.

201. Papadimitrakopoulou V, Soria JC, Douillard JY, et al. A phase II study of RAD001 (everolimus) monotherapy in patients with advanced non-small cell lung cancer failing prior platinum-based chemotherapy of prior chemotherapy and EGFR inhibitors. J Clin Oncol 2007;25(suppl). Abstract 7589.

202. Kris MG, Riely GJ, Azzoli CG, et al. Combined inhibtion of mTOR and EGFR with everolimus (RAD001) and gefitinib in patients with non-small cell lung cancer who have smoked cigarettes: a phase II trial. J Clin Oncol 2007;25(suppl). Abstract 7575.

203. Lara PN Jr, Gandara DR, Wurz GT, et al. High-dose toremifene as a cisplatin modulator in metastatic non-small cell lung cancer: targeted plasma levels are achievable clinically. Cancer Chemother Pharmacol 1998;42(6):504–8.

204. Bepler G, Oh Y, Burris A, et al. A phase II study of enzastaurin as second- or third-line treatment of non-small cell lung cancer. J Clin Oncol 2007;25(suppl). Abstract 7543.

205. Fanucchi MP, Fossella FV, Belt R, et al. Randomized phase II study of bortezomib alone and bortezomib in combination with docetaxel in previously treated advanced non-small-cell lung cancer. J Clin Oncol 2006;24(31):5025–33.

206. Govindan R, Crowley J, Schwartzberg L, et al. Phase II trial of bexarotene capsules in patients with advanced non-small-cell lung cancer after failure of two or more previous therapies. J Clin Oncol 2006;24(30):4848–54.

207. Dragnev KH, Petty WJ, Shah S, et al. Bexarotene and erlotinib for aerodigestive tract cancer. J Clin Oncol 2005;23(34):8757–64.

208. Edelman MJ, Smith R, Hausner P, et al. Phase II trial of the novel retinoid, bexarotene, and gemcitabine plus carboplatin in advanced non-small-cell lung cancer. J Clin Oncol 2005;23(24):5774–8.

209. Khuri FR, Rigas JR, Figlin RA, et al. Multi-institutional phase I/II trial of oral bexarotene in combination with cisplatin and vinorelbine in previously untreated patients with advanced non-small-cell lung cancer. J Clin Oncol 2001;19(10):2626–37.

210. Blumenschein G, Khuri FR, Gatzemeier U, et al. A randomized phase III trial comparing bexarotene/carbo-platin/paclitaxel versus carboplatin/paclitaxel in chemotherapy-naive patients with advanced or metastatic non-small cell lung cancer. J Clin Oncol 2005;23(suppl). Abstract 7001.

211. Csiki I, Morrow JD, Sandler A, et al. Targeting cyclooxygenase-2 in recurrent non-small cell lung cancer: a phase II trial of celecoxib and docetaxel. Clin Cancer Res 2005;11(18):6634–40.

212. Gasparini G, Meo S, Comella G, et al. The combination of the selective cyclooxygenase-2 inhibitor celecoxib with weekly paclitaxel is a safe and active second-line therapy for non-small cell lung cancer: a phase II study with biological correlates. Cancer J 2005;11(3):209–16.

213. Liao Z, Komaki R, Milas L, et al. A phase I clinical trial of thoracic radiotherapy and concurrent celecoxib for patients with unfavorable performance status inoperable/unresectable non-small cell lung cancer. Clin Cancer Res 2005;11(9):3342–8.

214. Altorki NK, Keresztes RS, Port JL, et al. Celecoxib, a selective cyclo-oxygenase-2 inhibitor, enhances the response to preoperative paclitaxel and carboplatin in early-stage non-small-cell lung cancer. J Clin Oncol 2003;21(14):2645–50.

215. Gadgeel SM, Ruckdeschel JC, Heath EI, et al. Phase II study of gefitinib, an epidermal growth factor receptor tyrosine kinase inhibitor (EGFR-TKI), and celecoxib, a cyclooxygenase-2 (COX-2) inhibitor, in patients with platinum refractory non-small cell lung cancer (NSCLC). J Thorac Oncol 2007;2(4):299–305.

216. Ross HJ, Hart LL, Swanson PM, et al. A randomized, multicenter study to determine the safety and efficacy of the immunoconjugate SGN-15 plus docetaxel for the treatment of non-small cell lung carcinoma. Lung Cancer 2006;54(1):69–77.

8 Targeted Therapy in Lymphoma

Amanda Wedgwood, MSN, RN, CNS
and Anas Younes, MD

CONTENTS

ABSTRACT

Advances in lymphoma biology and immunology have begun an exciting new era in cancer therapy. Standard therapy for lymphoma still consists of chemotherapy and radiotherapy, which are associated with short- and long-term toxicity. Emerging novel therapies, such as small molecules and antibodies that preferentially target tumor cells while potentially sparing normal cells, bring new hope to patients with lymphoma. This chapter discusses targeted therapy for non-Hodgkin's lymphoma and Hodgkin's lymphoma.

Key Words: Antibody, Lymphoma, Antigen, Receptor, Inhibitor, Kinase

1. INTRODUCTION

The CHOP regimen (cyclophosphamide, doxorubicin, vincristine, and prednisone) that was first described in 1976 remains the most widely used regimen for the treatment of non-Hodgkin's lymphoma (NHL) *(1)*. Similarly, the ABVD regimen (adriamycin, bleomycin, vinblastine, and dacarbazine) that was introduced during the 1970s is currently considered the standard of care for the treatment of Hodgkin's lymphoma (HL). These empirically designed regimens do not, however, take into consideration the biology of NHL and HL. Much progress is being made in expanding treatment options that are rationally designed to target specifically well defined pathways that contribute to lymphoma cell survival and/or resistance to cell death. This new, personalized, approach includes novel antibodies that target lineage-specific antigens and receptors and small molecules that inhibit intracellular signaling proteins (Fig. 1).

From: *Current Clinical Oncology: Targeted Cancer Therapy*
Edited by: R. Kurzrock and M. Markman © Humana Press, Totowa, NJ

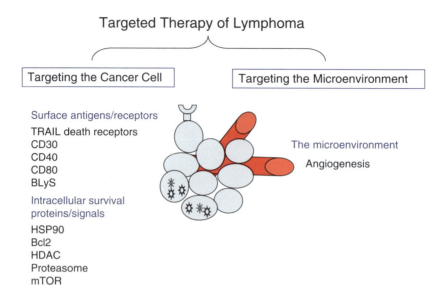

Fig. 1. Simplified model of drug development for lymphoma. Drugs can target tumor cells (by targeting cell surface proteins/receptors or intracellular survival proteins), or can target the microenvironment, such as angiogenesis.

2. TARGETING SURFACE ANTIGENS

2.1. CD20

Several antigens and receptors have been identified as potential targets for monoclonal antibodies (Fig. 2). CD20, a B cell-specific phosphoprotein, is expressed by 95% of B-cell lymphomas, making it an ideal target for antibody therapy *(2)*. Rituximab (Rituxan) was

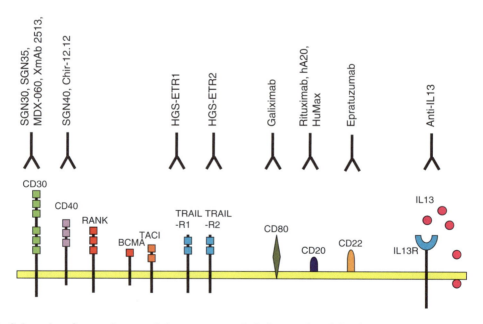

Fig. 2. Selected surface antigens and that are currently being explored for the treatment of lymphoma.

the first anti-CD20 antibody to be approved by the U.S. Food and Drug Administration (FDA) for the treatment of B-cell NHL. Because rituximab is a mouse/human chimeric antibody, it is frequently associated with an infusion reaction, including fever and chills. Based on its single-agent activity in various B-cell lymphomas and its excellent safety profile, it was rapidly combined with various chemotherapy regimens, including CHOP, CVP (cyclophosphamide, vincristine, and prednisone), and fludarabine-based regimens *(3–8)* These rituximab-based combinations have consistently demonstrated superiority in terms of event-free survival or overall survival when compared with chemotherapy alone in randomized trials *(9)*. Furthermore, several studies demonstrated its benefit when used as maintenance therapy after chemotherapy *(10)*.

In addition to rituximab, second-generation humanized and fully human monoclonal antibodies targeting CD20 (hA20 and HuMax-CD20) are being evaluated in Phase I and Phase II clinical trials for the treatment of NHL (Table 1). The potential advantages of these new antibodies are that they may be infused within a shorter period of time and may also be more effective at mediating antibody-dependent cellular cytotoxicity (ADCC) than first-generation targeted therapies.

Building on the success of rituximab, anti-CD20 antibodies have been conjugated with radioisotopes of yttrium (^{90}Y) or iodine (^{131}I) *(11)*. Theoretically, these agents have the capacity to target CD20-positive cells directly via the antibody and indirectly through crossfire irradiation, which may kill CD20-negative cells and CD20-positive cells that did not bind the antibody. Both antibodies are approved by the FDA for the treatment of patients with indolent lymphomas that are refractory to treatment with rituximab and/or chemotherapy *(11)*.

2.2. CD22

Expression of the human CD22 antigen is restricted to B cells. The safety and efficacy of the unconjugated CD22-targeted humanized immunoglobulin G1 (IgG1) antibody, epratuzumab, has been shown to be safe and effective when given alone and in combination with rituximab in Phase I and II clinical trials *(12,13)* (Table 2). Furthermore, CD22 is an ideal target for immunotoxin therapy as it is rapidly internalized when bound to a natural ligand or antibody and then induces proapoptotic signals within NHL-B cell lines. This approach has been examined using *Pseudomonas* and calicheamicin immunotoxin conjugates. BL22 has an antibody-derived domain that recognizes CD22 and has a truncated *Pseudomonas* exotoxin domain, which allows it to inhibit protein synthesis. It has proven

Table 1
Summary of single-agent activity of unconjugated monoclonal antibodies targeting CD20

Antibody	Protein component	Disease histology	Prior rituximab	No.	CR	OR	Ref.
Rituximab	Chimeric	Indolent	No	151	9 (6%)	71 (50%)	9
hA20	Humanized	Indolent and aggressive	Yes	23	6 (23%)	14 (61%)	196
HuMax-CD20	Fully human	Follicular	Yes	36	7 (19%)	15 (42%)	197

Rituximab has demonstrated variable single-agent activity against all CD20-expressing lymphomas
CR, complete response; OR, odds ratio

Table 2
Summary of selected monoclonal antibodies in lymphoma

Target	Antibody	Disease type	No.	CR/CRu	ORR	Ref
CD22	Epratuzumab	Aggressive B-cell lymphoma	56	3 (5%)	5 (10%)	12
CD22 + CD20	Epratuzumab + rituximab	B-cell lymphoma	23	12 (52%)	14 (61%)	13
CD22	BL22	B-cell malignances	46	19 (41%)	25 (54%)	198
CD22	CMC-544	B-cell lymphoma	28	Not reported	12 (43%)	199
CD80	Galiximab	Follicular lymphoma	37	2 (5%)	4 (11%)	55
CD80 + CD20	Galiximab + rituximab	Follicular lymphoma	64	20 (31%)	41 (64%)	200
TRAIL-R1	Mapatumumab	B-cell lymphoma	40	1 (3%)	3 (8%)	67
CD52	Alemtuzumab	Low grade lymphoma	50	2 (4%)	10 (20%)	201
CD52	Alemtuzumab	T-cell lymphoma	10	2 (20%)	6 (60%)	202
VEGF	Bevacizumab	Aggressive lymphoma	44	0	2 (5%)	190

CR/CRu, Complete remission/Complete remission unconfirmed; ORR, Overall response rate

effective in leukemia, and cell cycle arrest has been reported in mantle cell lymphoma cell lines (14,15).

CMC-544 is a humanized anti-CD22 antibody that is conjugated to calicheamicin (16). CMC-544 was administered intravenously every 4 weeks at the maximum tolerated dose of 1.8 mg/m^2 in a Phase I dose escalation trial. The objective response rate (RR) was 69% for follicular lymphoma (FL) and 33% for diffuse large B-cell lymphoma (DLBCL) (16). Combination treatment trials combining anti-CD20 antibody with anti-CD22 antibody report promising efficacy. Rituximab combined with CMC-544, compared to each agent given alone, showed improved median survival in in vivo studies (17,18). Finally, ^{90}Y-radiolabeled epratuzumab, a monocolonal antibody, demonstrated an overall RR of 62% with only minor toxicity in patients with B-cell lymphoma when administered in 3 weekly infusions (19).

2.3. CD19

CD19 is a surface receptor on B cells during all phases of development, which include the malignant NHL B cells. Patients whose disease is refractory to rituximab therapy could potentially benefit from alternative B cell-specific targeted therapies. The activity of humanized anti-CD19 antibody (XmAb CD19) is comparable to rituximab in lymphoma cell lines and in some instances has demonstrated superiority. The data suggest that anti-CD19 antibodies could provide a promising treatment option for rituximab-refractory NHL (20).

2.4. CD40

Unlike CD20 and CD20 antigens, which are restricted to B cells, CD40 is expressed by normal and malignant hematopoietic epithelial and endothelial cells *(21,22)*. CD40L is important for priming dendritic cells to activate CD8+ cytotoxic T cells so they mature and become cytotoxic T cells, in B-cell selection and survival, and in immunoglobulin isotype switching (*isotype switching* is the DNA recombination mechanism by which antibody genes diversify immunoglobulin effector functions). CD40L is detected in the serum of patients with lymphoma, chronic lymphocytic leukemia (CLL), autoimmune disease, and essential thrombocythemia (which results in the overproduction of platelet-forming cells, or megakaryocytes, in the marrow) *(23–25)*. This antigen is predominantly expressed by activated T lymphocytes. There are conflicting reports of CD40L activity against a variety of cultured and primary cancer cells *(26,27)*. However, several independent studies demonstrated that CD40 activation may promote B-cell lymphoma survival and resistance to chemotherapy *(21)*. Because CD40L and CD40 can be co-expressed by several types of B-cell malignancies, an autocrine–paracrine CD40L/CD40 survival loop has been proposed as playing a fundamental role in the pathogenesis and survival of some instances of B-cell lymphoma and CLL *(28)*. Clinical trials are currently being conducted using two different antibodies to the CD40 receptor in patients with B-cell NHL, CLL, and multiple myeloma *(29,30)*. Because CD40 is widely expressed and has diverse physiologic functions, it is important to establish the safety of this novel approach before exploring the efficacy of these novel antibodies.

SGN-40 is a humanized antibody that induces apoptosis against CD40+ NHL B-cell lines. Phase I results recently reported for SGN-40 in patients with NHL showed an objective response rate of 37.5% in diffuse large B-cell lymphoma (DLBCL) with additional responses seen in a patient with mantle cell lymphoma (MCL) and one with marginal zone lymphoma (MZL) *(31,32)*. No grade 4 toxicities were reported. Similar results were seen with two partial responses (PR) at the 3 mg/kg dose (one MZL and 1 DLBCL) and one PR at the 4 mg/kg dose in a relapsed DLBCL patient *(33)*. Dose escalation is continuing, and data are presented from additional cohorts in these studies in addition to Phase II studies. A study combining CHOP with SGN-40 or using SGN-40 alone in a lymphoma xenograft model demonstrated significantly more activity in the combination group *(34)*. CHIR12.12 has shown efficacy as a potent anti-CD40 antibody in NHL cell lines, and Phase I clinical trials are ongoing with B-cell malignancies.

2.5. CD30

CD30, a transmembrane cytokine receptor belonging to the tumor necrosis factor (TNF) receptor superfamily, is expressed on HRS (Hodgkin and Reed-Sternberg) cells and on anaplastic large-cell lymphoma (ALCL) cells *(21,35)*. Only a small number of activated B and T lymphocytes express CD30 in healthy individuals. Phase I results of two naked anti-CD30 antibodies in patients with CD30+ hematologic malignancies were recently reported. A chimeric antibody (SGN-30; Seattle Genetics, Bothell, WA, USA) was found to induce cell cycle arrest and apoptosis in Hodgkin's-derived cell lines in vitro *(36)*. SGN-30 was used in a Phase II study to treat relapsed or refractory CD30+ ALCL patients with a dose of 6 or 12 mg/kg/week for 6 consecutive weeks. SGN-30 exhibited good tolerability and antitiumor activity with an overall RR (ORR) of 21%: two complete remissions (CRs) and 6 PRs *(37)*. A different, fully human, monoclonal anti-CD30 antibody (MDX-060; Medarex,

Princeton, NJ, USA) was also evaluated in a Phase I/II study of CD30+ malignancies *(38)* in 48 patients (40 HL, 6 ALCL, 2 other CD30+ lymphomas). The patients were treated with a dosage escalation scheme (range 0.1–10 mg/kg), with weekly doses for 4 consecutive weeks in the Phase I portion. In the Phase II portion patients were administered MDX-060 at dosages of 10 or 15 mg/kg weekly for 4 weeks. Two patients achieved a CR and three a PR *(39)*. Stable disease was observed in 17 patients. At the present time, clinical trials are being conducted for NHL using various anti-CD30-based combination regimens, such as CHOP plus anti-CD30 antibody in newly diagnosed patients with ALCL.

An iodine-131 (^{131}I)-labeled murine anti-CD30 monoclonal antibody was administered to refractory HL patients based on the HRS cell expression of CD30 antigen in large amounts *(40)*. Responses included one complete remission, five partial remissions, and three minor responses lasting for an average of 4 months.

The efficacy of anti-CD30 antibodies might be reduced because CD30 is shed in a soluble form and can be detected in sera of patients with CD30+ lymphoma *(41)*. Recent data suggest that soluble CD30 may lack specific epitopes associated with membrane-bound CD30, thus allowing monoclonal antibodies to be engineered that preferentially target CD30+ cells without being neutralized by soluble CD30 *(42)*. The activity of these antibodies could be improved by enhancing antigen binding and Fcγ receptor affinity and specificity *(43)*. For example, chimeric anti-CD30 antibody can be humanized by human string content optimization that improves antigen binding. Compared to other anti-CD30 antibodies, the humanized anti-CD30 compound XmAb2513 demonstrated an approximately threefold higher efficacy than the parent antibody *(41)*.

In a different approach, SGN-30 was conjugated to the antimiotic agent monomethyl auristatin E (MMAE), yielding the antibody–drug conjugate SGN-35 *(44,45)*. In vitro experiments demonstrated that SGN-35 had potent and selective in vitro activity for CD30+ cell lines, compared with CD30-negative cells *(44,45)*. Based on these promising data, SGN-35 is currently being evaluated in a Phase I trial in patients with relapsed HL and ALCL.

2.6. CD80

CD80 is a membrane-bound co-stimulatory molecule that is involved in regulating T-cell activation *(46,47)*. CD80 is transiently expressed in healthy individuals on the surface of activated B cells, dendritic cells, and T cells *(48)* and in various lymphoid malignancies *(49–53)*. CD80 was recently identified as a potential target for lymphoid malignancies because of its rather restricted expression. Preclinical studies demonstrated that anti-CD80 antibodies can inhibit lymphoma cell proliferation and induce antibody-dependent cell-mediated cytotoxicity (ADCC).

Galiximab is a primatized, anti-CD80 (IgG1λ) monoclonal antibody with human constant regions and primate (cynomologous macaque) variable regions *(54)*. The single-agent activity of galiximab was recently examined in a multicenter Phase I/II study in patients with relapsed or refractory follicular B-cell lymphoma *(55)* (Table 2). Therapy was relatively safe, with no major side effects observed. Although the response rate (CR + PR) was only 11%, approximately 50% of the patients had decreased tumor measurements. Interestingly, some responses were delayed, and the time to best response was seen up to 1 year later. The delayed response cannot be explained by a direct passive antibody effect, as the half-life is measured in a few weeks, which raises the possibility that galiximab may induce an active immune response. Unlike the chimeric antibody rituximab, which had a relatively short half-life, the half-life of galiximab was 2 to 3 weeks. After almost 2 years, some patients had no evidence of progression.

In a Phase II study, response rates of more than 60% were observed when galiximab (500 mg/m^2 q week × 4 weeks) was combined with standard-dose Rituxan (375 mg/m^2 q week × 4 weeks) *(56)*. Progression-free survival was longer in patients treated with galiximab and Rituxan (12.1 months) compared to treatment with Rituxan alone (9.4 months). Toxicity and tolerability were similar to that seen with rituximab alone.

2.7. CD2

CD2 antigen expression is restricted to T lymphocytes and natural killer (NK) cells, making it a potentially good target in the treatment of T-cell lymphoma. MEDI-507 is a humanized IgG1κ monoclonal antibody that binds to the CD2 receptor on human T and NK cells *(40,57)*. Preclinical studies demonstrated that MEDI-507 kills target cells by an ADCC mechanism. Survival of mice bearing adult human T-cell leukemia/lymphoma cells was significantly prolonged after treatment with MEDI-507 *(58)*. A Phase I trial in patients with relapsed/refractory CD2-positive T-cell lymphoma/leukemia was conducted with MEDI-507 (Siplizumab). Results showed a response in NK-cell large granular lymphocytic leukemia (LGL) and in peripheral T-cell lymphoma (PTCL), both at doses of 3.4 mg/kg *(57)*. Combination trials with chemotherapy will be evaluated in the future should this antibody prove to be safe and active.

2.8. CD52

CD52 is expressed by B cells, T cells, monocytes, and macrophages. Campath-1H is a human IgG1 anti-CD52 monoclonal antibody. A 14% PR rate was revealed in a Phase II trial conducted in patients with B-cell lymphoma when 30 mg was administered intravenously three times weekly for a maximum of 12 weeks *(59)* (Table 2). In patients with mycosis fungoides, two complete remissions were seen. The most profound results were observed in the blood and marrow in 16 of 17 patients (94%), with lymphoma cells being removed from blood and a 32% CR in the bone marrow. Anti-CD52 monoclonal antibody was given to patients with peripheral and cutaneous T-cell lymphoma at a dose of 10 mg 3 times weekly for 4 consecutive weeks in a Phase II study. Two of ten patients (20%) achieved a CR, and four had a PR (40%) *(60)*.

2.9. Interleukin-13

More than 70% of classic HL lymph node primary HRS cells express interleukin-13 (IL-13). Detectable levels of IL-13 have been found in the sera of 10% of newly diagnosed HL patients and in 16% of patients with relapsed HL *(61)*. An IL-13 autocrine mechanism in HRS cells suggests that these cells produce IL-13 and stimulate HRS cell growth. IL-13 may play a role in providing survival signals to HRS cells, and its signal interruption may prove beneficial for those with HL. A Phase I trial in patients with relapsed classic HL is currently enrolling patients using an anti-IL-13 monoclonal antibody.

3. TARGETING SURFACE RECEPTORS

3.1. Anti-TRAIL Death Receptors

TRAIL (Apo2 ligand) is a death protein that is expressed predominantly by activated T cells and natural killer cells. TRAIL has four exclusive receptors: TRAIL-R1 (DR4),

TRAIL-R2 (DR5, KILLER, TRICK2), TRAIL-R3 (DcR1, TRID, LIT), and TRAIL-R4 (DcR2 TRUNDD) *(26,62,63)*. TRAIL also binds to osteoprotegerin although with lower affinity *(64)*. TRAIL-R1 and TRAIL-R2 are death receptors that are preferentially expressed by HL cell lines, whereas TRAIL-R3 and TRAIL-R4 are decoy receptors *(65)*. TRAIL preferentially kills cancer cells expressing TRAIL-R1 and TRAIL-R2, whereas normal cells do not, protecting them from TRAIL-induced apoptosis. Thus, TRAIL is a potentially useful target for cancer therapy. In fact, TRAIL demonstrates a degree of antitumor activity against most human cancer cell lines, including lymphoma *(26)*. Anti-TRAIL-R1 and anti-TRAIL-R2 antibodies and Apo2L/TRAIL protein antibodies can induce cell death in HL cell lines by activating extrinsic and intrinsic mitochondrial apoptotic pathways *(66)*. Both anti-TRAIL-R1 and anti-TRAIL-R2 have demonstrated activity against a wide variety of cultured and primary lymphoma cells in vitro *(66)*. Preliminary data from a Phase II study using a therapeutic monoclonal antibody targeting TRAIL-R1 in NHL appears promising *(67)*. Three patients (8%) had a response, with one CR and two PRs after a maximum of six cycles—more than 30% of patients having stable disease. Therapy was tolerated well, with no subjects discontinuing treatment due to toxicity. Thus, the safety and promising clinical activity of this antibody warrants further investigation in combination with other active agents.

3.2. BAFF and its Receptors

BAFF (also known as BLyS, TALL-1, ZANK, zTNF4, and TNFS 13B) is a member of the TNF ligand family that is expressed by macrophages, monocytes and dendritic cells but not by benign B or T lymphocytes *(68)*. BAFF binds to three receptors: TACI (transmembrane activator and calcium modulator and cyclophylin ligand interactor); BAFF-R (also known as BR-3); and BCMA (B-cell maturation antigen). TACI and BCMA are also shared with a related TNF family member called APRIL (a proliferation-inducing ligand; also called TRDL-1 or TALL-2), which binds to both TACI and BCMA receptors *(69,70)*. These three receptors are almost exclusively expressed by B lymphocytes, although TACI transcripts have been observed in T lymphocytes. APRIL, a secreted soluble protein that is expressed in monocytes, macrophages, dendritic cells, and T lymphocytes, shares the highest sequence homology with BAFF *(69,70)*. BAFF is an important survival factor for both benign and malignant B lymphocytes *(68,71,72)*. Several malignant B cells aberrantly express BAFF and APRIL and their receptors, suggesting that a BAFF-mediated autocrine survival loop may contribute to the pathogenesis of B-cell lymphoid malignancies *(73–77)*.

Belimumab (LymphoStat-B) is a fully human antibody directed against BLyS protein. Monkeys showed significant decreases in peripheral blood B lymphocytes with decreases also seen in spleen and lymph node B lymphocytes *(78)*. These results supported continued clinical development of belimumab. Lymphorad-131 (LR131) is a radioconjugate consisting of BLyS protein labeled with iodine-131. A Phase I dose escalation trial showed that two of eight patients had an unconfirmed complete remission; two others had a PR, and one had stabilized disease. This agent was well tolerated, with only mild to moderate, reversible toxicity *(79)*. Strategies to interrupt BAFF signaling are currently being explored in patients with autoimmune disease and B-cell malignancies using monoclonal antibodies and soluble receptors.

Both BAFF and APRIL are expressed by reactive cells surrounding HRS cells. Primary HRS cells express BAFF and APRIL, independently of Epstein-Barr virus infection *(80)*. Patients with HL have elevated levels of serum BAFF, which is associated with a poor prognosis *(81)*. BAFF and APRIL rescued HRS cells from spontaneous or induced apoptosis through nuclear factor kappa B (NFκB) pathway activation, up-regulation of the pro-survival Bcl-2 and Bcl-X$_L$ proteins, and down-regulation of the proapoptotic BAX protein. The survival of HRS cells is thought to be supported by BAFF and APRIL through both autocrine and paracrine pathways. These data suggest that targeting this survival loop may be of therapeutic value for treating HL in addition to B-cell lymphoid malignancies.

3.3. RANK Ligand (RANKL) and its Receptors

RANK and osteoprotegerin (OPG) are two receptors of RANKL (also called TRANCE), which is expressed primarily by activated T cells and osteoblasts *(26,82,83)*. RANK receptor is expressed by dendritic cells, T lymphocytes, and osteoclast precursor cells *(84)*. OPG is a secreted receptor that binds to both RANKL and TRAIL *(85)*. Cancer cells may secrete several cytokines and hormones that can up-regulate RANKL expression on benign osteoblasts, leading to lytic bone lesions, whereas malignant cells may express RANKL, which directly activates osteoclasts *(26,35)*. The OPG receptor is frequently elevated in the sera of HL patients and has been shown to express RANKL, RANK, and OPG. Blocking the RANK/RANKL pathway can be therapeutically achieved by blocking antibodies to RANKL or RANK or by using a soluble OPG receptor. There are currently no trials investigating the targeting of the RANK/RANKL pathway in HL.

4. TARGETING LYMPHOMA CELLS WITH SMALL MOLECULES

4.1. Proteasome Inhibitors

Bortezomib is a small-molecule proteasome inhibitor that is currently approved by the FDA for the treatment of multiple myeloma (MM) and MCL *(86–88)*. Bortezomib inhibits the activation of NFκB by inhibiting the degradation of cytoplasmic IκBα and alters the expression of several survival and cell cycle regulatory proteins (p21, p27, Bcl-2, Bax, XIAP, survivin, p53), leading to cell cycle arrest and apoptosis in several tumor types, including lymphoma *(89,90)*. Bortezomib activity was recently evaluated in patients with relapsed NHL and demonstrated significant antitumor activity in patients with relapsed MCL *(91–93)*. In a study treating patients with relapsed MCL and other types of NHL with bortezomib, 41% of patients with MCL achieved PR or CR, compared to 19% of patients with other types of NHL *(92)*. Responses were seen in heavily pretreated patients, including those who had previously received autologous stem cell transplants. The most common toxic effects were thrombocytopenia and neuropathy.

O'Connor et al. showed an ORR of 58% when using the same dose and treatment schedule of bortezomib to treat 26 patients with relapsed NHL *(91)*. Of the nine patients with FL, seven (77%) achieved a major clinical response, and 5 of the 10 (50%) patients with MCL also achieved PR or CR. Belch et al. treated 24 patients with bortezomib, all with MCL, of whom 10 had not received prior chemotherapy, resulting in an ORR of 30%. Responses were similar among those who did and did not receive prior treatment *(94)*. In a fourth study, Strauss et al. treated 32 patients with relapsed NHL and HL. Of the 11 patients with MCL, 4 (36%) achieved PR or CR *(95)*. A recent multicenter trial confirmed that bortezomib has significant single-agent activity in patients with relapsed MCL, which led to its approval by the FDA *(87)*. Similar activity was recently confirmed in a multicenter study with bortezomib, demonstrating a 40% response rate in patients with relapsed MCL *(96)*. Bortezomib-based combination trials with rituximab and various chemotherapy regimens, including R-CHOP (rituximab, cytoxan, adriamycin, vincristine, prednisone) and R-Hyper-CVAD, are currently being explored in Phase I and Phase II studies.

Based on encouraging preclinical data that demonstrated bortezomib's significant antiproliferative activity in HL-derived cell lines (90), a pilot study was recently conducted in patients with relapsed and refractory classic HL. Fourteen patients, who were all heavily pretreated and refractory to their last treatment regimens were given bortezomib intravenously. Only one patient had a PR and two had minor responses. Thus, in heavily pretreated patients with treatment-refractory, relapsed classic HL, bortezomib has minimal single-agent activity (97). This was confirmed in a recently reported Phase II study treating patients who had relapsed HL with bortezomib (98). No response was observed for the 12 patients included in the study, and 2 discontinued the study due to toxicities. Whether proteasome inhibitors has a better response rate in patients with less refractory disease remains to be determined.

4.2. mTOR Inhibitors

Inhibition of PI3K, AKT, or mTOR kinases has been shown to confer an antiproliferative effect and apoptosis in various tumor types in vitro. The phosphoinositide 3-kinase (PI3K) signaling pathway plays a major role in regulating cell growth and survival (99–101). PI3K is a lipid kinase that phosphorylates phosphatidylinositol-4,5-bisphosphate (PI-4,5-P_2, also called PIP2) to generate the second messenger PI-3,4,5-P_3 (PIP3). A growth factor engages with its receptor protein tyrosine kinase, activating PI3K (Fig. 3). This leads to activation of a downstream serine/threonine (Ser/Thr) kinase called AKT, or protein kinase B (PKB). Active AKT phosphorylates critical proteins such as Bad, caspase-9, inhibitor of NFκB kinase (IKK), and mammalian target of rapamycin (mTOR). Active AKT regulates cell survival and growth and several cellular proteins critical to cell cycle progression and survival. This pathway is negatively regulated by a PIP3 phosphatase called PTEN (phosphatase and tensin homologue deleted on chromosome 10, also called MMAC1), which dephosphorylates PIP3 to PIP2. Aberrant expression, deletion, and mutations in many components of this pathway have been observed in various human cancers, including lymphoma (99,101–103). mTOR inhibitors are currently being evaluated in clinical trials.

mTOR (also called FRAP, RAFT1, or SEPT) is a Ser/Thr kinase that regulates protein translation (104–106). Rapamycin, a bacterially derived natural product, was the first mTOR inhibitor showing anticancer activity (105,106). The binding site of rapamycin is located upstream of the kinase domain and is referred to as the FKBP12-rapamycin binding (FRB) domain (Fig. 3b). Rapamycin binds to FK506-binding protein (FKBP12), which presents rapamycin to mTOR in a conformation that favors interacting with the FRB domain. Several downstream targets have been identified, including protein translation regulators S6K-1 and 4EBP1. In some tumor types, inhibiting the function of mTOR induces cell cycle arrest by inhibiting cyclin D1 translation, which promotes cell cycle progression from G_1 to S phase (107). CCI-779, RAD001, and AP23573, three mTOR inhibitors, are currently being studied in clinical trials for the treatment of cancer, including lymphoma (105,108–110). CCI-779 is a water-soluble rapamycin ester that is administered by intravenous infusion or orally. A Phase II study of CCI-779 in patients with relapsed MCL resulted in a 44% response rate (111) (Table 3). CCI-779 is currently being assessed in a large international randomized study in patients with relapsed MCL.

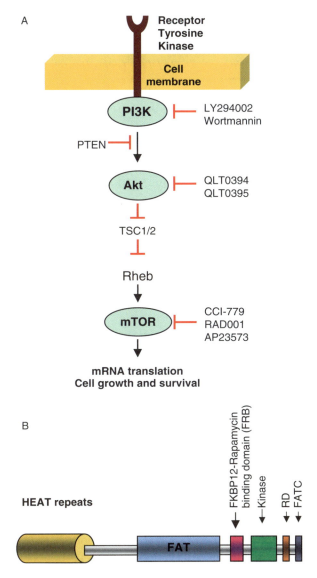

Fig. 3. a Simplified scheme of the PI3K/AKT/mTOR pathway. Activation of a receptor protein tyrosine kinase (RTK) by a growth factor leads to activation of PI3K, with subsequent activation of downstream kinases such as AKT and mTOR. Activate mTOR enhances mRNA translation of several cell cycle proteins including cyclin D. Inhibition of mTOR by a variety of small molecules induces cell cycle arrest. **b** Molecular structure of mTOR. The rapamycin analogues CC1-779 and RAD001 inactivate mTOR by binding to the FRB domain.

RAD001 is an orally bioavailable hydroxyethyl ether of rapamycin *(105,108–110)*. It is currently being evaluated in clinical trials in patients with relapsed leukemia and lymphoma. Phase I trials in hematologic malignancies are now being conducted.

AP23573, a rapamycin analogue, is very stable in several media. Phase II studies in patients with solid tumors and hematologic malignancies are underway *(112)*.

The importance of the PI3K pathway as a potential target for HL therapy is further enhanced by studies on primary lymph node sections *(113)*. Primary HRS cells showed activated pAkt in approximately 65% of HL lymph nodes. Differences in PTEN or pPTEN

Table 3
Summary of Clinical Results of mTOR Inhibitors in Hematologic Malignancies

Drug	CCI-779 (Sirolimus)	RAD001 (everolimus)	AP23573
Study	Witzig (111)	Yee (203)	Feldman (112)
Institution	Mayo/NCCTG	UTMDACC	Multicenter
Phase	II	I	II
Malignancy	Mantle cell lymphoma	Hematologicmalignancy	Hematologicmalignancy
No. of patients	47	15	12
Dose	250 or 25 mg	Daily: 5, 10 mg	12.5 mg
Schedule	IV, weekly	Oral	IV, daily, 5 days every other week
PR + CR	38–58%	7%	0%
Stable disease	—	14%	55%

PR, partial response; CR, complete response

expression levels (which have not been examined in primary HRS cells), could explain why one-third of the cases do not express pAKT. This phenomenon could also be explained by differences in cytokine expression (e.g., CD30 ligand) but is unrelated to Epstein-Barr virus infection (114).

4.3. Heat Shock Protein Inhibitors

Heat shock proteins (Hsps) are cellular chaperone proteins that are required for essential cell housekeeping functions such as protein folding, assembly, and transportation (115,116). Hsp90 interacts with and stabilizes several key survival signaling proteins—AKT, MEK, components of the NFkB signaling pathways—all of which are known to promote HRS cell survival (117). Hsps are required for the maintenance and function of various client proteins that regulate the cell cycle, cell survival, and apoptosis (118). In benign unstressed cells, Hsp90 exists in an inactive form. Activation by an ATP-dependent mechanism and the formation of multiprotein complexes and co-chaperones are required for functional Hsp90 (Fig. 4).

Primarily cancer cells express the active form of Hsp90, which has an increased affinity to Hsp inhibitors, therefore making cancer cells more sensitive to Hsp inhibition than are normal cells (118,119). Several Hsp90 inhibitors have been identified, some of which have already entered clinical trials (120–125). 17-Allylamino-17-demethoxy-geldanamycin (17-AAG) is a geldanamycin analogue that inhibits Hsp90 function, causing cell cycle arrest and apoptosis in various tumor types (117,126). 17-AAG has a higher affinity to tumor Hsp90 and preferentially inhibits tumor growth (119).

Inhibiting Hsp90 is potentially an attractive strategy for the treatment of HL. Recent studies demonstrated that Hsp90 is overexpressed in primary and cultured HL cells (127). Inhibition of Hsp90 function by 17-AAG in HL cell lines induced cell cycle arrest in the G_0/G_1 or G_2M phase followed by induction of apoptosis. 17-AAG has been shown to potentiate the killing effect of chemotherapy and antibodies. Phase II single-agent trials with 17-AAG are ongoing for several tumor types, including NHL and HL.

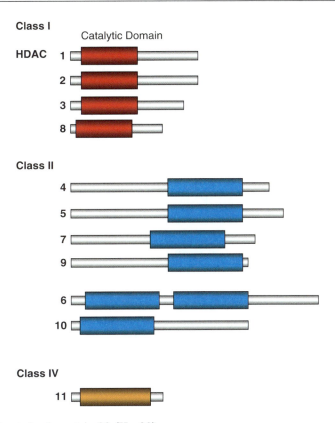

Fig. 4. Structure of heat shock protein 90 (Hsp90).

4.4. Histone Deacetylases Inhibitors

The human genome is packaged in the nucleus in the form of chromatin, which is made up of repetitive units of DNA, histones, and nonhistone proteins termed nucleosomes *(8,12)*. Eight histone molecules arranged in four histone partners make up each nucleosomal core unit (Fig. 5). This is surrounded by a piece of DNA, which coils twice around the nucleosome core. The four nucleosomal histones are H3, H4, H2A, and H2B, with their C-terminal domains located inside the nucleosome core and the N-terminal tail located outside of the nucleosome. The tails of H3 and H4 histones can be targeted for posttranslational modifications by acetylation and methylation. This, in turn, regulates chromatin condensation. Histone acetylation is mediated by histone acetyltransferases (HATs), leading to DNA relaxation. This enables transcription factors to have greater access to DNA, subsequently increasing gene transcription. Repression of gene expression and condensation of chromatin decrease histone acetylation by histone deacetylases (HDACs) *(129)*. HATs are opposed by HDACs. Abnormalities in the function of both HATs and HDACs have been observed in various cancers, including lymphoma.

Mammalian HDACs are grouped in four major classes: Class I includes HDACs 1, 2, 3, 8; class II includes HDACs 4, 5, 6, 7, 9, and 10; class III includes homologues of yeast Sir2; and class IV consists of HDAC II (Fig. 4). Altered expression of cell cycle regulatory genes, including p21, p27, p53, Rb, BCL6, BCL2, BCL-XL, MCL-1, cyclin D1, and Hsp90, can inhibit these HDACs by synthetic compounds *(130)*. Furthermore, HDAC inhibitors

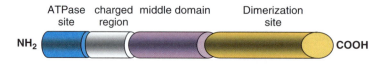

Fig. 5. Classification of histone deacetylases demonstrating the four major domains.

can induce apoptosis by caspase-dependent and caspase-independent mechanisms *(131)*. Preclinical testing has shown that HDAC inhibitors are active against lymphoma cells *(132)*.

Several HDAC inhibitors are currently being evaluated in clinical trials in patients with cancer, including SAHA (vorinostat), PXD101, LAQ824, valproic acid, MGCD0103, and depsipeptide *(130,133,134)* (Table 4). SAHA was recently evaluated in two Phase I studies in patients with solid tumors and hematologic malignancies *(135,136)*. One trial showed minor responses of HL in patients who were given intravenous SAHA *(135)*. In the second trial, an oral formulation was used *(136)*. Nineteen patients with HL and NHL were included in the study. Two patients with DLBCL achieved remissions (one PR, one CR), and four patients had stable disease. Two patients with refractory HL had tumor reduction and disappearance of their symptoms *(136)*. Phase II studies of oral vorinostat are continuing in patients with various types of lymphoma. A 24% response rate was demonstrated in patients with cutaneous T-cell lymphoma when given oral SAHA in a Phase II study *(137)*. Of the 33 patients, 8 had a PR and an additional 11 had pruritic relief. Clinical benefit was demonstrated in 58% of patients. These data led to the approval of vorinostat for the treatment of relapsed cutaneous T-cell lymphoma.

Depsipeptide is a natural product produced by *Chromobacterium violaceum* that demonstrated antitumor activity in vitro and in xenograft tumor models *(138)*. This prodrug inhibits class I HDAC enzymes and is activated intracellularly by reduction *(138)*. Three Phase I studies of depsipeptide were recently completed in patients with advanced solid tumors and leukemia *(140–142)*. Reversible electrocardiographic changes with ST/T wave flattening were frequently observed in patients on the study. Although depsipeptide induced an increase in histone acetylation and p21 protein expression in a study with CLL and acute myeloid leukemia, no objective clinical responses were observed *(140)*. A Phase II study of depsipeptide in patients with relapsed T-cell lymphoma demonstrated encouraging results *(143)*. Fifty percent of patients with cutaneous T-cell lymphoma and 24% patients with peripheral T-cell lymphoma achieved PRs and CRs that lasted for as long as 34 months.

Vorinostat (SAHA) and MGCD0103 are currently being evaluated in patients with relapsed HL in Phase II studies. The rationale for evaluating HDAC inhibitors in HL is based on several observations that implicate the role of epigenetics in the HRS phenotype, including B cell-specific gene silencing *(144–146)*. Vorinostat (SAHA) produced antiproliferative activity in vitro against HL-derived cell lines, presumably by dephosphorylating AKT, ERK, and STAT6 *(147)*.

MGCD0103 is a novel oral inhibitor of HDACs, with selectivity for HDACs 1, 2, 3, and 11 isoforms *(148)*. In a recent Phase I study, MGCD0103 was evaluated in patients with relapsed solid tumors or NHL *(149)*. The most common side effects were fatigue, nausea, anorexia, vomiting, and diarrhea. Whereas other HDAC inhibitors have demonstrated cardiac and/or significant hematologic toxicity, this was not observed with MDGC0103. The clinical activity of vorinostat and MGCD0103 is currently being examined in Phase II clinical trials in patients with relapsed HL.

Table 4
Selected List of HDAC Inhibitors in Clinical Development

HDAC inhibitor group and compound	Clinical formulation	Phase of clinical development
Hydroxamic acid compounds		
SAHA (vorinostat)	IV or PO	I, II
TSA		
CBHA		
ABHA		
NVP-LAQ824	IV	I
LBH589	PO	I
Oxamflatin		
PXD101	IV	I
Scriptaid		
Pyroxamide		
Cyclic tetrapeptides		
Depsipeptide	IV	I, II
Apicidine		
Trapoxin		
HC toxin		
Chlamydocin		
Depudesin		
CHAPS		
Short-chain fatty acids		
Valproic acid		
Phenylbutyrate	IV or PO	I
Phenylacetate	IV	I, II
Sodium butyrate		
AN-9	IV	I, II
Ketones		
Trifluoromethyl ketone		
α-Ketomides		
Benzamide derivatives		
CI-994	PO	I
MS-275	PO	I
Rational design		
MGCD0103	PO	I

Voinostat is the only compound approved for the treatment of lymphoma (cutaneous T-cell type)

4.5. Bcl-2

Antiapoptotic proteins of the Bcl-2 family are overexpressed in lymphomas *(150)*. These proteins are involved in oncogenesis and chemoresistance and are important regulators of the apoptotic pathway. Several studies demonstrated that HRS cells frequently express Bcl-2 protein, which correlates with a poor treatment outcome. Several Bcl-2 family members can now be pharmacologically targeted by antisense and various small molecules. GX15-070 is a small-molecule antagonist, which occupies the BH3 groove on the surface of antiapoptotic members of the Bcl-2 family. GX15-070 induces apoptosis by inhibiting the interaction between pro- and antiapoptotic proteins. Phase I results show GX15-070MS activity in patients with relapsed CLL *(151)* as well as in three MCL cell lines. GX15-70MS is currently being evaluated in Phase II clinical trials of various malignancies, including patients with relapsed classic HL. It is possible that GX15-070MS acts synergistically in combination with doxorubicin or proteasome inhibitors *(150)*.

4.6. BCL6

The BCL6 proto-oncogene encodes a transcriptional repressor whose expression is deregulated by chromosomal translocations in approximately 40% of DLBCLs. Deregulation of the BCL6 proto-oncogene is one of the genetic abnormalities observed in DLBCL *(152–154)*. This proto-oncogene regulates germinal center formation and lymphoma genesis by transcriptional suppression of target genes that control B-cell activation and differentiation by p53-dependent chromosome segregation-dependent mechanisms *(155,156)*. Mice deficient in BCL6 failed to form germinal centers in response to antigen stimulation *(157)*. In contrast, mice that constitutively express BCL6 in their B cells displayed increased germinal center formation and developed B cell lymphoproliferative disorders that frequently evolved into DLBCL *(158)*. Treatment with peptides that specifically bind BCL6 and block its function induce lymphoma cell apoptosis and cell cycle arrest *(159)*. Small-molecule inhibitors of BCL6 could be tested in clinical trials to investigate this potential further for clinical applicability.

4.7. Mitotic Kinases

For mitosis to take place, centrosome maturation, chromosome condensation, centrosome separation, bipolar spindle assembly, and perfect chromosome segregation must occur. These highly coordinated events are regulated by a group of Ser/Thr kinases called mitotic kinases. The only mitotic target used for cancer therapy for many years was the microtubule, which forms a critical part of the mitotic spindle. However, recent advances in cell biology identified new kinases involved in regulating cell division and mitosis that can serve as targets for cancer therapy. Targeting mitotic kinases is a rapidly evolving field, with many small molecules being identified and evaluated for cancer therapy. These small-molecule inhibitors have the potential to act as effective targets for therapy for managing aggressive lymphoma due to their fundamental effect on dividing cells. Aurora kinases, polo-like kinases, and cyclin-dependent kinases, three classes of mitotic kinase, are currently being evaluated in clinical trials for the treatment of cancer *(160–162)*.

4.7.1. AURORA KINASES

Aurora kinases are Ser/Thr kinases that regulate several components of cell division. Three associated kinases have been identified—A, B, C—which share highly conserved catalytic domains *(160)*. (Fig. 6a). Aurora A and B have coordinated functions in regulating cell cycle progression from G_2 through cytokinesis, although the precise function of aurora C remains poorly understood. Aurora A is required for spindle assembly, whereas aurora B is required for chromosome segregation and cytokinesis. It was suggested that the aurora A gene *(STK15)* is involved in the malignant process and it is overexpressed in aggressive NHL *(163)*. Several substrates have been reported for aurora A and B, including CPEB, Eg5, TACC, Ajuba, TPX2, CENP-A, p53, histone H3, INCENP, and Rec8, among others *(164–166)*. To date, at least eight aurora kinase inhibitors have been described, some of which are already in clinical trials for the treatment of cancer. Examples are ZM447439 (AstraZeneca, Grafenau, Switzerland), a compound that inhibits both aurora A and B and

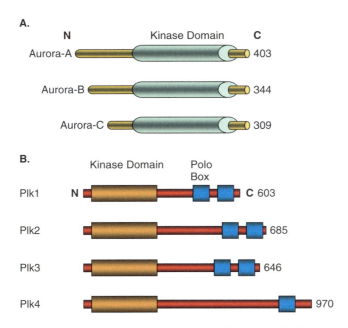

Fig. 6. Structure of selected mitotic kinases. **a** Aurora kinase family. **b** Plk family.

has antiproliferative activity against cancer cells in vitro; Hesperadin (Bohringer Ingelheim, Mannheim, Germany), a small molecule that inhibits aurora B; and VX-680 (Vertex Pharmaceuticals, Cambridge, MA, USA), which inhibits aurora A *(167–169)*. Because these compounds target dividing cells, cytopenia is expected to be the dose-limiting toxicity.

Polo-like kinases (Plks) are essential for successful cell division. In humans, four Plks have been identified *(170)*. Plks are Ser/Thr kinases that contain two conserved domains: an N-terminal kinase domain that closely resembles aurora kinase domains and a C-terminal polo-box domain (Fig. 6b). The *Plk* genes are expressed on different chromosomes and are differentially expressed during normal cell cycle progression *(171,172)*. Tissues with actively proliferating cells, such as hematopoietic sites, testis, ovary, and other cancers such as NHL *(172)*, highly express Plk1. In contrast, nondividing tissues such as kidney and brain express Plk1 at very low or undetectable levels. Plk1 is primarily expressed during late G_2 and M phases of the cell cycle, whereas Plk2 is primarily expressed in early G_1, illustrating that these kinases regulate entry into different parts of the cell cycle. Plk1 expression was found to be higher in aggressive NHL compared with indolent NHL. Plk1 demonstrated superiority over Ki-67 as an index of cell proliferation *(172)*. In B-cell malignancies Plk2 is frequently down-regulated by gene methylation *(173)*. Collectively, these data suggest that inhibiting Plk1 can help abrogate tumorigenesis in some cancers. In fact, several preclinical experiments in discrete tumor types demonstrated that inhibiting Plk1 may induce G_2M cell cycle arrest followed by apoptosis *(174)*. A Phase I study of Plk1 inhibitor (Bohringer-Ingelheim) is currently enrolling patients with aggressive NHL.

4.7.2. Cyclin-Dependent Kinases

Cyclin-dependent kinases (CDKs) are also being targeted for cancer therapy *(162)*. (162). Examples of CDK inhibitors include flavopiridol (Alvocidib), UCN-01, E7070, R-Roscovitine (CYC202), and BMS387032, which have been tested in clinical trials *(162)*. The initial evaluation of flavopiridol in patients with MCL was disappointing; but with a new schedule it was shown to be highly effective in lymphocytic leukemia *(175)*. This activity warrants reexamining the efficacy of these compounds in patients with NHL *(176)*. UCN-01 was also evaluated in a Phase I study in which one patient with large-cell lymphoma achieved a PR *(177)*. Further exploration into the role of CDK inhibitors in the treatment of NHL is needed.

4.8. Protein Kinase (CPKC)-β

The PKC family consists of 12 Ser/Thr kinases with involvement in signal transduction pathways that regulate cell proliferation, apoptosis, and growth factor response *(178)*. PKCβ can be overexpressed in DLBCL, correlating with poor survival *(179,180)*. PKCβ may serve as a potential therapeutic target for B-cell malignancies as it is specifically required for B-cell receptor-mediated NFκB activation, and inhibition of PKCβ promoted cell death in B lymphocytes *(181)*. Results from clinical trials evaluating the use of PKCβ inhibitors in patients with DLBCL are ongoing.

4.9. Extracellular Signal-Regulated Kinase

The mitogen-activated protein kinases (MAPKs), Ser/Thr kinases that mediate signal transduction from the cell surface to the nucleus, are activated in response to various extracellular stimuli. The active phosphorylated form of MAPK/ERK (p44/42) is expressed in primary HRS cells *(182)*. The small-molecule UO126 inhibits ERK phosphorylation and inhibits the upstream MAPK kinase (also called MEK), thereby inhibiting the growth of HL-derived cell lines *(182)*. Mechanistically, UO126 down-regulated the expression of key antiapoptotic proteins, including Bcl-2, Mcl-1, and cFLIP, resulting in enhanced sensitivity to Apo2L/TRAIL and chemotherapy-induced cell death. Up-regulation of ERK in HL could be induced by activating CD30, CD40, and RANK receptors *(182)*, suggesting that inhibiting the MEK/ERK pathway may have a therapeutic value in HL.

5. TARGETING TUMOR ANGIOGENESIS

In cancer, angiogenesis factors are typically produced by benign hematopoietic cells in the tumor microenvironment, including monocytes, lymphocytes, dendritic cells, neutrophils, and mast cells, but they can also be produced by tumor cells. Angiogenesis is a complex, multistep process that requires several growth factors, including acidic and basic fibroblast growth factor (FGF), IL-8, transforming growth factor-α and -β (TGFα, TGFβ), hepatocyte growth factor (HGF), tumor necrosis factor-α (TNFα), epidermal growth factor (EGF), angiogenin, angiopoietin-1, platelet-derived growth factor (PDGF), and vascular endothelial growth factor (VEGF).

5.1. Targeting VEGF and its Receptors

VEGF (also called VEGF-A), a secreted dimeric protein that promotes the growth and survival of embryonic and newly formed endothelial cells in adults, belongs to a gene family that includes VEGF-B, -C, and -D. VEGF-C and -D are involved in regulating lymphangiogenesis, whereas VEGF primarily regulates angiogenesis *(183,184)*. VEGF binds to two receptors, VEGFR-2 (also known as KDR or Flk-1) and VEGFR-1 (also known as FLT1), whereas VEGF-B binds only to VEGFR-1 *(185)*. Both VEGFR-1 and VEGFR-2 are expressed on most endothelial cells. VEGF-C and -D bind to VEGFR-3, which is expressed on lymphatic endothelial cells.

The role of angiogenesis was studied by examining microvessel density and the expression of several angiogenesis factors in response to tumor-associated inflammation *(186–188)*. Furthermore, several studies have reported that correlations may exist between poor treatment outcomes and high levels of soluble angiogenic factors found in the sera of patients with lymphoma *(189)*. A Phase II study of bevacizumab (recombinant antibody to VEGF) was recently completed in patients with relapsed aggressive lymphoma *(190)* and showed only minor single-agent activity. A Phase II trial for the treatment of relapsed aggressive NHL with single-agent bevacizumab (Avastin; Genentech, South San Francisco, CA, USA) treated 46 patients, with 2 (5%) patients achieving PR and 8 with stable disease. Grade 3 toxicities were observed in 15 patients. Ongoing trials are currently evaluating bevacizumab in combination with rituximab and chemotherapy *(190)*. This combination and other clinical trials will hopefully provide more background for the potential utility of antiangiogenesis therapy in patients with aggressive and other types of lymphoma, including HL.

Thalidomide, an oral sedative that targets angiogenesis, has antiinflammatory and immunosuppressive properties. It has minor single-agent activity in patients with recurrent or refractory lymphoma *(191)*. Significant antitumor activity of thalidomide plus rituximab was observed in patients with relapsed or refractory MCL *(192)*. This observation is currently being confirmed in a randomized study in Europe.

Lenalidomide (Revlimid) is a chemical derivative of thalidomide *(193)*. It is indicated in the treatment of myelodysplastic syndrome, transfusion-dependent anemia, and multiple myeloma. As does thalidomide, lenalidomide inhibits the secretion of proinflammatory cytokines and increases the secretion of antiinflammatory cytokines in addition to having antiangiogenesis properties. In Phase II studies conducted to assess its activity in NHL *(194,195)*, 32% of patients exhibited an objective response, with two CRs and 5 PRs. Studies are planned to assess further its role in HL and NHL.

REFERENCES

1. McKelvey EM, et al. Hydroxyldaunomycin (Adriamycin) combination chemotherapy in malignant lymphoma. Cancer 1976;38(4):1484–93.
2. Stashenko P, et al. Characterization of a human B lymphocyte-specific antigen. J Immunol 1980;125(4): 1678–85.
3. Czuczman MS, et al. Prolonged clinical and molecular remission in patients with low-grade or follicular non-Hodgkin's lymphoma treated with rituximab plus CHOP chemotherapy: 9-year follow-up. J Clin Oncol 2004;22(23):4711–6.
4. Coiffier B, et al. CHOP chemotherapy plus rituximab compared with CHOP alone in elderly patients with diffuse large-B-cell lymphoma. N Engl J Med 2002;346(4):235–42.
5. Feugier P, et al. Long-term results of the R-CHOP study in the treatment of elderly patients with diffuse large B-cell lymphoma: a study by the Groupe d'Etude des Lymphomes de l'Adulte. J Clin Oncol 2005;23(18):4117–26.
6. Pfreundschuh M, et al. Two-weekly or 3-weekly CHOP chemotherapy with or without etoposide for the treatment of elderly patients with aggressive lymphomas: results of the NHL-B2 trial of the DSHNHL. Blood 2004;104(3):634–41.
7. Pfreundschuh M, et al. Six, not eight cycles of bi-weekly CHOP with rituximab (R-CHOP-14) is the preferred treatment for elderly patients with diffuse large B-cell lymphoma (DLBCL): results of the RICOVER-60 trial of the German high-grade non-Hodgkin lymphoma study group (DSHNHL). ASH Annu Meet Abstr 2005;106(11):13.
8. McLaughlin P, et al. Stage IV indolent lymphoma: a randomized study of concurrent vs. sequential use of FND chemotherapy (fludarabine, mitoxantrone, dexamethasone) and rituximab (R) monoclonal antibody therapy, with interferon maintenance. Proc Am Soc Clin Oncol 2003;22:564. Asbtract 2269.
9. McLaughlin P, et al. Rituximab chimeric anti-CD20 monoclonal antibody therapy for relapsed indolent lymphoma: half of patients respond to a four-dose treatment program. J Clin Oncol 1998;16(8):2825–33.

10. Witzens-Harig M, et al. Rituximab maintenenance therapy in CD20+ B-cell non-Hodgkin-lymphoma: results of a multicenter prospective randomised phase II study. ASH Annu Meet Abstr 2006;108(11):4704.

11. Witzig TE. Radioimmunotherapy for B-cell non-Hodgkin lymphoma. Best Pract Res Clin Haematol 2006;19(4):655–68.

12. Leonard JP, et al. Epratuzumab, a humanized anti-CD22 antibody, in aggressive non-Hodgkin's lymphoma: phase I/II clinical trial results. Clin Cancer Res 2004;10(16):5327–34.

13. Leonard JP, et al. Combination antibody therapy with epratuzumab and rituximab in relapsed or refractory non-Hodgkin's lymphoma. J Clin Oncol 2005;23(22):5044–51.

14. Decker T, et al. BL22, a recombinant anti-CD22 immunotoxin, induces cell cycle arrest and apoptosis in B-cell lymphoma. ASH Annu Meet Abstr 2004;104(11):4613.

15. Kreitman R, et al. Phase I trial of recombinant immunotoxin RFB4(dsFv)-PE38 (BL22) in patients with B-cell malignancies. J Clin Oncol 2005;23(27):6719–29.

16. Fayad L, et al. Clinical activity of the immunoconjugate CMC-544 in B-cell malignancies: preliminary report of the expanded maximum tolerated dose (MTD) cohort of a phase 1 study. ASH Annu Meet Abstr 2006;108(11):2711.

17. Hernandez-Ilizaliturri FJ, et al. Targeting CD20 and CD22 with rituximab in combination with CMC-544 results in improved anti-tumor activity against non-Hodgkin's lymphoma (NHL) pre-clinical models. ASH Annu Meet Abstr 2005;106(11):1473.

18. DiJoseph JF, et al. Antitumor efficacy of a combination of CMC-544 (inotuzumab ozogamicin), a CD22-targeted cytotoxic immunoconjugate of calicheamicin, and rituximab against non-Hodgkin's B-cell lymphoma. Clin Cancer Res 2006;12(1):242–9.

19. Linden O, et al. Dose-fractionated radioimmunotherapy in non-Hodgkin's lymphoma using DOTA-conjugated, 90Y-radiolabeled, humanized anti-CD22 monoclonal antibody, epratuzumab. Clin Cancer Res 2005;11(14):5215–22.

20. Zhukovsky EA, et al. Fc engineered anti-CD19 monoclonal antibodies with enhanced in vitro efficacy against multiple lymphoma cell lines. ASH Annu Meet Abstr 2006;108(11):4747.

21. Younes A, Carbone A. CD30/CD30 ligand and CD40/CD40 ligand in malignant lymphoid disorders. Int J Biol Markers 1999;14(3):135–43.

22. Van Kooten C, Banchereau J. CD40-CD40 ligand. J Leukoc Biol 2000;67(1):2–17.

23. Kato K, et al. The soluble CD40 ligand sCD154 in systemic lupus erythematosus. J Clin Invest 1999;104(7):947–55.

24. Viallard JF, et al. Increased soluble and platelet-associated CD40 ligand in essential thrombocythemia and reactive thrombocytosis. Blood 2002;99(7):2612–4.

25. Younes A, et al. Elevated levels of biologically active soluble CD40 ligand in the serum of patients with chronic lymphocytic leukaemia. Br J Haematol 1998;100(1):135–41.

26. Younes A, Kadin ME. Emerging applications of the tumor necrosis factor family of ligands and receptors in cancer therapy. J Clin Oncol 2003;21(18):3526–34.

27. Fiumara P, Younes A. CD40 ligand (CD154) and tumour necrosis factor-related apoptosis inducing ligand (Apo-2L) in haematological malignancies. Br J Haematol 2001;113(2):265–74.

28. Younes A. The dynamics of life and death of malignant lymphocytes. Curr Opin Oncol 1999;11(5):364–9.

29. Weng W, et al. A fully human anti-CD40 antagonistic antibody, CHIR-12.12, inhibit the proliferation of human B cell non-Hodgkin lymphoma. Blood 2004;104:3279. Abstract.

30. Drachman JG, et al. A humanized anti CD40 monoclonal antibody (SGN-40) demonstrates antitumor activity in non-Hodgkin lymphoma: initiation of a phase-I clinical trial. J Clin Oncol 2005;23(16S):6572.

31. Advani R, et al. SGN-40 (anti-huCD40 mAb) monotherapy induces durable objective responses in patients with relapsed aggressive non-Hodgkin's lymphoma: evidence of antitumor activity from a phase I study. ASH Annu Meet Abstr 2006;108(11):695.

32. Advani RH, et al. Phase I study of humanized anti-CD40 immunotherapy with SGN-40 in non-Hodgkin's lymphoma. Blood 2005;106(11):1504. Abstract.

33. Forero-Torres A, et al. A humanized antibody against CD40 (SGN-40) is well tolerated and active in non-Hodgkin's lymphoma (NHL): results of a phase I study. J Clin Oncol 2006;24(suppl):7534.

34. Lewis TS, et al. The humanized anti-CD40 antibody, SGN-40, promotes apoptosis signaling and is effective in combination with standard therapies in lymphoma xenograft models. ASH Annu Meet Abstr 2006;108(11):2499.

35. Younes A, Aggarwall BB. Clinical implications of the tumor necrosis factor family in benign and malignant hematologic disorders. Cancer 2003;98(3):458–67.

36. Wahl AF, et al. SGN-30, a chimeric antibody to CD30, for the treatment of Hodgkin's disease. Proc Am Assoc Cancer Res 2002;43:4979a.

37. Forero-Torres A, et al. SGN-30 (anti-CD30 mAb) has a single-agent response rate of 21% in patients with refractory or recurrent systemic anaplastic large cell lymphoma (ALCL). ASH Annu Meet Abstr 2006;108(11):2718.

38. Ansell SM, et al. Phase I/II study of a fully human anti-CD30 monoclonal antibody (MDX-060) in Hodgkin's disease (HD) and anaplastic large cell lymphoma (ALCL). Blood 2003;102(11):632. Abstract.

39. Carbone A, et al. Expression of functional CD40 antigen on Reed-Sternberg cells and Hodgkin's disease cell lines. Blood 1995;85(3):780–9.

40. Schnell R, et al. Treatment of refractory Hodgkin's lymphoma patients with an iodine-131-labeled murine anti-CD30 monoclonal antibody. J Clin Oncol 2005;23(21):4669–78.

41. Hammond PW, et al. A humanized anti-CD30 monoclonal antibody, XmAbTM2513, with enhanced in vitro potency against CD30-positive lymphomas mediated by high affinity Fc-receptor binding. Blood 2005;106(11):1470.

42. Nagata S, et al. Cell membrane-specific epitopes on CD30: potentially superior targets for immunotherapy. Proc Natl Acad Sci U S A 2005;102(22):7946–51.

43. Lazar GA, et al. Engineered antibody Fc variants with enhanced effector function. Proc Natl Acad Sci U S A 2006;103(11):4005–10.

44. Hamblett KJ, et al. SGN-35, an anti-CD30 antibody-drug conjugate, exhibits potent antitumor activity for the treatment of CD30+ malignancies. Blood 2005;106(11):610.

45. Okeley NM, et al. Specific tumor targeting and potent bystander killing with SGN-35, an anti-CD30 antibody drug conjugate. ASH Annu Meet Abstr 2006;108(11):231.

46. Schultze J, et al. B7-mediated costimulation and the immune response. Blood Rev 1996;10(2):111–27.

47. June CH, et al. The B7 and CD28 receptor families. Immunol Today 1994;15(7):321–31.

48. Vyth-Dreese FA, et al. Localization in situ of the co-stimulatory molecules B7.1, B7.2, CD40 and their ligands in normal human lymphoid tissue. Eur J Immunol 1995;25(11):3023–9.

49. Dorfman DM, et al. In vivo expression of B7–1 and B7–2 by follicular lymphoma cells can prevent induction of T cell anergy but is insufficient to induce significant T cell proliferation. Blood 1997;90:4297–306.

50. Trentin L, et al. B lymphocytes from patients with chronic lymphoproliferative disorders are equipped with different costimulatory molecules. Cancer Res 1997;57(21):4940–7.

51. Vooijs WC. et al. B7–1 (CD80) as target for immunotoxin therapy for Hodgkin's disease. Br J Cancer 1997;76(9):1163–9.

52. Nozawa Y, et al. Costimulatory molecules (CD80 and CD86) on Reed-Sternberg cells are associated with the proliferation of background T cells in Hodgkin's disease. Pathol Int 1998;48(1):10–4.

53. Munro JM, et al. In vivo expression of the B7 costimulatory molecule by subsets of antigen-presenting cells and the malignant cells of Hodgkin's disease. Blood 1994;83(3):793–8.

54. Younes A, et al. Initial trials of anti-CD80 monoclonal antibody (galiximab) therapy for patients with relapsed or refractory follicular lymphoma. Clin Lymphoma 2003;3(4):257–9.

55. Czuczman MS, et al. Phase I/II study of galiximab, an anti-CD80 antibody, for relapsed or refractory follicular lymphoma. J Clin Oncol 2005;23(19):4390–8.

56. Friedberg JW, et al. Updated results from a phase II study of galiximab (anti-CD80) in combination with rituximab for relapsed or refractory, follicular NHL. ASH Annu Meet Abstr 2005;106(11):2435.

57. Casale DA, et al. A phase I open label dose escalation study to evaluate MEDI-507 in patients with CD2-positive T-cell lymphoma/leukemia. ASH Annu Meet Abstr 2006;108(11):2727.

58. Zhang Z, et al. Effective therapy for a murine model of adult T-cell leukemia with the humanized anti-CD2 monoclonal antibody, MEDI-507. Blood 2003;102(1):284–8.

59. Lundin J, et al. CAMPATH-1H monoclonal antibody in therapy for previously treated low- grade non-Hodgkin's lymphomas: a phase II multicenter study; European Study Group of CAMPATH-1H Treatment in low-grade non-Hodgkin's lymphoma. J Clin Oncol 1998;16(10): 3257–63.

60. Zinzani PL, et al. Phase II study of alemtuzumab treatment in patients with pretreated T-cell lymphoma. ASH Annu Meet Abstr 2004;104(11):4605.

61. Kapp U, et al. Interleukin 13 is secreted by and stimulates the growth of Hodgkin and Reed-Sternberg cells. J Exp Med 1999;189(12):1939–46.

62. Ashkenazi A. Targeting death and decoy receptors of the tumour-necrosis factor superfamily. Nat Rev Cancer 2002;2(6):420–30.

63. Bhardwaj A, Aggarwal BB. Receptor-mediated choreography of life and death. J Clin Immunol 2003;23(5):317–32.

64. Emery JG, et al. Osteoprotegerin is a receptor for the cytotoxic ligand TRAIL. J Biol Chem 1998;273(23):14363–7.

65. Degli-Esposti M. To die or not to die—the quest of the TRAIL receptors. J Leukoc Biol 1999;65(5):535–42.

66. Georgakis GV, et al. Activity of selective fully human agonistic antibodies to the TRAIL death receptors TRAIL-R1 and TRAIL-R2 in primary and cultured lymphoma cells: induction of apoptosis and enhancement of doxorubicin- and bortezomib-induced cell death. Br J Haematol 2005;130(4):501–10.

67. Younes A, et al. Results of a phase 2 trial of HGS-ETR1 (agonistic human monoclonal antibody to TRAIL receptor 1) in subjects with relapsed/refractory non-Hodgkin's lymphoma (NHL). Blood 2005;106(11):489.

68. Schneider P, Tschopp J. BAFF and the regulation of B cell survival. Immunol Lett 2003;88(1):57–62.

69. Medema JP, et al. The uncertain glory of APRIL. Cell Death Differ 2003;10(10):1121–5.

70. Mackay F, et al. BAFF AND APRIL: a tutorial on B cell survival. Annu Rev Immunol 2003;21:231–64.

71. Mackay F, et al. Mice transgenic for BAFF develop lymphocytic disorders along with autoimmune manifestations. J Exp Med 1999;190(11):1697–710.

72. Khare SD, et al. Severe B cell hyperplasia and autoimmune disease in TALL-1 transgenic mice. Proc Natl Acad Sci U S A 2000;97(7):3370–5.

73. Kern C, et al. Involvement of BAFF and APRIL in the resistance to apoptosis of B-CLL through an autocrine pathway. Blood 2004;103(2):679–88.

74. Novak AJ, et al. Aberrant expression of B-lymphocyte stimulator by B chronic lymphocytic leukemia cells: a mechanism for survival. Blood 2002;100(8):2973–9.

75. Moreaux J, et al. BAFF and APRIL protect myeloma cells from apoptosis induced by IL-6 deprivation and dexamethasone. Blood 2004;103:3148–57.

76. Novak AJ, et al. Expression of BCMA, TACI, and BAFF-R in multiple myeloma: a mechanism for growth and survival. Blood 2004;103(2):689–94.

77. He B, et al. Lymphoma B cells evade apoptosis through the TNF family members BAFF/BLyS and APRIL. J Immunol 2004;172(5):3268–79.

78. Halpern WG, et al. Chronic administration of belimumab, a BLyS antagonist, decreases tissue and peripheral blood B-lymphocyte populations in cynomolgus monkeys: pharmacokinetic, pharmacodynamic, and toxicologic effects. Toxicol Sci 2006;91(2):586–99.

79. Belch A, et al. Tumor targeting, dosimetry and clinical response data for lymphorad-131 (LR131; iodine I-131 labeled B-lymphocyte stimulator) in patients with relapsed/refractory non-Hodgkin's lymphoma. Blood 2004;104:750.

80. Chiu A, et al. The TNF family members BAFF and APRIL play an important role in Hodgkin lymphoma. Blood 2005;106(11):22.

81. Oki Y, et al. Serum BLyS level as a prognostic marker in patients with lymphoma. Blood 2005;106(11):1926.

82. Khosla S. Minireview: the OPG/RANKL/RANK system. Endocrinology 2001;142(12):5050–5.

83. Wong BR, et al. TRANCE is a TNF family member that regulates dendritic cell and osteoclast function. J Leukoc Biol 1999;65(6): 715–24.

84. Wong BR, et al. The TRAF family of signal transducers mediates NF-kappaB activation by the TRANCE receptor. J Biol Chem 1998;273(43):28355–9.

85. Yasuda H, et al. Identity of osteoclastogenesis inhibitory factor (OCIF) and osteoprotegerin (OPG): a mechanism by which OPG/OCIF inhibits osteoclastogenesis in vitro. Endocrinology 1998;139(3):1329–37.

86. Richardson PG, et al. Bortezomib (PS-341): a novel, first-in-class proteasome inhibitor for the treatment of multiple myeloma and other cancers. Cancer Control 2003;10(5):361–9.

87. Fisher RI, et al. Multicenter phase II study of bortezomib in patients with relapsed or refractory mantle cell lymphoma. J Clin Oncol 2006;24(30):4867–74.

88. Kane RC, et al. United States Food and Drug Administration approval summary: bortezomib for the treatment of progressive multiple myeloma after one prior therapy. Clin Cancer Res 2006;12(10):2955–60.

89. Adams J. Potential for proteasome inhibition in the treatment of cancer. Drug Discov Today 2003;8(7): 307–15.

90. Zheng B, et al. Induction of cell cycle arrest and apoptosis by the proteasome inhibitor PS-341 in Hodgkin disease cell lines is independent of inhibitor of nuclear factor-kappaB mutations or activation of the CD30, CD40, and RANK receptors. Clin Cancer Res 2004;10(9):3207–15.

91. O'Connor OA, et al. Phase II clinical experience with the novel proteasome inhibitor bortezomib in patients with indolent non-Hodgkin's lymphoma and mantle cell lymphoma. J Clin Oncol 2005;23(4):676–84.

92. Goy A, et al. Phase II study of proteasome inhibitor bortezomib in relapsed or refractory B-cell non-Hodgkin's lymphoma. J Clin Oncol 2005;23(4):667–75.

93. Assouline S, et al. A phase II study of bortezomib in patients with mantle cell lymphoma. Blood 2003;102(11):3358. Abstract.

94. Beland JL, et al. Recombinant CD40L treatment protects allogeneic murine bone marrow transplant recipients from death caused by herpes simplex virus-1 infection. Blood 1998;92(11):4472–8.

95. Strauss SJ, et al. Phase II clinical study of bortezomib (Velcade) in patients with relapsed/refractory non-Hodgkin lymphoma and Hodgkin disease. Blood 2004;104:1386. Abstract.

96. Goy A, et al. Bortezomib in patients with relapsed or refractory mantle cell lymphoma: preliminary results of the PINNACLE study. J Clin Oncol 2005;23(16S):6563.

97. Younes A, et al. Experience with bortezomib for the treatment of patients with relapsed classical Hodgkin lymphoma. Blood 2006;107(4):1731a-2.

98. Trelle S, et al. Bortezomib is not active in patients with relapsed Hodgkin's lymphoma: results of a prematurely closed phase II study. ASH Annu Meet Abstr 2006;108(11):2477.

99. Fresno Vara JA, et al. PI3K/Akt signalling pathway and cancer. Cancer Treat Rev 2004;30(2):193–204.

100. Lu Y, et al. Targeting PI3K-AKT pathway for cancer therapy. Rev Clin Exp Hematol 2003;7(2):205–28.

101. Abbott RT, et al. Analysis of the PI-3-Kinase-PTEN-AKT pathway in human lymphoma and leukemia using a cell line microarray. Mod Pathol 2003;16(6):607–12.

102. Xu G, et al. Pharmacogenomic profiling of the PI3K/PTEN-AKT-mTOR pathway in common human tumors. Int J Oncol 2004;24(4):893–900.

103. Paez J, Sellers WR. PI3K/PTEN/AKT pathway: a critical mediator of oncogenic signaling. Cancer Treat Res 2003;115:145–67.

104. Dutcher JP. Mammalian target of rapamycin (mTOR) Inhibitors. Curr Oncol Rep 2004;6(2):111–5.

105. Huang S, Houghton PJ. Targeting mTOR signaling for cancer therapy. Curr Opin Pharmacol 2003;3(4):371–7.

106. Sawyers CL. Will mTOR inhibitors make it as cancer drugs? Cancer Cell 2003;4(5):343–8.

107. Gao N, et al. G1 cell cycle progression and the expression of G1 cyclins are regulated by PI3K/AKT/mTOR/p70S6K1 signaling in human ovarian cancer cells. Am J Physiol Cell Physiol 2004;287(2):C281–91.

108. Vignot S, et al. mTOR-targeted therapy of cancer with rapamycin derivatives. Ann Oncol 2005;16(4):525–37.

109. Chan S. Targeting the mammalian target of rapamycin (mTOR): a new approach to treating cancer. Br J Cancer 2004;91(8):1420–4.

110. Dancey JE. Inhibitors of the mammalian target of rapamycin. Expert Opin Invest Drugs 2005;14(3):313–28.

111. Witzig TE, et al. Phase II trial of single-agent temsirolimus (CCI-779) for relapsed mantle cell lymphoma. J Clin Oncol 2005;23(23):5347–56.

112. Feldman E, et al. A phase 2 clinical trial of AP23573, an mTOR inhibitor, in patients with relapsed or refractory hematologic malignancies. J Clin Oncol 2005;23(16S):6631.

113. Georgakis GV, et al. Inhibition of the phosphatidylinositol-3 kinase/Akt promotes G1 cell cycle arrest and apoptosis in Hodgkin lymphoma. Br J Haematol 2006;132(4):503–11.

114. Morrison JA, et al. Differential signaling pathways are activated in the Epstein-Barr virus-associated malignancies nasopharyngeal carcinoma and Hodgkin lymphoma. Cancer Res 2004;64(15):5251–60.

115. Neckers L. Heat shock protein 90 inhibition by 17-allylamino-17- demethoxygeldanamycin: a novel therapeutic approach for treating hormone-refractory prostate cancer. Clin Cancer Res 2002;8(5):962–6.

116. Beere HM. Death versus survival: functional interaction between the apoptotic and stress-inducible heat shock protein pathways. J Clin Invest 2005;115(10):2633–9.

117. Georgakis GV, Younes A. Heat-shock protein 90 inhibitors in cancer therapy: 17AAG and beyond. Future Oncol 2005;1(2):273–81.

118. Sreedhar AS; Csermely P. Heat shock proteins in the regulation of apoptosis: new strategies in tumor therapy: a comprehensive review. Pharmacol Ther 2004;101(3):227–57.

119. Kamal A, et al. A high-affinity conformation of Hsp90 confers tumour selectivity on Hsp90 inhibitors. Nature 2003;425(6956):407–10.

120. Rowlands MG. et al. High-throughput screening assay for inhibitors of heat-shock protein 90 ATPase activity. Anal Biochem 2004;327(2):176–83.

121. Workman P. Altered states: selectively drugging the Hsp90 cancer chaperone. Trends Mol Med 2004;10(2):47–51.

122. Workman P. Overview: translating Hsp90 biology into Hsp90 drugs. Curr Cancer Drug Targets 2003;3(5):297–300.

123. Uehara Y. Natural product origins of Hsp90 inhibitors. Curr Cancer Drug Targets 2003;3(5):325–30.

124. Neckers L. Development of small molecule Hsp90 inhibitors: utilizing both forward and reverse chemical genomics for drug identification. Curr Med Chem 2003;10(9):733–9.

125. Isaacs JS, et al. Heat shock protein 90 as a molecular target for cancer therapeutics. Cancer Cell 2003;3(3):213–7.

126. Ramanathan RK, et al. Phase I pharmacokinetic-pharmacodynamic study of 17-(allylamino)-17-demethoxygeldanamycin (17AAG, NSC 330507), a novel inhibitor of heat shock protein 90, in patients with refractory advanced cancers. Clin Cancer Res 2005;11(9):3385–91.

127. Georgakis GV, et al. Inhibition of heat shock protein 90 function by 17-allylamino-17-demethoxy-geldanamycin in Hodgkin's lymphoma cells down-regulates Akt kinase, dephosphorylates extracellular signal-regulated kinase, and induces cell cycle arrest and cell death. Clin Cancer Res 2006;12(2):584–90.

128. Monneret C. Histone deacetylase inhibitors. Eur J Med Chem 2005;40(1):1–13.

129. Hess-Stumpp H. Histone deacetylase inhibitors and cancer: from cell biology to the clinic. Eur J Cell Biol 2005;84(2–3):109–21.

130. Drummond DC, et al. Clinical development of histone deacetylase inhibitors as anticancer agents. Annu Rev Pharmacol Toxicol 2005;45:495–528.

131. Shao Y, et al. Apoptotic and autophagic cell death induced by histone deacetylase inhibitors. Proc Natl Acad Sci U S A 2004;101(52):18030–5.

132. Sakajiri S, et al. Histone deacetylase inhibitors profoundly decrease proliferation of human lymphoid cancer cell lines. Exp Hematol 2005;33(1):53–61.

133. McLaughlin F, La Thangue NB. Histone deacetylase inhibitors open new doors in cancer therapy. Biochem Pharmacol 2004;68(6):1139–44.

134. Acharya MR, et al. Rational development of histone deacetylase inhibitors as anticancer agents: a review. Mol Pharmacol 2005;68(4):917–32.

135. Kelly WK, et al. Phase I clinical trial of histone deacetylase inhibitor: suberoylanilide hydroxamic acid administered intravenously. Clin Cancer Res 2003;9(10 Pt 1):3578–88.

136. Kelly WK, et al. Phase I study of an oral histone deacetylase inhibitor, suberoylanilide hydroxamic acid, in patients with advanced cancer. J Clin Oncol 2005;23:3923–31.

137. Duvic M, et al. Phase 2 trial of oral vorinostat (suberoylanilide hydroxamic acid, SAHA) for refractory cutaneous T-cell lymphoma (CTCL). Blood 2007;109(1):31–9.

138. Ueda H, et al. FR901228, a novel antitumor bicyclic depsipeptide produced by Chromobacterium violaceum no. 968. III. Antitumor activities on experimental tumors in mice. J Antibiot (Tokyo) 1994;47(3):315–23.

139. Furumai R, et al. FK228 (depsipeptide) as a natural prodrug that inhibits class I histone deacetylases. Cancer Res 2002;62(17):4916–21.

140. Byrd JC, et al. A phase 1 and pharmacodynamic study of depsipeptide (FK228) in chronic lymphocytic leukemia and acute myeloid leukemia. Blood 2005;105(3):959–67.

141. Sandor V, et al. Phase I trial of the histone deacetylase inhibitor, depsipeptide (FR901228, NSC 630176), in patients with refractory neoplasms. Clin Cancer Res 2002;8(3):718–28.

142. Marshall JL, et al. A phase I trial of depsipeptide (FR901228) in patients with advanced cancer. J Exp Ther Oncol 2002;2(6):325–32.

143. Piekarz R, et al. Update on the phase II trial and correlative studies of depsipeptide in patients with cutaneous T-cell lymphoma and relapsed peripheral T-cell lymphoma. J Clin Oncol 2004;22(14S):3028.

144. Ushmorov A, et al. Epigenetic processes play a major role in B-cell-specific gene silencing in classical Hodgkin lymphoma. Blood 2006;107(6):2493–500.

145. Ushmorov A, et al. Epigenetic silencing of the immunoglobulin heavy-chain gene in classical Hodgkin lymphoma-derived cell lines contributes to the loss of immunoglobulin expression. Blood 2004;104(10):3326–34.

146. Doerr JR, et al. Patterned CpG methylation of silenced B cell gene promoters in classical Hodgkin lymphoma-derived and primary effusion lymphoma cell lines. J Mol Biol 2005;350(4):631–40.

147. Georgakis GV, et al. The histone deacetylase inhibitor vorinostat (SAHA) induces apoptosis and cell cycle arrest in hodgkin lymphoma (HL) cell lines by altering several survival signaling pathways and synergizes with doxorubicin, gemcitabine and bortezomib. ASH Annu Meet Abstr 2006;108(11):2260.

148. Kalita A, et al. Pharmacodynamic effect of MGCD0103, an oral isotype-selective histone deacetylase (HDAC) inhibitor, on HDAC enzyme inhibition and histone acetylation induction in phase I clinical trials in patients (pts) with advanced solid tumors or non-Hodgkin's lymphoma (NHL). J Clin Oncol 2005;23(suppl):9631.

149. Gelmon K, et al. Phase I trials of the oral histone deacetylase (HDAC) inhibitor MGCD0103 given either daily or 3× weekly for 14 days every 3 weeks in patients (pts) with advanced solid tumors. ASCO Meet Abstr 2005;23(suppl):3147.

150. Yazbeck VY, et al. Inhibition of the Pan-Bcl-2 family by the small molecule gx15–070 induces apoptosis in mantle cell lymphoma (MCL) cells and enhances the activity of two proteasome inhibitors (NPI-0052 and bortezomib), and doxorubicin chemotherapy. ASH Annu Meet Abstr 2006;108(11):2532.

151. O'Brien S, et al. A phase I trial of the small molecule Pan-Bcl-2 family inhibitor GX15–070 administered intravenously (IV) every 3 weeks to patients with previously treated chronic lymphocytic leukemia (CLL). Blood 2005;106(11):446.

152. Ye BH, et al. Alterations of a zinc finger-encoding gene, BCL-6, in diffuse large-cell lymphoma. Science 1993;262(5134):747–50.

153. Ye BH, et al. Cloning of bcl-6, the locus involved in chromosome translocations affecting band 3q27 in B-cell lymphoma. Cancer Res 1993;53(12):2732–5.

154. Lo Coco F, et al. Rearrangements of the BCL6 gene in diffuse large cell non-Hodgkin's lymphoma. Blood 1994;83(7):1757–9.

155. Phan RT, et al. BCL6 interacts with the transcription factor Miz-1 to suppress the cyclin-dependent kinase inhibitor p21 and cell cycle arrest in germinal center B cells. Nat Immunol 2005;6(10):1054–60.

156. Phan RT, Dalla-Favera R, The BCL6 proto-oncogene suppresses p53 expression in germinal-centre B cells. Nature 2004;432(7017):635–9.

157. Ye BH, et al. The BCL-6 proto-oncogene controls germinal-centre formation and Th2-type inflammation. Nat Genet 1997;16(2):161–70.

158. Cattoretti G, et al. Deregulated BCL6 expression recapitulates the pathogenesis of human diffuse large B cell lymphomas in mice. Cancer Cell 2005;7(5):445–55.

159. Polo JM, et al. Specific peptide interference reveals BCL6 transcriptional and oncogenic mechanisms in B-cell lymphoma cells. Nat Med 2004;10(12):1329–35.

160. Marumoto T, et al. Aurora-A—a guardian of poles. Nat Rev Cancer 2005;5(1):42–50.

161. Van Vugt MA, Medema RH. Polo-like kinase-1: activity measurement and RNAi-mediated knockdown. Methods Mol Biol 2005;296:355–69.

162. Benson C, et al. Clinical anticancer drug development: targeting the cyclin-dependent kinases. Br J Cancer 2005;92(1):7–12.

163. Hamada M, et al. Aurora2/BTAK/STK15 is involved in cell cycle checkpoint and cell survival of aggressive non-Hodgkin's lymphoma. Br J Haematol 2003;121(3):439–47.

164. Ditchfield C, et al. Aurora B couples chromosome alignment with anaphase by targeting BubR1, Mad2, and Cenp-E to kinetochores. J Cell Biol 2003;161(2):267–80.

165. Sessa F, et al. Mechanism of Aurora B activation by INCENP and inhibition by hesperadin. Mol Cell 2005;18(3):379–91.

166. Morrow CJ, et al. Bub1 and aurora B cooperate to maintain BubR1-mediated inhibition of APC/CCdc20. J Cell Sci 2005;118(Pt 16):3639–52.

167. Gadea BB, Ruderman JV. Aurora kinase inhibitor ZM447439 blocks chromosome-induced spindle assembly, the completion of chromosome condensation, and the establishment of the spindle integrity checkpoint in Xenopus egg extracts. Mol Biol Cell 2005;16(3):1305–18.

168. Harrington EA, et al. VX-680, a potent and selective small-molecule inhibitor of the Aurora kinases, suppresses tumor growth in vivo. Nat Med 2004;10(3):262–7.

169. Hauf S, et al. The small molecule Hesperadin reveals a role for Aurora B in correcting kinetochore-microtubule attachment and in maintaining the spindle assembly checkpoint. J Cell Biol 2003;161(2):281–94.

170. Lowery DM, et al. Structure and function of Polo-like kinases. Oncogene 2005;24(2):248–59.

171. Winkles JA, Alberts GF. Differential regulation of polo-like kinase 1, 2, 3, and 4 gene expression in mammalian cells and tissues. Oncogene 2005;24(2):260–6.

172. Mito K, et al. Expression of Polo-like kinase (PLK1) in non-Hodgkin's lymphomas. Leuk Lymphoma 2005;46(2):225–31.

173. Syed N, et al. Transcriptional silencing of Polo-like kinase 2 (Snk/Plk2) is a frequent event in B cell malignancies. Blood 2006;107:250–6.

174. Eckerdt F, et al. Polo-like kinases and oncogenesis. Oncogene 2005;24(2):267–76.

175. Lin TS, et al., Seventy-two hour continuous infusion flavopiridol in relapsed and refractory mantle cell lymphoma. Leuk Lymphoma 2002;43(4):793–7.

176. Byrd JC, et al. Treatment of relapsed chronic lymphocytic leukemia by 72-hour continuous infusion or 1-hour bolus infusion of flavopiridol: results from Cancer and Leukemia Group B study 19805. Clin Cancer Res 2005;11(11):4176–81.

177. Sausville EA, et al. Phase I trial of 72-hour continuous infusion UCN-01 in patients with refractory neoplasms. J Clin Oncol 2001;19(8):2319–33.

178. Guo B, et al. Protein kinase C family functions in B-cell activation. Curr Opin Immunol 2004;16(3):367–73.

179. Shipp MA, et al. Diffuse large B-cell lymphoma outcome prediction by gene-expression profiling and supervised machine learning. Nat Med 2002;8(1):68–74.

180. Hans CP, et al. Expression of PKC-beta or cyclin D2 predicts for inferior survival in diffuse large B-cell lymphoma. Mod Pathol 2005;18(10):1377–84.

181. Su TT, et al. PKC-beta controls I kappa B kinase lipid raft recruitment and activation in response to BCR signaling. Nat Immunol 2002;3(8):780–6.

182. Zheng B, et al. MEK/ERK pathway is aberrantly active in Hodgkin disease: a signaling pathway shared by CD30, CD40, and RANK that regulates cell proliferation and survival. Blood 2003;102(3):1019–27.

183. Ferrara N, et al. The biology of VEGF and its receptors. Nat Med 2003;9(6):669–76.

184. Plate K. From angiogenesis to lymphangiogenesis. Nat Med 2001;7(2):151–2.
185. Olofsson B, et al. Vascular endothelial growth factor B (VEGF-B) binds to VEGF receptor-1 and regulates plasminogen activator activity in endothelial cells. Proc Natl Acad Sci U S A 1998;95(20):11709–14.
186. Ribatti D, et al. Angiogenesis induced by B-cell non-Hodgkin's lymphomas: lack of correlation with tumor malignancy and immunologic phenotype. Anticancer Res 1990;10(2A):401–6.
187. Ribatti D, et al. Angiogenesis and mast cell density with tryptase activity increase simultaneously with pathological progression in B-cell non-Hodgkin's lymphomas. Int J Cancer 2000;85(2):171–5.
188. Vacca A, et al. Angiogenesis in B cell lymphoproliferative diseases: biological and clinical studies. Leuk Lymphoma 1995;20(1–2):27–38.
189. Salven P, et al. Simultaneous elevation in the serum concentrations of the angiogenic growth factors VEGF and bFGF is an independent predictor of poor prognosis in non-Hodgkin lymphoma: a single-institution study of 200 patients. Blood 2000;96(12):3712–8.
190. Stopeck AT, et al. Phase II trial of single agent bevacizumab in patients with relapsed, aggressive non-Hodgkin's lymphoma (NHL): Southwest Oncology Group study S0108. J Clin Oncol 2005;23(16S):6529.
191. Pro B, et al. Thalidomide for patients with recurrent lymphoma. Cancer 2004;100(6):1186–9.
192. Drach J, et al. Marked anti-tumor activity of rituximab plus thalidomide in patients with relapsed/resistant mantle cell lymphoma. Blood 2002;100(11):606. Abstract.
193. Richardson PG, et al. A randomized phase 2 study of lenalidomide therapy for patients with relapsed or relapsed and refractory multiple myeloma. Blood 2006;108(10):58–3464.
194. Wiernik PH, et al. Preliminary results from a phase II study of lenalidomide monotherapy in relapsed/refractory aggressive non-Hodgkin's lymphoma. ASH Annu Meet Abstr 2006;108(11):531.
195. Witzig TE, et al. Early results from a phase II study of lenalidomide monotherapy in relapsed/refractory indolent non-Hodgkin's lymphoma. ASH Annu Meet Abstr 2006;108(11):2482.
196. Morshhauser F, et al. Phase I/II results of a second-generation humanized anti-CD20 antibody, IMMU-106 (hA20), in NHL. J Clin Oncol 2006;24(18S):7530.
197. Hagenbeek A, et al. HuMax-CD20, a novel fully human anti-CD20 monoclonal antibody: results of a phase I/II trial in relapsed or refractory follicular non-Hodgkins's lymphoma. Blood 2005;106:4760.
198. Kreitman R, et al. Phase I trial of recombinant immunotoxin RFB4(dsFv)-PE38 (BL22) in patients with B-cell malignancies J Clin Oncol 2005;23(27):6719–29.
199. Advani A, et al. Preliminary report of a phase 1 study of CMC-544, an antibody-targeted chemotherapy agent, in patients with B-cell non-Hodgkin's lymphoma (NHL). Blood 2005;106:230.
200. Friedberg J, et al. Updated results from a phase II study of galiximab (anti-CD80) in combination with rituximab for relapsed or refractory, follicular NHL. Blood 2005;106:2435.
201. Lundin J, et al. CAMPATH-1H monoclonal antibody in therapy for previously treated low- grade non-Hodgkin's lymphomas: a phase II multicenter study; European Study Group of CAMPATH-1H treatment in low-grade non-Hodgkin's lymphoma. J Clin Oncol 1998;16:3257–63.
202. Zinzani P, et al. Phase II study of alemtuzumab treatment in patients with pretreated T-cell lymphoma. Blood 2004;104:4605.
203. Yee K, et al. A phase I/II study of the oral mTOR inhibitor RAD001 in patients with advanced hematologic malignancies. J Immunother 2004;27(6):S35.

9   Targeted Therapy in Melanoma

Michael Davies, MD, PhD, Sunil Patel, MD, and Kevin B. Kim, MD

CONTENTS

SUMMARY

Melanoma is notorious for its resistance to cytotoxic and radiation therapy, and patients with advanced melanoma has a poor prognosis. Despite development of new cytotoxic drugs, immunotherapies, and treatment strategies combining the two, overall survival of patients with metastatic melanoma has not improved significantly. Recent studies provide a modicum of optimism regarding our understanding of the biology of melanoma and potentially regarding targeted therapy for this disease. Genomic mutations in N-Ras, B-Raf, and PTEN have demonstrated intimate involvement in the progression, invasion, and survival of neoplastic cells in most cutaneous melanomas. An increasing number of drugs inhibit the signal transduction pathways activated by these aberrations, and recent clinical studies have shown cautiously promising responses to these drugs. Many of these studies are also elucidating the role of angiogenesis and immunoregulation in melanoma, opening the door to a wide variety of new strategies for tumor environment modulation and immunostimulation for more effective melanoma therapy. Because of the complicated signal transduction pathways in melanoma cells and the complex interactions of these tumors with the surrounding environment and immune system, combining these drugs with other targeted therapies, cytotoxic agents, or immunotherapies will likely be required for successful treatment of melanoma.

From: *Current Clinical Oncology: Targeted Cancer Therapy*
Edited by: R. Kurzrock and M. Markman © Humana Press, Totowa, NJ

Key Words: Melanoma, Signal transduction, Receptor kinase, B-Raf, N-Ras, PTEN, MAP kinase, NFκB, Angiogenesis, Immunotargeting

1. INTRODUCTION

Melanoma is the most aggressive form of skin cancer. An estimated 59,940 cases of melanoma will be diagnosed in the United States in 2007, and approximately 8110 patients will die of the disease *(1)*. Patients with metastatic melanoma have a median survival of approximately 6 months, and fewer than 10% live 5 years after diagnosis *(2)*. Two agents have been approved by the U.S. Food and Drug Administration (FDA) for the treatment of metastatic melanoma: dacarbazine and high-dose bolus interleukin 2 (IL-2). Dacarbazine elicits a clinical response in fewer than 20% of patients, the median duration of response is 1.5 to 2.0 months, and it yields no improvement over supportive care in overall survival *(3)*. High-dose bolus IL-2 has a response rate of approximately 15% to 20%, but it appears to result in durable complete remissions in approximately 6% of patients *(4)*. However, high-dose bolus IL-2 is a highly toxic therapy that must be administered under intensive care unit (ICU)-level care or in a closely monitored unit and thus is not broadly applicable. Trials of numerous single-agent treatment, or combination chemotherapy regimens have failed to improve patient outcomes significantly over dacarbazine alone *(3)*.

The development of improved therapies for melanoma is likely to become an increasingly important public health issue. A review of the Surveillance Epidemiology and End Results (SEER) database from 1950 to 2000 showed that the annual incidence of malignant melanoma increased 619%, more than any other malignancy *(5)*. The failures of multiple single-agent and combination cytotoxic chemotherapy regimens, which generally target DNA and/or its replicative machinery, suggest that new therapeutic approaches are necessary. One approach that is showing promise is the use of inhibitors against proteins that become dysregulated in cancer, often referred to as targeted therapy. This approach has yielded promising results in a number of diseases that had traditionally demonstrated poor responsiveness to cytotoxic chemotherapy, including chronic myelogenous leukemia (CML), gastrointestinal stromal tumors (GISTs), and clear cell renal cell carcinoma *(6–8)*. For each of these diseases, developing an appropriate and effective therapy depended on identifying a molecular target that was dysregulated and highly prevalent *(9)*.

Targeted therapies have also proven beneficial when applied to appropriately selected subpopulations of cancer patients. The most dramatic example is the success of trastuzumab (Herceptin), a monoclonal antibody directed against the growth factor receptor HER2/NEU. Trastuzumab has dramatically improved outcomes of patients with breast cancer in both adjuvant and metastatic settings *(10–12)*. It appears, however, that this benefit is limited to patients who have tumors characterized by amplification of the *HER2/neu* gene, and that no significant benefit is seen in the absence of this molecular event *(13)*.

Thus, a better understanding of the molecular pathogenesis of melanoma is likely required before targeted therapies can be developed rationally. This chapter reviews some of the recent insights into the molecular events that characterize this disease and some of the early clinical experiences with targeted therapies for melanoma. This includes approaches to the regulation of signal transduction, angiogenesis, and the immune response to cancer.

2. SIGNALING PATHWAYS

2.1. RAS/RAF/MAPK Pathway

The RAS/RAF/MAPK pathway is one of the most common targets of genetic aberrations in melanoma. This pathway, which includes a cascade of serine-threonine kinases, is initiated by activation of the RAS family GTPases, a family of guanine-nucleotide binding proteins embedded in the inner surface of the cell membrane *(14,15)*. The RAS family includes three isoforms: N-RAS, K-RAS, and H-RAS. Activation of the RAS proteins, which can be induced by stimulation of a variety of membrane-bound receptor tyrosine kinases, changes these proteins from a GDP-bound state to the active GTP-bound state. The activated forms of RAS are then able to activate various pathways, with selectivity often dependent on cellular context. One important downstream pathway is the mitogen-activated protein kinase (MAPK) cascade, which has been demonstrated to have an important role in regulating cellular proliferation and survival in multiple models *(16)*. This pathway is triggered when GTP-bound RAS interacts with and activates the serine-threonine protein kinase RAF, which similarly has three isoforms: A-RAF, B-RAF, and C-RAF (RAF-1) *(17)*. The cascade propagates when activated RAF phosphorylates the MAPK/ERK kinase (MEK) protein kinases MEK1 and MEK2, thereby activating their serine-threonine protein kinase activity. Activated MEK then phosphorylates the p44/42 MAPK serine/threonine protein kinases (ERK1 and ERK2), which in turn activate a number of substrates that are effectors of this pathway, including transcription factors, cytosolic proteins, and other kinases *(16)*. Measurement of phosphorylated ERK1/2 is frequently used as a surrogate measurement for the activation status of this pathway.

Experiments have demonstrated that the RAS/RAF/MAPK pathway is frequently constitutively active in melanomas *(18)*. The predominant mechanism of activation appears to be genetic mutation of components of the pathway (Fig. 1). Whereas mutations of Ras family members are common in a number of malignancies, they appear to be relatively infrequent, and limited to the N-Ras isoform, in melanoma *(19,20)*. N-*Ras* mutations are detected in approximately 15% of melanomas; K-*Ras* and H-*Ras* mutations are rare *(21–23)*. The predominant mechanism of activation of the RAS/RAF/MAPK pathway in cutaneous melanoma is mutation of B-*Raf* *(24)*. In 2002, the Sanger Institute reported the results of an ambitious study in which B-*raf* mutational status was determined for more than 500 cell lines and clinical specimens of various cancers. Mutations of *B-raf* were detected more frequently in melanoma than in any other tumor type *(25)*. B-*raf* mutations were present in 59% of the melanoma cell lines, 80% of the melanoma short-term cultures, and 67% of the melanoma clinical specimens examined. Like N-*RAS*, B-*RAF* is selectively altered in melanoma, being the only RAF isoform mutated in this cancer; no mutations in A-*RAF* or C-*RAF* have been reported.

The mutations in *B-raf* are predominantly localized to the kinase domain; one single-substitution mutation (V600E[1]) accounts for more than 80% of the detected mutations *(25)*. This mutation results in constitutive activation of the kinase activity of B-RAF, and expression of the V600E mutant form of B-RAF in melanoma cells produces constitutive phosphorylation of MAPK *(25)*. Interestingly, subsequent studies have demonstrated that the

---

[1]The initial analysis of *B-raf* mutations identified the amino acid residue most commonly mutated as being at position 599 (V599E). This nomenclature was actually incorrect, and the mutation affects the amino acid residue 600 (V600E).

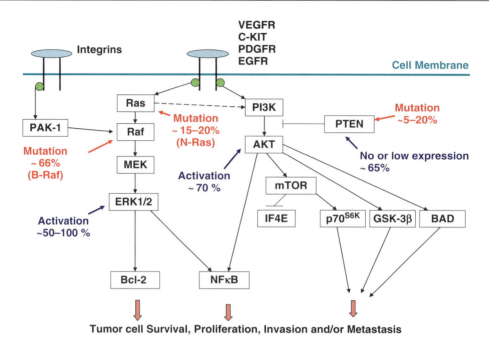

Fig. 1. Complicated signal pathways for melanomas. Genomic mutations in the Ras/Raf/MEK and PTEN /PI3K/AKT pathways are frequent.

prevalence of this mutation varies considerably in melanomas arising from different anatomic sites. Although the V600E mutation occurs in approximately 60% of cutaneous melanomas arising from sites with intermittent sun exposure, only 11% of cutaneous melanomas with evidence of chronic sun damage, fewer than 10% of mucosal melanomas, and no uveal melanomas appear to harbor the V600E B-*raf* mutation *(26–29)*. B-*raf* mutations have been identified in as many as 80% of common nevi *(30,31)*. Thus, although the high prevalence of *B-raf* mutations in melanoma suggests that they have a role in this disease, such mutation alone does not appear to be sufficient to induce tumor formation. Consistent with this, expression of the V600E mutant form of B-RAF in zebrafish resulted in abnormal melanocyte proliferation, but not transformation; tumors were seen only when the mutant was expressed in a p53-null genetic background *(32)*.

The RAS/RAF/MAPK pathway also may be activated by the autocrine secretion of growth factors, which characterizes melanoma progression *(33)*. Taken together, these data suggest that because multiple alterations that are highly prevalent in melanoma activate this pathway, the pathway may be critical to melanoma cellular proliferation and therefore may represent a potential therapeutic target.

In preclinical studies of melanoma cell lines, inhibition of V600E B-RAF function by small inhibitory RNA (siRNA) resulted in decreased mitogenic signaling, inhibition of cellular proliferation, and induction of programmed cell death *(34)*. This functional evidence, combined with the high prevalence of activating mutations, rapidly led to clinical trials testing the hypothesis that inhibition of B-RAF would produce clinical benefit in patients with metastatic melanoma.

The first B-RAF inhibitor used in clinical trials was sorafenib (Nexavar), also known as BAY43-9006 *(35)*. Sorafenib is a small-molecule inhibitor of C-RAF, wild-type B-RAF, and to a lesser degree, mutant (V600E) B-RAF kinase activity. It also inhibits the kinase activity of a number of other kinases, including vascular endothelial growth factor receptor 2 (VEGFR-2), VEGFR-3, platelet-derived growth factor receptor (PDGFR), FLT3, and c-Kit at nanomolar concentrations *(35)*. Sorafenib was well tolerated in Phase I studies, and a dose of 400 mg twice daily was recommended for Phase II studies *(36)*. The initial Phase II single-agent study in patients with metastatic melanoma yielded disappointing results *(37)*. Among 34 patients evaluable for response, there was no response, and seven patients (19%) had stable disease. This contrasts with the efficacy of sorafenib in metastatic renal cell carcinoma, in which sorafenib improved progression-free survival in a pivotal Phase III trial *(38)*, leading to FDA approval for this disease. However, more promising results in melanoma were observed when sorafenib was combined with cytotoxic chemotherapy. A Phase I/II trial has been reported describing the treatment of 35 patients who had metastatic melanoma with paclitaxel, carboplatin, and sorafenib *(39)*. In this study, 11 patients (31%) achieved a partial response by Response Evaluation Criteria in Solid Tumors (RECIST) and 19 patients (54%) had stable disease. Interestingly, clinical benefit did not correlate with the presence of *B-raf* mutations. As the regimen of paclitaxel and carboplatin, particularly at the doses used in this trial, is not a widely used or well characterized regimen for metastatic melanoma, it is possible that the promising results were due to the chemotherapy alone. Alternatively, the inhibition of kinases other than B-RAF, such as VEGFR2, by sorafenib may contribute to the activity of this regimen.

A number of other sorafenib-based combination regimens have been tried in melanoma. In a Phase II trial of the combination of sorafenib and dacarbazine in patients with metastatic melanoma, 4 (12%) of 32 treated patients had a partial response, and 17 (53%) had stable disease *(40)*. In another study in which patients were randomized to either dacarbazine alone or the combination of dacarbazine and sorafenib in a phase II study setting, the overall response rate was 24%, and the progression-free survival at day 180 was 41% in the combination arm *(41)*. In a Phase II trial of the combination of sorafenib and temozolomide, the disease control rate was 72% (30% partial response, 6% minor response, 36% stable disease) among 47 patients without brain metastases who had not previously been treated with temozolomide *(42)*. These results suggest that although sorafenib is not clinically active as a single agent it can potentiate the clinical benefit of cytotoxic chemotherapy drugs in patients with metastatic melanoma. The additive activity of sorafenib in combination with cytotoxic agents is being addressed by a randomized Phase III trial in which patients with metastatic melanoma receive paclitaxel and carboplatin with or without sorafenib.

As a drug with multiple targets, sorafenib can result in undesirable side effects in patients. To minimize toxicity and increase clinical activity by targeting melanoma cells more selectively, more specific inhibitors of mutated B-RAF kinase have been developed. Three such potent small-molecule inhibitors (RAF265, PLX4032, SB590885) are currently being tested in Phase I trials. These drugs inhibit the kinase activity of mutated B-RAF at a nanomolar range. In preclinical studies, the reduction of tumor burden with treatment with these drugs was more striking in melanoma cells with the V600E B-*raf* mutation than in those with wild-type B-*raf* or mutated N-*ras*.

Other therapeutic approaches to inhibiting the RAS/RAF/MAPK pathway are also likely to be feasible in patients. Farnesyltransferase inhibitors theoretically block RAS from associating with the cell membrane and thus inhibit downstream signaling pathways. These agents were generally well tolerated in Phase I clinical trials, and a number of them are currently under investigation in Phase II studies *(43)*. Small-molecule inhibitors of MEK, the kinase activated by B-RAF, are also in clinical trials and are similarly well tolerated *(44–47)*.

Interestingly, in patients with advanced solid tumors enrolled in a Phase I trial of PD0325901, a potent specific MEK inhibitor, two of the responders were being treated for metastatic melanoma *(47)*. After 15 days of treatment, the expression of p-ERK1/2 was significantly decreased in samples of those patients' tumors. A phase II study of AZD6244, another potent specific MEK inhibitor, in patients with metastatic melanoma is near completion to patient accrual.

2.2. PI3K/AKT/mTOR Pathway

The PI3K/AKT cascade, an evolutionarily conserved pathway involved in numerous important physiologic processes, is activated by various growth factor receptor proteins and cell–cell contacts *(48)*. Upon activation of RAS proteins induced by these extracellular signals or constitutive activation of cell surface receptor kinases, phosphoinositide-3 kinase (PI3K) phosphorylates membrane phosphatidylinositol on the 3′-hydroxyl group of the inositol ring to create polyphosphoinositides that recruit a number of pleckstrin homology (PH) domain–containing proteins to the cell membrane, including AKT. AKT (also known as protein kinase B, or PKB) is serine/threonine protein kinase and is a well characterized main effector of PI3K. Activated PI3K effectively recruits AKT to the plasma membrane, where AKT is phosphorylated at two critical residues (Thr^{308} and Ser^{473}), thereby activating its full kinase activity. Melanomas rarely harbor mutations in either the *PI3K* or the *Akt* gene, and thus activation of the PI3K/AKT pathway appears to be dependent on activation of the upstream signaling molecules *(49)*. AKT regulates a wide range of proteins, including forkhead transcription factors *(50)*, NFκB *(51,52)*, BAD *(53)*, mTOR *(54)*, and GSK-3β *(55)*. The ability of AKT to control such proteins, which influence many important cellular processes such as apoptosis, proliferation, invasion, and angiogenesis, suggests its role as an essential molecule in the development and progression of cancers such as melanoma.

The AKT protein kinase family consists of three members, AKT1 (PKBα), AKT2 (PKBβ), and AKT3 (PKBγ), which share extensive structural similarity *(56)*. Although all three AKT isoforms are activated through similar mechanisms, each isoform may be regulated in a distinct manner in different cell types *(56–60)*. In melanoma, dysregulation of AKT3 appears to play a significant role in the survival of melanoma cells and the progression of disease *(61)*. Stahl and his colleagues demonstrated that the level of p-AKT was diminished after treatment with siRNA against AKT3 but not after treatment with siRNA against AKT1 or AKT2 *(61)*. They also showed that, compared to AKT1 or AKT2, both total and phosphorylated AKT3 are preferentially overexpressed in metastatic melanoma lesions. It has not yet been shown, however, whether overexpression of p-AKT by itself can transform normal melanocytes into melanoma cells.

AKT is negatively regulated by tumor suppressor phosphatase and tensin homologue (PTEN). PTEN, also known as MMAC1 (mutated in multiple advanced cancers 1) or TEP1 (telomerase-associated protein 1), is a dual-function lipid and protein phosphatase that dephosphorylates phosphatidylinositol 3,4,5-trisphosphate, the product of PI3K *(62,63)*. Accordingly, aberrance in PTEN function results in up-regulation of p-AKT, leading to decreased apoptosis and increased cell growth. Numerous preclinical studies have demonstrated that PTEN is a critical negative regulator of AKT activity *(64–66)*. Hwang and colleagues demonstrated that ectopic expression of PTEN reduced melanoma tumorigenicity and metastasis in PTEN-deficient melanoma cells *(67)*. PTEN has been shown to be absent from many tumor types and to be correlated with increased AKT activation in these cells *(68,69)*.

In melanoma, mutations in *PTEN* have been identified by various groups *(70–76)*. Earlier studies revealed *PTEN* mutation in 30% to 40% of melanoma cell lines and 10% of melanoma lesions *(72,77)*. In addition to mutation, an epigenetic PTEN silencing phenomenon is observed rather frequently in melanoma. Zhou et al. reported that 15% of melanoma lesions have no expression of PTEN, and that 50% of melanoma lesions have a low level of PTEN expression, shown by immunostaining analysis *(78)*. These genetic and epigenetic studies suggest that nonfunctional PTEN might play an important role in as many as 60% of sporadic melanomas *(70–78)*. In addition to loss of negative regulation by *PTEN* mutation or down-expression, AKT also can be activated by kinase-activating mutations of N-*Ras (49)*. Mutations in N-*Ras* and *PTEN* are mutually exclusive in most cases; concomitant mutations in *PTEN* and B-*Raf* are found more frequently in a given melanoma cell *(23,79)*.

The association between activation of the PI3K/AKT pathway and melanoma progression has been examined by a number of investigators. By using immunohistochemical staining, Dhawan and her colleagues showed in their series of 29 melanoma samples that as many as 66% of severely dysplastic nevi and metastatic melanomas expressed p-AKT, whereas no significant AKT activation was detected in normal or slightly dysplastic nevi *(52)*. Stahl et al. reported strong staining patterns of p-AKT expression in 12%, 53%, and 67% of dysplastic nevi, primary melanomas, and metastatic melanomas, respectively *(61)*. In a larger series of 292 melanoma specimens, analyzed by immunohistochemical staining, Dai et al. found a significant correlation between the level of strong p-AKT expression and melanoma progression and also an inverse relation between p-AKT expression and survival of patients with primary melanoma. In their study, 77% of metastatic melanoma lesions had strong expression of p-AKT, as did 43% and 49% of dysplastic nevi and primary melanomas, respectively *(80)*. Considering the important role of PI3K/AKT in melanoma survival and progression, inhibition of the PI3K/AKT pathway appears to be a logical approach to melanoma therapy.

Clinical development of drugs directly targeting the PI3K or AKT protein has progressed slowly. Perifosine (KRX-0401) is a synthetic alkylphospholipid that inhibits AKT by interfering with its recruitment to the cell membrane *(81)*. A Phase II trial of perifosine in chemotherapy-naive patients with metastatic melanoma revealed that none of 17 treated patients had an objective response, and only 21% of patients had stable disease for at least two cycles. The drug was relatively well tolerated at a loading dose of 900 mg on day 1 of the first cycle and a daily maintenance dose of 150 mg for 3 weeks (of a 4-week cycle), followed by a loading dose of 300 mg on day 1 and the same maintenance dose in subsequent cycles *(82)*. Whether a higher dose of perifosine or combinations with cytotoxic or other targeted agents might result in superior clinical efficacy has not been tested. A number of other small-molecule AKT or PI3K inhibitors, such as BEZ235 or PI-103, are currently being tested in early-phase clinical studies.

Small-molecule agents that inhibit the activation of mTOR (mammalian target of rapamycin), an important effector of AKT, have been tested more extensively in patients with cancer. One of these potent, selective mTOR inhibitors, temsirolimus (CCI-779), is an ester of the macrocyclic immunosuppressive agent rapamycine (sirolimus) and a cytostatic cell cycle inhibitor with antitumor properties. CCI-779 inhibits tumor growth and survival in cell lines in which the PI3K pathway is activated *(83)*. In vivo studies in nude mice have demonstrated that CCI-779 has activity against human tumor xenografts of diverse histologic types, including gliomas, pancreatic tumors, and breast tumors *(83)*. Phase I and II studies demonstrated that CCI-779 is well tolerated and, unlike rapamycin, has no immunosuppressive effects when administered on an intermittent schedule. Adverse effects are manageable and reversible at doses up to 220 mg/m^2 given weekly by intravenous infusion (84). Margolin and her colleagues conducted a Phase II trial of temsirolimus in patients with metastatic melanoma (85). The trial was designed to detect a median time to progression of longer than 18 weeks using a weekly dose of 250 mg of temsirolimus administered intravenously; the actual median time to disease progression was only 10 weeks in this study. Of 33 treated patients, 1 (3%) had a partial response, which lasted 2 months. Because of its minimal activity in this trial, further studies of temsirolimus as a single agent are not warranted in unselected patients with metastatic cutaneous melanoma. Currently, RAD-001, an orally administered mTOR kinase inhibitor, is under clinical investigation in patients with advanced melanoma, and the results of this study will be available shortly.

2.3. NFκB

Nuclear factor-kappa B (NFκB) is an inducible transcription factor that regulates genes involved in the normal immune response of human cells and has emerged as a key regulator of oncogenesis in many types of cancer cells (86). NFκB is actually a family of five structurally related proteins: p65 (RelA), RelB, Rel (c-Rel), p50/p105, and p52/p100. These proteins share a common 300-amino-acid N-terminal domain known as the Rel homology (RH) domain. This domain is critical for DNA binding, dimerization of family members, and interactions with the regulatory protein inhibitor of NFκB (IκB). The subunits normally exist as homodimers or heterodimers that are sequestered in the cytoplasm and are thus inactive as transcription factors. The most common functional transcription factor is a heterodimer composed of the p50 and p65 subunits; by convention, this is referred to as NFκB. NFκB is regulated by sequestration in the cytoplasm by an interaction with IκB, which binds to its nuclear localization sequence. The transcriptional activity of NFκB requires degradation of IκB. This is achieved when IκB is phosphorylated by the IκB kinase (IKK) complex, which leads to ubiquitination and proteasome-mediated degradation of IκB. The degradation of IκB releases NFκB from its cytoplasmic sequestration and allows it to translocate to the nucleus to carry out its transcriptional activity. Thus, whereas transcription factors have been difficult to inhibit with small molecules, the mechanism of NFκB regulation provides a number of potential therapeutic targets to block its activity.

NFκB is constitutively activated in many cancers, including pancreatic, colon, and breast carcinomas and melanoma (86). NFκB regulates many genes that may contribute to the malignant phenotype, including many encoding antiapoptotic proteins, autocrine growth factors, or proteases (87–89). In preclinical models, NFκB activity promotes cellular survival, invasion, angiogenesis, and chemotherapy resistance in cancer cells (86,90). NFκB activity is greater in primary melanomas than in normal melanocytes (91,92). This increase in activity appears to be maintained throughout melanoma progression, implicating NFκB as a potentially important factor in melanoma pathogenesis (93). A number of mechanisms have been proposed as contributing to the activation of NFκB in melanoma. AKT/PKB, which is activated in melanoma by both activating N-Ras mutations and PTEN loss of function, increases IKK activity and also directly phosphorylates NFκB (52,94,95). Activation of the RAS/RAF/MAPK pathway, which is common in melanoma, also activates NFκB, although the mechanism by which it occurs is less clear (96,97). Moreover, the NFκB-inducing kinase (NIK) is frequently overexpressed in melanoma (52). NIK induces activation of NFκB as a consequence of activation of cytokine receptors.

The frequent activation of NFκB in melanoma has led to diverse therapeutic approaches attempting to inhibit this pathway. The activation of NFκB requires proteasome-mediated degradation of IκB. Bortezomib (Velcade), also known as PS-341, is a proteasome inhibitor that has demonstrated significant clinical activity in multiple myeloma and mantle cell lymphoma and is now approved by the FDA for use in both of these diseases (98,99). A total of 27 chemotherapy-naive patients with metastatic melanoma were treated in a Phase II trial of bortezomib as a single agent (100). No clinical responses were observed, and the median time to progression was only 1.5 months. Because of its lack of efficacy, the trial was stopped at the first planned interim analysis, and it is unlikely that borte-zomib has much of a role as a single-agent regimen for this disease. In preclinical studies, however, bortezomib demonstrated dramatic synergy with temozolomide, suggesting that it may be effective in combination with cytotoxic chemotherapy (86). This combination is being evaluated currently in ongoing clinical trials, as are other bortezomib combinations (http://www.clinicaltrials.gov).

Another therapeutic approach undergoing clinical evaluation is direct inhibition of IKK, which should similarly block activation of NFκB. Small-molecule inhibitors of IKK potently inhibit melanoma cells in vitro (101), but the safety and efficacy of these compounds in patients is not yet known. Finally, therapies inhibiting pathways that result in activation of NFκB, such as the RAS/RAF/MAPK and PI3K/AKT/PKB pathways, may provide insight into the role of these pathways in melanoma. This will require specific evaluation of the effects of such pharmacologic approaches on the status of NFκB.

3. RECEPTOR TYROSINE KINASE INHIBITORS

Imatinib (Gleevec) is a small molecule that inhibits a number of protein tyrosine kinases, including the Bcr-Abl fusion protein, C-ABL, abl-related gene (ARG), PDGFRα, PDGFRβ, and the C-KIT tyrosine kinase receptor (102–104). The potent clinical activity of imatinib in patients with CML through the inhibition of Bcr-Abl fusion protein, and in patients with GIST through inhibition of c-Kit and/or PDGFRα, has been well documented. On the basis of its ability to inhibit these receptor tyrosine kinases, there has been great interest in investigating the clinical efficacy of imatinib in patients with various solid tumors.

Human melanoma cells have been reported to contain more tyrosine phosphate than normal melanocytes (105). Platelet-derived growth factor (PDGF) is secreted by melanoma cell lines and by metastatic melanomas, as shown in vivo. PDGF has also been reported to stimulate the development of tumor stroma and new blood vessels. Barnhill et al. studied the expression of PDGF and its receptors in primary and metastatic melanomas and in normal skin specimens (106). Both primary and metastatic melanomas exhibited significant expression of PDGF-AA, PDGF-BB, and PDGFRα, shown in both immunohistochemical and in situ hybridization analysis, whereas only background expression was detected in normal skin. Their results suggest that PDGF may function as an autocrine growth factor, as well as an angiogenesis factor, in melanoma development.

In paraffin-embedded human melanoma specimens, Shen et al. demonstrated differential expression of receptor tyrosine kinases in metastatic melanomas (107). Among 31 metastatic melanoma specimens examined by his group, 17 (54.8%) were positive for c-Kit, 30 (96.8%) were positive for PDGFRα, 21 (67.7%) were positive for PDGFRβ, 23 (74.2%) were positive for ARG, and 27 (87.1%) were positive for C-ABL by immunohistochemical staining. This finding suggests that a subset of patients with metastatic melanoma may have appropriate imatinib targets in their tumors.

The clinical efficacy of imatinib in patients with metastatic melanoma has been tested in two Phase II trials *(108,109)*. In both trials, imatinib was given orally at 400 mg twice a day. In a study by Wyman et al., 26 patients were enrolled, 62% of whom had received as many as three prior systemic treatments *(108)*. The treatment was unexpectedly toxic, causing grade 3 or 4 adverse events, including fatigue, thrombosis, hyponatremia, anemia, and gastrointestinal and neurologic toxic effects. Among the 25 patients evaluable for response, there was no objective response, and only 2 patients had disease stabilization for at least 8 weeks. A median time to progression among all patients was 54 days.

In a study by Eton and his colleagues at The University of Texas M. D. Anderson Cancer Center, enrollment was limited only to patients whose tumor cells, when subjected to immunohistochemical analysis, stained at least 25% for PDGFRα, PDGFRβ, c-Kit, C-ABL, or ARG *(109)*. None of the patients had received more than one prior systemic treatment. Among 21 patients treated with imatinib, 1 patient had a partial response, and 4 others had disease stabilization. The responder had major tumor regression in the lung, inguinal lymph nodes, and multiple cutaneous metastatic lesions and remained free of disease progression for more than 1 year. Interestingly, this patient's tumor had strong expression of c-Kit in more than 75% of the tumor cells, the strongest staining pattern observed in the pretreatment samples of all patients in the study. With only one patient achieving a clinical response, a definite association could not be made between the baseline levels of receptor kinase expression and clinical activity. Imatinib treatment was well tolerated in this study; fatigue and edema were the only grade 3 or 4 adverse events that occurred in more than 10% of the patients.

It is apparent that the criteria used for patient selection in this trial did not predict the clinical benefit of imatinib. It is possible that the complex signal pathways of melanoma cells easily induce mechanisms of resistance to imatinib. It also can be speculated that the expression levels of phosphorylated receptor kinases, rather than of total kinases, may be more predictive of imatinib's clinical activity. Tissue analyses of phosphorylated receptor kinases in these patient tumor samples are ongoing at this time.

Sunitinib (Sutent) is another potent small-molecule inhibitor of multiple receptor kinases, including VEGFRs and PDGFRs, c-Kit, RET, and FLT3 *(85,110,111)*. Its effectiveness in patients with advanced renal cell carcinoma, mostly due to its inhibitory effect on VEGF receptors, earned FDA approval for its use in patients with this cancer *(112,113)*. It has also shown efficacy in imatinib-refractory GIST *(114)*. Sunitinib as a single agent has not been tested in patients with metastatic melanoma, but phase I/II studies of the combination of sunitinib and temozolomide and also, separately, the combination of sunitinib and dacarbazine, are currently accruing patients.

4. PROAPOTOTIC PATHWAYS

4.1. Bcl-2

Bcl-2 (B-cell lymphoma gene-2) was one of the first oncogenes to be implicated in the regulation of an apoptosis pathway *(115)*. It was cloned from the chromosome breakpoint of the t(14;18) translocation in B-cell follicular lymphoma, which results in constitutive expression of Bcl-2, which in turn inhibits the induction of apoptosis *(116,117)*. In gene transfection experiments, overexpression of *Bcl-2* can render neoplastic cells resistant to the induction of apoptosis by a variety of chemotherapeutic drugs *(118)*. Down-regulation of

Bcl-2 protein has been shown to reverse chemotherapy resistance in a number of experimental systems *(118–120)*. One of the ways to down-regulate Bcl-2 expression is through the use of antisense RNA, which hybridizes to the respective target RNA bases and leads to selective decreases in concentrations of both the RNA and the protein product. Oblimersen (G3139, Genasense) is an 18-base phosphorothioate oligonucleotide antisense to the first six codons of *bcl-2* mRNA, which causes a decrease in Bcl-2 protein translation and thereby significantly reduces levels of Bcl-2 protein in various tumor systems, including melanoma *(121)*. Jansen et al. demonstrated that treatment with the *bcl-2* antisense RNA improves the chemosensitivity of human melanoma in SCID mice *(121)*.

Overexpression of Bcl-2 was demonstrated in human melanoma specimens by several groups. Utikal et al. showed that 27 of 30 metastatic melanoma specimens and 24 of 34 tumors expressed Bcl-2, as determined through the polymerase chain reaction (PCR) and immunohistochemical analysis, respectively *(122,123)*. Bcl-2 was strongly expressed in 87.5% of metastatic melanomas and in 53%, 46%, and 43% of primary melanomas, melanocytic nevi, and normal tissue samples, respectively *(124)*.

The results of a Phase I/II study of the combination of oblimersen and dacarbazine in patients with stage IV melanoma—which suggested that oblimersen might improve clinical response to dacarbazine—were consistent with the preclinical data *(125)*. Daily oblimersen doses of 1.7 mg/kg or higher resulted, by day 5, in a median decrease of 40% in Bcl-2 expression in melanoma samples compared to baseline and to an increase in tumor cell apoptosis.

On the basis of the encouraging early clinical data, a randomized Phase III study in patients with metastatic melanoma was conducted *(126)*. In this multinational, multicenter trial, 771 patients were randomly assigned to receive dacarbazine (1000 mg/m^2 intravenously for 60 minutes), either alone or in combination with oblimersen (7 mg/kg/day by continuous intravenous infusion for 5 days) every 3 weeks. When evaluated after a minimum follow-up of 24 months, the overall response rate, complete response rate, durable response rate, and median progression-free survival duration were all better in the combination group than in the dacarbazine only group ($p < 0.05$) (Table 1). However, overall survival duration, a primary objective of the trial, was not significantly longer in the combination group than in the dacarbazine group. Interestingly, in a multivariate analysis of 508 patients with normal baseline serum lactate dehydrogenase (LDH) levels in this study, a significant difference

Table 1
Comparison of Clinical Benefit in Intent-to-Treat Analysis for All Patients

Parameter	Dacarbazine (n = 385)[a]	Oblimersen + dacarbazine (n = 386)[a]	p
Overall response rate	7.5%	13.5%	0.007
Complete response rate	0.8%	2.8%	—
Durable response rate[b]	3.6%	7.3%	0.027
Progression-free survival (median)	1.6 months	2.6 months	<0.001
Overall survival (median)	7.8 months	9.0 months	0.077

LDH, lactate dehydrogenase
[a]Represents intent-to-treat analysis
[b]Response lasting ≥ 6 months from the date response was first documented

was observed, favoring the combination group, for all efficacy endpoints. Because of the equivocal overall survival benefit, however, oblimersen was not approved for treatment of metastatic melanoma by the FDA. Currently, a randomized Phase III study comparing the same two arms is underway in patients with serum LDH levels in the normal range.

5. POLY(ADP-RIBOSE) POLYMERASE INHIBITORS

An ability to detect and repair DNA damage is critical for maintaining genomic integrity. One of the immediate eukaryotic cellular responses to DNA breakage induced by noxious stress such as ionizing radiation, alkylating agents, or oxidants is poly(ADP-ribose) synthesis, in which the enzyme poly(ADP-ribose) polymerase (PARP) catalyzes the successive transfer of ADP-ribose units from NAD^+ to nuclear proteins. PARP activation induced by DNA damage leads to mediation of DNA repair *(127,128)*, modulation of p53 stability and function *(129,130)*, and regulation of apoptosis *(131)*. Apoptosis is associated with dramatic changes in PARP. Proteolytic cleavage of PARP by activated caspase-3 has been found during the execution phase of apoptosis; therefore, PARP cleavage is generally regarded as a biochemical marker of cell apoptosis *(132)*.

With its functional involvement in cell survival after DNA damage, PARP has been regarded as a promising target for inhibitors, which would potentiate the antitumor effect of chemotherapeutic agents. After DNA damage by alkylating agents, such as temozolomide, biochemical blockage of PARP inhibits the repair of DNA strand breaks and enhances cytotoxicity in vitro *(127)*. The combination of temozolomide and a PARP inhibitor, NU1025, resulted in marked reduction of tumor growth and a significant improvement in survival of mice injected with lymphoma cells intracranially, compared with temozolomide treatment alone *(133)*.

The first-generation PARP inhibitors, such as nicotinamide and benzamide, were not clinically useful because of their low solubility and limited specificity. However, new compounds with potent PARP-inhibitory activity have been developed recently. At least two PARP inhibitors are now in clinical trials. Plummer and his colleagues reported the result of a Phase I dose-escalating study of AG-014699 in combination with temozolomide in patients with solid tumors *(134)*. The combination was well tolerated at doses of intravenous AG-014699 as high as 12 mg/m^2 and of oral temozolomide at 200 mg/m^2 for 5 days in 28-day cycles; 90% of the median tumor PARP inhibition was achieved at 5 hours of treatment with AG-014699 12 mg/m^2. Of 18 patients with metastatic melanoma, 4 had a partial response, and at least 2 of them had a durable response for more than 8 months. A dose-escalation Phase I trial of another PARP inhibitor, INO-1001, in combination with temozolomide in patients with advanced melanoma is currently ongoing.

6. ANTIANGIOGENESIS STRATEGIES

Melanoma is known to be a highly vascular tumor, and evidence that melanoma progression requires induction of angiogenesis, is mounting *(135–141)*. As melanoma progresses from the radial to the vertical growth phase, neovascularization takes place *(136–138)*. Moreover, greater microvessel density in primary melanomas has been correlated with a higher probability of metastasis *(139–142)*. Melanoma cells, like other types of cancer cellA, have been demonstrated to produce and secrete a wide variety of angiogenic factors, including vascular endothelial growth factor (VEGF) *(143–146)*, basic fibroblast growth factor (bFGF) *(147–149)*, and interleukin-8 (IL-8) *(89,150)*. VEGF, also known as vascular permeability factor, is a key growth factor during vascular development and stimulates endothelial cell proliferation and migration through its receptors, especially KDR (VEGFR-2) *(151,152)*. A hepatic binding cytokine, bFGF plays an important role as an autocrine mediator of mitogenesis of endothelial cells *(153–155)*. IL-8, also known as CXCL-8, a member of the CXC chemokine family, promotes angiogenesis by directly enhancing endothelial cell proliferation and survival *(156,157)*. Rofstad and Halsor demonstrated that multiple angiogenic factors, such as VEGF, IL-8, bFGF, and platelet-derived epidermal growth factor (PDEGF), are expressed in melanoma cells; and each of these angiogenic factors can promote metastasis of these cells in vivo *(158)*. Furthermore, there is evidence that repeated treatment with cytotoxic drugs such as dacarbazine can induce chemoresistance by increasing the transcriptional up-regulation of angiogenic factors such as IL-8 and VEGF in melanoma cells, leading to the selection of much more aggressive clones of melanoma cells *(159,160)*. These findings underscore the significance of angiogenesis in the progression and metastasis of melanoma cells. Therefore, antiangiogenic and antivascular therapy may benefit patients with advanced melanoma.

6.1. VEGF Targeting

VEGF plays an important role in angiogenesis and progression in malignant melanoma. The soluble isoform of VEGF, a dimeric glycoprotein of 36 to 46 kDa, binds to two specific tyrosine kinase receptors, VEGFR-1 (FLT1) and VEGFR-2 (KDR/flk-1), which are selectively expressed in vascular endothelium and promote angiogenesis in cancer *(161–164)*. VEGF is expressed and secreted by melanomas, and its expression has been found to be associated with tumor progression and a worse overall prognosis *(137,165–171)*. Aberrant expression of VEGF receptors also has been shown in human melanoma cells and melanoma specimens, supporting the hypothesis that VEGF stimulates melanoma growth and progression in an autocrine and/or paracrine fashion *(132,172)*.

Bevacizumab (Avastin) was the first drug to be tested as a selective inhibitor of VEGF signaling in melanoma. Bevacizumab is a monoclonal antibody that specifically binds to VEGF and blocks the binding of VEGF to its receptors. A Phase II study of bevacizumab with or without low-dose interferon-α was conducted to examine the clinical efficacy of bevacizumab as a single agent and as part of that combination regimen *(173)*. A preliminary analysis of 16 chemotherapy-naive patients with metastatic melanoma who were randomized to receive either bevacizumab or the combination showed that two patients in the combination arm had clinical responses and one had prolonged disease stabilization, whereas three patients in the bevacizumab-only arm had disease stabilization lasting more than 24 weeks. There was no association between serum VEGF level and clinical response. Currently, a number of Phase II trials are underway in which bevacizumab is combined with various cytotoxic drugs, including paclitaxel and carboplatin or kinase inhibitors such as erlotinib, temsirolimus, or sorafenib.

6.2. Thalidomide and Immunomodulatory Drugs

Initially developed as a sedative and an antiemetic to treat morning sickness in pregnant women, thalidomide suffered a great misfortune when it was found to cause a worldwide epidemic of serious birth defects during the late 1950s and early 1960s. With the persistence of dedicated scientists, however, thalidomide has reemerged as a treatment for many cancers and dermatologic diseases. It has been shown to inhibit angiogenesis induced by bFGF or VEGF *(174,175)*. Although its antiangiogenic activity appears to play a major role in its anticancer action, thalidomide also has a number of antiinflammatory and immunomodulatory activities. Thalidomide was shown to reduce tumor necrosis factor-α (TNFα) production from macrophages; to modulate natural killer (NK) cell and T-lymphocyte activity, affecting both CD8+ and CD4+ T cells; and to increase production of T-helper-1 cytokines, including IL-2 and interferon-γ (176–178). It also has been demonstrated to interfere with the DNA-binding activity of NFκB through a mechanism of IκB activity inhibition in vitro (179).

In a finding consistent with the promising preclinical data, thalidomide was proven to be an effective agent for multiple myeloma (180–182). It has only minimal activity, however, as a single agent in patients with metastatic melanoma. Eisen et al. reported a Phase II study of thalidomide in patients with advanced cancers (183). In this trial, 17 patients with metastatic melanoma who were treated with 100 mg of oral thalidomide were evaluable for a clinical response; there was no clinical response, and only one patient had disease stabilization lasting longer than 3 months. In another Phase II study of thalidomide, at daily doses as high as 800 mg the clinical activity was minimal in patients whose metastatic disease was progressive while receiving standard therapies; there was no objective response, and only 7 of 20 patients (35%) achieved disease stabilization as a best response (184). Likewise, Reiriz et al., in their Phase II trial with 14 patients, concluded that thalidomide has poor clinical activity in patients with advanced melanoma (185).

Thalidomide has shown some promise when it is combined with temozolomide. Hwu and her colleagues at Memorial Sloan-Kettering Cancer Center reported that the combination of extended-dose temozolomide (75 mg/m^2 daily for 6 weeks followed by 2 weeks of rest, repeating every 8 weeks) and thalidomide at daily doses as high as 400 mg yielded an objective response rate of 32% (1 complete response, 11 partial responses), with a median survival duration of 9.5 months among 38 chemotherapy-naive patients (163). In a separate study, they showed that 3 of 26 treated patients (12%) with progressive metastatic brain metastases had either a complete or a partial response, and 7 others had a minor response or stable disease in the brain (186). However, this regimen has limited clinical efficacy in previously treated patients. In a Phase II study of the combination regimen, only 3 patients had a clinical response (12%) among 26 who were extensively treated with prior systemic therapies, and only 5 patients had stable disease (187). Although this combination regimen appeared to have significant activity in brain metastases initially, a follow-up multicenter Phase II trial yielded no objective responses among 16 patients with brain metastases (188). Because of the convenient oral dosage form and schedule, the combination of thalidomide and temozolomide has been used widely in the United States. However, a crucial Phase III randomized study comparing this combination regimen to standard treatment has not been conducted.

Because of the undesirable side effects of thalidomide, analogues with less severe side effects have been developed. A class of these analogues, called immunomodulatory drugs (IMiDs), is more potent than thalidomide in antiangiogenic, immunomodulatory, and direct antitumor property (176,189). One of these analogues, lenalidomide (Revlimid), was recently approved for treatment of multiple myeloma and myelodysplastic syndrome. In a Phase I trial by Bartlett et al., lenalidomide was well tolerated; most of the adverse events were confined to grade 1 or 2, and there was one partial response among 13 patients with metastatic melanoma (190). Following the Phase I trial, two randomized Phase III trials were conducted in the United States and Europe to test the clinical benefit of lenalidomide as a single agent. Disappointingly, both trials were stopped after unblinded interim analysis because of the lack of difference between high-dose and low-dose lenalidomide and between lenalidomide and placebo. The combination of lenalidomide and dacarbazine is being investigated in patients with metastatic melanoma at this time.

6.3. Anti-integrins

Integrins are heterodimers composed of α- and β-subunit transmembrane glycoproteins that are noncovalently linked. Each α-subunit can form a heterodimer with various β-subunits, and each β-subunit can, in turn, form functional receptors with various α-subunits, which determines ligand specificity. Integrins adhere to extracellular matrix proteins, such as vitronectin, fibronectin, laminin, and collagen, to promote endothelial cell attachment, migration, and survival (191,192). Integrins are essential in endothelial cell proliferation and tumor angiogenesis, and they are widely expressed in endothelial cells in progressing melanoma lesions (193).

The integrin $\alpha_v\beta_3$ is one of the most extensively studied in melanoma. It is expressed not only on endothelial cells but also on melanoma cells, and its expression has been shown to correlate with the vertical growth phase of human melanoma, suggesting an important role in melanoma progression (194). This integrin is expressed in 60% and 80% of lymph node metastases and cutaneous metastatic lesions, respectively (195). Furthermore, $\alpha_v\beta_3$ expression in melanoma lesions was found to be associated with poor prognosis in patients with this cancer (195).

The function of the integrins may also be closely related to those of other angiogenic factors. For example, VEGF has been shown to activate integrins, including $\alpha_v\beta_3$ and $\alpha_v\beta_5$, through KDR, leading to enhanced adhesion of human umbilical vein endothelial cells to vitronectin and augmentation of cell migration (196). In accordance with the role of $\alpha_v\beta_3$ in tumor endothelial cell proliferation and adhesion, angiogenesis can be inhibited by blocking $\alpha_v\beta_3$ (191).

Another integrin, $\alpha_5\beta_1$, is also intimately involved in tumor angiogenesis. The expression of $\alpha_5\beta_1$ is significantly up-regulated on endothelium during angiogenesis, whereas it is not expressed by quiescent endothelium (197). Interaction between $\alpha_5\beta_1$ and fibronectin in the extracellular matrix was shown to promote the survival of endothelial cells, and blockage of this interaction resulted in inhibition of endothelial proliferation and survival (198). These findings suggest that drugs that block the ligation of $\alpha_5\beta_1$ to fibronectin can be useful as a cancer therapy by reversing the process of tumor angiogenesis.

At least three Phase II trials have evaluated novel drugs that target integrins in patients with metastatic melanoma. MEDI-522 (Vitaxin) is a humanized version of the LM609 monoclonal antibody, which has specificity for the $\alpha_v\beta_3$ integrin. A multicenter study was conducted to evaluate the antitumor activity and safety of MEDI-522 (8 mg/kg/week) with or without dacarbazine (1000 mg/m^2 once every 3 weeks) in patients with stage IV melanoma (199). No patient had received prior systemic therapy, except for adjuvant immunotherapy. A total of 112 patients were randomized to receive either MEDI-522 alone ($n = 57$) or the combination of MEDI-522 and dacarbazine ($n = 55$). Sixty percent of the patients in this trial had stage M1c disease. Although these treatments were well tolerated, there was no clinical response among patients who received MEDI-522 only, and the early disease progression rate (at the first tumor evaluation) was 49%, whereas 13% of patients who received the combination regimen had an objective clinical response, and the early disease progression rate was 38%.

EMD121974 (Cilengitide) is an inner salt of a cyclized pentapeptide that is a potent and selective antagonist of $\alpha_v\beta_3$ integrin. To evaluate the clinical activity of EMD121974, a

Table 2
Comparison of Different Integrin-Targeting Studies

Parameter	EMD121974	MEDI-522	MEDI-522 + dacarbazine	Volociximab + dacarbazine
Complete response rate[a]	0	0	0	0
Partial response rate[a]	4%	0%	14%	3%
Stable disease rate[a]	12%	47%	44%	60%
Duration of progression-free survival (days), median	< 56	42	78	72
Overall survival duration (months), median	—	11.8	9.3	7.9

[a]Response evaluation was performed according to the RECIST criteria

Phase II study was conducted at M. D. Anderson Cancer Center (Table 2) *(200)*. In this trial, patients with advanced melanoma (stage IV or unresectable or recurrent stage III) were randomized to receive one of two doses of EMD121974. Among 29 patients enrolled in the study, 26 were randomized and treated; 14 received 500 mg twice weekly and 12 received 2000 mg twice weekly. The treatment was well tolerated, and there were no grade 3 or 4 adverse events except in one patient with grade 3 lymphopenia at the 2000 mg dose level; however, only 3 of 26 patients had their disease controlled for at least 8 weeks. Only one patient at the 2000 mg dose level had a prolonged partial response, which lasted 1 year.

Volociximab (M200) is a high-affinity chimeric immunoglobulin G4 (IgG4) monoclonal antibody, which specifically binds $\alpha_5\beta_1$ integrin. Forty patients with metastatic melanoma, including 22 patients (55%) with stage M1c disease, were enrolled and treated with the combination of intravenous volociximab 10 mg/kg every 2 weeks and dacarbazine 1000 mg/m^2 monthly in a Phase II study of volociximab *(201)*. Of 37 patients evaluable for a clinical response, 1 (3%) had a partial response, and 22 (60%) had disease stabilization for at least 8 weeks, with a median time to progression of 72 days in all 37. Because of the good tolerability and modest clinical efficacy of the 10 mg/kg biweekly dosing, a higher dose of volociximab is currently being evaluated. The results of these trials of integrin-targeting drugs suggest that a combination of an integrin-targeting drug with a cytotoxic drug is more efficacious than a single agent, and further studies should be conducted to find the optimal combinations with these agents.

7. ANTI-CTLA-4 ANTIBODY

Because both spontaneous and immunotherapy-induced disease regressions are known to occur in melanoma, it is considered an important model of tumor immunology *(85,202)*. Proof of this principle is provided by immunotherapeutic approaches, such as high-dose IL-2, which results in durable disease remissions in a subset of patients (approximately 5%–15%) *(85)*. Such sustained remissions reflect the promise of immune-based approaches in treating melanoma, but improvements are needed to broaden efficacy and reduce toxicity.

Vaccine-based approaches aimed at augmenting antimelanoma effector T-cell responses have now been tested extensively in both the adjuvant and metastatic settings. Although such strategies are typically able to elicit significant numbers of antigen-specific cytotoxic T cells in the bloodstream and/or tumors of vaccinated patients, they have met with little clinical success *(203)*. These findings suggest that tumor antigen-specific T-cell responses are actively attenuated in vivo. Precisely how tumor cells are able to circumvent the immune response remains an area of intense investigation, but existing data suggest that tumors use a diverse array of tools to escape immune surveillance *(204)*. Immunotherapeutic targeting of these escape mechanisms may allow improved activity of antitumor T cells and, ultimately, immune-mediated clearance of tumor.

One of the key mechanisms of tumor escape is induction of immune tolerance to tumor-associated antigens *(205)*. T-cell activation is a two-step process that first requires presentation of antigens by host cells or, more commonly, by antigen-presenting cells (APCs). The APC presents degraded peptide antigens as a complex with major histocompatibility complex (MHC) class I or class II molecules, and this complex is recognized by clonal T-cell receptors. The interaction between the T-cell receptor and peptide–MHC complexes determines the specificity of the immune response, but by itself it is typically insufficient for activation of naive T cells *(206)*. A second, antigen-independent co-stimulatory signal is required to trigger downstream events that regulate clonal T-cell expansion and activation of the effector phenotype. Absence of co-stimulatory signaling typically results in T-cell anergy or tolerance *(207)*.

The archetypal co-stimulatory signal is provided by CD28, which resides on the surface of T cells and is recruited to the immunologic synapse upon binding of the peptide–MHC complex with the T-cell receptor. CD28 has two known ligands, B7.1 and B7.2 (also known as CD80 and CD86, respectively), both of which are found almost exclusively on APCs. Upon binding of CD28 to either B7 ligand, signaling cascades are triggered, resulting in increased proliferation, suppression of apoptosis, secretion of proinflammatory cytokines such as IL-2, and increased metabolism to support lymphocyte activation *(208,209)*. Other co-stimulatory molecules have been identified, including inducible T-cell co-stimulator, which is a CD28 homologue, as well as members of the TNF-receptor superfamily such as 4-1BB and OX40 *(210)*. As a mechanism of immune homeostasis and innate protection against autoimmunity, corresponding ligands for these co-stimulatory molecules are typically restricted to APCs and other immune cells. As tumor cells do not express these co-stimulatory ligands, presentation of tumor-associated antigens by tumor cells often results in T-cell anergy and tolerance *(207)*.

As a critical checkpoint in immune function, co-stimulation of T-cell activation is regulated by co-inhibitory molecules that bear structural homology to their stimulatory counterparts. The key co-inhibitor of T-cell activation is cytotoxic T-lymphocyte antigen 4 (CTLA-4), which shares B7.1 and B7.2 as ligands with CD28, albeit with significantly greater binding affinity *(211)*. Binding of CTLA-4 to B7.1 or B7.2 at the immunologic synapse results in down-regulation of T-cell activation by outcompeting CD28 for B7 ligands and also by triggering downstream signal transduction events, resulting in cell cycle arrest and decreased IL-2 production *(212)*. The role of CTLA-4 as a key inhibitor of CD28-dependent T-cell activation is demonstrated in CTLA-4 knockout mice, which develop a rapidly lethal lymphoproliferative disease within weeks of birth *(213,214)*. CTLA-4 is also expressed on regulatory T cells (CD4+ CD25+ FoxP3+ T-cells, or T_{reg} cells), although its functional role in this cell type remains unclear. Data from both mouse and human tumors suggest that T_{reg} cells, though first identified for their role in suppressing autoimmunity *(215,216)*, are also involved in suppression of tumor immunity *(216–218)*.

Given the role of CTLA-4 as a negative regulator of T-cell activation as well as its expression on immunosuppressive T_{reg} cells, inhibition of CTLA-4 has been viewed as an opportunity to shift the balance of tumor immunity from immune tolerance toward immune activation. In mouse models, monoclonal antibodies to CTLA-4 enhance T-cell proliferation in response to a variety of antigens, including peptide antigens, superantigens, and parasites *(219)*. Moreover, infusion of anti-CTLA-4 antibody resulted in disease exacerbation in murine models of autoimmune disease *(219)*. In murine tumor models, including lymphoma and colon, prostate, and renal carcinomas, anti-CTLA-4 antibody induced tumor rejection and augmented tumor-specific T-cell responses *(220–222)*. Intrinsic immunogenicity of the tumor directly correlated with the efficacy of anti-CTLA-4 therapy, such that less-immunogenic tumors, such as melanoma B16, exhibited minimal responses to anti-CTLA-4 monotherapy *(223)*.

Combinatorial approaches in the preclinical setting demonstrated improved efficacy of anti-CTLA-4, particularly in less immunogenic tumors. One such approach examined anti-CTLA-4 in combination with an irradiated granulocyte-macrophage colony-stimulating factor (GM-CSF)-producing tumor cell vaccine. Because of the ability of these agents to attract bone marrow-derived APCs, the GM-CSF–producing tumor vaccine worked synergistically with anti-CTLA-4 antibody to enhance immune responses to melanoma B16 tumors *(223)*. Combining anti-CTLA-4 therapy with other therapeutic modalities, including radiotherapy, chemotherapy, and other novel immunotherapies, demonstrated improved efficacy in cases where single-agent therapy was ineffective *(224–228)*.

As a result of the promising preclinical data observed in animal models, two humanized anti-CTLA-4 monoclonal antibodies have been developed: ipilimumab (also known as MDX-010) and ticilimumab (also known as CP-675,206). Both antibodies block the binding of CTLA-4 to B7.1 and B7.2; they differ from one another primarily by immunoglobulin subtype and serum half-life. In the first human Phase I trial of anti-CTLA-4 therapy, a single dose of ipilimumab (3 mg/kg) was administered to nine previously vaccinated patients with advanced melanoma or ovarian cancer *(229)*. Although no objective tumor regression was identified, biopsies of tumor lesions in three of seven melanoma patients exhibited leukocytic infiltration and tumor necrosis. Notably, in the five patients who were previously treated with a GM-CSF–secreting tumor cell vaccine, all demonstrated either histopathologic or serologic (CA-125 levels) evidence of immune response, whereas the remaining four patients, who had been treated previously with tumor antigen vaccines, had no such responses.

In the Phase I trial of ticilimumab, 39 patients (34 with melanoma, 4 with renal cell carcinoma, 1 with colon cancer) were treated on a dose-escalation protocol, resulting in two complete responses and two partial responses, all in melanoma patients and all remarkably durable (> 24 months) *(230)*. Further studies with ipilimumab and ticilimumab as monotherapy in variably pretreated patients with melanoma and renal cell carcinoma have demonstrated response rates ranging from 5% to 13%. Notably, responses have been seen in patients with both visceral and central nervous system metastases *(206)*.

Given the modest response rates seen with anti-CTLA-4 monotherapy and the preclinical data supporting the rationale for combinatorial approaches, a number of Phase II trials have been performed to explore the expected synergism between vaccine-based immunotherapeutic approaches and ipilimumab. In combination with a melanoma antigen vaccine, ipilimumab given every 3 weeks at two dose levels resulted in overall responses in 7 of 56 patients treated: 4 in the high-dose group and 3 in the low-dose group *(231)*. An ongoing trial comparing vaccine alone, ipilimumab alone, and combination therapy should address the question of synergism more accurately.

As with vaccine therapy, combining anti-CTLA-4 therapy with chemotherapy has demonstrated synergism in preclinical models. A Phase II study in 70 patients with unresectable melanoma compared ipilimumab (3 mg/kg monthly for 4 months) alone with a combination of ipilimumab (3 mg/kg monthly for 4 months) and dacarbazine (250 mg/m^2 on days 1–5 for a maximum of six cycles) (232). Of the 35 patients in the combination arm, 6 were responders (two complete responses, four partial responses), whereas there were 2 responders among the 35 patients in the monotherapy arm (two partial responses). Moreover, the combination arm had a significantly longer overall survival duration than the monotherapy arm (14.2 vs. 11.2 months). Both arms demonstrated better overall survival than historical controls, who received dacarbazine alone (6.4 months). Trials are ongoing to identify synergy between anti-CTLA-4 therapy and other established chemotherapies for melanoma. Combination of high-dose IL-2 with ipilimumab demonstrated an overall response rate of 22%, suggesting that combination therapy has an additive effect but not a clearly synergistic effect (233).

Adverse events related to anti-CTLA-4 therapy are tied closely to its presumed role in breaking T cell-mediated tolerance. Transient elevations in autoimmune serologic markers (e.g., antinuclear antibodies) have been reported, typically in the absence of overt autoimmune or rheumatologic symptomatology, suggesting a release of the immunologic "brake" on recognition of self-antigens (229). The most common adverse effects manifest as skin and gastrointestinal disturbances, usually with histopathologic evidence of neutrophilic and lymphocytic infiltrates suggestive of an autoimmune etiology. Skin manifestations typically include vitiligo, pruritus, and/or eczematous dermatitis; and grade 3/4 skin reactions have been reported in 2% to 5% of patients (229–231). Gastrointestinal manifestations include diarrhea and colitis in approximately 20% of patients, with clinical and pathologic similarity to both intestinal graft-versus-host disease and inflammatory bowel disease. Colonic perforation is perhaps the most feared complication of anti-CTLA-4 therapy, occurring in 4 of the 41 patients who developed colitis in the largest cohort reported to date (234). Other significant adverse effects include hypophysitis, hepatitis, nephritis, uveitis, and arthritis, all of which are presumed to be related to tissue infiltration with inflammatory T cells (230,235–237). Development of immune-mediated adverse effects does not seem to correlate with timing of anti-CTLA-4 therapy and can occur early or late in the treatment course. Treatment of adverse effects typically includes cessation of antibody therapy and institution of high-dose steroids. Anti–TNFα antibody (infliximab) has been used in cases of steroid-refractory colitis with good results (234). Interestingly, the incidence of immune-mediated adverse effects seems to correlate with response to therapy. Overall response rates in melanoma and renal cell carcinoma patients who developed colitis were approximately 36% and 35%, respectively, whereas they were 11% and 2% in patients who did not develop colitis (234).

Anti-CTLA-4 therapy has shown promise in early clinical trials for melanoma and renal cell carcinoma, with durable responses observed in small proportions of patients. Trials of combination therapy with both established and novel treatment modalities may reveal new synergies and lend further mechanistic insight; and laboratory-based correlative studies should shed light on markers predictive of clinical response. Small trials in other tumor types, including prostate, colon, and ovarian carcinomas, suggest some response to anti-CTLA-4 therapy, hinting that immunotherapy may have activity in cancers previously thought to be beyond the control of the immune system (229,238). Perhaps most importantly, anti-CTLA-4 therapy may serve as a platform on which other rationally designed agents can be added.

Activating antibodies that bind co-stimulatory molecules such as 4-1BB and OX40 are currently in clinical development, as are antibodies directed against novel co-inhibitors such as PD-1. As our understanding of tumor immunology advances, treatment modalities designed to harness the latent power of host immunity will continue to emerge.

8. FUTURE DIRECTIONS

Successful targeted therapy should involve the development of potent and selective drugs against clinically relevant target proteins or genes and identification of appropriate patient populations with proper targets for the drugs. In this way, the therapy will greatly benefit cancer patients by providing prolonged tumor control, palliation of disabling symptoms by tumor reduction, and extension of the life span without significant undesirable adverse events. Despite much enthusiasm and hopes for targeted therapy in melanoma, we are still facing a number of challenges that must be overcome.

One of the most urgent challenges is to identify predictive markers for targeted drugs. For some drugs, the predictive markers may seem obvious. For example, the V600E B-*raf* mutation is likely an appropriate marker for specific small-molecule inhibitors of mutated B-Raf. Unfortunately, predictive markers are not well established for most small kinase inhibitors. Is total expression of $\alpha_v\beta_3$ integrin or the phosphorylated forms of its downstream effector kinases, such as focal adhesion kinase, a better predictive marker for $\alpha_v\beta_3$ antagonists? For inhibitors of VEGFR, should we select patients with overexpression of p-VEGFR or *Vegfr* mutation in their tumors? Is an increased copy number of the c-*kit* gene a good marker for imatinib? Identification of such predictive markers may be achieved only through well designed correlative studies during the clinical investigation of drugs. The fact that melanoma tends to metastasize to skin and superficial lymph nodes, which are easy to access for tumor biopsy, makes it possible to conduct translational trials in patients with melanoma.

The discouraging results of recent clinical trials of targeted drugs as single agents in patients with metastatic melanoma underscore the complexity of signal transduction pathways in melanoma cells and their interaction with the surrounding environment. Unlike the clear-cell type of renal cell carcinoma containing aberrant hypoxia-induced factor-1 or GIST with mutated c-*kit* and/or *Pdgfr-α*, a predominant signal pathway for melanoma progression and survival has not been found. A recent finding reported by Curtin, Bastian, and their colleagues on genetic alteration in different types of melanoma is encouraging for targeted therapy for melanoma *(27,239)*. These investigators found that c-*kit* mutation and/or aberration is more common and relevant than B-*Raf/N-Ras* mutation in acral lentiginous, mucosal melanoma, or cutaneous melanoma on chronically sun-damaged skin, whereas the opposite is true for cutaneous melanoma on skin without chronic sun damage. This type of study is necessary to define further the role of certain signal pathways in subsets of melanoma and potentially to improve clinical outcomes by investigating targeted drugs in the right subsets of patients.

For successful targeted therapy of melanoma, which has complex interactions of signal proteins at multiple levels and with multiple pathways, combinations of targeted therapies, rather than a single agent, will likely be required for most patients. Identification of rational combinations is urgently needed. With more targeted drugs being approved for other types of cancer and becoming commercially available, an increased number of trials of combination therapies are to be anticipated. Moreover, recent important initiatives by the Cancer Therapy and Evaluation Program of the National Cancer Institute to facilitate the combination of promising drugs by working closely with the pharmaceutical industry will accelerate the research on targeted therapy in melanoma.

REFERENCES

1. Jemal A, Siegel R, Ward E, et al. Cancer statistics, 2007. CA Cancer J Clin 2007;57:43–66.
2. Balch CM, Soong SJ, Gershenwald JE, et al. Prognostic factors analysis of 17,600 melanoma patients: validation of the American Joint Committee on Cancer melanoma staging system. J Clin Oncol 2001;19:3622–34.
3. Tsao H, Atkins MB, Sober AJ. Management of cutaneous melanoma. N Engl J Med 2004;351:998–1012.
4. Atkins MB, Kunkel L, Sznol M, et al. High-dose recombinant interleukin-2 therapy in patients with metastatic melanoma: long-term survival update. Cancer J Sci Am 2000;6(Suppl 1):S11–4.
5. National Cancer Institute. 51-year trends in U.S. cancer death rates. In SEER cancer statistics review -AD, 2007, at http://seer.cancer.gov/csr/1975_2000/results_merged/topic_inc_mor_trends.pdf.
6. Demetri GD, von Mehren M, Blanke CD, et al. Efficacy and safety of imatinib mesylate in advanced gastrointestinal stromal tumors. N Engl J Med 2002;347:472–80.
7. Druker BJ, Talpaz M, Resta DJ, et al. NB Efficacy and safety of a specific inhibitor of the BCR-ABL tyrosine kinase in chronic myeloid leukemia. N Engl J Med 2001;344:1031–7.
8. Choueiri TK, Bukowski RM, Rini BI. The current role of angiogenesis inhibitors in the treatment of renal cell carcinoma. Semin Oncol 2006;33:596–606.
9. Davies M, Hennessy B, Mills GB. Point mutations of protein kinases and individualised cancer therapy. Expert Opin Pharmacother 2006;7:2243–61.
10. Piccart-Gebhart MJ, Procter M, Leyland-Jones B, et al. Trastuzumab after adjuvant chemotherapy in HER2-positive breast cancer. N Engl J Med 2005;353:1659–72.
11. Romond EH, Perez EA, Bryant J, et al. Trastuzumab plus adjuvant chemotherapy for operable HER2-positive breast cancer. N Engl J Med 2005;353:1673–84.
12. Slamon DJ, Leyland-Jones B, Shak S, et al. Use of chemotherapy plus a monoclonal antibody against HER2 for metastatic breast cancer that overexpresses HER2. N Engl J Med 2001;344:783–92.
13. Mass RD, Press MF, Anderson S, et al. Evaluation of clinical outcomes according to HER2 detection by fluorescence in situ hybridization in women with metastatic breast cancer treated with trastuzumab. Clin Breast Cancer 2005;6:240–6.
14. Colicelli J. Human RAS superfamily proteins and related GTPases. Sci STKE 2004;2004:RE13.
15. Giehl K. Oncogenic Ras in tumour progression and metastasis. Biol Chem 2005;386:193–205.
16. Rubinfeld H, Seger R. The ERK cascade: a prototype of MAPK signaling. Mol Biotechnol 2005;31:151–74.
17. Wellbrock C, Karasarides M, Marais R. The RAF proteins take centre stage. Nat Rev Mol Cell Biol 2004;5:875–85.
18. Cohen C, Zavala-Pompa A, Sequeira JH, et al. Mitogen-actived protein kinase activation is an early event in melanoma progression. Clin Cancer Res 2002;8:3728–33.
19. Lebedeva IV, Sarkar D, Su ZZ, et al. Molecular target-based therapy of pancreatic cancer. Cancer Res 2006;66:2403–13.
20. Grady WM, Markowitz SD. Genetic and epigenetic alterations in colon cancer. Annu Rev Genomics Hum Genet 2002;3:101–28.
21. Smalley KS. A pivotal role for ERK in the oncogenic behaviour of malignant melanoma? Int J Cancer 2003;104:527–32.
22. Goydos JS, Mann B, Kim HJ, et al. Detection of B-RAF and N-RAS mutations in human melanoma. J Am Coll Surg 2005;200:362–70.
23. Goel VK, Lazar AJ, Warneke CL, et al. Examination of mutations in BRAF, NRAS, and PTEN in primary cutaneous melanoma. J Invest Dermatol 2006;126:154–60.
24. Gray-Schopfer VC, da Rocha Dias S, Marais R. The role of B-RAF in melanoma. Cancer Metastasis Rev 2005;24:165–83.
25. Davies H, Bignell GR, Cox C, et al. Mutations of the BRAF gene in human cancer. Nature 2002;417:949–54.
26. Rimoldi D, Salvi S, Lienard D, et al. Lack of BRAF mutations in uveal melanoma. Cancer Res 2003;63:5712–15.
27. Curtin JA, Fridlyand J, Kageshita T, et al. Distinct sets of genetic alterations in melanoma. N Engl J Med 2005;353:2135–47.
28. Wong CW, Fan YS, Chan TL, et al. BRAF and NRAS mutations are uncommon in melanomas arising in diverse internal organs. J Clin Pathol 2005;58:640–4.

29. Zuidervaart W, van Nieuwpoort F, Stark M, et al. Activation of the MAPK pathway is a common event in uveal melanomas although it rarely occurs through mutation of BRAF or RAS. Br J Cancer 2005;92:2032–8.

30. Pollock PM, Harper UL, Hansen KS, et al. High frequency of BRAF mutations in nevi. Nat Genet 2003;33:19–20.

31. Yazdi AS, Palmedo G, Flaig MJ, et al. Mutations of the BRAF gene in benign and malignant melanocytic lesions. J Invest Dermatol 2003;121:1160–2.

32. Patton EE, Widlund HR, Kutok JL, et al. BRAF mutations are sufficient to promote nevi formation and cooperate with p53 in the genesis of melanoma. Curr Biol 2005;15:249–54.

33. Lazar-Molnar E, Hegyesi H, Toth S, et al. Autocrine and paracrine regulation by cytokines and growth factors in melanoma. Cytokine 2000;12:547–54.

34. Hingorani SR, Jacobetz MA, Robertson GP, et al. Suppression of BRAF(V599E) in human melanoma abrogates transformation. Cancer Res 2003;63:5198–202.

35. Strumberg D. Preclinical and clinical development of the oral multikinase inhibitor sorafenib in cancer treatment. Drugs Today (Barc) 2005;41:773–84.

36. Strumberg D, Voliotis D, Moeller JG, et al. Results of phase I pharmacokinetic and pharmacodynamic studies of the Raf kinase inhibitor BAY 43–9006 in patients with solid tumors. Int J Clin Pharmacol Ther 2002;40:580–1.

37. Eisen T, Ahmad T, Flaherty KT, et al. Sorafenib in advanced melanoma: a Phase II randomised discontinuation trial analysis. Br J Cancer 2006;95:581–6.

38. Escudier B, Eisen T, Stadler WM, et al. Sorafenib in advanced clear-cell renal-cell carcinoma. N Engl J Med 2007;356:125–34.

39. Flaherty KT, Brose M, Schuchter L, et al. Phase I/II trial of BAY 43–9006, carboplatin (C) and paclitaxel (P) demonstrates preliminary antitumor activity in the expansion cohort of patients with metastatic melanoma. In Proceedings of Am Soc Clin Oncol; New Orleans, LA. 2004: No 14S (July 15 Supplement), 7507.

40. Lorigan P, Corrie P, Chao D, et al. Phase II trial of sorafenib combined with dacarbazine in metastatic melanoma patients. In Proceedings of Am Soc Clin Oncol; Atlanta, GA. 2006: No 18S (June 20 Supplement), 8012.

41. McDermott DF, Sosman JA, Hodi FS, et al. Randomized phase II study of dacarbazine with or without sorafenib in patients with advanced melanoma. In Proceedings of Am Soc Clin Oncol; Chicago, IL. 2007: No 18S (June 20 Supplement), 8511.

42. Amaravadi RK, Schuchter LM, Kramer A, et al. Preliminary results of a randomized phase II study comparing two schedules of temozolomide in combination with sorafenib in patients with advanced melanoma. In Proceedings of Am Soc Clin Oncol; Atlanta, GA. 2006: No 18S (June 20 Supplement), 8009.

43. Caponigro F, Casale M, Bryce J. Farnesyl transferase inhibitors in clinical development. Expert Opin Investig Drugs 2003;12:943–54.

44. Rinehart J, Adjei AA, Lorusso PM, et al. Multicenter phase II study of the oral MEK inhibitor, CI-1040, in patients with advanced non-small-cell lung, breast, colon, and pancreatic cancer. J Clin Oncol 2004; 22:4456–62.

45. Lorusso PM, Adjei AA, Varterasian M, et al. Phase I and pharmacodynamic study of the oral MEK inhibitor CI-1040 in patients with advanced malignancies. J Clin Oncol 2005;23:5281–93.

46. Wallace EM, Lyssikatos JP, Yeh T, et al. Progress towards therapeutic small molecule MEK inhibitors for use in cancer therapy. Curr Top Med Chem 2005;5:215–29.

47. Lorusso P, Krishnamurthi S, Rinehart JR, et al. A phase I-II clinical study of a second generation oral MEK inhibitor, PD 0325901 in patients with advanced cancer. In Proceedings of Am Soc Clin Oncol; Orlando, FL. 2005.

48. Downward J. PI 3-kinase, Akt and cell survival. Semin Cell Dev Biol 2004;15:177–82.

49. Robertson GP. Functional and therapeutic significance of Akt deregulation in malignant melanoma. Cancer Metastasis Rev 2005;24:273–85.

50. Brunet A, Bonni A, Zigmond MJ, et al. Akt promotes cell survival by phosphorylating and inhibiting a Forkhead transcription factor. Cell 1999;96:857–68.

51. Romashkova JA, Makarov SS. NF-kappaB is a target of AKT in anti-apoptotic PDGF signalling. Nature 1999;401:86–90.

52. Dhawan P, Singh AB, Ellis DL, et al. Constitutive activation of Akt/protein kinase B in melanoma leads to up-regulation of nuclear factor-kappaB and tumor progression. Cancer Res 2002;62:7335–42.

53. Datta SR, Dudek H, Tao X, et al. Akt phosphorylation of BAD couples survival signals to the cell-intrinsic death machinery. Cell 1997;91:231–41.

54. Sekulic A, Hudson CC, Homme JL, et al. A direct linkage between the phosphoinositide 3-kinase-AKT signaling pathway and the mammalian target of rapamycin in mitogen-stimulated and transformed cells. Cancer Res 2000;60:3504–13.

55. Cross DA, Alessi DR, Cohen P, et al. Inhibition of glycogen synthase kinase-3 by insulin mediated by protein kinase B. Nature 1995;378:785–9.
56. Datta SR, Brunet A, Greenberg ME. Cellular survival: a play in three Akts. Genes Dev 1999;13:2905–27.
57. Testa JR, Bellacosa A. AKT plays a central role in tumorigenesis. Proc Natl Acad Sci U S A 2001; 98:10983–5.
58. Scheid MP, Woodgett JR. Unravelling the activation mechanisms of protein kinase B/Akt. FEBS Lett 2003;546:108–12.
59. Bellacosa A, Testa JR, Staal SP, et al. A retroviral oncogene, akt, encoding a serine-threonine kinase containing an SH2-like region. Science 1991;254:274–7.
60. Brazil DP, Park J, Hemmings BA. PKB binding proteins. Getting in on the Akt. Cell 2002;111:293–303.
61. Stahl JM, Sharma A, Cheung M, et al. Deregulated Akt3 activity promotes development of malignant melanoma. Cancer Res 2004;64:7002–10.
62. Maehama T, Dixon JE. The tumor suppressor, PTEN/MMAC1, dephosphorylates the lipid second messenger, phosphatidylinositol 3,4,5-trisphosphate. J Biol Chem 1998;273:13375–8.
63. Lin H, Bondy ML, Langford LA, et al. Allelic deletion analyses of MMAC/PTEN and DMBT1 loci in gliomas: relationship to prognostic significance. Clin Cancer Res 1998;4:2447–54.
64. Stambolic V, Suzuki A, de la Pompa JL, et al. Negative regulation of PKB/Akt-dependent cell survival by the tumor suppressor PTEN. Cell 1998;95:29–39.
65. Davies MA, Lu Y, Sano T, et al. Adenoviral transgene expression of MMAC/PTEN in human glioma cells inhibits Akt activation and induces anoikis. Cancer Res 1998;58:5285–90.
66. Davies MA, Koul D, Dhesi H, et al. Regulation of Akt/PKB activity, cellular growth, and apoptosis in prostate carcinoma cells by MMAC/PTEN. Cancer Res 1999;59:2551–6.
67. Hwang PH, Yi HK, Kim DS, et al. Suppression of tumorigenicity and metastasis in B16F10 cells by PTEN/MMAC1/TEP1 gene. Cancer Lett 2001;172:83–91.
68. Dahia PL, Aguiar RC, Alberta J, et al. PTEN is inversely correlated with the cell survival factor Akt/PKB and is inactivated via multiple mechanismsin haematological malignancies. Hum Mol Genet 1999;8:185–93.
69. Cheney IW, Johnson DE, Vaillancourt MT, et al. Suppression of tumorigenicity of glioblastoma cells by adenovirus-mediated MMAC1/PTEN gene transfer. Cancer Res 1998;58:2331–4.
70. Boni R, Vortmeyer AO, Burg G, et al. The PTEN tumour suppressor gene and malignant melanoma. Melanoma Res 1998, 8:300–302.
71. Celebi JT, Shendrik I, Silvers DN, Peacocke M. Identification of PTEN mutations in metastatic melanoma specimens. J Med Genet 2000;37:653–7.
72. Guldberg P, thor Straten P, Birck A, et al. Disruption of the MMAC1/PTEN gene by deletion or mutation is a frequent event in malignant melanoma. Cancer Res 1997;57:3660–3.
73. Robertson GP, Furnari FB, Miele ME, et al. In vitro loss of heterozygosity targets the PTEN/MMAC1 gene in melanoma. Proc Natl Acad Sci U S A 1998;95:9418–9423.
74. Birck A, Ahrenkiel V, Zeuthen J, et al. Mutation and allelic loss of the PTEN/MMAC1 gene in primary and metastatic melanoma biopsies. J Invest Dermatol 2000;114:277–80.
75. Reifenberger J, Wolter M, Bostrom J, et al. Allelic losses on chromosome arm 10q and mutation of the PTEN (MMAC1) tumour suppressor gene in primary and metastatic malignant melanomas. Virchows Arch 2000;436:487–93.
76. Poetsch M, Dittberner T, Woenckhaus C. PTEN/MMAC1 in malignant melanoma and its importance for tumor progression. Cancer Genet Cytogenet 2001;125:21–6.
77. Tsao H, Zhang X, Benoit E, et al. Identification of PTEN/MMAC1 alterations in uncultured melanomas and melanoma cell lines. Oncogene 1998;16:3397–402.
78. Zhou XP, Gimm O, Hampel H, et al. Epigenetic PTEN silencing in malignant melanomas without PTEN mutation. Am J Pathol 2000;157:1123–8.
79. Tsao H, Goel V, Wu H, et al. Genetic interaction between NRAS and BRAF mutations and PTEN/MMAC1 inactivation in melanoma. J Invest Dermatol 2004;122:337–41.
80. Dai DL, Martinka M, Li G. Prognostic significance of activated Akt expression in melanoma: a clinicopathologic study of 292 cases. J Clin Oncol 2005;23:1473–82.
81. Kondapaka SB, Singh SS, Dasmahapatra GP, et al. Perifosine, a novel alkylphospholipid, inhibits protein kinase B activation. Mol Cancer Ther 2003;2:1093–103.
82. Ernst DS, Eisenhauer E, Wainman N, et al. Phase II study of perifosine in previously untreated patients with metastatic melanoma. Invest New Drugs 2005;23:569–75.
83. Investigators Brochure CCI-779. Wyeth.
84. Raymond E, Alexandre J, Faivre S, et al. Safety and pharmacokinetics of escalated doses of weekly intravenous infusion of CCI-779, a novel mTOR inhibitor, in patients with cancer. J Clin Oncol 2004;22:2336–47.

85. Atkins MB, Lotze MT, Dutcher JP, et al. High-dose recombinant interleukin 2 therapy for patients with metastatic melanoma: analysis of 270 patients treated between 1985 and 1993. J Clin Oncol 1999; 17:2105–16.

86. Amiri KI, Richmond A. Role of nuclear factor-kappa B in melanoma. Cancer Metastasis Rev 2005; 24:301–13.

87. Wang CY, Mayo MW, Korneluk RG, et al. NF-kappaB antiapoptosis: induction of TRAF1 and TRAF2 and c-IAP1 and c-IAP2 to suppress caspase-8 activation. Science 1998;281:1680–3.

88. Catz SD, Johnson JL. Transcriptional regulation of bcl-2 by nuclear factor kappa B and its significance in prostate cancer. Oncogene 2001;20:7342–51.

89. Kunz M, Hartmann A, Flory E, et al. Anoxia-induced up-regulation of interleukin-8 in human malignant melanoma. A potential mechanism for high tumor aggressiveness. Am J Pathol 1999;155:753–63.

90. Cusack JC, Liu R, Baldwin AS. NF-kappa B and chemoresistance: potentiation of cancer drugs via inhibition of NF-kappa B. Drug Resist Updat 1999;2:271–3.

91. Meyskens FL, Jr., Buckmeier JA, McNulty SE, et al. Activation of nuclear factor-kappa B in human metastatic melanomacells and the effect of oxidative stress. Clin Cancer Res 1999;5:1197–202.

92. McNulty SE, Tohidian NB, Meyskens FL, Jr. RelA, p50 and inhibitor of kappa B alpha are elevated in human metastatic melanoma cells and respond aberrantly to ultraviolet light B. Pigment Cell Res 2001;14:456–65.

93. McNulty SE, del Rosario R, Cen D, et al. Comparative expression of NFkappaB proteins in melanocytes of normal skin vs. benign intradermal naevus and human metastatic melanoma biopsies. Pigment Cell Res 2004;17:173–80.

94. Koul D, Yao Y, Abbruzzese JL, et al. Tumor suppressor MMAC/PTEN inhibits cytokine-induced NFkappaB activation without interfering with the IkappaB degradation pathway. J Biol Chem 2001;276:11402–8.

95. Madrid LV, Mayo MW, Reuther JY, et al. Akt stimulates the transactivation potential of the RelA/p65 Subunit of NF-kappa B through utilization of the Ikappa B kinase and activation of the mitogen-activated protein kinase p38. J Biol Chem 2001;276:18934–40.

96. Troppmair J, Hartkamp J, Rapp UR. Activation of NF-kappa B by oncogenic Raf in HEK 293 cells occurs through autocrine recruitment of the stress kinase cascade. Oncogene 1998;17:685–90.

97. Jo H, Zhang R, Zhang H, et al. NF-kappa B is required for H-ras oncogene induced abnormal cell proliferation and tumorigenesis. Oncogene 2000;19:841–9.

98. Belch A, Kouroukis CT, Crump M, et al. A phase II study of bortezomib in mantle cell lymphoma: the National Cancer Institute of Canada Clinical Trials Group trial IND.150. Ann Oncol 2007;18:116–21.

99. Richardson PG, Hideshima T, Anderson KC. Bortezomib (PS-341): a novel, first-in-class proteasome inhibitor for the treatment of multiple myeloma and other cancers. Cancer Control 2003;10:361–9.

100. Markovic SN, Geyer SM, Dawkins F, et al. A phase II study of bortezomib in the treatment of metastatic malignant melanoma. Cancer 2005;103:2584–9.

101. Yang J, Amiri KI, Burke JR, et al. BMS-345541 targets inhibitor of kappaB kinase and induces apoptosis in melanoma: involvement of nuclear factor kappaB and mitochondria pathways. Clin Cancer Res 2006, 12:950–60.

102. Druker BJ, Lydon NB. Lessons learned from the development of an abl tyrosine kinase inhibitor for chronic myelogenous leukemia. J Clin Invest 2000, 105:3–7.

103. Okuda K, Weisberg E, Gilliland DG, et al. ARG tyrosine kinase activity is inhibited by STI571. Blood 2001, 97:2440–8.

104. Schindler T, Bornmann W, Pellicena P, et al. Structural mechanism for STI-571 inhibition of abelson tyrosine kinase. Science 2000, 289:1938–42.

105. Easty DJ, Bennett DC. Protein tyrosine kinases in malignant melanoma. Melanoma Res 2000, 10:401–11.

106. Barnhill RL, Xiao M, Graves D, et al. Expression of platelet-derived growth factor (PDGF)-A, PDGF-B and the PDGF-alpha receptor, but not the PDGF-beta receptor, in human malignant melanoma in vivo. Br J Dermatol 1996, 135:898–904.

107. Shen SS, Zhang PS, Eton O, et al. Analysis of protein tyrosine kinase expression in melanocytic lesions by tissue array. J Cutan Pathol 2003, 30:539–47.

108. Wyman K, Atkins MB, Prieto V, et al. Multicenter Phase II trial of high-dose imatinib mesylate in metastatic melanoma: significant toxicity with no clinical efficacy. Cancer 2006, 106:2005–11.

109. Eton O, Billings L, Kim K, et al. Phase II trial of imatinib mesylate (STI-571) in metastatic melanoma (MM). In Proceedings of Am Soc Clin Oncol; New Orleans, LA. 2004: No.14S (July 15 Supplement), 7528.

110. Mendel DB, Laird AD, Xin X, et al. In vivo antitumor activity of SU11248, a novel tyrosine kinase inhibitor targeting vascular endothelial growth factor and platelet-derived growth factor receptors: determination of a pharmacokinetic/pharmacodynamic relationship. Clin Cancer Res 2003, 9:327–37.

111. O'Farrell AM, Abrams TJ, Yuen HA, et al. SU11248 is a novel FLT3 tyrosine kinase inhibitor with potent activity in vitro and in vivo. Blood 2003, 101:3597–605.

112. Motzer RJ, Hutson TE, Tomczak P, et al. Sunitinib versus interferon alfa in metastatic renal-cell carcinoma. N Engl J Med 2007, 356:115–24.

113. Atkins M, Jones CA, Kirkpatrick P. Sunitinib maleate. Nat Rev Drug Discov 2006, 5:279–80.

114. Demetri GD, van Oosterom AT, Garrett CR, et al. Efficacy and safety of sunitinib in patients with advanced gastrointestinal stromal tumour after failure of imatinib: a randomised controlled trial. Lancet 2006, 368:1329–38.

115. Vaux DL, Cory S, Adams JM. Bcl-2 gene promotes haemopoietic cell survival and cooperates with c-myc to immortalize pre-B cells. Nature 1988, 335:440–2.

116. Tsujimoto Y, Finger LR, Yunis J, et al. Cloning of the chromosome breakpoint of neoplastic B cells with the t(14;18) chromosome translocation. Science 1984, 226:1097–99.

117. Bakhshi A, Jensen JP, Goldman P, et al. Cloning the chromosomal breakpoint of t(14;18) human lymphomas: clustering around JH on chromosome 14 and near a transcriptional unit on 18. Cell 1985, 41:899–906.

118. Konopleva M, Zhao S, Xie Z, et al. Apoptosis. Molecules and mechanisms. Adv Exp Med Biol 1999, 457:217–36.

119. Maung ZT, MacLean FR, Reid MM, et al. The relationship between bcl-2 expression and response to chemotherapy in acute leukaemia. Br J Haematol 1994, 88:105–09.

120. Bedner E, Li X, Gorczyca W, et al. Analysis of apoptosis by laser scanning cytometry. Cytometry 1999, 35:181–95.

121. Jansen B, Schlagbauer-Wadl H, Brown BD, et al. Bcl-2 antisense therapy chemosensitizes human melanoma in SCID mice. Nat Med 1998, 4:232–4.

122. Utikal J, Leiter U, Udart M, et al. Expression of c-myc and bcl-2 in primary and advanced cutaneous melanoma. Cancer Invest 2002, 20:914–21.

123. Korsmeyer SJ. BCL-2 gene family and the regulation of programmed cell death. Cancer Res 1999, 59:1693s–1700s.

124. Leiter U, Schmid RM, Kaskel P, et al. Antiapoptotic bcl-2 and bcl-xL in advanced malignant melanoma. Arch Dermatol Res 2000, 292:225–32.

125. Jansen B, Wacheck V, Heere-Ress E, et al. Chemosensitisation of malignant melanoma by BCL2 antisense therapy. Lancet 2000, 356:1728–33.

126. Bedikian AY, Millward M, Pehamberger H, et al. Bcl-2 antisense (oblimersen sodium) plus dacarbazine in patients with advanced melanoma: the Oblimersen Melanoma Study Group. J Clin Oncol 2006, 24:4738–45.

127. Boulton S, Pemberton LC, Porteous JK, et al. Potentiation of temozolomide-induced cytotoxicity: a comparative study of the biological effects of poly(ADP-ribose) polymerase inhibitors. Br J Cancer 1995, 72:849–56.

128. Trucco C, Oliver FJ, de Murcia G, et al. DNA repair defect in poly(ADP-ribose) polymerase-deficient cell lines. Nucleic Acids Res 1998, 26:2644–9.

129. Malanga M, Pleschke JM, Kleczkowska HE et al. Poly(ADP-ribose) binds to specific domains of p53 and alters its DNA binding functions. J Biol Chem 1998, 273:11839–43.

130. Agarwal ML, Agarwal A, Taylor WR, et al. Defective induction but normal activation and function of p53 in mouse cells lacking poly-ADP-ribose polymerase. Oncogene 1997, 15:1035–41.

131. Pieper AA, Verma A, Zhang J, et al. Poly (ADP-ribose) polymerase, nitric oxide and cell death. Trends Pharmacol Sci 1999, 20:171–81.

132. Burkle A. Physiology and pathophysiology of poly(ADP-ribosyl)ation. Bioessays 2001, 23:795–806.

133. Tentori L, Leonetti C, Scarsella M, et al. Combined treatment with temozolomide and poly(ADP-ribose) polymerase inhibitor enhances survival of mice bearing hematologic malignancy at the central nervous system site. Blood 2002, 99:2241–44.

134. Plummer R, Lorigan P, Evans J, et al. First and final report of a phase II study of the poly(ADP-ribose) polymerase (PARP) inhibitor, AG014699, in combination with temozolomide (TMZ) in patients with metastatic malignant melanoma (MM). In Proceedings of Am Soc Clin Oncol; Atlanta, GA. 2006: No. 18S (June 20 Supplement), 8013.

135. Srivastava A, Laidler P, Hughes LE, et al. Neovascularization in human cutaneous melanoma: a quantitative morphological and Doppler ultrasound study. Eur J Cancer Clin Oncol 1986, 22:1205–9.

136. Marcoval J, Moreno A, Graells J, et al. Angiogenesis and malignant melanoma. Angiogenesis is related to the development of vertical (tumorigenic) growth phase. J Cutan Pathol 1997, 24:212–8.

137. Straume O, Akslen LA. Expresson of vascular endothelial growth factor, its receptors (FLT-1, KDR) and TSP-1 related to microvessel density and patient outcome in vertical growth phase melanomas. Am J Pathol 2001, 159:223–35.

138. Erhard H, Rietveld FJ, van Altena MC, et al. Transition of horizontal to vertical growth phase melanoma is accompanied by induction of vascular endothelial growth factor expression and angiogenesis. Melanoma Res 1997, 7 Suppl 2:S19–26.

139. Srivastava A, Laidler P, Davies RP, et al. The prognostic significance of tumor vascularity in intermediate-thickness (0.76–4.0 mm thick) skin melanoma. A quantitative histologic study. Am J Pathol 1988, 133: 419–23.

140. Denijn M, Ruiter DJ. The possible role of angiogenesis in the metastatic potential of human melanoma. Clinicopathological aspects. Melanoma Res 1993, 3:5–14.

141. Graham CH, Rivers J, Kerbel RS, et al. Extent of vascularization as a prognostic indicator in thin (< 0.76 mm) malignant melanomas. Am J Pathol 1994, 145:510–4.

142. Demirkesen C, Buyukpinarbasili N, Ramazanoglu R, et al. The correlation of angiogenesis with metastasis in primary cutaneous melanoma: a comparative analysis of microvessel density, expression of vascular endothelial growth factor and basic fibroblastic growth factor. Pathology 2006, 38:132–7.

143. Potgens AJ, Lubsen NH, van Altena MC, et al. Vascular permeability factor expression influences tumor angiogenesis in human melanoma lines xenografted to nude mice. Am J Pathol 1995, 146:197–209.

144. Oku T, Tjuvajev JG, Miyagawa T, et al. Tumor growth modulation by sense and antisense vascular endothelial growth factor gene expression: effects on angiogenesis, vascular permeability, blood volume, blood flow, fluorodeoxyglucose uptake, and proliferation of human melanoma intracerebral xenografts. Cancer Res 1998, 58:4185–92.

145. Claffey KP, Brown LF, del Aguila LF, et al. Expression of vascular permeability factor/vascular endothelial growth factor by melanoma cells increases tumor growth, angiogenesis, and experimental metastasis. Cancer Res 1996, 56:172–81.

146. Rofstad EK, Danielsen T. Hypoxia-induced angiogenesis and vascular endothelial growth factor secretion in human melanoma. Br J Cancer 1998, 77:897–902.

147. Halaban R, Kwon BS, Ghosh S, et al. bFGF as an autocrine growth factor for human melanomas. Oncogene Res 1988, 3:177–86.

148. Becker D, Meier CB, Herlyn M. Proliferation of human malignant melanomas is inhibited by antisense oligodeoxynucleotides targeted against basic fibroblast growth factor. Embo J 1989, 8:3685–91.

149. Li J, Yen C, Liaw D, Podsypanina K, et al. PTEN, a putative protein tyrosine phosphatase gene mutated in human brain, breast, and prostate cancer. Science 1997, 275:1943–7.

150. Zachariae CO, Thestrup-Pedersen K, Matsushima K. Expression and secretion of leukocyte chemotactic cytokines by normal human melanocytes and melanoma cells. J Invest Dermatol 1991, 97:593–599.

151. Dvorak HF, Brown LF, Detmar M, et al. Vascular permeability factor/vascular endothelial growth factor, microvascular hyperpermeability, and angiogenesis. Am J Pathol 1995, 146:1029–39.

152. Ferrara N. Vascular endothelial growth factor. Eur J Cancer 1996, 32A:2413–22.

153. Slavin J. Fibroblast growth factors: at the heart of angiogenesis. Cell Biol Int 1995, 19:431–44.

154. Ellis LM, Fidler IJ. Angiogenesis and metastasis. Eur J Cancer 1996, 32A:2451–60.

155. Bikfalvi A, Klein S, Pintucci G, et al.. Biological roles of fibroblast growth factor-2. Endocr Rev 1997, 18:26–45.

156. Bar-Eli M. Role of interleukin-8 in tumor growth and metastasis of human melanoma. Pathobiology 1999, 67:12–8.

157. Li A, Dubey S, Varney ML, et al. IL-8 directly enhanced endothelial cell survival, proliferation, and matrix metalloproteinases production and regulated angiogenesis. J Immunol 2003, 170:3369–76.

158. Rofstad EK, Halsor EF. Vascular endothelial growth factor, interleukin 8, platelet-derived endothelial cell growth factor, and basic fibroblast growth factor promote angiogenesis and metastasis in human melanoma xenografts. Cancer Res 2000, 60:4932–8.

159. Lev DC, Ruiz M, Mills L, et al. Dacarbazine causes transcriptional up-regulation of interleukin 8 and vascular endothelial growth factor in melanoma cells: a possible escape mechanism from chemotherapy. Mol Cancer Ther 2003, 2:753–63.

160. Lev DC, Onn A, Melinkova VO, et al. Exposure of melanoma cells to dacarbazine results in enhanced tumor growth and metastasis in vivo. J Clin Oncol 2004, 22:2092–100.

161. Terman BI, Dougher-Vermazen M, Carrion ME, et al. Identification of the KDR tyrosine kinase as a receptor for vascular endothelial cell growth factor. Biochem Biophys Res Commun 1992, 187:1579–86.

162. de Vries C, Escobedo JA, Ueno H, et al. The fms-like tyrosine kinase, a receptor for vascular endothelial growth factor. Science 1992, 255:989–91.

163. Hwu WJ, Krown SE, Menell JH, et al. Phase II study of temozolomide plus thalidomide for the treatment of metastatic melanoma. J Clin Oncol 2003, 21:3351–6.

164. Kaipainen A, Korhonen J, Pajusola K, et al. The related FLT4, FLT1, and KDR receptor tyrosine kinases show distinct expression patterns in human fetal endothelial cells. J Exp Med 1993, 178:2077–88.

165. Salven P, Heikkila P, Joensuu H. Enhanced expression of vascular endothelial growth factor in metastatic melanoma. Br J Cancer 1997, 76:930–4.

166. Bayer-Garner IB, Hough AJ, Jr., Smoller BR. Vascular endothelial growth factor expression in malignant melanoma: prognostic versus diagnostic usefulness. Mod Pathol 1999, 12:770–4.

167. Birck A, Kirkin AF, Zeuthen J, et al. Expression of basic fibroblast growth factor and vascular endothelial growth factor in primary and metastatic melanoma from the same patients. Melanoma Res 1999, 9:375–81.

168. Lacal PM, Failla CM, Pagani E, et al. Human melanoma cells secrete and respond to placenta growth factor and vascular endothelial growth factor. J Invest Dermatol 2000, 115:1000–7.

169. Simonetti O, Lucarini G, Brancorsini D, et al. Immunohistochemical expression of vascular endothelial growth factor, matrix metalloproteinase 2, and matrix metalloproteinase 9 in cutaneous melanocytic lesions. Cancer 2002, 95:1963–70.

170. Ugurel S, Rappl G, Tilgen W et al. Increased serum concentration of angiogenic factors in malignant melanoma patients correlates with tumor progression and survival. J Clin Oncol 2001, 19:577–83.

171. Vlaykova T, Laurila P, Muhonen T, . Prognostic value of tumour vascularity in metastatic melanoma and association of blood vessel density with vascular endothelial growth factor expression. Melanoma Res 1999, 9:59–68.

172. Gitay-Goren H, Halaban R, Neufeld G. Human melanoma cells but not normal melanocytes express vascular endothelial growth factor receptors. Biochem Biophys Res Commun 1993, 190:702–708.

173. Carson WE, Biber J, Shah N, et al. A phase 2 trial of a recombinant humanized monoclonal anti-vascular endothelial growth factor (VEGF) antibody in patients with malignant melanoma In Proceedings of Am Soc Clin Oncol; Chicago, IL. 2003: (abstr 2873).

174. D'Amato RJ, Loughnan MS, Flynn E, et al.. Thalidomide is an inhibitor of angiogenesis. Proc Natl Acad Sci U S A 1994, 91:4082–5.

175. Kruse FE, Joussen AM, Rohrschneider K, et al. Thalidomide inhibits corneal angiogenesis induced by vascular endothelial growth factor. Graefes Arch Clin Exp Ophthalmol 1998, 236:461–6.

176. Marriott JB, Clarke IA, Dredge K, et al. Thalidomide and its analogues have distinct and opposing effects on TNF-alpha and TNFR2 during co-stimulation of both CD4(+) and CD8(+) T cells. Clin Exp Immunol 2002, 130:75–84.

177. Shannon EJ, Sandoval F. Thalidomide increases the synthesis of IL-2 in cultures of human mononuclear cells stimulated with Concanavalin-A, Staphylococcal enterotoxin A, and purified protein derivative. Immunopharmacology 1995, 31:109–16.

178. Verbon A, Juffermans NP, Speelman P, et al. A single oral dose of thalidomide enhances the capacity of lymphocytes to secrete gamma interferon in healthy humans. Antimicrob Agents Chemother 2000, 44:2286–90.

179. Keifer JA, Guttridge DC, Ashburner BP, et al. Inhibition of NF-kappa B activity by thalidomide through suppression of IkappaB kinase activity. J Biol Chem 2001, 276:22382–7.

180. Cavenagh JD, Oakervee H. Thalidomide in multiple myeloma: current status and future prospects. Br J Haematol 2003, 120:18–26.

181. Dimopoulos MA, Anagnostopoulos A, Weber D. Treatment of plasma cell dyscrasias with thalidomide and its derivatives. J Clin Oncol 2003, 21:4444–54.

182. Glasmacher A, Hahn C, Hoffmann F, et al. A systematic review of phase-II trials of thalidomide monotherapy in patients with relapsed or refractory multiple myeloma. Br J Haematol 2006, 132:584–93.

183. Eisen T, Boshoff C, Mak I, et al. Continuous low dose Thalidomide: a phase II study in advanced melanoma, renal cell, ovarian and breast cancer. Br J Cancer 2000, 82:812–7.

184. Pawlak WZ, Legha SS. Phase II study of thalidomide in patients with metastatic melanoma. Melanoma Res 2004, 14:57–62.

185. Reiriz AB, Richter MF, Fernandes S, et al. Phase II study of thalidomide in patients with metastatic malignant melanoma. Melanoma Res 2004, 14:527–31.

186. Hwu WJ, Lis E, Menell JH, et al. Temozolomide plus thalidomide in patients with brain metastases from melanoma: a phase II study. Cancer 2005, 103:2590–7.

187. Laber DA, Okeke RI, Arce-Lara C, et al. A phase II study of extended dose temozolomide and thalidomide in previously treated patients with metastatic melanoma. J Cancer Res Clin Oncol 2006, 132:611–6.

188. Krown SE, Niedzwiecki D, Hwu WJ, et al. Phase II study of temozolomide and thalidomide in patients with metastatic melanoma in the brain: high rate of thromboembolic events (CALGB 500102). Cancer 2006, 107:1883–90.

189. Raje N, Anderson KC. Thalidomide and immunomodulatory drugs as cancer therapy. Curr Opin Oncol 2002, 14:635–40.

190. Bartlett JB, Michael A, Clarke IA, et al. Phase I study to determine the safety, tolerability and immunostimulatory activity of thalidomide analogue CC-5013 in patients with metastatic malignant melanoma and other advanced cancers. Br J Cancer 2004, 90:955–61.

191. Brooks PC, Montgomery AM, Rosenfeld M, et al. Integrin alpha v beta 3 antagonists promote tumor regression by inducing apoptosis of angiogenic blood vessels. Cell 1994, 79:1157–64.
192. Varner JA, Cheresh DA. Tumor angiogenesis and the role of vascular cell integrin alphabeta3. In Important Adv Oncol. Edited by De Vita VT, Hellman S, Rosenberg SA. Philadelphia, PA: Lippincott-Raven; 1996: 69–87.
193. Varner JA, Cheresh DA. Integrins and cancer. Curr Opin Cell Biol 1996, 8:724–30.
194. Albelda SM, Mette SA, Elder DE, et al. Integrin distribution in malignant melanoma: association of the beta 3 subunit with tumor progression. Cancer Res 1990, 50:6757–64.
195. Natali PG, Hamby CV, Felding-Habermann B, et al. Clinical significance of alpha(v)beta3 integrin and intercellular adhesion molecule-1 expression in cutaneous malignant melanoma lesions. Cancer Res 1997, 57:1554–60.
196. Byzova TV, Goldman CK, Pampori N, et al. A mechanism for modulation of cellular responses to VEGF: activation of the integrins. Mol Cell 2000, 6:851–60.
197. Kim S, Bell K, Mousa SA, Varner JA. Regulation of angiogenesis in vivo by ligation of integrin alpha5beta1 with the central cell-binding domain of fibronectin. Am J Pathol 2000, 156:1345–62.
198. Kim S, Bakre M, Yin H, et al. Inhibition of endothelial cell survival and angiogenesis by protein kinase A. J Clin Invest 2002, 110:933–41.
199. Hersey P, Sosman J, O'Day S, et al. A phase II, randomized, open-label study evaluating the antitumor activity of MEDI-522, a humanized monoclonal antibody directed against the human alpha v beta 3 (avb3) integrin, ± dacarbazine (DTIC) in patients with metastatic melanoma (MM) In Proceedings of Am Soc Clin Oncol; Orlando, FL. 2005: No. 16S, Part I of II (June 11 Supplement), 7507.
200. Kim KB, Diwan AH, Papadopoulos NE,et al. A randomized phase II study of EMD 121974 in patients (pts) with metastatic melanoma (MM). In Proceedings of Am Soc Clin Oncol; Chicago, IL. 2007: No 18S (June 20 Supplement), 8548.
201. Cranmer LD, Bedikian AY, Ribas A, et al. Phase II study of volociximab (M200), an α5β1 anti-integrin antibody in metastatic melanoma. In Proceedings of Am Soc Clin Oncol; Atlanta, GA. 2006: No. 18S (June 20 Supplement), 8011.
202. Nathanson L.Spontaneous regression of malignant melanoma: a review of the literature on incidence, clinical features, and possible mechanisms. Natl Cancer Inst Monogr 1976, 44:67–76.
203. Rosenberg SA, Yang JC, Restifo NP. Cancer immunotherapy: moving beyond current vaccines. Nat Med 2004, 10:909–15.
204. Rivoltini L, Canese P, Huber V, et al. Escape strategies and reasons for failure in the interaction between tumour cells and the immune system: how can we tilt the balance towards immune-mediated cancer control? Expert Opin Biol Ther 2005, 5:463–76.
205. Banchereau J, Steinman RM. Dendritic cells and the control of immunity. Nature 1998, 392:245–52.
206. Korman AJ, Peggs KS, Allison JP. Checkpoint blockade in cancer immunotherapy. Adv Immunol 2006, 90:297–39.
207. Schwartz RH. A cell culture model for T lymphocyte clonal anergy. Science 1990, 248:1349–56.
208. Acuto O, Michel F. CD28-mediated co-stimulation: a quantitative support for TCR signalling. Nat Rev Immunol 2003, 3:939–51.
209. Alegre ML, Frauwirth KA, Thompson CB. T-cell regulation by CD28 and CTLA-4. Nat Rev Immunol 2001, 1:220–8.
210. Melero I, Hervas-Stubbs S, Glennie M, et al. Immunostimulatory monoclonal antibodies for cancer therapy. Nat Rev Cancer 2007, 7:95–106.
211. Collins AV, Brodie DW, Gilbert RJ, et al. The interaction properties of costimulatory molecules revisited. Immunity 2002, 17:201–10.
212. Peggs KS, Quezada SA, Korman AJ, et al. Principles and use of anti-CTLA4 antibody in human cancer immunotherapy. Curr Opin Immunol 2006, 18:206–13.
213. Chambers CA, Sullivan TJ, Allison JP. Lymphoproliferation in CTLA-4-deficient mice is mediated by costimulation-dependent activation of CD4+ T cells. Immunity 1997, 7:885–95.
214. Waterhouse P, Penninger JM, Timms E, et al. Lymphoproliferative disorders with early lethality in mice deficient in Ctla-4. Science 1995, 270:985–8.
215. Sakaguchi S, Sakaguchi N, Asano M, et al. Immunologic self-tolerance maintained by activated T cells expressing IL-2 receptor alpha-chains (CD25). Breakdown of a single mechanism of self-tolerance causes various autoimmune diseases. J Immunol 1995, 155:1151–64.
216. Wang HY, Lee DA, Peng G, et al. Tumor-specific human CD4+ regulatory T cells and their ligands: implications for immunotherapy. Immunity 2004, 20:107–18.
217. Kronenberg M, Rudensky A. Regulation of immunity by self-reactive T cells. Nature 2005, 435:598–604.

218. Sakaguchi S. Naturally arising Foxp3-expressing CD25+CD4+ regulatory T cells in immunological tolerance to self and non-self. Nat Immunol 2005, 6:345–52.

219. Thompson CB, Allison JP. The emerging role of CTLA-4 as an immune attenuator. Immunity 1997, 7:445–50.

220. Leach DR, Krummel MF, Allison JP. Enhancement of antitumor immunity by CTLA-4 blockade. Science 1996, 271:1734–6.

221. Kwon ED, Hurwitz AA, Foster BA, et al. Manipulation of T cell costimulatory and inhibitory signals for immunotherapy of prostate cancer. Proc Natl Acad Sci U S A 1997, 94:8099–103.

222. Sotomayor EM, Borrello I, Tubb E, et al. In vivo blockade of CTLA-4 enhances the priming of responsive T cells but fails to prevent the induction of tumor antigen-specific tolerance. Proc Natl Acad Sci U S A 1999, 96:11476–81.

223. van Elsas A, Hurwitz AA, Allison JP. Combination immunotherapy of B16 melanoma using anti-cytotoxic T lymphocyte-associated antigen 4 (CTLA-4) and granulocyte/macrophage colony-stimulating factor (GM-CSF)-producing vaccines induces rejection of subcutaneous and metastatic tumors accompanied by autoimmune depigmentation. J Exp Med 1999, 190:355–66.

224. Hurwitz AA, Foster BA, Kwon ED, etal. Combination immunotherapy of primary prostate cancer in a transgenic mouse model using CTLA-4 blockade. Cancer Res 2000, 60:2444–8.

225. Sutmuller RP, van Duivenvoorde LM, van Elsas A, et al. Synergism of cytotoxic T lymphocyte-associated antigen 4 blockade and depletion of CD25(+) regulatory T cells in antitumor therapy reveals alternative pathways for suppression of autoreactive cytotoxic T lymphocyte responses. J Exp Med 2001, 194:823–32.

226. Demaria S, Kawashima N, Yang AM, et al. Immune-mediated inhibition of metastases after treatment with local radiation and CTLA-4 blockade in a mouse model of breast cancer. Clin Cancer Res 2005, 11:728–34.

227. Mokyr MB, Kalinichenko T, Gorelik L, et al. Realization of the therapeutic potential of CTLA-4 blockade in low-dose chemotherapy-treated tumor-bearing mice. Cancer Res 1998, 58:5301–4.

228. Davila E, Kennedy R, Celis E. Generation of antitumor immunity by cytotoxic T lymphocyte epitope peptide vaccination, CpG-oligodeoxynucleotide adjuvant, and CTLA-4 blockade. Cancer Res 2003, 63:3281–88.

229. Hodi FS, Mihm MC, Soiffer RJ, et al. Biologic activity of cytotoxic T lymphocyte-associated antigen 4 antibody blockade in previously vaccinated metastatic melanoma and ovarian carcinoma patients. Proc Natl Acad Sci U S A 2003, 100:4712–7.

230. Ribas A, Camacho LH, Lopez-Berestein G, et al. Antitumor activity in melanoma and anti-self responses in a phase I trial with the anti-cytotoxic T lymphocyte-associated antigen 4 monoclonal antibody CP-675,206. J Clin Oncol 2005, 23:8968–77.

231. Attia P, Phan GQ, Maker AV, et al. Autoimmunity correlates with tumor regression in patients with metastatic melanoma treated with anti-cytotoxic T-lymphocyte antigen-4. J Clin Oncol 2005, 23:6043–53.

232. Fischkoff SA, Hersh E, Weber J, et al. Durable responses and long-term progression-free survival observed in a phase II study of MDX-010 alone or in combination with dacarbazine (DTIC) in metastatic melanoma. In Proceedings of Am Soc Clin Oncol; Orlando, FL. 2005: No. 16S, Part I of II (June 11 Supplement), 7525.

233. Maker AV, Phan GQ, Attia P, et al. Tumor regression and autoimmunity in patients treated with cytotoxic T lymphocyte-associated antigen 4 blockade and interleukin 2: a phase I/II study. Ann Surg Oncol 2005, 12:1005–16.

234. Beck KE, Blansfield JA, Tran KQ, et al. Enterocolitis in patients with cancer after antibody blockade of cytotoxic T-lymphocyte-associated antigen 4. J Clin Oncol 2006, 24:2283–9.

235. Phan GQ, Yang JC, Sherry RM, et al. Cancer regression and autoimmunity induced by cytotoxic T lymphocyte-associated antigen 4 blockade in patients with metastatic melanoma. Proc Natl Acad Sci U S A 2003, 100:8372–7.

236. Robinson MR, Chan CC, Yang JC, et al. Cytotoxic T lymphocyte-associated antigen 4 blockade in patients with metastatic melanoma: a new cause of uveitis. J Immunother 2004, 27:478–9.

237. Blansfield JA, Beck KE, Tran K, et al. Cytotoxic T-lymphocyte-associated antigen-4 blockage can induce autoimmune hypophysitis in patients with metastatic melanoma and renal cancer. J Immunother 2005, 28:593–8.

238. Small EJ, Tchekmedyian NS, Rini BI, et al. A pilot trial of CTLA-4 blockade with human anti-CTLA-4 in patients with hormone-refractory prostate cancer. Clin Cancer Res 2007, 13:1810–5.

239. Curtin JA, Busam K, Pinkel D, et al. Somatic activation of KIT in distinct subtypes of melanoma. J Clin Oncol 2006, 24:4340–6.

10 Targeted Therapy in Multiple Myeloma

Yuhong Zhou, MD, Raymond Alexanian, MD, and Michael Wang, MD

CONTENTS

ABSTRACT

Multiple myeloma is a plasma cell malignancy that is incurable with existing conventional and/or high-dose chemotherapy. However, increased understanding of the molecular pathogenesis of myeloma has allowed for the development of novel targeted approaches based on identification of genetic and signaling pathway abnormalities and interaction between multiple myeloma cells and their microenvironment in the development, progression, and drug resistance and bone disease of multiple myeloma. These studies were rapidly translated from the bench to the bedside as clinical applications, including the use of thalidomide and its more potent multiple myeloma immunomodulatory analogues (IMiDs): lenalidomide. the proteasome inhibitor bortezomib. and arsenic trioxide (As_2O_3). Furthermore, numerous agents directed to both multiple myeloma cells and the bone marrow microenvironment, including farnesyltransferase inhibitors, histone deacetylase inhibitors, Bcl-2 antisense oligonucleotide, heat shock protein inhibitors, and inhibitors of vascular endothelial growth factor (VEGF) or its receptor and inhibitors of insulin-like growth factors and their receptor (IGF-1R) have also been identified and are in early clinical trials. Furthermore, genomics, proteomics, and cell signaling studies have provided the rationale for incorporating these novel agents into existing therapies or into a targeted therapy approach in combination. In the future, these approaches will improve outcomes of patients with multiple myeloma, overcome drug resistance, and finally change the natural history of this disease.

Key Words: Multiple myeloma, Molecular pathogenesis, Microenvironment, Targeted therapy

From: *Current Clinical Oncology: Targeted Cancer Therapy*
Edited by: R. Kurzrock and M. Markman © Humana Press, Totowa, NJ

1. INTRODUCTION

Multiple myeloma (MM) is a malignant plasma dyscrasia characterized by excessive numbers of abnormal plasma cells in the bone marrow and overproduction of intact monoclonal immunoglobulins (IgG, IgA, IgD, IgE) or Bence-Jones protein (free light chains) *(1)*. In the United States, the estimated incidence of MM in 2006 is 16,5705, with approximately 11,310 deaths (http://www.leukemia-lymphoma.org/attachments/National/br_1152629053/). Despite the use of conventional or intensive chemotherapy followed by stem cell transplantation, classic cytotoxic agents cannot suppress the inevitable relapses of this tumor, and myeloma remains incurable. Recent advances in the understanding of the mechanisms that mediate MM cell homing, proliferation, survival, drug resistance, and bone disease have facilitated the development of novel targeted approaches. Insight into intracellular signaling pathways as well as interactions in the MM cell–host bone marrow microenvironment through cell adhesion molecules and the secretion of cytokines has identified multiple novel therapeutic targets. Importantly, identification of genetic changes associated with progression of monoclonal gammopathy of unclear significance (MGUS) to MM will provide novel therapeutic targets as well as stratify patients who have diverse risk and prognostic implications. Novel targeted agents, especially those used in combination to improve patient outcome and overcome drug resistance, represent the future of MM therapy. In this chapter, we describe recent data obtained from laboratory research as well as the clinical utility of targeted therapy approaches in multiple myeloma.

2. MOLECULAR PATHOGENESIS OF MULTIPLE MYELOMA

Multiple myeloma is a clonal plasma cell neoplasm of transformed plasmablasts with somatic hypermutation and immunoglobulin H (IgH) switching during B-cell development in the germinal center or transformed terminally differentiated plasma cells in the bone marrow *(2)*. MM can be preceded by several premalignant stages, including monoclonal gammopathy of undetermined significance (MGUS) and smoldering myeloma. The application of extensive molecular, cytogenetic, and chromosomal comparative genomic hybridization (CGH) techniques have identified sequential genetic changes during MGUS progression to MM and those that lead to further progression to plasma cell leukemia (PCL) *(3–6)*. Moreover, it has been demonstrated that most of the gradual changes in gene expression were in the transformation of normal cells to MGUS plasma cells, with only a relatively small list of differentially expressed genes being perturbed in the progression of MGUS to MM *(4)*. These findings improved DNA-based classification by delineating distinct prognostic implications and the ability to provide new therapeutic targets in MM. Attempting to better understand this multistep transformation process, Davies et al. defined the differentially expressed genes in MM by different functional groups, including oncogenes/tumor-suppressor genes, cell-signaling genes, DNA-binding and transcription factor genes, and developmental genes *(4)* (Fig. 1).

Nearly all MGUS and MM patients have numeric and/or structural chromosome abnormalities *(7)*. Two major subtypes of ploidy categories characterize MM: hyperdiploid and nonhyperdiploid. The biologic basis of hyperdiploid MM involves multiple trisomies of chromosomes 3, 5, 7, 9, 11, 15, 19, and 21, whereas nonhyperdiploid MM is associated with primary IgH translocations at the 14q32 locus *(5,8)*. At present, the ploidy categories of myeloma can be detected by karyotype analysis, intracytoplasmic immunoglobulin fluorescence in situ hybridization (cIg-FISH), gene expression profiling, or the proliferation index

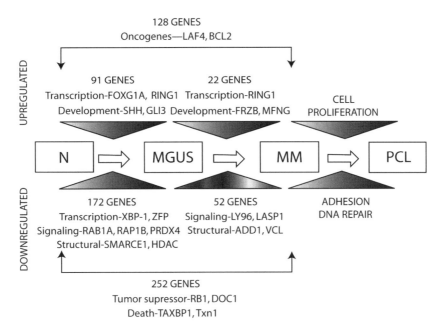

Fig. 1. Multistep pathogenesis with different gene expression in the transition from normal plasma cells to myeloma *(4)*.

(PI) DNA (through flow cytometry). Ploidy level often affects the prognosis in patients with MM: Hyperdiploid MM is associated with a better survival than is nonhyperdiploid MM, despite a similar response to treatment for patients with both types. Survival is negatively affected by IgH translocations, especially those involving unknown chromosomal partners *(8,9)*. Deletion of chromosome 13 is commonly observed in nonhyperdiploid MM and is associated with a higher risk of recurrence and shorter survival *(10–12)*. However, Chng et al. found that the presence of chromosome 13 deletion as determined by FISH did not significantly affect patient survival (median survival 50 vs. 47 months, log-rank $p = 0.47$) *(9)*.

Recently, a novel translocation/cyclin D expression (TC) classification of MM based on early pathogenic DNA expression profiling has been proposed. IgH is usually reciprocally translocated with with recurrent chromosomal loci, including 11q13 (*CCND1*), 4p16 (*FGFR3/WHSC1*), 6p21 (*CCND3*), 16q23 (*c-MAF*), and 20q11 (*MAFB*), resulting in dysregulated expression of these target genes in MM cells *(13)*. There are eight proposed molecular subgroups of MM (11q13, 6p21, 4p16, maf, D1, D1+D2, D2, none) characterized by diverse biologic and clinical correlates *(13)*. Patients who have t(4; 14) (TC4) and t(14; 16) (TC5) translocations have substantially shortened survivals and a poorer prognosis, whereas patients with a t(11; 14) translocation (TC1) appear to have marginally better survival following conventional chemotherapy and better survival following intense therapy *(5,12)*. Although all IgH translocations detected in MM are also seen in MGUS, the prevalence of chromosome partners may differ for MGUS versus MM. The significance of these differences remains to be defined and determined *(14)*. Numerous other genetic abnormalities, including activating mutations of *KRAS* and *NRAS* oncogenes and inactivating mutations or deletion of *p53* and inactivation of *PTEN* tumor suppressor genes (TSGs), are also involved in progression of the disease. Secondary translocations involving other chromosomes (e.g., *c-myc* translocation)

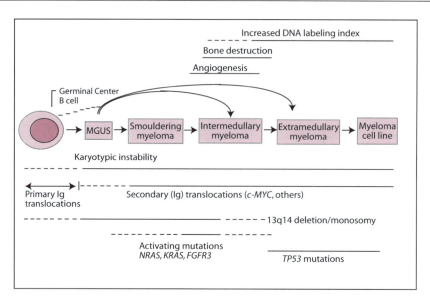

Fig. 2. Molecular pathogenesis of myeloma *(16)*. Developing multiple myeloma (MM) either occurs from a monoclonal gammopathy of unclear significance (MGUS) or arises from a normal germinal center B cell. Oncogenesis occurs in MGUS and throughout the course of MM, such as karyotypic instability, primary and secondary immunoglobulin (Ig) translocations, chromosome deletion, and gene mutation.

usually correlate with advanced stages of the disease and a poorer prognosis *(7,15,16)*. Figure 2 describes the molecular pathogenesis of myeloma in detail *(16)*.

Recently, Carrasco and colleagues used a high-resolution aCGH oligonucleotide methodology to stratify MM into specific subgroups in a nonnegative matrix factorization-based (NMF) classification of the MM genome in which the classic hyperdiploid MM was further subdivided into two subgroups with distinct clinical outcomes. These insights into the pathogenesis and clinical behavior of MM provide an impetus for future cancer-relevant targeted studies *(8)*.

The critical role of cyclin D dysregulation in the pathogenesis of MM suggests that there may be a therapeutic window in targeting this pathway for all molecular subtypes of MM. This seems to be especially true in the case of the t(4;14) chromosomal translocation in which two enzymes are overexpressed: FGFR3 (fibroblast growth factor receptor 3), a tyrosine kinase receptor, and MMSET, which shares sequence homology with histone methyltransferases *(17)*. Preclinical studies have validated FGFR3 as a therapeutic target in t(4;14) MM *(18)*. PKC412 and CHIR-258 are small-molecule RTK inhibitors with antiproliferative and proapoptotic activity in in vitro and in vivo animal models *(19,20)*. A Phase I trial of CHIR-258 has recently been initiated *(21)*. Studies are also underway to validate IgH/MMSET as a target in t(4;14) MM by inhibitors of histone methyltransferases. In myeloma, the genomic aberrations del(13), t(4;14), nonhyperdiploidy, and del(17p) negatively affected event-free and overall survival, whereas t(11;14) and *Myc* translocations did not influence prognosis. Novel agents such as the proteasome inhibitor bortezomib and the thalidomide analogue lenalidomide have demonstrated the ability to overcome high-risk cytogenetic abnormalities, including t(4;14), del(17p), and del(13q14) *(22,23)*. With the advent of oncogenomics, risk stratification factors and tailored therapeutic approaches have been better identified, and studies to pinpoint individual prognostic factors that can predict patient outcome have become especially important areas of investigation. The future will reveal additional intracellular targets and candidate gene products and will allow better designed combination trials that can improve overall survival and evade drug resistance, one of the biggest obstacles in personalized medicine today.

3. ROLE OF THE MYELOMA CELL AND ITS MICROENVIRONMENT

The pathogenesis of MM depends on mutual interactions among MM cells and components of their bone marrow (BM) microenvironment. Among these microenvironment components are extracellular matrix (ECM) protein, BM stromal cells (BMSCs), and osteoblasts/osteoclasts. The interaction between MM cells with ECM protein and BMSCs via adhesion molecules and/or cytokines is crucial in the process of MM cells homing to BM as well as for growth, survival, drug resistance, bone disease, and BM angiogenesis. These components are potential therapeutic targets for MM (Fig. 3) *(24)*.

3.1. Multiple Myeloma Cells and Adhesion Molecules

The significance of functional molecules—e.g., CD20, CD56, CD59, CD138, Ku86, caveolae, insulin-like growth factor (IGF)-1R, CD40—on the MM cell surface and specific molecules such as NFκB, telomerase, p38MAPK, and AKT within MM cells have been

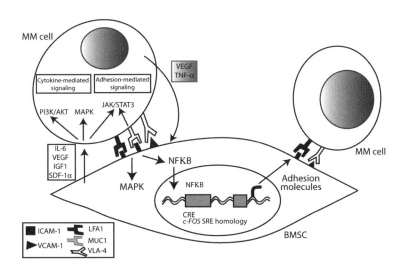

Hideshima T & Anderson KC, Nat Rev Cancer 2002;2:927-37

Fig. 3. Interaction of MM cells and their microenvironment. MM cells are dependent on mutual interactions with cells and extracellular matrix (ECM) protein, bone marrow (BM) stromal cells (BMSCs) for growth and survival. Initially, MM cells home to the bone marrow and adhere to ECM protein and BMSCs. Adhesion of MM cells to the ECM confers cell-adhesion-mediated drun resistance and triggers the production of bone-destroying cytokines.

characterized *(25)*. Adhesion molecules CD44, integrin α_4 β_1(VLA-4) and α_5 β_1 (VLA-5), syndecan-1 (CD138), and MCP-1 are involved in MM cell homing to the BM. Subsequently, MM cells adhere to ECM proteins. An example is fibronectin adhesion by MM cells through integrin, which inhibits Fas-induced apoptosis and protects MM cells from drug-induced DNA damage *(26,27)*; whereas MM cell binding to BMSCs triggers transcription and secretion of cytokines, which allows malignant plasma cells to localize in the BM microenvironment, conferring a growth and survival advantage *(28)*. Adhesion of MM cells to BMSCs localizes MM cells in the marrow microenvironment and triggers interleukin-6 (IL-6) secretion by BMSCs and related MM cell proliferation. The NFκB site is one of the essential regulatory elements for MM cell adhesion-induced IL-6 transcription in BMSCs *(29)*.

Adhesion is itself a dynamic process. CD40 activation of MM cells both augments expression of β_1 and β_2 integrins and induces translocation of new molecules (Ku86) to the cell surface, which augments MM cell binding to both fibronectin and BMSCs, triggering mitogen-activated protein kinase (MAPK) activation and proliferation in MM cells *(30,31)*. Moreover, IL-6 secretion is up-regulated by CD40 activation. Importantly, various studies show that cytokines in the BM microenvironment also affect adhesion. Interactions between adhesion molecules and extracellular protein matrix up-regulate the NFκB pathway, further enhancing adhesion molecule expression, antiapoptotic pathways, and cytokine secretion. Tumor necrosis factor-α (TNF-α) induces NFκB-dependent up-regulation in cell surface expression of adhesion molecules on both MM cells and BMSCs, which results in increased binding and related induction of IL-6 transcription and secretion in BMSCs *(29,32)*. VEGF has been proven to be produced in the bone marrow microenvironment and further induced by MM cell adhesion to BM stromal cells and CD40 activation *(33,34)*. Other important adhesion molecules involved in myeloma bone disease are the integrins $\alpha_v\beta_3$ *(35)* and $\alpha_4\beta_1$ expressed on myeloma cells, and their interaction with specific ECM proteins and the vascular cell adhesion molecule (VCAM-1) present on BMSCs*(36)* increases osteoclastogenesis activity and bone resorption.

3.2. Cytokines

Adhesion of MM cells to BMSCs induces increased transcription and secretion of cytokines, including IL-6, VEGF, IGF-1, TNF-α, SDF-1α, IL-1β, MIP-1α and MIP-1β *(37)*. IL-6, the most important cytokine in MM biology, is produced by MM and stromal cells and is up-regulated in MM cells by CD40 activation and in BMSCs either by adhesion of MM cells or cytokines (TNF-α, VEGF, IL-1β). IL-6 and IL-6 receptors (IL-6/IL-6R) play a major role in the autocrine/paracrine growth regulation of myeloma cells via the MAPK pathway *(38,39)*. IL-6 acts as both a growth and survival factor for myeloma cells. Clinically, serum IL-6 /IL-6Rs are prognostic factors in MM in addition to other systemic manifestations. Modulation of the IL-6/IL-6R cytokine feedback loop thus represents a rational therapeutic approach. Treatment strategies targeting IL-6 include antibodies to IL-6 and IL-6R, as well as IL-6 superantagonists that compete for IL-6R binding. To date, however, only transient responses have been observed *(2)*.

Emerging evidence suggests that VEGF may play an important role in the pathogenesis of myeloma. VEGF promotes angiogenesis, augments IL-6 production, and hampers the antigen-presenting cell (APC) function of dendritic cells *(40,41)*. VEGF triggers phosphorylation of VEGFR-1, resulting in downstream activation of the MEK/MAPK pathway, inducing proliferation of myeloma cells *(40)*. These direct effects of VEGF on MM cells and BM angiogenesis suggest the potential for using novel therapies to target VEGF. Pazopanib, a VEGF receptor inhibitor that targets myeloma and endothelial cells, has already demonstrated promise in preclinical studies, and a Phase I trial is ongoing *(42)*.

Tumor necrosis factor-α is secreted by MM cells and BMSCs. Although TNF-α does not induce growth, survival, or drug resistance in tumor cells, it increases expression of adhesion molecules such as VLA-4, LFA1, VCAM-1, and ICAM-1 and induction of cytokine [IL-6, insulin-like growth factor-1 (IGF-1), VEGF] secretion in BMSCs. TNF-α confers protection against apoptotic stimuli via NFκB activation and up-regulation of antiapoptotic proteins [i.e., Bcl-xL, XIAP, inhibitor of apoptosis protein (IAP)] *(43)*. This mechanism provides the basis for combining TNFα inhibition with NFκB blockade as a therapeutic approach. Novel agents, including thalidomide, bortezomib, and immunomodulatory agents (IMiDs), act against MM, at least in part, by inhibiting sequelae of those induced cytokines *(44)*.

Stromal cell derived factor-1 (SDF-1) and IGF-1 are produced by malignant plasma cells and stromal cells. In vitro studies have demonstrated that the interaction between IGFs and their receptor IGF-1R promotes MM cell growth, survival, migration, and drug resistance via activation of RAS/MAPK and PI3K/AKT pathways. IGF-1 up-regulates intracellular antiapoptotic proteins such as FLIP, survivin, cIAP-2, and XIAP (X-linked mammalian inhibitor of apoptosis) as well as NFκB activation *(45–47)*. These potential targets suggest that inhibiting IGF-1R by a specific monoclonal antibody, antagonistic peptides, or selective IGF-1R kinase inhibitors may suppress MM tumor growth. A12, a fully human anti-IGF-IR antibody has demonstrated modest to significant activity as monotherapy or in combination with other drugs (bortezomib, melphalan) in various MM models or by suppressing IGF-I-induced secretion of VEGF *(48)*. SDF-1 also promotes MM cell growth, survival, protection against apoptosis, and migration by up-regulating VLA-4–mediated MM cell adhesion and secretion of IL-6 and VEGF via activation of ERK, PI3K/AKT, and NFκB signaling cascades *(44)*.

Adhesion of MM cells to BMSCs induces the production of several other cytokines such as transforming growth factor-beta (TGFβ), IL-1β, receptor activator of NFκB ligand (RANKL), parathyroid hormone-related protein (PTHrP), macrophage inflammatory protein 1-α (MIP-1α), and MIP-1β *(49)*. Most patients with MM present with osteoporosis, osteolytic lesions, and/or pathologic fractures. The bone destruction characteristic of MM results from osteoclast activation regulated by many cytokines, such as IL-1β, IL-6, bFGF, IGF-1, TNF-α, MIP-1α, and MIP-1β. However, a central role in abnormal bone resorption is played by the receptor activator of the NFκB (RANK)/RANK-ligand (RANKL)/osteoprotegerin (OPG) axis. When RANKL binds to its functional receptor RANK, osteoclasts are activated. OPG, a soluble decoy receptor secreted by stromal cells, prevents osteoclast activation by competing with RANKL binding to its functional receptor RANK. Binding of MM cells with stromal cells determines a marked imbalance between OPG and RANKL that suppresses OPG levels and favors osteoclastogenesis *(50)*. In vitro and in vivo studies are targeting this system with recombinant OPG or soluble RANK constructs to prevent bone disease *(51)*. Denosumab (AMG 162), a fully human monoclonal antibody that can bind and inhibit human RANKL in a way that mimics the natural bone-protecting actions of OPG, is currently in development *(52)*.

3.3. Signaling Cascades in the Development of Multiple Myeloma

Binding of myeloma cell to bone marrow stromal cells via adhesion molecules induces the secretion of cytokines that mediate myeloma cell proliferation, survival, drug resistance, and migration by activating an array of intracellular signaling pathways. The proliferation signaling cascades are mediated via RAS/MEK/MAPK, whereas survival signaling is via the JAK/STAT3 pathway. Drug resistance signaling is via PI3K/AKT, and migration takes place through phosphokinase-C (PKC)-dependent signaling cascades. Moreover, apoptotic signaling has also been shown to be involved in these signaling cascades *(44)*. Targeted strategies aimed at simultaneously hitting these pathways to prevent myeloma cells from escaping drug effects are being investigated.

In summary, we have now characterized pathways that are dysregulated in the biology of MM. Potential mechanisms for future development of targeted therapies include the mechanisms responsible for inducing G_1 growth arrest and apoptosis; those underlying the inhibition of MM–BMSC adhesion; mechanisms that function to decrease cytokine production and its sequelae in the bone marrow environment; and mechanisms responsible for decreasing angiogenesis and inducing host anti-MM immunity.

4. THERAPIES TARGETING MM CELLS IN THE BONE MARROW MICROENVIRONMENT

In vitro and in vivo animal models have been used in the development of several promising biologically based therapies that can directly or indirectly target MM cells and their BM microenvironment and thereby overcome classic drug resistance. These novel agents, which were rapidly translated from the bench to the bedside, include thalidomide and its more potent IMiD analogues lenalidomide, the proteasome inhibitor bortezomib, and arsenic trioxide (As_2O_3). These agents are being integrated into myeloma management (1) as single agents; (2) in combination for relapsed/refractory MM; (3) as first-line agents for MM induction therapy; (4) with stem cell transplantation; or (5) as maintenance therapy for a posttransplant CR.

4.1. Thalidomide and its IMiD Analogues

4.1.1. MECHANISMS

Thalidomide is an immunomodulatory agent that has been shown to be highly active in the management of MM. It appears to have multiple effects that may account for its activity against myeloma, including the following *(51)*.

- Inhibiting angiogenesis in the milieu, induced by VEGF and bFGF
- Activating apoptotic pathways through caspase-8-mediated cell death
- Inhibiting the cytokine circuit involved in the growth and survival of myeloma cells
- Altering the expression of adhesion molecules located on the surface of tumor cells and bone marrow stromal cells, which trigger the release of cytokines that induce tumor cell growth and drug resistance
- Enhancing the host immune response by stimulating T cells to produce IL-2 and interferon-γ (IFNγ); altering natural killer (NK) cell numbers and function, thus augmenting the activity of NK-dependent cytotoxicity

Lenalidomide (CC-5013, Revlimid) and Actimid (CC-4047) are its two immunomodulatory analogues (IMiDs) that enhance anticancer and immunomodulation properties and minimize the side effects associated with thalidomide. Lenalidomide is more potent than thalidomide for inhibiting the release of cytokines (e.g., IL-6, VEGF, TNF) required for growth and survival of myeloma cells *(53,54)*. Lenalidomide produces no significant constipation, neuropathy, or sedation as does thalidomide; however, myelosuppression is more common.

4.1.2. CLINICAL STUDIES

4.1.2.1. Use of Thalidomide in Patients with Relapsed/Refractory Disease.
Thalidomide, first employed as a single agent in previously treated patients with refractory

MM, had a response rate of 32%, of whom 10% demonstrated a complete or nearly complete response *(55)*. Barlogie et al. reported ≥ 50% reduction of the monoclonal paraprotein in 30%, and a near-CR in 14% of 169 heavily pretreated and MM patients with refractory disease *(56)*. Its efficacy as a single agent was confirmed in other smaller trials *(57–61)*. The addition of dexamethasone to thalidomide (Thal-Dex) increased its response rate, which ranges from 41% to 62% *(62–64)*. Yakoub-Agha et al. compared two doses of thalidomide (100 mg vs. 400 mg) with dexamethasone (40 mg/day given on days 1–4) in relapsed/refractory MM patients with no inferiority of effect from the lower dose of thalidomide. The lower dose of thalidomide was significantly better tolerated, with less high-grade somnolence, less constipation, and less peripheral neuropathy than the higher dose *(65)*.

4.1.2.2. Use of Thalidomide in Previously Untreated Patients. The efficacy of thalidomide as salvage treatment prompted exploring its use in patients with untreated MM. Thalidomide in combination with dexamethasone for first-line myeloma therapy has been highly effective, most recently in randomized Phase III trials (MM-003, E1A00). One study compared thalidomide/dexamethasone (TD) with dexamethasone alone for newly diagnosed MM patients. TD demonstrated a significantly superior response [overall response rate (ORR): 63% vs. 41%, $p = 0.0017$]*(66)* with a statistically significant improvement in time to progression (TTP) of 22.4 vs. 6.5 months ($p < 0.0001$); and the overall survival (OS) with TD was not yet reached versus 32 months with dexamethasone alone *(67)*. However, TD was associated with higher toxicities than dexamethasone alone; deep vein thrombosis (DVT) was 17% vs. 3% ($p < 0.001$), and grade 3 or higher peripheral neuropathy was 7% vs. 4%, respectively *(66)*. A recent recommendation to prevent the occurrence of DVT is to use anticoagulation with warfarin, low-molecular-weight heparin, or a low dose of aspirin; or to minimize DVT by reducing the dose of dexamethasone and avoiding combining erythropoietin or a separation of doxorubicin therapy with thalidomide. A retrospective case–control analysis also demonstrated that TD was more active than VAD (vincristine/doxorubicin/dexamethasone) for induction therapy prior to autologous stem cell transplantation (ASCT) (ORR = 76% vs. 52%; $p = 0.0004$) *(68)*.

4.1.2.3. Other Thalidomide-Based Combination Regimens. Apart from thalidomide/ dexamethasone, a number of thalidomide-based combination regimens have been evaluated as first-line or salvage therapy with demonstrated efficacy in clinical trials. These regimens include BTD (clarithromycin-biaxin/thalidomide/dexamethasone) *(69)*, VTD (bortezomib/thalidomide/dexamethasone) *(70)*, DVd-T (liposomal doxorubicin/vincristine/ dexamethasone/thalidomide) *(71)*, TAD *(72)*, AD-TD (doxorubicin/dexamethasone followed by thalidomide/dexamethasone) *(73)*, CTD (cyclophosphamide/thalidomide/dexamethasone) *(74)*, MPT (melphalan/prednisone/thalidomide) *(75,76)*, ThaDD (thalidomide/pegylated liposomal doxorubicin/dexamethasone) *(77)*, and others. In the IFM 99-06 trial, Facon and colleagues enrolled a cohort of patients between the ages of 65 and 75 years and compared melphalan plus prednisone (MP) to MP/thalidomide and tandem autologous transplantation utilizing two courses of intermediate-dose melphalan (100 mg/m^2) after induction therapy with VAD. The median progression-free survival (PFS) was observed to be 17.1, 27.6, and 19.4 months among patients in the MP, MPT, and melphalan 100 mg/m^2 groups, respectively. This advantage of MPT also translated to a substantial benefit in terms of overall survival, which was 53.6 months versus 32.2 months for MPT and 38.6 months for intermediate melphalan *(75)*.

4.2. Thalidomide Maintenance Therapy

Prednisone, dexamethasone, and IFNα have mainly been used as maintenance therapy for MM patients after achieving remission or stable disease. At present, thalidomide is being considered as a new therapeutic option in several studies investigating maintenance therapy. Thalidomide maintenance after ASCT improved the 4-year event-free survival and overall survival to 50% and 87%, respectively *(78)*.

4.2.1. LENALIDOMIDE (REVLIMID)

4.2.1.1. Relapsed/Refractory Patients. In a Phase I dose-escalation study, lenalidomide as a single agent for relapsed/refractory MM demonstrated activity of 71% in 24 evaluable relapsed MM patients, 11 of whom had received treatment with thalidomide previously. The maximum tolerated dose (MTD) was 25 mg in this population, with no significant somnolence, constipation, or neuropathy. Reversible myelosuppression was identified as the dose-limiting toxicity *(79)*.

A Phase II trial of lenalidomide as salvage monotherapy in MM demonstrated a 25% response rate in relapsed/refractory MM, with the 30 mg daily dosage being better tolerated than 15 mg twice daily *(80)*.

Based on the finding that lenalidomide induced caspase-8-mediated apoptosis, whereas dexamethasone enhanced caspase-9-mediated apoptosis of MM cells in BM in vitro, several Phase I to III clinical trials were initiated and demonstrated the synergistic activity of the lenalidomide/dexamethasone combination. Two similar large-scale, multicenter, double-blinded Phase III trials (MM-009, MM-010) compared dexamethasone with dexamethasone plus lenalidomide in patients with relapsing or resistant myeloma. Patients were randomized to receive dexamethasone 40 mg/day on days 1 to 4, 9 to 12, and 17 to 20 every 28 days with or without lenalidomide 25 mg/day on days 1 to 21. The results showed superior response rates, a longer time to disease progression, and longer survival with lenalidomide/dexamethasone than with dexamethasone alone. However, the combination therapy has been associated with increased risk of thromboembolism and a greater degree of myelosuppression *(81,82)*.

4.2.1.2. Previously Untreated Patients. Lenalidomide has been assessed in a Phase II frontline trial in combination with dexamethasone *(83)*. This regimen has shown remarkable activity—CR + VGPR (complete response + very good partial response) + PR (partial response) of 91%—with durable disease control and encouraging overall survival. A recent multicenter Phase III trial (ECOG EA403) compared lenalidomide combined with high-dose or low-dose dexamethasone in 445 newly diagnosed, untreated MM patients. Lenalidomide combined with high-dose dexamethasone (40 mg on days 1–4, 9–12, and 17–20 with a 28-day cycle) was more toxic and had a higher mortality rate than when it was combined with low-dose dexamethasone (40 mg on days 1, 8, 15, and 22 with a 28-day cycle). Overall survival at 1 year was 96.4% in the low-dose dexamethasone arm, which was significantly higher than 84.6% for the high-dose dexamethasone arm *(84)*. However, the risk of DVT is high with lenalidomide plus dexamethasone, suggesting that all patients should receive some form of anticoagulation prophylaxis.

4.3. Other Lenalidomide-Based Combination Regimens

4.3.1. R-MP

MP currently remains the reference treatment for older patients with MM. In a multicenter Phase I/II study, patients > 65 years with newly diagnosed symptomatic MM received lenalidomide (5–10 mg/day for 21 days), melphalan (0.18–0.25 mg/kg/day) and prednisone (2 mg/kg/day) for 4 days, every 4 to 6 weeks for a maximum of nine cycles *(85)*. Total responses (CR + VGRP + PR) with this regimen totaled 81% (CR 24%, VGPR 24%, PR 33%). More importantly, lenalidomide may overcome the adverse prognostic impact associated with high-risk factors such as a 13q deletion and a t(4; 14) translocation.

4.3.2. REV-VEL

Preclinical studies indicate that lenalidomide may sensitize MM cells to bortezomib via dual apoptotic signaling pathways *(86)*. Apoptosis induced by bortezomib is mediated primarily via caspase-9 and by lenalidomide via caspase-8. A Phase I/II trial demonstrated that most patients who were refractory to either agent alone may respond to the combination. The overall response to the combination of lenalidomide with bortezomib ± dexamethasone was 58% (CR + PR + MR), including a 6% CR. When dexamethasone was given to patients with progressive disease, a PR or Minor response (MR) was achieved by 40% of the patients. The primary adverse events were neutropenia (90%) and thrombocytopenia (85%); the most common nonhematologic toxicities were fatigue (40%) and peripheral neuropathy (30%) *(87)*.

4.3.3. RAD

Another Phase I/II trial is evaluating the safety and efficacy of the combination of lenalidomide, adriamycin, and dexamethasone for relapsed MM patients. Preliminary results suggest that this regimen (lenalidomide 25 mg on days 1–21; adriamycin 9 mg/m^2 on days 1–4; dexamethasone 40 mg on days 1–4 and 17–20; and pegfilgrastim 6 mg every 4 weeks) can be used as a new salvage protocol for patients with relapsed MM, as indicated by an overall response rate of 84%. The toxicity profile is manageable. Neutropenia and infection/fever were the most frequent grade 3 or 4 adverse events *(88)*.

There are many trials of lenalidomide in combination with cytotoxic agents, such as lenalidomide plus pegylated liposomal doxorubicin, vincristine, and dexamethasone (Dvd-R) *(89)*. Other rationally based combination therapies being tested include lenalidomide plus anti-CD40 antibody SGN-40 or an mTOR inhibitor. Lenalidomide is also in an ongoing Phase III trial to evaluate its efficacy in maintenance therapy after ASCT.

4.4. Proteasome Inhibitors and NFκB as a Therapeutic Target: Bortezomib (PS-341, Velcade)

In an orderly fashion, the proteasome, a multienzyme complex found in all eukaryotic cells, degrades more than 80% of ubiquitin-tagged cellular proteins. These proteins control cellular division, growth, function, and death. The ubiquitin–proteasome pathway has been validated as a therapeutic target in myeloma. Bortezomib, a dipeptidyl boronate, is a potent and selective proteasome inhibitor that has been approved by the U.S. Food and Drug Administration (FDA) for MM therapy and has showed excellent results.

4.4.1. MECHANISM OF ACTION OF BORTEZOMIB

One of the potential mechanisms of action for bortezomib involves regulation of the NFκB/IκBα complex. In MM, NFκB is involved in up-regulating IL-6 transcription. TNF-α activates NFκB in BMSCs and MM cells, mediating further IL-6 secretion and expression of adhesion molecules (ICAM-1, VCAM-1) and resulting in increased MM cell–BMSC interaction. NFκB also activates the expression of various antiapoptotic molecules (e.g., Bcl-2, XIAP, survivin) and down-regulates the proapoptotic molecule BAX. In vitro experiments

Bortezomib Targets MM Cells in the BM Microenvironment

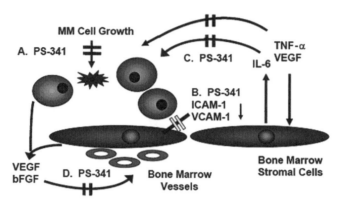

Fig. 4. Mechanisms of bortezomib

show that NFκB activation promotes the growth, survival, and drug resistance of MM cells, making it an important therapeutic target. Normally, NFκB is maintained in the cytosol where, bound to its inhibitor IκBα, it is inactive. Once IκBα is tagged and degraded by the proteasome, NFκB is activated, which turns on a number of prosurvival pathways, including an increased number of angiogenic factors (VEGF, bFGF), increased antiapoptotic proteins, up-regulation of cellular adhesion molecules, and increased autocrine/paracrine IL-6 production and secretion *(90)*.

4.4.1.1. Mechanisms Mediating the Antimyeloma Activity of Bortezomib at the Molecular Level. Analysis of the gene expression profile of bortezomib-treated MM cell lines and patient MM cells showed up-regulation of p53 and MDM2, activation of JNK, activation of caspase-8 and caspase-3, and subsequent cleavage of DNA-PK and ATM, which likely limits the DNA repair mechanism *(91–94)* (Fig. 4). This finding may partially explain the synergy observed when bortezomib is combined with DNA-damaging agents.

4.4.2. Clinical Studies

4.4.2.1. Bortezomib as a Single Agent for Advanced Refractory/Relapsed MM.

Phase II SUMMIT Trial. In a Phase II trial, called S̲tudy of U̲ncontrolled M̲yeloma M̲anagement with Proteasome I̲nhibitor T̲herapy (SUMMIT), patients with relapsed or refractory MM were given bortezomib 1.3 mg/m^2 twice weekly 2 weeks out of every 3 weeks for a maximum of eight cycles. The response rate was 27% as a single agent in a heavily pretreated patient population *(95)*.

Phase II CREST Trial. A second Phase II study of two doses of single-agent bortezomib (C̲linical R̲esponse and E̲fficacy S̲tudy of Bortezomib in the T̲reatment of Refractory Myeloma: CREST) showed response rates of 38% at 1.3 mg/m^2 and 30% at 1.0 mg/m^2 in patients with relapsed or refractory MM *(96)*.

Phase III APEX Trial. In the international, multicenter Phase III trial, called A̲ssessment of P̲roteasome I̲nhibition for E̲xtending R̲emissions (APEX) trial, 669 patients with relapsed

MM despite having received one to three previous therapies were randomized to receive bortezomib 1.3 mg/ m^2 biweekly on a 3-week schedule or high-dose dexamethasone. The results in the bortezomib arm were superior to those in the high-dose dexamethasone arm. The overall response rate was 43% for bortezomib and 18% for dexamethasone ($p < 0.001$); median time to progression was 6.2 months for bortezomib and 3.5 months for dexamethasone ($p < 0.001$); median overall survival was 29.8 months (vs. 23.7 months, $p = 0.0272$). Survival rates at 1 year were 80% for bortezomib and 67% for dexamethasone ($p = 0.003$). Grade 3 adverse events with bortezomib were thrombocytopenia (26%), neutropenia (12%), anemia (9%), peripheral neuropathy (7%), and diarrhea (7%). The grade 4 and serious adverse events as well as treatment discontinuations because of adverse events were similar in the two treatment arms *(97)*. Importantly, the efficacy of bortezomib was maintained in patients ≥ 65 years of age at high risk (β_2-microglobulin level > 2.5 mg/L)*(98)*; and it appears that this agent has the ability to overcome the adverse prognostic impact of a chromosome 13 deletion *(99)*.

4.4.2.2. Bortezomib as a Single Agent in First-Line Therapy. A Phase II trial of bortezomib monotherapy demonstrated efficacy, with an overall response of 40% and a CR of 10%, even in patients with high-risk myeloma *(100,101)*. Important side effects of bortezomib include an increased risk of peripheral neuropathy and reactivation of varicella zoster. Prophylaxis with once-daily valacyclovir is recommended.

4.4.2.3. Bortezomib-Based Combination Regimens in MM. Bortezomib has demonstrated additive anti-MM activity in vitro when combined with other antineoplastic agents such as dexamethasone, doxorubicin, or melphalan, as well as investigational agents such as histone deacetylase inhibitors or lenalidomide *(102–108)*. Many bortezomib-based combination regimens following preclinical production of an in vitro synergistic effect on MM cells are under investigation for the treatment of both previously untreated and relapsed/refractory MM patients. In different trials, the use of bortezomib has resulted in high response rates in newly diagnosed patients when combined with dexamethasone (Vel-Dex), MP (VMP), or MPT (VMPT) and successfully combined with TD (VTD) or AD as an induction regimen prior to autologous stem cell transplantation. A Phase III trial (IFM 2005-01) suggested that bortezomib in combination with dexamethasone (Vel-Dex) demonstrated superiority over VAD in newly diagnosed patients with MM (82% vs. 67%), and the difference is mostly due to a higher CR/nCR (near complete response) rate in the Vel-Dex arm *(107)*. A Phase I/II trial of bortezomib with pegylated liposomal doxorubicin resulted in overall result rate of 72% with a CR/nCR rate of 36% and significantly improved time to progression in relapsed/refractory patients with MM compared to bortezomib alone ($p = 0.02$) *(108)*. Recently, a multicenter Phase I/II study evaluated a four-drug combination regimen composed of bortezomib (Velcade), melphalan, prednisone, and thalidomide (VMPT) in patients with relapsed and/or refractory MM. An ongoing randomized, multicenter Phase III trial is evaluating VMPT in earlier-stage disease *(109)*. However, the best bortezomib combination has not yet been defined. Testing of many bortezomib-based combination regimens is ongoing.

Recent advances in gene array technology, proteomics, and studies of the mechanisms of cell signaling provide the preclinical rationale for combing bortezomib with other novel targeted agents, such as heat shock protein-90 (Hsp90) inhibitor, DNA damaging agents, the AKT inhibitor alkylphospholipid perifosine, and a p38 MAPK inhibitor. Histone deacetylase inhibitors such as tubacin or LBH-589 can block protein degradation via an aggresome autophagy pathway (the aggresome accumulates misfolded proteins destined for degradation by the ubiquitin–proteasome pathway), whereas blockade of the proteasome with bortezomib can up-regulate aggresome activity. Combining these agents will likely enhance tumor cytotoxicity.

4.5. Arsenic Trioxide

Arsenic trioxide (ATO), is a potent drug in the treatment of acute promyelocytic leukemia (APL) and has been shown to induce differentiation and apoptosis of APL cells in vitro and in vivo in animal models (110). Early results with this agent demonstrate promising clinical responses and safety in patients with MM.

4.5.1. MECHANISMS OF ACTION OF ARSENIC TRIOXIDE

Multiple events involved in the pathogenesis of MM coincide with pathways targeted by ATO, although the precise mechanism of ATO-induced apoptosis in MM cells is not yet known. Changes in cellular redox status, as measured by increases in free reactive oxygen species (ROS), are a common feature of ATO-induced cell death in cell lines and patient tissues. Preliminary research showed that activation of caspase-3, caspase-9, and caspase-8. R1 and R2 Apo2/TRAIL (TNF-related apoptosis-inducing ligand), and c-jun-N-terminal kinase (JNK) are critical in ATO-induced apoptosis in MM cell lines. ATO may functionally alter diverse signaling pathways by inhibiting MAPK phosphatases and NFκB activation. ATO may also induce antitumor activity through an immunologic mechanism by increasing lymphokine-activated killers (111–117).

4.5.2. CLINICAL STUDIES INVOLVING ARSENIC TRIOXIDE

Single-agent ATO has shown promising results, with an overall response rate of 21% to 33% in patients with relapsed or refractory MM (118,119), but the median duration of response was short. The generation of ROS, with subsequent accumulation of hydrogen peroxide, augments ATO-induced apoptosis, but glutathione potentially attenuates this effect (120), providing the rationale for augmenting its activity with ascorbic acid and reducing glutathione (121). Two Phase II trials of the combination of ATO, dexamethasone, and ascorbic acid in patients with relapsed or refractory MM yielded overall response rates of 40% and 30%, respectively. The regimen was well tolerated, and most adverse events were mild or moderate. The most common adverse events were hyperglycemia, bacterial infections, peripheral edema, reactivation of herpes zoster, neuropathy, neutropenia, thrombocytopenia, and malaise (122,123). It was recently shown that ATO might increase the sensitivity of MM cells to melphalan or bortezomib (124). Another combination therapy in patients with relapsed or refractory MM is melphalan, ATO, and ascorbic acid (MAC). Objective responses occurred in 31 of 65 (48%) patients, demonstrating a 3% CR, 23% PR, and a 22% median duration of response. Median progression-free survival and overall survival were 7 and 19 months, respectively. Specific grade 3/4 hematologic or cardiac adverse events were rare. Grade 3/4 nonhematologic adverse events included fever/chills (15%), pain (8%) and fatigue (6%). This steroid-free regimen showed efficacy and was well tolerated in the heavily pretreated patient group (125).

Despite relative safety, results with ATO-based regimens are inferior to those of other new agents such as bortezomib and lenalidomide. Ongoing studies include ATO in combination with other chemotherapy and biologic agents such as thalidomide.

5. OTHER TARGETED AGENTS IN EARLY DVELOPMENT

Because the signaling cascades and molecular mechanisms that mediate MM cell homing and adhesion to BM, as well as pathways mediating cytokine-induced growth, survival, and drug resistance in the BM milieu have been defined, more and more therapeutic approaches targeting these molecules and cytokines have been developed. In addition to IMiD analogues of thalidomide, lenalidomide, and the proteasome inhibitor bortezomib have been translated into clinical use and showed remarkable activity in MM (Table 1) with other agents in clinical trials. Efforts to identify new targets in MM are being made. Novel targeted therapies in early development include agents targeting tumor cell surface molecules or receptors, feedback loops mediating MM cell growth and survival, intracellular molecules or signaling pathway components, and the mechanisms of interaction between MM cells and the BM microenvironment (Table 2)

5.1. RAS as a Therapeutic Target and Farnesylation Inhibitors

Several studies indicate that when RAS-dependent signaling pathways in MM cells are activated tumor cell proliferation and viability are promoted. These pathways may be

Table 1
2007 NCCN Guidelines for Myeloma, Revised Based on Novel Active Agents

Primary induction therapy for transplant candidates
    Vincristine/doxorubicin/dexamethasone (VAD)
    Dexamethasone
    Thalidomide/dexamethasone (TD)
    Liposomal doxorubicin/vincristine/dexamethasone (DVD)
    Lenalidomide/doxorubicin (category 2B)
    Bortezomib/dexamethasone (category 2B)
    Bortezomib/doxorubicin/dexamethasone (category 2B)
Primary induction therapy for non-transplant candidates
    Melphalan/prednisone (MP)
    Melphalan/prednisone/thalidomide (MPT) (category 1)
    Melphalan/prednisone/bortezomib (MPB) (category 2B)
    Vincristine/doxorubicin/dexamethasone (VAD)
    Dexamethasone
    Thalidomide/dexamethsone (TD)
    Liposomal doxorubicin/vincristine/dexamethasone (DVD) (category 2B)
Salvage therapy
    Repeat primary induction therapy (if relapse at > 6 months)
    Bortezomib (category 1)
    Thalidomide
    Thalidomide/dexamethasone
    Bortezomib/dexamethasone
    Lenalidomide/dexamethasone
    Lenalidomide (single agent)
    Dexamethasone (single agent)
    Cyclophosphamide-VAD
    High-dose cyclophosphamide
    Dexamethasone/thalidomide/cisplatine/doxorubicin/cyclophosphamide/etoposide
    (DT-PACE)

Table 2
Novel Therapies Targeting Myeloma Cells in the BM Microenvironment

Targeting MM cell surface receptors
    Anti-CD40: SGN-40
    Anti-CD56
    Anti-CD20
    IGF-1R inhibitor
    TNF-related apoptosis-inducing ligand (TRAIL)/Apo2 ligand
Targeting feedback loops mediating MM cells growth and survival
    VEGF receptor tyrosine kinase inhibitor
    FGFR3 inhibitor
    Farnesyl transferase inhibitor
    Histone deacetylase inhibitor
    Heat shock protein-90 inhibitor
    Telomerase inhibitor rapamycin
    Smac mimetics
Targeting MM cells and interaction of MM cells with the BM microenvironment
    Thalidomide and its analog (lenalidomide)
    Proteasome inhibitor (bortezomib)
    Arsenic trioxide (As_2O_3)
    IκB kinase inhibitor (PS-1145)
    Atiprimod
    2-ME2
    bcl-2 antisense oligodeoxynucleotide
Targeting the bone marrow microenvironment
    P38 MAPK inhibitor
    TFGβ receptor inhibitor
Targeting bone destruction pathway
    Recombinant construct of OPG
    Soluble RANK construct

hyperactive due to continual stimulation with IL-6 or constitutively active mutated *ras* genes *(126–128)*. Thus, targeting *ras* processing and *ras*-dependent signaling pathways is feasible.

R115777 (tipifarnib), a nonpeptidomimetic farnesyltransferase inhibitor, has demonstrated an ability to induce significantly dose-dependent growth inhibition and time-dependent apoptosis of myeloma cell lines and bone marrow mononuclear cells from patients with MM *(129,130)*. In the large Phase II trial carried out by Alsina et al., in which tipifarnib was used to treat relapsed myeloma, there were no objective responses, although disease stabilization (defined as a 0%–25% decrease in serum paraprotein concentration) was achieved in 64% of the 43 patients enrolled. The median time to progression was 4 months (range 2–26 months). The treatment was well tolerated, with fatigue being the most common adverse event *(131)*.

5.2. Bcl-2 as a Therapeutic Target

Most malignant plasma cells overexpress Bcl-2, which contributes to resistance against apoptosis. G3139, an antisense oligonucleotide that specifically binds to Bcl-2 mRNA, decreases production of Bcl-2 protein in human myeloma cell lines as well as purified myeloma cells and restores the sensitivity of myeloma cells to dexamethasone and doxorubicin *(132)*. G3139, in combination with thalidomide/dexamethasone *(133)* or VAD *(134)* Bcl-2, treatment was feasible and well tolerated.

5.3. Heat Shock Protein-90 as a Therapeutic Target: KOS-953

Heat shock protein-90 (Hsp90) is one of the major molecular chaperones involved in maintaining appropriate folding and the conformation of many functional cellular proteins in regulation of the cell cycle, growth, survival, apoptosis, and oncogenesis *(135,136)*. The *Hsp90* gene and protein are overexpressed in MM. Recent studies utilizing 17-allylamino-17-demethoxygeldanamycin (17AAG), an inhibitor of Hsp90, demonstrated that 17AAG inhibited cytokine (IGF-1, IL-6, VEGF) production and exhibited antiangiogenic properties by directly suppressing the ability of endothelial cells to respond to these cytokines. Therefore, Hsp90 inhibitors could abrogate BMSC-derived protection of MM cells and sensitize them to other anticancer agents *(137)*. Microarray profiling shows that bortezomib induces Hsp90 gene transcripts in human MM cells, providing the rationale for combining bortezomib with 17AAG. Combining an Hsp90 inhibitor and bortezomib induces synergistic cytotoxicity and overcomes bortezomib resistance in vitro and in vivo. KOS-953, an Hsp90 inhibitor, is being studied in a Phase I clinical trial in combination with bortezomib *(138)*.

5.4. Histone Deacetylase as a Therapeutic Target: SAHA

Histone deacetylases (HDACs) affect cell growth at the transcriptional level by regulating the acetylation status of nucleosomal histones. By primarily targeting the regulation of gene expression, HDAC inhibitors, such as suberoylanilide hydroxamic acid (SAHA), affect MM cells and how they interact with their microenviroment, including down-regulating transcripts for members of the IGF/IGF-1 receptor axis and the IL-6 receptor signaling cascades, as well as suppressing antiapoptotic molecules (e.g., caspase inhibitors), oncogenic kinases, the synthesis of DNA repair enzymes, and transcription factors (e.g., XBP-1, E2F-1) implicated in MM pathophysiology *(139)*. Importantly, SAHA enhances MM cell sensitivity to proteasome inhibition by bortezomib (PS-341) and other proapoptotic agents, including dexamethasone, cytotoxic chemotherapy, thalidomide analogues and Hsp90 inhibitors *(140)*. These findings provide the framework for future clinical applications of SAHA to improve patient outcomes in MM. A Phase II trial of the HDAC inhibitor depsipeptides (FK228) is presently ongoing.

Many other promising targeted agents that have been developed include 2-methoxyestradiol (2ME2) *(141)*, atiprimod *(142,143)*, the MEK inhibitor AZD6244 *(144)*, the VEGF-receptor inhibitor pazopanib *(145)*, and cyclin D1 inhibitor P276-00 *(146)*, a novel and potent proteasome inhibitor NPI-0052 *(147)*.

A sustained proliferation of cancer cells requires telomerase to maintain telomeres that regulate chromosomal stability and cellular mitosis. Telomerase inhibitors are being studied in vitro and in vivo *(148)*. 2ME2, a natural endogenous product of estradiol metabolism, has demonstrated significant activity against myeloma cell lines and primary myeloma cells in vitro and in an animal model *(141)*. 2ME2 also induces apoptosis in MM cells resistant to conventional therapies, including melphalan, doxorubicin, and dexamethasone *(149)*. Atiprimod [N,N'-diethyl-8,8-dipropyl-2-azaspiro(4,5) decane-2-propanamine] is a novel orally bioavailable cationic amphiphilic agent that has been studied for its antiinflammatory and anticancer properties. Reports suggest that the compound exhibits antiproliferative and antiangiogenic activities, induces apoptosis vià activation of caspase-3 and caspase-9, reduces production of IL-6 and VEGF, and inhibits phosphorylation of AKT and

STAT (signal transducers and activators of transcription)-3 in vitro and in an in vivo animal model *(142,143)*. Atiprimod is being tested in an early clinical trial with a favorable side effect profile.

6. CONCLUSION AND FUTURE

Multiple myeloma is not yet a curable disease despite advances in conventional chemotherapy and a wider applicability of high-dose chemotherapy with stem cell transplantation. Biologic studies have provided new treatment paradigms on the basis of identifying genetic abnormalities, modulating growth and survival of nonhyperdiploidy cells in the bone marrow microenvironment, triggering apoptotic signaling cascades, enhancing antimyeloma immunity, and characterizing new myeloma antigens for serotherapy. Given the encouraging results with thalidomide, lenalidome, and bortezomib, additional clinical trials with combinations of agents as well as traditional cytotoxic therapies will continue to be explored. The best combinations and courses of therapy still need to be determined. Future efforts will find novel, more potent targeted agents and move them from the bench to the bedside and back. Importantly, gene array technology, proteomics, and cell signaling studies have aided in understanding the in vivo mechanisms of action and drug resistance and will help select patients most likely to respond to specific therapies, leading to new designs for clinical trials.

REFERENCES

1. Raje N, Hideshima T, Anderson KC. Plasma cell tumors. In: Kufe DW, Pollock RE, Weichselbaum RR, et al (eds) Cancer Medicine 6. Hamilton, Ontario: BC Decker; 2003. p. :2219–44.
2. Hideshima T, Bergsagel PL, Kuehl WM, et al. Advances in biology of multiple myeloma: clinical applications. Blood 2004;104:607–18.
3. Hallek M, Bergsagel PL, Anderson KC. Multiple myeloma: increasing evidence for a multistep transformation process. Blood 1998;91:3–21.
4. Davies FE, Dring AM, Li C, et al. Insights into the multistep transformation of MGUS to myeloma using microarray expression analysis. Blood 2003;102(13):4504–11.
5. Bergsagel PL, Kuehl WM. Molecular pathogenesis and a consequent classification of multiple myeloma. J Clin Oncol 2005;23:6333–8.
6. Carrasco DR, Tonon G, Huang Y, et al. High-resolution genomic profiles define distinct clinico-pathogenetic subgroups of multiple myeloma patients. Cancer Cell 2006;9:313–25.
7. Kuehl WM, Bergsagel PL. Multiple myeloma: evolving genetic events and host interactions. Nat Rev Cancer 2002;2:175–87.
8. Carrasco DR, Tonon G, Huang Y, et al. High-resolution genomic profiles define distinct clinico-pathogenetic subgroups of multiple myeloma patients. Cancer Cell 2006;9:313–25.
9. Chng WJ, Santana-Dávila R, Van Wier SA, et al. Prognostic factors for hyperdiploid-myeloma: effects of chromosome 13 deletions and IgH translocations. Leukemia 2006;20:807–13.
10. Tricot G, Sawyer J, Jagannath S, et al. Poor prognosis in multiple myeloma is associated with partial or complete deletions of chromosome-13 or abnormalities involving 11q and not with other karyotype abnormalities. Exp Hematol 1995;23:867.
11. Fonseca R, Oken MM, Harrington D, et al. Deletions of chromosome 13 in multiple myeloma identified by interphase FISH usually denote large deletions of the q arm or monosomy. Leukemia 2001;15:981–6.
12. Fonseca R, Blood E, Rue M, et al. Clinical and biologic implications of recurrent genomic aberrations in myeloma. Blood 2003;101:4569–75
13. Bergsagel PL, Keuhl WM, Zhan F, et al. Cyclin D dysregulation: an early and unifying pathogenic event in multiple myeloma. Blood 2005;106:296–303.
14. Fonseca R, Barlogie B, Bataille R, et al. Genetics and cytogenetics of multiple myeloma: a workshop report. Cancer Res 2004;64:1546–58
15. Bezieau S. Devilder MC, Avet-Loiseau H, et al. High incidence of N and K-Ras activating mutations in multiple myeloma and primary plasma cell leukemia at diagnosis. Hum Mutat 2001;18:212–24

16. Sirohi B, Powles R. Multiple myeloma. Lancet 2004;363:875–87.
17. Chesi M, Nardini E, Lim RSC. et al. The t(4;14) translocation in myeloma dysregulates both FGFR3 and a novel gene, MMSET, resulting in IgH/MMSET hybrid transcripts. Blood 1998;92:3025–34.
18. Trudel S, Ely SA, Farooqi Y, et al. Inhibition of fibroblast growth factor 3 induces differentiation and apoptosis in t (4;14) myeloma. Blood 2004;103:3521–8.
19. Chen J, Lee BH, Williams IR, et al. FGFR3 as a therapeutic target of the small molecule inhibitor PKC412 in hematopoietic malignancies. Oncogene 2005;24:8259–67.
20. Xin X, Abrams TJ, Hollenbach PW, et al. CHIR-258 is efficacious in a newly developed fibroblast growth factor receptor 3-expressing orthotopic multiple myeloma model in mice. Clin Cancer Res 2006;12(16): 4908–15.
21. Trudel S, Li ZH, Wei E, et al. CHIR-258, a novel, multitargeted tyrosine kinase inhibitor for the potential treatment of t(4;14) multiple myeloma. Blood 2005;105(7):2941–8.
22. Avet-Loiseau H , Attal M, Moreau P, et al. Genetic abnormalities and survival in multiple myeloma: the experience of the Intergroupe Francophone du Myelome. Blood 2007;109(8):3489–95.
23. Jagannath S, Richardson PG, Sonneveld P, et al. Bortezomib appears to overcome poor prognosis conferred by chromosome 13 deletion in phase 2 and 3 trials. J Clin Oncol 2005;24:560s. Abstract 6501.
24. Hideshima T, Anderson KC. Molecular mechanisms of novel therapeutic approaches for multiple myeloma. Nat Rev Cancer 2002;2:927–37.
25. Anderson KC. Targeted thearpy of multiple myeloma based upon tumor-microenvironmental interaction. Exp Hematol 2007;35:155–62.
26. Damiano JS, Cress AE, Hazlehurst LA, et al. Cell adhesion mediated drug resistance (CDM-DR): role of integrins and resistance to apoptosis in human myeloma cell lines. Blood 1999;93:1658–67.
27. Shain KH, Landowski TH, Dalton WS. Adhesion-mediated intracellular redistribution of c-Fas-associated death domain-like IL-1-converting enzyme-like inhibitory protein-long confers resistance to CD95-induced apoptosis in hematopoietic cancer lines. J Immunol 2002;268:2544–53.
28. Hayashi T, Hideshima T, Anderson KC. Novel therapies for multiple myeloma. Br J Haematol 2003; 120:10–7.
29. Chauhan D, Uchiyama H, Akbarali Y, et al. Multiple myeloma cell adhesion-induced interleukin-6 expression in bone marrow stromal cells involves activation of NF-κB. Blood 1996;87:1104–12.
30. Urashima M, Chauhan D, Uchiyama H, et al. Reduction in drug-induced DNA double strand breaks associated with β1 integrin mediated adhesion correlates with drug resistance in U937 cells. Blood 98: 1897–903.
31. Tai YT, Podark, Wang FC, et al. Translocation of Ku86/Ku70 to the multiple myeloma membrane: functional implications. Exp Hematol 2002;30:212–20.
32. Uchiyama H, Barut BA, Mohrbacher AF, et al. Adhesion of human myeloma derived cell lines to bone marrow stromal cells stimulates interleukin-6 secretion. Blood 1993;82:3712–20.
33. Gupta D, Treon SP, Shima Y, et al. Adherence of multiple myeloma cells to bone marrow stromal cells upregulates vascular endothelial growth factor secretion: therapeutic applications. Leukemia 2001;15: 1950–61.
34. Tai YT, Podar K, Gupta D, et al. CD40 activation induces p53-dependent vascular endothelial growth factor secretion in human multiple myeloma cells. Blood 2002;99:1419–27.
35. Carron CP, Myer DM, Engleman VW, et al. Peptidomimetic antagonist of $\alpha_v \beta_3$ inhibit bone resorption by inhibting osteoclast bone resorptive activity, not osteoclast adhesion to bone. J Endocrinol 2000;165:587–98.
36. Michigami T, Shimizu N, Williams PJ, et al. Cell-cell contact between marrow stromal cells and myeloma cells via VCAM-1 and α4β1-integrin enhances production of osteoclast-stimulating activity. Blood 2000;96:1953–60.
37. Chng WJ, Lau LG, Yusof N, et al. Targeted therapy in multiple myeloma. Cancer Control 2005;12(2): 91–104.
38. Ogata A, Chauhan D, Teoh G, et al. Interleukin-6 triggers cell growth via the ras dependent mitogen activated protein kinase (MAPK) cascade. J Immunol 1997;159:2212–21.
39. Ogata A, Chauhan D, Urashima M, et al. Blockade of MAPK signaling in interleukin-6 independent multiple myeloma cells. Clin Cancer Res 1997;3:1017–22.
40. Podar K, Tai YT, Davies FE, et al. Vascular endothelial growth factor triggers signaling cascades mediating multiple myeloma cell growth and migration. Blood 2001;98:428–35.
41. Dankbar B, Padro T, Leo R, et al. Vascular endothelial growth factor and interleukin-6 in paracrine tumor–stromal cell interactions in multiple myeloma. Blood 2000;95:2630–6.
42. Podar K,Tonon G, Sattler M, et al The small-molecule VEGF receptor inhibitor pazopanib (GW786034B) targets both tumor and endothelial cells in multiple myeloma. Proc Natl Acad Sci U S A 2006;103:19478–83.
43. Mitsiades N, Misiades CS, Poulaki V, et al. Biologic sequelae of nuclear factor-kappaB blockade in multiple myeloma: therapeutic applications. Blood 2002;99:4079–86.

44. Podar K , Hideshima T, Chauhan D, et al. Targeting signalling pathways for the treatment of multiple myeloma. Expert Opin Ther Targets 2005;9 (2):359-81.

45. Tu Y, Gardner A, Lichtenstein A, et al. The phosphatidylinositol 3-kinase/AKT kinase pathway in multiple myeloma plasma cells: roles in cytokine-dependent survival and proliferative status. Cancer Res 2000;60:6763–70.

46. Qiang YW, Kopantzev E, Rudikoff S. Insulin-like growth factor 1 signaling in multiple myeloma: downstream elements, functional correlates, and pathway cross-talk. Blood 2002;99:4138–46.

47. Mitsiades C, Mitsiades N, Poulaki V, et al. Activation of NF-κB and upregulation of intracellular anti-apoptotic proteins via IGF-1/Akt signaling in human multiple myeloma cells: the therapeutic implication. Oncogene 2002;21:5673–83.

48. Bruno B, Giaccone L, Rotta M, et al. Novel targeted drugs for the treatment of multiple myeloma: from bench to bedside. Leukemia 2005;19:1729–38.

49. Giuliani N, Bataille R, Mancini C, et al. Myeloma cells induce imbalance in the osteoprote-gerin/osteoprotegerin ligand system in the human bone marrow environment. Blood 2001;98:3527–33.

50. Vanderkerken K, Asosingh K, Croucher P, et al. Multiple myeloma biology: lessons from the 5TMM models. Immunol Rev 2003;194:196–206.

51. Richardson P, Anderson K. Immunomodulatory analogs of thalidomide: an emerging new therapy in myeloma. J Clin Oncol 2004;22(16):3212–4.

52. Body JJ, Facon T, Coleman RE, et al. A study of the biological receptor activator of nuclear factor-kappaB ligand inhibitor, denosumab, in patients with multiple myeloma or bone metastases from breast cancer. Clin Cancer Res 2006;12(4):1221–8.

53. Mitsiades N, Mitsiades CS, Poulaki V, et al. Apoptotic signaling induced by immunomodulatory thalidomide analogs in human multiple myeloma cells: therapeutic implications. Blood 2002; 99:4525–30.

54. Dredge K, Marriott JB, Macdonald DC, et al. Novel thalidomide analogues display anti-angiogenic activity independently of immunomodulatory effects. Br J Cancer 2002;87:1166–72.

55. Singhal S, Mehta J, Desikan R, et al. Antitumor activity of thalidomide in refractory multiple myeloma. N Engl J Med 1999;341:1565–71.

56. Barlogie B, Desikan R, Eddlemon P, et al. Extended survival in advanced and refractory multiple myeloma after single-agent thalidomide: identification of prognostic factors in a phase 2 study of 169 patients. Blood 2001;98(2):492–4.

57. Rajkumar SV, Fonseca R, Dispenzieri A, et al. Thalidomide in the treatment of relapsed multiple myeloma. Mayo Clin Proc 2000;75:897–901.

58. Hus M, Dmoszynska A, Soroka-Wojtaszko M, et al. Thalidomide treatment of resistant or relapsed multiple myeloma patients. Haematologica 2001;86: 404–8.

59. Neben K, Moehler T, Benner A, et al. Dose-dependent effect of thalidomide on overall survival in relapsed multiple myeloma. Clin Cancer Res 2002;8:3377–82.

60. Tosi P, Zamagni E, Cellini C, et al. Salvage therapy with thalidomide in patients with advanced relapsed/refractory multiple myeloma. Haematologica 2002;87:408–14.

61. Mileshkin L, Biagi JJ, Mitchell P, et al. Multicenter phase 2 trial of thalidomide in relapsed/refractory multiple myeloma: adverse prognostic impact of advanced age. Blood 2003;102:69–77.

62. Palumbo A, Giaccone L, Bertola A, et al. Low-dose thalidomide plus dexamethasone is an effective salvage therapy for advanced myeloma. Haematologica 2001;86:399–403.

63. Dimopoulos MA, Zervas K, Kouvatseas G, et al. Thalidomide and dexamethasone combination for refractory multiple myeloma. Ann Oncol 2001;12:991–5.

64. Alexanian R, Weber D, Giralt S, et al. Consolidation therapy of multiple myeloma with thalidomide-dexamethasone after intensive chemotherapy. Ann Oncol 2002;13(7):1116–9.

65. Yakoub-Agha, Doyen C, Hulin C, et al. A multicenter prospective randomized study testing non-inferiority of thalidomide 100 mg/day as compared with 400 mg/day in patients with refractory/relapsed multiple myeloma: results of the final analysis of the IFM 01–02 study. J Clin Oncol 2006;24(18S):187.

66. Rajkumar SV, Blood E, Vesole D, et al. Phase III clinical trial of thalidomide plus dexamethasone compared with dexamethasone alone in newly diagnosed multiple myeloma: a clinical trial coordinated by the Eastern Cooperative Oncology Group. J Clin Oncol 2006;24(3):431–6.

67. Rajkumar SV, Hussein M, Catalano, et al. A randomized, double-blinded, placebo-controlled trial of thalidomide plus dexamethasone versus dexamethasone alone as primary therapy for newly diagnosed multiple myeloma. Blood 2006;108(11):238a.

68. Cavo M, Zamagni E, Tosi P, et al. Superiority of thalidomide and dexamethasone over vincristine-doxorubicin dexamethasone (VAD) as primary therapy in preparation for autologous transplantation for multiple myeloma. Blood 2005;106 (1):35–9.

69. Coleman M, Leonard J, Lyons L, et al. BLT-D (clarithromycin [Biaxin], low-dose thalidomide, and dexamethasone) for the treatment of myeloma and Waldenstrom's macroglobulinemia. Leuk Lymphoma 2002;43(9):1777–82.

70. Wang LM, Weber, DM, Delasalle KB, et al. Rapidly control of previously untreated multiple myeloma with bortezomib-thalidomide-dexamethasone followed by early intensive therapy. Blood 2005;106:231a. Abstract 784.

71. Agrawal NR, Hussein MA, Elson P, et al. Pegylated doxorubicin (D), vincristine (V), reduced frequency dexamethasone (D) and thalidomide (T) (DVdT) in newly diagnosed (Nmm) and relapsed/refractory (Rmm) multiple myeloma patients. Blood 2003;102:237a. Abstract 831.

72. Breitkreutz I, Benner A, Cremer FW, et al. No influence of previous thalidomide administration on peripheral blood stem cell collection in patients with multiple myeloma. Blood 2004;104:307b. Abstract 4902.

73. Hassoun H, Reich L, Klimek VM, et al. Doxorubicin and dexamethasone followed by thalidomide and dexamethasone is an effective well tolerated initial therapy for multiple myeloma. Br J Haematol 2006;132(2):155–61.

74. Suvannasankha A, Fausel C, Juliar BE, et al. Final report of a phase II study of oral cyclophosphamide, thalidomide, and prednisone (CTP) for patients with relapsed or refractory multiple myeloma: a Hoosier Oncology Group trial: HEM01–21. J Clin Oncol 2005;23(16S):6591.

75. Facon T, Mary JY, Hulin C, et al. Major superiority of melphalan–prednisone (MP) + thalidomide (THAL) over MP and autologous stem cell transplantation in the treatment of newly diagnosed elderly patients with multiple myeloma. Blood 2005;106. Abstract 780.

76. Palumbo A, Bringhen S, Caravita T, et al. Oral melphalan and prednisone chemotherapy plus thalidomide compared with melphalan and prednisone alone in elderly patients with multiple myeloma: randomised controlled trial. Lancet 2006;367:825–31.

77. Offidani M, Corvatta L, Piersantelli M, et al. Thalidomide, dexamethasone and pegylated liposomal doxorubicin (ThaDD) for newly diagnosed multiple myeloma patients over 65 years. Blood 2006;108(7):2159–64.

78. Attal M, Harousseau JL, Leyvraz S, Doyen C, et al. Maintenance therapy with thalidomide improves survival in patients with multiple myeloma. Blood 2006;108(10):3289–94.

79. Richardson PG, Schlossman RL, Weller E, et al. Immunomodulatory drug CC-5013 overcomes drug resistance and is well tolerated in patients with relapsed multiple myeloma. Blood 2002;100:3063–7.

80. Richardson PG, Blood E, Mitsiades CS. A randomized phase 2 study of lenalidomide therapy for patients with relapsed or relapsed and refractory multiple myeloma. Blood 2006;108(10):3458–64.

81. Weber D, Chen C, Niesvizky R, et al. A multicenter, randomized, parallel-group, double-blinded, placebo-controlled study of lenalidomide plus dexamethasone versus dexamethasone alone in previously treated subjects with multiple myeloma. Haematologica 2005;90(suppl 1):155. Abstract 738.

82. Dimopoulos MA, Spencer A, Attal M, et al. Study of lenalidomide plus dexamethasone versus dexamethasone alone in relapsed or refractory multiple myeloma (MM): results of a phase 3 study (MM-010). Blood 2005;106(11):6a.

83. Lacy M, Gertz M, Dispenzieri A, et al. Lenalidomide plus dexamethasone (rev/dex) in newly diagnosed myeloma: response to therapy, time to progression, and survival. Blood 2006;108:239a. Abstract 798.

84. Rajkumar SV, Jacobus S, Callander N, et al. A randomized phase III trial of lenalidomide plus high-dose dexamethasone versus lenalidomide plus low-dose dexamethasone in newly diagnosed multiple myeloma (E4A03): a trial coordinated by the Eastern Cooperative Oncology Group. Blood 2006;108(11):239a.

85. Palumbo A, Falco P, Benevolo G, et al. Oral lenalidomide plus melphalan and prednisone (R-MP) for newly diagnosed multiple myeloma. Blood 2006;108:240a.

86. Mitsiades N, Mitsiades CS, Poulaki V, et al. Apoptotic signaling induced by immunomodulatory thalidomide analogs in human multiple myeloma cells: therapeutic implications. Blood 2002;99(12): 4525–30.

87. Richardson PG, Jagannath S, Avigan DE, et al. Lenalidomide plus bortezomib (Rev-Vel) in relapsed and/or refractory multiple myeloma (MM): final results of a multicenter phase I trial. Blood 2006;108;124a. Abstract 405.

88. Knop S Gerecke C, Topp MS, et al. Lenalidomide (Revlimid™), adriamycin and dexamethasone chemotherapy (RAD) is safe and effective in treatment of relapsed multiple myeloma: first results of a German multicenter phase I/II trial. Blood 2006;108(11). Abstract 408.

89. Baz R, Walker R, Karam MA, et al. Lenalidomide and pegylated liposomal doxorubicin-based chemotherapy for relapsed or refractory multiple myeloma: safety and efficacy. Ann Oncol 2006;17(12):1766–71.

90. Hideshima T, Richardson P, Chauhan D, et al. The proteasome inhibitor PS-341 inhibits growth, induces apoptosis, and overcomes drug resistance in human multiple myeloma cells. Cancer Res 2001;61:3071–6.

91. Hideshima T, Mitsiades C, Akiyama M, et al. Molecular mechanisms mediating antimyeloma activity of proteasome inhibitor PS-341. Blood 2003;101:1530–4.

92. Hideshima T, Chauhan D, Richardson P, et al. NF-kappa B as a therapeutic target in multiple myeloma. J Biol Chem. 2002;277:16639–47.
93. Mitsiades N, Mitsiades CS, Poulaki V, et al. Biologic sequelae of NF-κB blockade in multiple myeloma: therapeutic applications. Blood 2002;99:4079–86.
94. Hideshima T, Chauhan D, Schlossman R, et al. The role of tumor necrosis factor alpha in the pathophysiology of human multiple myeloma: therapeutic applications. Oncogene 2001;20:4519–27.
95. Richardson PG, Barlogie B, Berenson J, et al. A phase 2 study of bortezomib in relapsed, refractory myeloma. N Engl J Med 2003;26(348):2609–17.
96. Jagannath S, Barlogie B, Berenson J, et al. A phase 2 study of two doses of bortezomib in relapsed or refractory myeloma. Br J Haematol 2004;127(2):165–72.
97. Richardson PG, Sonneveld P, Schuster MW, et al. Bortezomib or high-dose dexamethasone for relapsed multiple myeloma. N Engl J Med 2005;352(24):2487–98.
98. Richardson PG, Sonneveld P, Schuster MW, et al. Safety and efficacy of bortezomib in high-risk and elderly patients with relapsed myeloma. J Clin Oncol 2005;23(16s):6533.
99. Jagannath S, Richardson PG, Sonneveld P, et al. Bortezomib appears to overcome poor prognosis conferred by chromosome 13 deletion in phase 2 and 3 trials. J Clin Oncol 2005;23(16s):6501.
100. Anderson K, Richardson P, Chanan-Khan A, et al. Single-agent bortezomib in previously untreated multiple myeloma (MM): results of a phase II multicenter study. J Clinl Oncol 2006;24(18S):7504.
101. Dispenzieri A, Zhang L, Fonseca R, et al. Single agent bortezomib is associated with a high response rate in patients with high risk myeloma: a phase II study from the Eastern Cooprative Oncology Group (E2A02). Blood 2006;108(11):1006a.
102. Ma MH, Yang HH, Parker K, et al. The proteasome inhibitor PS-341 markedly enhances sensitivity of multiple myeloma tumor cells to chemotherapeutic agents. Clin Cancer Res 2003;9:1136–44.
103. Mitsiades N, Mitsiades CS, Richardson PG, et al. The proteasome inhibitor PS-341 potentiates sensitivity of multiple myeloma cells to conventional chemotherapeutic agents: therapeutic applications. Blood 2003;101:2377–80.
104. Hideshima T, Bradner JE, Wong J, et al. Small-molecule inhibition of proteasome and aggresome function induces synergistic antitumor activity in multiple myeloma. Proc Natl Acad Sci U S A 2005;102:8567–72.
105. Pei XY, Dai Y, Grant S. Synergistic induction of oxidative injury and apoptosis in human multiple myeloma cells by the proteasome inhibitor bortezomib and histone deacetylase inhibitors. Clin Cancer Res 2004;10:3839–52.
106. Richardson PG, Schlossman RL, Munshi N, et al. Phase I study of the safety and efficacy of bortezomib (Velcade) in combination with CC-5013 (Revlimid) in relapse and refractory multiple myeloma (MM): the revel study. Blood 2005;106:110a. Abstract 365.
107. Harousseau J, Marit G, Caillot D, et al. Velcade/dexamethasone (Vel/Dex) versus VAD in induction treatment prior to autologous stem cell transplantation (ASCT) in newly diagnosed multiple myeloma (MM): an interim analysis of the IFM 2005–01 randomized multicenter phase III trial. Blood 2006;108(11):21a.
108. Orlowski RZ, Zhuang SH, Parekh T, et al. The Doxil-MMY-3001 Study Investigators: the combination of pegylated liposomal doxorubicin and bortezomib significantly improves time to progression of patients with relapsed/refractory multiple myeloma compared with bortezomib alone: results from a planned interim analysis of a randomized phase III study. Blood 2006;108(11):124a.
109. Palumbo A, Ambrosini MT, Benevolo G, et al. Bortezomib, melphalan, prednisone, and thalidomide for relapsed multiple myeloma. Blood 2007;109(7):2767–72.
110. Soignet SL, Maslak P, Wang ZG, et al. Complete remission after treatment of acute promyelocytic leukemia with arsenic trioxide. N Engl J Med 1998;339:1341–8.
111. Cai X, Shen YL, Zhu Q, et al. Arsenic trioxide-induced apoptosis and differentiation are associated respectively with mitochondrial transmembrane potential collapse and retinoic acid signaling pathways in acute promyelocytic leukemia. Leukemia 2000;14:262–70.
112. Grad JM, Bahlis NJ, Reis I, et al. Ascorbic acid enhances arsenic trioxide-induced cytotoxiciy in multiple myeloma. Blood 2001;98:805–13.
113. Liu Q, Hilsenbeck S, Gazitt Y. Arsenic trioxide-induced apoptosis in myeloma cells: p53-dependent G1 or G2/M cell cycle arrest, activation of caspase-8 or caspase-9, and synergy with APO2/TRAIL. Blood 2003;101(10):4078–87.
114. Kajiguchi T, Yamamoto K, Iida S, et al. Sustained activation of c-jun-N-terminal kinase plays a critical role in arsenic trioxide-induced cell apoptosis in multiple myeloma cell lines. Cancer Sci 2006;97(6):540–5.
115. Cavigelli M, Li WW, Lin A, et al. The tumor promoter arsenite stimulates AP-1 activity by inhibiting a JNK phosphatase. EMBO J 1996;15:6269–79.
116. Kapahi P, Takahashi T, Natoli G, et al. Inhibition of NF-kappa B activation by arsenite through reaction with a critical cysteine in the activation loop of Ikappa B kinase. J Biol Chem 2000;275:36062–6.

117. Deaglio S, Canella D, Baj G,et al. Evidence of an immunologic mechanism behind the therapeutical effects of arsenic trioxide (As(2)O(3)) on myeloma cells. Leuk Res 2001;25(3):227–35.

118. Munshi NC, Tricot G, Desikan R. Clinical activity of arsenic trioxide for the treatment of multiple myeloma. Leukemia 2002;16(9):1835–7.

119. Hussein MA, Saleh M, Ravandi F, et al. Phase 2 study of arsenic trioxide in patients with relapsed or refractory multiple myeloma. Br J Haematol 2004;125:470–6.

120. Dai J, Weinberg RS, Waxman S, et al. Malignant cells can be sensitized to undergo growth inhibition and apoptosis by arsenic trioxide through modulation of the glutathione redox system. Blood 1999;93:268–7.

121. Bahlis NJ, McCafferty-Grad J, Jordan-McMurry I, et al. Feasibility and correlates of arsenic trioxide combined with ascorbic acid-mediated depletion of intracellular glutathione for the treatment of relapsed/refractory multiple myeloma. Clin Cancer Res 2002;8:3658–68.

122. Wu KL, Beksac M, van Droogenbroeck J, et al. Phase II multicenter study of arsenic trioxide, ascorbic acid and dexamethasone in patients with relapsed or refractory multiple myeloma. Haematologica 2006;91(12):1722–3.

123. Abou-Jawde RM, Reed J, Kelly M, et al. Efficacy and safety results with the combination therapy of arsenic trioxide, dexamethasone and ascorbic acid (AA) in multiple myeloma patients. Med Oncol 2006;23(2): 263–72.

124. Campbell RA, Chen H, Zhu D, et al. Arsenic trioxide shows synergistic anti-myeloma effects when combined with bortezomib and melphalan in vitro and helps overcome resistance of multiple myeloma cells to these treatments in vivo. Blood 2004;104. Abstract 2467.

125. Berenson JR, Boccia R, Siegel D, et al. Efficacy and safety of melphalan, arsenic trioxide and ascorbic acid combination therapy in patients with relapsed or refractory multiple myeloma: a prospective, multicentre, phase II, single-arm study. Br J Haematol 2006;135(2):174–83.

126. Ogata A, Chauhan D, Urashima M, et al. IL-6 triggers multiple myeloma cell growth via the Ras dependent mitogen activated protein kinase cascade. J Immunol 1997;159:2212–20.

127. Sepp-Lorenzino L, Ma Z, Rands E, et al. A peptidomimetic inhibitor of farnesyl:protein transferase blocks the anchorage-dependent and -independent growth of human tumor cell lines. Cancer Res1995; 55:5302–9.

128. Nagasu T, Yoshimatsu K, Rowell C, et al. Inhibition of human tumor xenograft growth by treatment with the farnesyltransferase inhibitor B956. Cancer Res 1995;55:5310–4.

129. Le Gouill S, Pellat-Deceunynck C, Rapp MJ, et al. Farnesyl transferase inhibitor R115777 induces apoptosis of human myeloma cells. Leukemia 2002;16(9):1664–7.

130. Beaupre DM, Cepero E, Obeng EA, et al. R115777 induces Ras-independent apoptosis of myeloma cells via multiple intrinsic pathways. Mol Cancer Ther 2004;3(2):179–86.

131. Alsina M, Fonseca R, Wilson EF, et al. Farnesyltransferase inhibitor tipifarnib is well tolerated, induces stabilization of disease, and inhibits farnesylation and oncogenic/tumor survival pathways in patients with advanced multiple myeloma. Blood 2004;103:3271–7.

132. Chanan-Khan AA. Bcl-2 antisense therapy in multiple myeloma. Oncology (Williston Park) 2004;18(suppl 10):21–4.

133. Badros AZ, Goloubeva O, Rapoport AP, et al. Phase II study of G3139, a Bcl-2 antisense oligonucleotide, in combination with dexamethasone and thalidomide in relapsed multiple myeloma patients. J Clin Oncol 2005;23(18):4089–99.

134. Van de Donk NWCJ, de Weerdt O, Veth G, et al. G3139, a Bcl-2 antisense oligodeoxynucleotide, induces clinical responses in VAD refractory myeloma. Leukemia 2004;18(6):1078–84.

135. Miyata Y. Molecular chaperone HSP90 as a novel target for cancer chemotherapy. Nippon Yakurigaku Zasshi 2003;121(1):33–42.

136. Solit DB, Rosen N. Hsp90: a novel target for cancer therapy. Curr Top Med Chem 2006;6(11):1205–14.

137. Mitsiades CS, Mitsiades NS, McMullan CJ, et al. Antimyeloma activity of heat shock protein-90 inhibition. Blood 2006;107(3):1092–100.

138. Richardson P, Chanan-Khan AA, Lonial S, et al. A multicenter phase I trial of tanespimycin (KOS-953) + bortezomib (BZ): encouraging activity and manageable toxicity in heavily pre-treated patients with relapsed refractory multiple myeloma (MM). Blood 2006;108(11):124a-5a.

139. Mitsides CS, Mitsides NS, McMullan CJ, et al. Transcriptional signature of histone deacetylase inhibition in multiple myeloma: biological and clinical implications. Proc Natl Acad Sci U S A 2004;101(2):540–5.

140. Mitsiades N, Mitsiades CS, Richardson PG, et al. Molecular sequelae of histone deacetylase inhibition in human malignant B cells. Blood 2003;101:4055–62.

141. Dingli D, Timm M, Russell SJ, et al. Promising preclinical activity of 2-methoxyestradiol in multiple myeloma. Clin Cancer Res 2002;8(12):3948–54.

142. Amit-Vazina M, Shishodia S, Harris D, et al. Atiprimod blocks STAT3 phosphorylation and induces apoptosis in multiple myeloma cells. Br J Cancer 2005;93(1):70–80.

143. Hamasaki M, Hideshima T, Tassone P, et al. Azaspirane (N-N-diethyl-8,8-dipropyl-2-azaspiro [4,5] decane-2-propanamine) inhibits human multiple myeloma cell growth in the bone marrow milieu in vitro and in vivo. Blood 2005;105(11):4470–6.

144. Tai YT, Tonon G, Li XF, et al. The MEK1/2 inhibitor AZD6244 (ARRY-142886) downregulates constitutive and adhesion-induced c-MAF oncogene expression and its downstream targets in human multiple myeloma. Blood 2006;108:988a.

145. Podar k, Tonon G, Sattler M, et al. The small-molecule VEGF receptor inhibitor pazopanib (GW786034b) targets both tumor and endothelial cells in multiple myeloma. Proc Natl Acad Sci U S A 2006;103(51):19478–83.

146. Raje N, Hideshima T, Vallet S, et al. Targeting cyclin D1 in the treatment of multiple myeloma: preclinical validation of a novel specific small molecule cyclin D1 inhibitor, P276-00. Blood 2006;108(11):985a-6a.

147. Chauhan D, Catley L, Li G, et al. A novel orally active proteasome inhibotor induces apoptosis in multiple myeloma cells with mechanisms distinct from bortezomib. Cancer Cell 2005;8(5):407–19.

148. Shammas MA, Reis, RJ, Li C, et al. Telomerase inhibition and cell growth arrest after telomestatin treatment in multiple myeloma. Clin Cancer Res 2004;10:770–6.

149. Chauhan D, Catley L, Hideshima T, et al. 2-Methoxyestradiol overcomes drug resistance in multiple myeloma cells. Blood 2002;100(6):2187–94.

11 Targeted Therapy in Myelodysplastic Syndrome

Alfonso Quintás-Cardama, MD, Hagop Kantarjian, MD, Guillermo Garcia-Manero, MD, and Jorge Cortes, MD

Contents

Abstract

Managing patients with myelodysplastic syndrome (MDS) is a highly challenging endeavor. MDS appears to arise from intrinsic or acquired genetic defects in stem cells that confer a proliferative advantage to the malignant clone over normal stem cells. Recurrent chromosomal abnormalities are present in 40% to 70% of patients at diagnosis and in 95% of patients with treatment-related MDS. Until now, allogeneic stem cell transplantation and occasionally high-dose chemotherapy have been viewed as possibly curative options for patients with MDS disorders, but they are limited by the advanced age of most patients, concomitant co-morbidities, and/or in the case of stem cell transplantation the lack of donors. The escalating unraveling of numerous pathogenetic pathways in MDS has spurred development of novel targeted approaches for the treatment of these complex disorders. The recognition of the importance that epigentic phenomena play in the regulation of gene transcription led to the development of methylation inhibitors and histone deacetylase inhibitors in hematologic malignancies. Currently, these agents constitute the mainstay of therapy for MDS. Several agents with antiangiogenic properties have also been evaluated for the treatment of MDS, and immunotherapeutic approaches are under investigation for patients with MDS. Identifying the genes that are associated with recurrent chromosomal deletions and numerical abnormalities in patients with MDS, including studies and tests for haplo-insufficiency, are important directions to pursue in the future.

Key Words: Myelodysplastic syndrome, Decitabine, DNA methylation, 5-Azacitidine, Lenalidomide, Targeted therapy

From: *Current Clinical Oncology: Targeted Cancer Therapy*
Edited by: R. Kurzrock and M. Markman © Humana Press, Totowa, NJ

1. BACKGROUND

Myelodysplastic syndrome (MDS) is a term commonly used to refer to a heterogeneous group of clonal disorders of the hematopoietic stem cell characterized by excessive apoptosis, maturation abnormalities of hematopoietic precursors manifested as dysplastic changes and ineffective hematopoiesis, and increased propensity to transform into acute myelogenous leukemia (AML). The annual incidence of MDS ranges from 2 to 12 cases per 100,000 people but increases to 35 to 50 cases per 100,000 among persons over 70 years of age *(1)*. It is estimated that more than 10,000 new cases of MDS are diagnosed in the United States each year *(2)*. Unlike other malignant hematologic disorders, the biologic hallmark of the stem cell in MDS is a limited ability for self-renewal and differentiation. Ultimately, in approximately 30% to 40% of patients MDS evolves into AML. Patients with AML evolving from MDS are usually refractory to standard chemotherapy-based therapies, and their prognosis is dismal, particularly those with therapy-related MDS *(3)*.

The survival of patients with MDS is variable, ranging from weeks to years. Accordingly, a number of taxonomic schemes have been designed in an attempt to stratify these syndromes more accurately regarding prognosis. The French, American, and British (FAB) consensus conference devised a classification that encompassed five categories of MDS: refractory anemia; refractory anemia with ringed sideroblasts; refractory anemia with excess blasts; chronic myelomonocytic leukemia; and refractory anemia with excess blasts in transformation (Table 1) *(4)*. Although useful, this classification system has been criticized for setting an arbitrary dividing line between MDS and AML at 30% of marrow blasts, which has proved both biologically inconsistent and clinically confusing, and by failing to incorporate the presence of cytogenetic abnormalities as a major prognostic component in its diagnostic and prognostic algorithm. Extensive evidence indicates that a significant number of patients who have refractory anemia with excess blasts in transformation and AML with MDS-related features share important biologic and clinical features. This prompted the development of a new classification of MDS by the World Health Organization (WHO) (Table 2) *(5)*. In this system, the blast threshold for the diagnosis of AML was reduced from 30% to 20% blasts in the blood or marrow *(5)*.

Still, this threshold can be considered equally arbitrary. In an attempt to incorporate clinical features associated with prognosis in MDS, the International Prognostic Scoring System (IPSS)

Table 1
French-American-British Classification of MDS

MDS type	Frequency(%)	Blasts (%)	Transformation to AML(%)	Other
RA	10–40	< 5	10–20	
RARS	10–20	< 5	10	> 15% RS
RAEB	25–30	5–20	40–50	
CMML	10–20	≤ 20	20	> 10^9 monocytes
RAEB-T	10–30	21–30	50–60	

AML, acute myelogenous leukemia; CMML, chronic myelomonocytic leukemia; MDS, myelodysplastic syndrome; RA, refractory anemia; RAEB, refractory anemia with excess blasts; RAEB-T, refractory anemia with excess blasts in transformation; RARS, refractory anemia with ringed sideroblasts; RS, ringed sideroblasts

Table 2
World Health Organization Classification of MDS

MDS type	Blood findings	BM findings
RA	Anemia, no or rare blasts	Erythroid dysplasia
RARS	Anemia, no blasts	Erythroid dysplasia, $\geq$ 15% ringed sideroblasts
RCMD	Cytopenias (2–3)	Dysplasia in $\geq$ 2 lineages
RCMD-RS	Cytopenias (2–3)	Dysplasia in $\geq$ 2 lineages and $\geq$ 15% ringed sideroblasts
RAEB-1	Cytopenias, < 5% blasts	Unilineage or multilineage dysplasia, 5%–9% blasts
RAEB-2	Cytopenias, 5%–19% blasts	Dysplasia, 10%–19% blasts
MDS-U	Cytopenias (1), rare blasts	Unilineage dysplasia in granulocytes or megakaryocytes
MDS, 5q-	Anemia, < 5% blasts	Normal to increased megakaryocytes with hypolobated nuclei

MDS-U, myelodysplastic syndromes, unclassified; RA, refractory anemia; RAEB, refractory anemia with excess blasts; RARS, refractory anemia with ringed sideroblasts; RCMD, refractory cytopenia with multilineage dysplasia; RCMD-RS, refractory cytopenia with multilineage dysplasia with ringed sideroblasts

was developed. This system identified the presence of specific cytogenetic aberrancies, the percentage of blasts in the bone marrow, and the number of cytopenias as the most important variables in disease outcome (Table 3) (6). Advanced age and male sex also were shown to affect survival adversely but were not incorporated in the final model. Patients were divided into four prognostic groups, with median survival times ranging from more than 5 years for patients with the best prognosis to less than 6 months for those with the worst prognosis (6).

Allogeneic stem-cell transplantation (SCT) has been frequently been thought to impart curative potential to patients with MDS. However, only about 8% of patients with MDS are eligible for allogeneic SCT due to advanced age, concomitant co-morbidities, and/or lack of donors (3). Traditionally, most patients are treated with supportive measures such

Table 3
Survival and Evolution to AML in Patients with MDS According to the International Prognostic Scoring System

Parameter	Survival and AML transformation score value				
Prognostic variable	0	0.5	1.0	1.5	2.0
Marrow blasts (%)	< 5	5–10	–	11–20	21–30
Karyotype[a]	Good	Intermediate	Poor		
Cytopenias[b]	0–1	2–3			
Risk category					
Low			0		
Int-1			0.5–1.0		
Int-2			1.5–2.0		
High			> 2.5		

[a]Good: normal [Y, del(5q), del(20q)]; Poor: complex ($\geq$ 3 abnormalities) or chromosome 7 aberrances; Intermediate: other abnormalities
[b]Neutrophils < 1.8 × 10^9/L; hemoglobin < 10 g/dl; platelets < 100 × 10^9/L Adapted from Greenberg et al (6).

Table 4
Targeted Agents for the Treatment of MDS

Class of targeted agent	Name of compound
Hypomethylating agents	5-Azacitidine (Vidaza)
	Decitabine (Dacogen)
Histone deacetylase inhibitors	Sodium phenylbutirate
	Depsipeptide (FK228)
	Valproic acid
	SAHA (Vorinostat)
	MGCD0103
	MS-275
Angiogenesis inhibitors	
IMIDs	Thalidomide
	Lenalidomide (Revlimid)
Anti-VEGF monoclonal antibodies	Bevacizumab (Avastin)
VEGFR tyrosine kinase inhibitors	SU5416
	SU11248
	PTK787/ZK222584
	AG-013736
Farnesyltransferase inhibitors	Tipifarnib (Zarnestra)
	Lonafarnib (Sarasar)
Tyrosine kinase inhibitors	Imatinib (Gleevec)
FLT3 inhibitors	Lestaurtinib (formerly CEP-701)
	Tandutinib (formerly MLN518/CT53518)
	PKC412
	Sorafenib (formerly BAY43-9006)
Proteasome inhibitors	Bortezomib (Velcade)
Arsenicals	Arsenic trioxide
	SGLU1 (ZIO-101)
Vaccines	PR1 vaccine
	WT1 vaccine

as erythropoietin, chronic transfusions, and chelating agents. AML-like chemotherapy has been used in some studies, resulting in a small percentage of long-term survivors. However, this therapy is associated with significant toxicity and is therefore also offered infrequently to patients with MDS, who are typically older. The unraveling of numerous pathogenetic pathways in MDS has spurred development of novel targeted approaches for the treatment of these complex disorders (Table 4). Single-agent therapy such as epigenetic modulators (i.e., decitabine, 5-azacitidine), tyrosine kinase inhibitors (TKIs), and antiangiogenic molecules) has provided encouraging results, based on which more active and tolerable therapeutic strategies for MDS are being developed.

2. MOLECULAR PATHOGENESIS OF MDS

MDS appears to arise from intrinsic or acquired genetic defects in stem cells that confer a proliferative advantage to the malignant clone over the normal stem cells. Recurrent chromosomal abnormalities are present in 40% to 70% of patients at diagnosis and in 95% of patients with treatment-related MDS (Table 5) (7). The most frequently observed cytogenetic

Table 5
Frequency of Recurrent Cytogenetic Abnormalities in Patients with MDS

	Abnormality	Frequency (%)
De novo MDS	−5/del(5q)	10–20
	+8	10
	−7/del(7q)	5–10
	−Y	10
	17p-	7
	del(20q)	5
	t(11q23)	5–6
	Complex	10–20
CMML	t(5;12)(q33;p12)	< 1
Therapy-related MDS	−5/del(5q) or −7/del(7q)	90
	+8	10
	t(11q23)	3
	Complex	90

CMML, chronic myelomonocytic leukemia

abnormalities observed in de novo MDS include +8, -5/del(5q), and -7/del(7q), which are frequently associated with other abnormalities in a complex kayotype *(7)*. In therapy-related MDS, the most frequently encountered abnormalities are -5/del(5q) as well as -7/del(7q) and complex karyotypes *(7)*. Loss of gene function is therefore frequent in MDS, which can occur through several mechanisms, including chromosomal loss or partial deletions, balanced translocations, point mutations, or by epigenetic transcriptional silencing via methylation of promoter-associated CpG islands and/or posttranslational deacetylation of histones *(8)*. Unlike AML, where many of the chromosomal aberrancies are balanced, in MDS it is more common to observe partial or complete chromosomal losses *(7)*. Commonly, these genomic losses involve tumor suppressor genes *(7)*. However, a few specific balanced translocations have been observed, including those involving 5q-, 17p-, and 3q21q26 *(7,9,10)*. Several molecular aberrations have also been frequently associated with MDS *(11)*. They include mutations in *NRAS*, rearrangements of *EVI1*, balanced translocation of nucleoporin 98 with homeobox D13 (*NUP98-HOXD13*), and hypermethylation of *CDKN2B*, which encodes for cyclin-dependent kinase inhibitor 2B (also known as $p15^{INK4b}$), as well as affected genes in inherited bone marrow failure syndromes *(12)*. Inappropriate activation of the *EVI1* gene located on chromosome 3q26 is a recurring abnormality in approximately 5% of cases of MDS. The *NPM1* gene on chromosome 5q35 is frequently deleted in primary and therapy-related MDS *(12)*.

Recent advances in the understanding of the pathogenesis of MDS have improved both our ability to diagnose and prognosticate patients with MDS and the rationale for developing targeted therapies with the potential for changing the natural history of MDS.

3. TARGETED AGENTS FOR THE TREATMENT OF MDS

3.1. Epigenetic Therapy

DNA methylation is an epigenetic phenomenon that leads to silencing of gene expression. Aberrant DNA methylation of CpG islands is frequent in leukemia. There is evidence implicating methylation of certain genes, such as the $p15^{INK4b}$ promoter and the suppressor of cytokine signaling-1 (*SOCS1*) gene, in the progression from MDS to AML *(13,14)*. Hence, targeting DNA hypermethylation with hypomethylating agents such as 5-azacitidine or decitabine has been suggested as an important strategy in MDS therapy in an attempt to induce reexpression of key tumor suppressor genes that would potentially lead to clinical responses (Table 6). In addition, histone acetylation plays a key role in gene transcription. A wide array of modifications occur at the amino-terminal "tails" of histones, including acetylation, methylation, phosphorylation, and glycosylation among others *(15)*. Acetylation of lysine residues by histone acetyltransferases (HATs) at the N-terminus of histone proteins results in local chromatin expansion, which facilitates the access of RNA polymerase and transcription factors to DNA promoter regions *(16)*. By contrast, histone deacetylases (HDACs) remove acetyl groups, leading to chromatin condensation and transcriptional repression. Because decreasing histone acetylation may also lead to gene silencing, a host of HDAC inhibitors are under development. The close link between histone acetylation and DNA methylation provides the rationale for the clinical development and optimization of combinatorial approaches for patients with MDS and AML.

3.1.1. DNA METHYLTRANSFERASE INHIBITORS

3.1.1.1. 5-Azacitidine. 5-Azacitidine is a pyrimidine analogue DNA methyltransferase inhibitor that induces reexpression of key tumor suppressor genes in MDS (Fig. 1). In a Phase III study, the Cancer and Leukemia Group (CALGB) undertook a randomized controlled trial in 191 patients with MDS to compare the activity of 5-azacitidine given subcutaneously at 75 mg/m^2 daily for 7 days every 28 days (*n* = 99) with best supportive care (*n* = 92) *(17)*. The dose of 5-azacitidine was increased in 33% of patients who demonstrated no benefit by day 57. Responses were observed in 60% of patients receiving 5-azacitidine, including 7% with a complete response (CR), 16% with a partial response (PR), and 37% with hematologic improvement (HI). In contrast, only 5% of patients in the supportive care arm responded (all HI) (*p* < 0.001). Trilineage responses were observed in 23% of patients receiving 5-azacitidine. The median duration of response was 15 months, and the median time to leukemic transformation or death was 21 months for 5-azacitidine-treated patients versus 13 months for those receiving supportive care only (*p* = 0.007). Transformation to AML was documented in 15% of patients receiving 5-azacitidine and in 38% receiving supportive care (*p* = 0.001) *(17)*. Furthermore, the quality of life indicators were superior among patients who received 5-azacitidine. However, there was only a trend for improved survival for those treated with 5-azacitidine (20 vs. 14 months; *p* = 0.10) *(17)*. This was probably due to the crossover design of the study. In fact, a landmark analysis 6 months after eliminating the confounding effect of early crossover to 5-azacitidine showed a median survival of an additional 18 months for 5-azacitidine and 11 months for supportive care (*p* = 0.03). These results led to the approval of 5-azacitidine by the U.S. Food and Drug Administration (FDA) for the treatment of patients with MDS *(18)*.

In a separate study involving patients with MDS who were anemic and/or thrombocytopenic, 5-azacitidine at a dose of 75 mg/m^2 daily was administered for 7 days in 28-day cycles *(19)*. A total of 48 patients were evaluable for response after having received at least one cycle. Of the 46 transfusion-dependent patients, 18 (39%) became transfusion-independent; the median duration of response was 7 months, with 3 patients still transfusion-independent after 2 years *(19)*.

Table 6

Clinical Outcome in Selected Studies of the Hypomethylating Agents 5-Azacitidine and Decitabine

Agent and study	No. of patients	Treatment	Response	OR	Median response duration (months)	Overall survival (months)
5- Azacitidine						
Silverman (17)	99	75 mg/m^2/d s.c. for 7 d every 28 d	CR: 7% PR: 16% HI: 37%	60 (60%)	15	20
Gryn (19)	48	75 mg/m^2/d s.c. for 7 d every 28 d	Transfusion-independence 39%	18 (39%)	7	–
Decitabine						
Wijermans (29)	66	15 mg/m^2 i.v. over 4 h every 8 h × 3 d every 6 weeks	CR: 13% PR: 3% HI: 16%	32 (49%)	8	15
Lubber (30)	115	50 mg/m^2/d c.i. for 3 d or 40 mg/m^2/d c.i. for 3 d or 15 mg/m^2 three times daily for 3 d	MCGR: 31% (60% in low-risk, 20% in intermediate-risk, and 38% in high-risk by IPSS)	19 (17%)	7.5	10.5 (24 for those with MCGR)
Kantarjian (32)	89	15 mg/m^2 i.v. over 3 h every 8 h x 3 d every 6 weeks	CR: 9%, PR: 8%, HI: 13%	27 (30%)	10	14
Kantarjian (33)	95	20 mg/m^2 i.v. × 5 d every 4 weeks or 20 mg/m^2 s.c. × 5 d every 4 weeks or 10 mg/m^2 i.v. × 10 d every 4 weeks	CR: 34% PR: 1% HI: 14% Marrow CR: 24%	69 (73%)	–	19

[a]Response in the study by Lubber refers to achievement of major cytogenetic responses (MCGR)

OR, overall response; d, daily; s.c., subcutaneous; i.v., intravenous; c.i., continuous infusion; CR, complete response; PR, partial response; HI, hematologic improvement

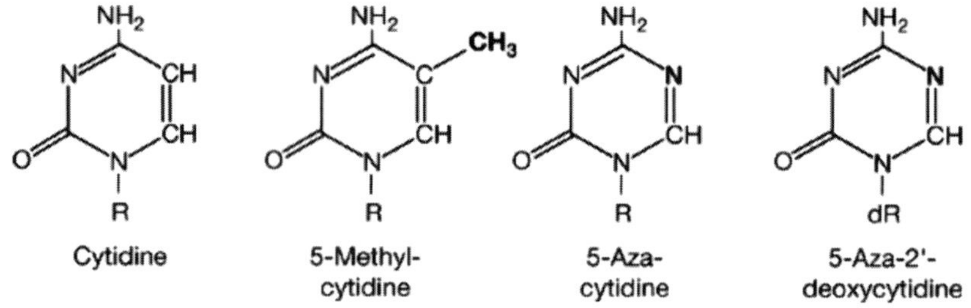

Fig. 1. Structure of cytidine, 5-methylcytidine, and methylation inhibitors azacitidine (5-azacytidine) and decitabine (5-aza-2'-deoxycytidine).

The impact of 5-azacitidine on survival and transformation to AML is currently being investigated in an international randomized Phase III trial of patients with intermediate- and high-risk MDS. Patients in the control arm are treated with supportive care, low-dose cytarabine arabinoside, or induction chemotherapy *(20)*. The Nordic MDS Group is evaluating the activity of 5-azacitidine given as long-term maintenance therapy for patients with high-risk MDS or AML following MDS who achieved a complete response after induction chemotherapy *(20)*.

3.1.1.2. Decitabine (5-Aza-2'-deoxycytidine). Decitabine [4-amino-1-(2-deoxy-β-D-erythro-pentofuranosyl)-1,3,5-triazin-2(1H)] is a deoxycytidine analogue with higher potency as a hypomethylating agent than 5-azacitidine (Fig. 1). Like cytosine arabinoside (ara-C), decitabine undergoes phosphorylation to its mono- (5-aza-dCMP), di- (5-aza-dCDP), and triphosphate (5-aza-dCTP) forms through a first rate-limiting step catalyzed by deoxy-cytidine kinase (dCK) *(21)*. Unlike 5-azacytidine, which is incorporated into both DNA and RNA, decitabine is incorporated only into DNA *(22)*. Decitabine has a bimodal mechanism of action. At high doses, decitabine-induced DNA-DNA methyltransferase (DNMT) adducts result in apoptosis *(23)*. In contrast, at lower doses, substitution of DNA with decitabine leads to covalent trapping of the enzyme, thereby depleting the cells of enzyme activity and resulting in DNA demethylation, activation of silent genes, decondensation of chromatin, and induction of cellular differentiation *(23)*.

Decitabine has been investigated in several Phase I studies of patients with acute leukemia or MDS. A maximum tolerated dose (MTD) was established at between 1500 and 2250 mg/m^2 *(24,25)* Another Phase I/II study included 10 patients with high-risk MDS randomized to receive 45 mg/m^2/day intravenously infused over 4 hours every 3 days and 50 mg/m^2/day via continuous infusion every 3 days. Decitabine therapy resulted in a significant increase in circulating neutrophils, platelets, and hemoglobin with respect to pretreatment values in more than 50% of patients, with 4 patients achieving a complete response that lasted for a median of 11 months (range 10–14 months) *(26)*. In a Phase I study aiming at establishing the lowest effective biologic dose that would optimize its hypomethylating potential, decitabine was administered intravenously over 1 hour to 35 patients with AML, 7 with MDS, 5 with chronic myelogenous leukemia (CML), and 1 with acute lymphoblastic leukemia (ALL). Decitabine doses ranged from 5 to 20 mg/m^2 for 10 to 20 days *(27)*. The overall response was 32%: 22% in AML, 58% in MDS, and 80% in CML. Of interest, response rates dropped at dose levels below or above 15 mg/m^2 daily for 10 days, thus highlighting the clinical impact of the dose and schedule used *(27)*. In some patients, recovery of normal hematopoiesis was observed after multiple cycles of therapy, suggesting a noncytotoxic mode of action.

The most commonly observed toxicity was myelosuppression with minimal extramedullary toxicity.

Several Phase II studies have been reported evaluating various decitabine schedules. A Phase II trial explored decitabine at a dose of 50 mg/m^2 administered as a 72-hour continuous infusion every 3 days once every 6 weeks in 29 patients with high-risk MDS *(28)*. Responses were observed in 54% of patients, with a complete response (CR) rate of 28%. In a subsequent multicenter Phase II trial, 66 patients with MDS received decitabine intravenously at a dose of 15 mg/m^2 over 4 hours every 8 hours daily for 3 days, once every 6 weeks *(29)*. The overall response rate was 49% [CR 20%, partial response (PR) 4%, HI 24%], and the induction mortality was 8%. The actuarial median response duration was 31 weeks *(30)*. Patients who achieved a complete cytogenetic response had a survival advantage over those with persistent aberrant clones (24 vs. 11 months; $p = 0.02$) *(30)*. Decitabine appears to be particularly effective in patients with thrombocytopenia. Follow-up of 162 patients treated with decitabine in three consecutive Phase II studies revealed that 69% of thrombocytopenic patients had a platelet response, 58% after only one cycle of therapy. Interestingly, platelet response strongly predicted overall survival ($p < 0.0001$) *(31)*.

In a multicenter Phase III study, 170 patients were randomized to receive either decitabine 15 mg/m^2 given intravenously over 3 hours every 8 hours for 3 days (at a dose of 135 mg/m^2 per course) and repeated every 6 weeks, or best supportive care *(32)*. Patients who received decitabine attained an overall response rate of 30% (9% CR, 8% PR, 13% HI) that was significantly higher than that achieved by patients receiving supportive care (0%) ($p < 0.001$). Responses were maintained for a median of 10.3 months and were associated with transfusion independence. No significant difference was observed regarding time to AML progression or death between the two arms (12.1 vs. 7.8 months; $p = 0.16$) *(32)*. However, significant differences were observed among patients with IPSS intermediate-2/high-risk disease (12.0 vs. 6.8 months; $p = 0.03$), those with de novo MDS (12.6 vs. 9.4 months; $p = 0.04$), and treatment-naive patients (12.3 vs. 7.3 months; $p = 0.08$). Grade 3 to 4 neutropenia and thrombocytopenia occurred in 87% and 85%, respectively, but these abnormalities decreased with continuation of therapy *(32)*. The results from this study led to the approval of decitabine for the treatment of patients with MDS in the United States.

With the intent of further optimizing the schedule of decitabine, a Phase II study using low-dose (100 mg/m^2 per course) decitabine was conducted at M. D. Anderson Cancer Center *(33)*. Patients were randomized based on a Bayesian adaptive randomization design to receive decitabine at either 20 mg/m^2 intravenously over 1 hour daily for 5 days, 20 mg/m^2 given in two subcutaneous doses daily for 5 days, or 10 mg/m^2 intravenously over 1 hour daily for 10 days. The 5-day intravenous schedule rendered the best responses, and thus 64 (67%) of 95 patients were enrolled in that arm. Therapy was administered every 4 weeks regardless of peripheral blood counts so long as patients demonstrated acceptable tolerance. The median number of cycles administered was six (range 1–18). Overall, 32 patients (34%) achieved a CR, and 69 (73%) had an objective response by the modified International Working Group criteria *(33)*. The 5-day intravenous schedule, which had the highest dose intensity, was selected as optimal; the CR rate in that arm was 39%, compared with 21% in the 5-day subcutaneous arm and 24% in the 10-day intravenous arm ($p < 0.05$). Hospitalization secondary to myelosuppression-related symptoms was required in 18% of cycles. The high-dose-intensity arm was also superior at inducing hypomethylation at day 5 and at activating *p15* expression at days 12 or 28 after therapy.

3.1.2. Histone Deacetylase Inhibitors

HDACs are typically divided into three families: class I, which includes the human HDACs 1, 2, 3, and 8; class II, which includes the human HDACs 5, 6, 7, 9, and 10; and class IV, defined by the recently identified human HDAC 11 *(34)*. Inhibition of HDACs can reverse aberrant epigenetic gene silencing and induce morphologic changes characteristic of apoptosis in cancer cells. Recognition of the importance that posttranslational modifications of histones play in gene transcription led to the development of HDAC inhibitors for hematologic malignancies. HDAC inhibitors are divided into various structural classes, including hydroxamates, cyclic peptides, aliphatic acids, benzamides, and electrophilic ketones (Fig. 2).

3.1.2.1. Phenylbutyrate. The first compound with HDAC inhibitory activity to be used in myeloid malignancies was the fatty acid phenylbutyrate *(35)*. Upon demonstration of the in vitro activity of the butyrate analogue sodium phenylbutyrate in growth arrest and differentiation of primary AML samples, a Phase I trial in which phenylbutyrate was administered as a 7-day continuous infusion was conducted in patients with MDS ($n = 11$) and AML ($n = 16$) *(36)*. The MTD was 375 mg/kg/day, and the dose-limiting toxicity (DLT) was encephalopathy. Although responses consisted of HI in four patients, this experience paved the way for the clinical development of more sophisticated HDAC inhibitors.

3.1.2.2. Depsipeptide (FK228). Depsipeptide is a potent inhibitor of class I HDAC enzymes. Depsipeptide was first investigated in a Phase I trial in patients with AML *(37)*. Nine patients received a dose of 13 mg/m^2 infused on days 1, 8, and 15 every 28 days. The median acetylation of histones H3 and H4 after 4 hours of treatment was 40% and 100%, respectively. A similar study failed to show any response in 10 patients with AML *(38)*. The development of progressive fatigue and nausea precluded repeated treatment.

3.1.2.3. Valproic Acid. Valprioc acid (VPA) is a short-chain fatty acid traditionally used as an oral anticonvulsant. However, VPA can induce differentiation of transformed hematopoietic progenitor cells and leukemic blasts from bone marrow and peripheral blood of patients with AML *(39)*. Recently, VPA has been shown to inhibit HDAC activity and to synergize with all-*trans* retinoic acid (ATRA) in the differentiation induction of AML

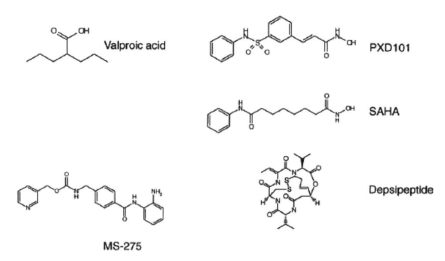

Fig. 2. Chemical structure of representative compounds from the major classes of histone deacetylases (HDACs). Small fatty acids (valproic acid), hydroxamic derivatives (PXD101, SAHA), nonhydroxamate small-molecule inhibitors (MS-275), and cyclic peptides (depsipeptide).

blasts in vitro. In a Phase I study, VPA monotherapy resulted in responses in 8 (44%) of 18 patients with high-risk MDS and AML secondary to MDS, including 1 PR and 7 HI *(40)*. In a recent Phase II trial, 20 elderly, poor-risk patients with relapsed or refractory AML or MDS received sequential VPA and ATRA therapy *(41)*. VPA was started at 10 mg/kg daily and escalated to achieve a serum concentration of 45 to 100 µg/ml. ATRA was then added at 45 mg/m^2 daily. Hematologic improvement was observed in 6 of 11 evaluable patients, although no significant blast count reduction was observed. The median duration of response was 189 days (range 63–550 days). Treatment with ATRA did not modify the response observed with VPA alone *(41)*.

3.1.2.4. Suberoylanilide Hydroxamic Acid. The potent HDAC inhibitor suberoylanilide hydroxamic acid (SAHA) contains the hydroxamic acid moiety that binds to the zinc-containing pocket in the catalytic site of class I and II HDAC enzymes and causes their reversible inhibition *(42)*. SAHA can be administered through oral and intravenous routes. The oral formulation of SAHA is rapidly absorbed by the gastrointestinal tract and excreted via the urinary and biliary systems. Peak acetylation is induced 4 to 8 hours after administration. Initial Phase I studies of SAHA in patients with lymphoma and solid tumors showed that the prolonged use of this drug is limited by the development of anorexia, vomiting, diarrhea, and dehydration, which were reversible upon drug discontinuation and typically occurred after 2 weeks of therapy *(43)*. In a Phase I study exclusively involving patients with relapsed or refractory MDS or leukemia, SAHA was administered at two dose schedules: orally 3 times daily for 14 days every 21 days or orally twice daily for 14 days every 21 days. A total of 41 patients were treated: 31 with AML, 4 with chronic lymphocytic leukemia, 3 with MDS, 2 with ALL, and 1 with CML *(44)*. The starting dose was 100 mg daily and was increased in 50-mg steps. The MTD was determined at either 200 mg three times daily or 200 mg twice daily for 14 days every 21 days. The disease-limiting toxicities (DLTs) were nausea, vomiting, and diarrhea. Overall, 9 (21%) patients (all with AML) obtained an objective response: 1 CR, 2 CRp (CR with incomplete platelet recovery), 1 PR, and 5 marrow responses (blasts < 5%). Histone acetylation was observed in all patients at all dose levels tested. On the basis of these data, the activity of SAHA is being explored further in combination with hypomethylating agents or chemotherapy for patients with MDS and AML.

3.1.2.5. MGCD0103. MGCD0103 is a novel, orally bioavailable sulfonamide anilide derivative isotype-specific HDAC inhibitor. MGCD0103 is a nonhydroxamate compound that targets HDAC isoforms 1, 2, 3, and 11 in vivo. In a recent Phase I, open-label, dose escalation study, MGCD0103 was administered three times weekly to patients with relapsed/refractory leukemia or MDS and to older patients with untreated AML or MDS *(45)*. A total of 20 patients were enrolled at four dose levels: 20, 40, 60, and 80 mg/m^2. The MTD was reached at 80 mg/m^2, with three of four patients developing grade 3 toxicity, mainly fatigue, nausea, vomiting, and diarrhea. Dose-dependent HDAC inhibition occurred in all patients. Two patients with multiple relapsed/refractory AML and one with MDS achieved a complete marrow response. The maximal HDAC inhibition was observed at the time of best response *(45)*. Studies are ongoing exploring the combination of MGCD0103 with hypomethylating agents.

3.1.2.6. Other HDAC Inhibitors. Several other potent HDAC inhibitors are currently under clinical investigation. One such agent, LBH589, has been assessed in a Phase I study involving 15 patients: 13 with AML, 1 with MDS, 1 with ALL *(46)*. Patients received LBH589 intravenously as a 30-minute infusion on days 1 to 7 of a 21-day cycle. In 8 of 11 patients with peripheral blasts, transient reductions occurred with a rebound following the 7-day treatment period. Other hydroxamic acid derivatives, such as LAQ824 and PXD101, are currently being explored in clinical studies *(47,48)*. MS-275 is a benzamide HDAC inhibitor that has been recently tested in a Phase I trial through oral administration to 39 adults with advanced acute leukemias. Although no responses were observed, MS-275 induced histone H3/H4 acetylation, p21 expression, and caspase-3 activation in bone marrow mononuclear cells *(49)*.

3.1.3. COMBINED EPIGENETIC STRATEGIES

Several combined approaches involving hypomethylating agents, HDAC inhibitors, and/or conventional chemotherapeutic agents have been investigated in an attempt to improve response rates. The rationale for the combination of hypomethylating agents and HDAC inhibitors is based on the fact that silencing of genes associated with methylated promoters is due, at least in part, to the recruitment of HDAC enzymes, thus leading to removal of acetyl groups from specific lysine residues in the tails of histones in nucleosomes associated with the methylated promoter. Because HDAC inhibitors per se cannot reactivate the expression of hypermethylated genes, sequential exposure to hypomethylating agents followed by HDAC inhibitors results in additive or synergistic reactivation of gene expression.

This concept has been explored in a Phase I trial evaluating various dosing regimens of 5-azacitidine followed by a 7-day infusion of phenylbutyrate (375 mg/kg/day by intravenous continuous infusion) in patients with MDS and AML *(50)*. Of 29 evaluable patients, 11 responded, including 4 with CRs and 1 with a PR; this correlated with reversed methylation of *p15* or *CDH-1* promoter genes *(50)*.

In a similar approach, Garcia-Manero et al. administered a fixed dose of decitabine (15 mg/m^2 daily) for 10 days along with escalating doses of VPA orally for 10 days to 54 patients with advanced leukemia *(51)*. A 50 mg/kg daily dose of VPA was found to be safe. Twelve (22%) patients responded, including 10 (19%) with a CR and 2 (3%) with a CRp, for a median of 7.2 months. Transient *p15* hypomethylation and global histone H3 and H4 acetylation were induced.

A Phase I study combining subcutaneous 5-azacitidine for 10 days in combination with the HDAC inhibitor MS-275 given on days 3 and 10 of a 28-day cycle was recently conducted in 31 patients with MDS and AML *(52)*. Of 27 evaluable patients, 12 (44%) responded, including 2 with CRs and 4 with PRs. H4 acetylation increased in 28 (96%) of 29 patients. The contribution of MS-275 to these responses is under examination in an ongoing study randomizing patients to 5-azacitidine and MS-275 versus 5-azacitidine alone *(52)*.

The recent demonstration of the additive activity of the combination of idarubicin with the HDAC inhibitors SAHA and VPA on the leukemia cell lines MOLT4 and HL60 has provided the rationale for clinical development of this combination for patients with MDS and AML *(53)*.

3.2. Antiangiogenesis Inhibitors

Deregulation of angiogenesis plays an important role in hematologic malignancies. Bone marrow microvascular density as well as production of several angiogenic factors such as vascular endothelial growth factor (VEGF) has been shown to be substantially increased in both MDS and AML *(54,55)*. VEGF is a potent angiogenic peptide that regulates hematopoietic stem cell development and inflammatory cytokine generation. VEGF contributes to leukemia progenitor self-renewal and inflammatory cytokine elaboration in

MDS *(56)*. Although elevated levels of VEGF have been linked to a worse prognosis in patients with AML, this association has not been confirmed in MDS *(57)*. Other cytokines such as basic fibroblast growth factor (bFGF), angiogenin, angiopoietin-1, platelet-derived growth factor (PDGF), hepatocyte growth factor (HGF), tumor necrosis factor-α (TNFα), and transforming growth factor-α (TGFα) have been shown to modulate angiogenesis in MDS in an autocrine fashion *(55)*. On these grounds, several agents with antiangiogenic properties have been evaluated for the treatment of MDS.

3.2.1. THALIDOMIDE

Thalidomide has been shown to inhibit bFGF- and VEGF-induced angiogenesis and is endowed with potent immunomodulatory activity, which leads to increased production of interleukin (IL)-2, interferon-γ (IFNγ), IL-5, and IL-10 by polarized Th1- and Th2-type CD4+ T cells and down-regulation of TNFα, IL-1β, IL-12, and IL-6 production *(58)*. These properties led to the hypothesis that thalidomide could have potential clinical benefit in MDS, which resulted in the initiation of several clinical trials of thalidomide in MDS *(59–63)* (Table 7).

In a Phase II study, 83 patients with MDS received thalidomide orally at doses between 100 and 400 mg daily *(59)*. By intention-to-treat analysis, 16 (19%) of 83 patients responded, but the response rate increased to as high as 31% when only evaluable patients (those who finished at least 12 weeks of therapy) were analyzed. In addition, 10 previously transfusion-dependent patients became transfusion-independent *(59)*. Similar results were observed in a multicenter trial of 72 patients with MDS in which thalidomide was administered at an initial dose of 200 mg daily and was escalated by 50 mg/week to a target dose of 1000 mg daily *(62)*. Combinations of thalidomide with either erythropoietin *(64)* or topotecan *(65)* have not significantly improved the response rates observed with single-agent thalidomide (Table 7). Overall, clinical trials of thalidomide in MDS have shown discrete response rates and poor tolerability.

3.2.2. LENALIDOMIDE

Lenalidomide (CC-5013) is a second-generation immunomodulatory drug (IMiD) with pleiotropic cytokine activity. Like other IMiDs, lenalidomide inhibits TNFα, having 10,000-fold increased potency compared with its parent compound thalidomide *(66)* and shows increased antiangiogenic activity in vivo *(67)*. In addition, lenalidomide potentiates signaling through the erythropoietin receptor. Lenalidomide exhibits a less severe toxicity profile than that of thalidomide, with significantly less neuropathy, sedation, and gastrointestinal side effects *(68)*. In addition, lenalidomide has no known teratogenicity. Interstitial 5q deletions are the most frequent chromosomal abnormalities in MDS and can be detected in 10% to 15% of patients as either the sole karyotypic abnormality or in association with other chromosomal abnormalities *(69)*. The 5q- syndrome is a distinct subtype of MDS, classically defined by the presence of an isolated interstitial deletion of chromosome 5q31, female predominance, less than 5% marrow blasts, refractory anemia with erythroblastopenia, mild leukopenia, and normal or high platelet counts *(70)*. Notably, lenalidomide inhibits the proliferation of chromosome 5-deleted hematopoietic tumor cell lines in vitro, whether from B-cell, T-cell, or myeloid lineage *(71)*. There is now evidence that the clinical course of patients with the 5q- syndrome may be modified with lenalidomide therapy.

In the landmark Phase I trial of lenalidomide in MDS, List et al. treated 43 patients who were either transfusion-dependent or had symptomatic anemia. Three oral dosing schedules

Table 7
Selected Studies of Thalidomide in Patients with MDS

Study design	No. of patients	Treatment	Response	Dropout rate (%)	Study
Phase II, thalidomide single-agent	83	100–400 mg daily in escalating doses	16 (19%) had HI, including 10 who became transfusion-independent	38	Raza (59)
Thalidomide single-agent	34	100–500 mg daily	19 (54%), including 4 transfusion independent, 9 PR, and 6 with minor response	15	Strupp (60)
Multicenter trial, thalidomide single-agent	72	Initial dose 200 mg daily, escalated by 50 mg weekly up to 1000 mg daily	6 (19%) patients responded, including 5 HI and 1 PR	54	Moreno-Aspitia (62)
Phase II, dose-escalating single-agent thalidomide	47	Initial dose 200 mg daily, escalated by 200 mg every 4 weeks	33 (59%) patients had HI	56	Bouscary (63)
Pilot study, thalidomide and rh-EPO	30	Thalidomide 200 mg daily and rh-EPO 40,000/U s.c. once-weekly for 12 weeks	7 (23%) patients had HI (erythroid responses)	10	Musto (64)
Phase II, thalidomide and topotecan	45	Thalidomide (100–300 mg daily) + topotecan 1.25 mg/m on days 1–5 of 21-day cycles	9 (24%) of 38 evaluable patients had HI	16	Raza (65)

HI. hematologic improvement; PR. partial response; rh-EPO. recombinant human erythropoietin

were sequentially evaluated: 25 mg daily, 10 mg daily, and 10 mg daily for 21 days of every 28-day cycle. Neutropenia and thrombocytopenia were the most frequent side effects, occurring in 65% and 74% of patients, respectively, necessitating treatment interruption or dose reduction in 25 (58%) patients. After 16 weeks of therapy, 24 (56%) patients achieved a response: 20 had sustained transfusion independence, 1 had an increase in the hemoglobin level of more than 2 g/dL, and 3 had more than a 50% reduction in the need for transfusions. Responses were significantly more frequent among patients with clonal interstitial deletion of chromosome 5q31.1 (83%), whether present as the sole chromosomal abnormality or associated with other abnormalities, compared to those with a normal karyotype (57%) or with other karyotypic abnormalities (12%) ($p = 0.007$). Interestingly, 10 (50%) of 20 patients with cytogenetic abnormalities had a complete cytogenetic response. After a median follow-up of 81 weeks, the median duration of transfusion independence had not been reached, and the median hemoglobin level was 13.2 g/dL (range 11.5–15.8 g/dL) *(72)*.

These impressive results prompted a subsequent multicenter Phase II trial of lenalidomide in patients with MDS carrying the 5q- aberration *(73)*. The study included 148 transfusion-dependent patients, 20% of whom had ≥ 5% marrow blasts; 74% had isolated 5q-, and 25% had one or more additional cytogenetic changes. Patients received 10 mg of lenalidomide daily either continuously or on a 3 weeks on/1 week off schedule. After 24 weeks of treatment, 112 (76%) patients had reduced their transfusion requirements, and 99 (67%) no longer required transfusions. Responses were observed at a similar rate regardless of the karyotype complexity. Most patients responded rapidly, achieving transfusion independence after a median of 4.6 weeks. After a median follow-up of 2.8 years, the median duration of transfusion independence was 2.2 years, with an ongoing response in 50 (44%) patients *(74)*. Notably, 81 of 115 (70%) assessable patients had cytogenetic improvement, being complete in 51 (44%). Also, a reduction in blast count by at least 50% was seen in 75% of evaluable patients, and responses fulfilling the criteria for a complete hematologic response were achieved in 36%. Moderate-to-severe transient neutropenia in 55% and thrombocytopenia in 44% of patients were the most common reasons for treatment interruption or dose adjustment of lenalidomide *(74)*.

The mechanism of action of lenalidomide in patients with a 5q chromosome deletion, including those with 5q- syndrome, remains an enigma. The clinical data available to date suggest that this drug predominantly targets the hematopoiesis derived from the 5q-clone. Achievement of complete cytogenetic responses, normalization of the marrow blast percentage and platelet counts, and significant erythroid responses are in agreement with this hypothesis. The activity of lenalidomide in patients with low-risk MDS without deleted 5q is currently being tested.

Lenalidomide has also been investigated in patients with MDS with no 5q- abnormalities. A total of 214 patients were treated with one of two schedules: 10 mg daily on a continuous schedule or 10 mg daily for 21 days of every 28-day cycle. All patients had MDS with a low or intermediate-1 IPSS score, and all were transfusion-dependent, with a minimum requirement of 2 units of packed red blood cell over the 8 weeks prior to enrollment. An erythroid response was achieved in 92 (43%) patients, with 56 (26%) becoming transfusion-independent. Responses were not as durable as those in patients with 5q- abnormalities, with a median duration of 41 weeks (range 8 to 136+ weeks). Interestingly, 22% of evaluable patients also achieved a cytogenetic response. Thus, although not as impressive as the responses achieved in patients with the 5q- abnormality, lenalidomide appears to be effective in some patients with MDS with no or other cytogenetic abnormalities. The mechanism of action in these instances is even less clear *(75)*.

3.2.3. OTHER ANGIOGENESIS INHIBITORS

Bevacizumab is a recombinant humanized monoclonal antibody directed against VEGF that has shown some antitumor activity and synergy with other treatment modalities in several types of tumor *(76)*. Bevacizumab was administered to 15 patients with MDS at an initial dose of 10 mg/kg intravenously every 2 weeks for 4 months with dose escalation to 15 mg/kg for an additional 2 months in nonresponders. Responses, mostly minor, were observed in 20% of patients only *(77)*. A different approach to inhibit VEGF signaling is to inhibit the VEGF receptor. AML and MDS precursors express these receptors specifically. A host of small-molecule inhibitors of VEGF receptor tyrosine kinase (RTK) are currently in development. All of these agents inhibit cell proliferation, suggesting a potential role in MDS therapy. SU5416 *(78)* and SU11248 *(79)* have been shown to inhibit VEGF-mediated cell growth. SU5416 has reached Phase II development in 22 high-risk MDS and 33 refractory AML patients, showing activity in 7% of them *(78)*. SU11248 is an RTK with considerable potency against KDR, PDGFR, and KIT *(79)*. A Phase I study of SU11248 administered orally to 29 patients with AML resulted in a significant reduction in peripheral blood blast counts in 5 of them. PTK787/ZK222584 *(80)* and AG-013736 *(81)* have been also tested in MDS, demonstrating, in general, disappointing results.

3.3. Signal Transduction Inhibitors

3.3.1. FARNESYL TRANSFERASE INHIBITORS

RAS mutations are encountered in 10% to 15% of patients with MDS; and although the prognostic implications of such mutations have been controversial, some studies suggest that they are associated with a worse outcome *(82)*. Hence, the development of inhibitors that target the activation of RAS family proteins (N-RAS, K-RAS, H-RAS) have been actively sought as therapy for MDS. Localization to the inner plasma membrane is critical in RAS activation. This process is accomplished through a posttranslational reaction termed prenylation, by which a 15-carbon isoprenyl (farnesyl) moiety is attached to the C-terminal cysteine residue by the enzyme farnesyltransferase (FTase) and to a lesser extent by geranyl-geranyl-protein transferases (GGPTases) *(83)*. Thus, the development of FTase inhibitors (FTIs) was initially pursued as a means of inhibiting RAS activation. However, FTIs probably do not inhibit RAS signaling in vivo *(84)*, and their antineoplastic activity is likely mediated through inhibition of other proteins that depend on prenylation such as RhoB *(83–85)*, Rab *(86)*, and CENP-E and CENP-F *(87)*.

The activity of one such FTI, tipifarnib, was evaluated in a Phase I study of 21 patients with MDS *(88)*. Tipifarnib was administered at 300 mg orally twice daily on a 3 weeks on/1 week off schedule for 8 weeks. The maximum tolerated dose was 400 mg by mouth twice a day. Responses were seen in 6 (30%) of 20 evaluable patients, including 1 with a CR, 2 with PRs, and 3 with HIs *(88)*. These results led to a Phase II study in which tipifarnib was given to 28 patients with MDS at 600 mg twice daily for 4 weeks in a 6-week cycle *(89)*. Responses were observed in 3 (2 CR, 1 PR) of 27 assessable patients. Altogether, 11 (41%) patients required dose reduction or tipifarnib interruptions, suggesting a dose of 300 mg twice daily as more appropriate for future use. Notably, there was no correlation between response to tipifarnib and *RAS* mutational status, supporting the notion that FTIs have a broader range of action.

The FTI lonafarnib was investigated in a Phase I/II study of 67 patients with advanced MDS *(90)*. Therapy was administered continuously at doses of 200 to 300 mg orally twice daily until development of grade 3 to 4 toxicity or disease progression. Responses occurred in 12 (29%) of 42 assessable patients, including 2 with CRs and 10 with HIs. Discontinuation of therapy owing to grade 3 to 4 toxicity was required in 17 (26%) patients *(90)*.

Another FTI, BMS-214662, has also been evaluated in a Phase I trial in patients with either AML or high-risk MDS *(91)*. BMS-214662 was well tolerated at doses as high as 118 mg/m^2 as a 1-hour infusion and showed activity in 5 (17%) of 30 assessable patients, including 1 with MDS.

The toxicity profile and the efficacy of FTIs in the treatment of MDS may be further improved by optimizing their dose and schedule. Because FTIs inhibit the farnesylation of multiple proteins other than RAS, the identification of the target(s) responsible for their clinical activity may facilitate a more rational use of these agents for the treatment of MDS and their potential use in combination with other targeted agents.

3.3.2. IMATINIB

Imatinib mesylate (Gleevec) was investigated in MDS because of its inhibitory activity against c-Kit, which is expressed nearly universally in patients with MDS. However, it has been largely unsuccessful for the treatment of MDS, both alone or in combination with low-dose ara-C *(92)*. However, therapy with this TKI has paid unexpected dividends in a small subset of patients with chronic myelomonocytic leukemia (CMML) carrying a reciprocal translocation that juxtaposes the PDGF receptor-β *(PDGFRβ)* gene on chromosome 5q33 to various fusion partners including, among others, *TEL (93)*, *HIP (94)*, and *H4/D10S170 (95)*, resulting in the constitutive activation of the tyrosine kinase activity of PDGFRβ. Imatinib can bind to the adenosine triphosphate-binding pocket of PDGFRβ. Treatment of four patients who had CMML with chromosomal translocations involving 5q33 with imatinib 400 mg daily resulted in a sustained complete cytogenetic response *(96)*. In another report, 12 patients with PDGFRβ fusion-positive, BCR-ABL-negative chronic myeloproliferative syndromes achieved prompt and durable hematologic and cytogenetic responses with imatinib therapy *(97)*.

3.3.3. FMS-LIKE TYROSINE KINASE 3

In 15% to 30% of patients, de novo AML aberrant proliferation is a consequence of a juxtamembrane mutation in the FMS-like tyrosine kinase 3 (FLT3) gene *(FLT3*-ITD), causing constitutive kinase activity. This effect can also be observed in 5% of patients with AML carrying *FLT3* point mutations, generally involving codon D835 *(98)*. Activating *FLT3* mutations have been associated with lower response rates and a worse prognosis *(98)*. These mutations can also be detected in some patients with therapy-related MDS but rarely in de novo MDS. Lestaurtinib (formerly CEP-701) is an orally available selective inhibitor of FLT3 autophosphorylation.

The activity of this compound has been evaluated in a Phase I/II trial in patients with refractory, relapsed, or poor-risk AML carrying FLT3-activating mutations *(99)*. Of 14 patients with AML, 5 had marked reductions in bone marrow and peripheral blood blasts that correlated with sustained FLT3 inhibition. In another Phase I trial, tandutinib (formerly MLN518/CT53518) was tested in 40 patients with either AML or high-risk MDS *(100)*. Tandutinib was given orally in doses ranging from 50 to 700 mg twice daily. The main DLTs were reversible generalized muscular weakness and fatigue. Two of five assessable patients with *FLT3*-ITD had decreases in both peripheral and bone marrow blasts, suggesting potential activity of tandutinib in this context. Stone's group *(100)* treated 20 patients, each with mutant *FLT3*-positive relapsed/refractory AML or high-grade MDS, with the potent oral FLT3 inhibitor PKC412 at a dose of 75 mg three times daily. The peripheral blast count decreased by 50% in 14 patients (70%), and bone marrow blast counts were decreased by at least 50% in 6 patients, including 2 with a reduction to < 5%. FLT3 autophosphorylation was inhibited in most responders, indicating in vivo target inhibition. Other agents with potent inhibitory activity against *FLT3* activating mutations, such as sorafenib, KRN383, and ABT-869, are being actively investigated in patients with MDS and AML.

3.3.4. Bortezomib

Nuclear factor-κ β (NF-κβ) inhibition by bortezomib results in the down-regulation of apoptosis-inhibitory NF-κβ target genes and subsequent cell death in AML cell lines and in bone marrow cells from patients with high-risk MDS that exhibited constitutive NF-κβ activation *(101)*. Hence, bortezomib may constitute a useful approach in MDS *(101)*. In a Phase II study, bortezomib rendered a PR rate of 35% among 32 patients with MDS *(102)*.

3.4. Targeting EVI1 Overexpression

The paracentric inversion inv(3) (q21;q26) and the reciprocal translocation t(3;3)(q21;q26) have been described in MDS *(9,10)*. These cytogenetic abnormalities define the so-called 3q21q26 syndrome in 0.5% to 2.0% of patients with MDS. The 3q21.2 chromosome band contains the *EVI1* (ecotropic virus insertion site) proto-oncogene, which has been implicated in the pathogenesis of MDS and AML *(9,10)*. Overexpression of *EVI1* in hematopoietic cells interferes with erythroid and myeloid development. In addition, some MDS patients without the 3q26 abnormality demonstrate overexpression of *EVI1*, which in turn has been associated with unfavorable cytogenetic abnormalities and transformation to AML. Notably, arsenic trioxide (ATO) has shown significant activity in patients with MDS with *EVI1* overexpression *(103)*.

In a recent Phase II study, single-agent ATO was given at 0.25 mg/kg daily on 5 consecutive days per week on a 2 weeks on/2 weeks off schedule to patients with MDS *(104)*. Among patients who completed two or more cycles ($n = 51$), the HI rates were 39% in lower-risk patients and 9% in higher-risk patients, including one who achieved a CR. Transfusion independence or reduction by $\geq$ 50% occurred in 33% of transfusion-dependent patients. The overall median duration of HI was 6.8 months (range 2–40 months). Hence, further investigation of ATO as well as other arsenic derivatives such as SGLU1 is warranted in patients with MDS, particularly in those with 3q21q26.

3.5. Vaccination Approaches for MDS

Antigens targeted for MDS and/or AML must ideally be preferentially expressed in myeloid neoplastic cells relative to normal hematopoietic progenitors. On the basis of this fundamental principle, several immunotherapeutic approaches are under investigation for patients with MDS.

3.5.1. PR1 Vaccine

Proteinase 3 (PR3) is a 26-kDa neutral serine protease found in primary azurophil granules of cells of the myeloid lineage *(83)*. PR1 is a nonapeptide (VLQELNVTV) derived from PR3 that is overexpressed in myeloid malignancies with variable frequency *(105)*. PR1 is presented through HLA-A2.1 molecules and can elicit cytotoxic T lymphocytes (CTLs) from HLA-A2.1+ normal donors in vitro *(106)*. PR1-specific CTLs show preferential cytotoxicity toward allogeneic HLA-A2.1+ myeloid leukemia cells over HLA-identical normal donor marrow *(105)*.

A Phase I trial of vaccination with PR1 peptide in an incomplete Freund's adjuvant and 75 mg of granulocyte-macrophage colony stimulating factor (GM-CSF) included 35 patients with myeloid malignancies who had failed prior therapies *(107)*. Patients were assigned to receive 0.25, 0.50, or 1.0 mg of PR1 peptide subcutaneously every 3 weeks for a total of three injections. Immune responses were elicited in 20 (60%) of 33 evaluable patients. Of 16 patients with relapsed/refractory AML, 4 (25%) had clinical responses (3 CR, 1 PR). Of

5 patients with MDS, 1 had a PR *(107)*. A Phase II trial of PR1 vaccination for patients with MDS is currently ongoing.

3.5.2. WILMS' TUMOR 1 VACCINE

The Wilms' tumor 1 gene (*WT1*) is a highly expressed tumor suppressor gene in myeloid neoplasms. It has very low expression in normal tissues and plays a key role in cell proliferation, making it an ideal candidate target. There is animal and in vitro evidence that WT1, an antigen commonly found overexpressed in MDS *(108)*, can generate leukemia-specific CTLs *(109)*, supporting a potential use for cancer immunotherapy.

Phase I/II studies of a 9-mer WT1 peptide have recently been opened, aiming at investigating the tolerability and immunogenicity of this vaccine in patients with MDS and AML. In a German study, one of the first four patients enrolled has achieved a CR, two had stable disease, and one progressed *(110)*. In a second trial, conducted in Japan, several patients with overt AML following MDS or MDS with myelofibrosis had, after only a single dose of WT1 vaccination, an increase in WT1-specific cytotoxic T lymphocytes, followed by a rapid reduction in WT1 levels as well as peripheral blood leukemic blast counts *(111)*. Severe leukopenia and local erythema at the injection sites of WT1 peptide were the most commonly observed adverse effects *(111)*.

Collectively, these results highlight the safety and promising activity of peptide-based vaccines for patients with MDS.

4. FUTURE DIRECTION OF MOLECULAR THERAPEUTICS IN MDS

Managing patients with MDS remains a challenge. Thus far, allogeneic SCT has been viewed as the only curative option for patients with these disorders. Unfortunately, only a small percentage of patients with MDS are eligible for allogeneic STC owing to limited donor availability and frequent significant co-morbidities, as patients with MDS are predominantly elderly. Until recently, therapy for most patients with MDS was fundamentally supportive and entailed the use of growth factors and transfusional support to ameliorate the hematologic deficits of blood production and palliate symptoms associated with them. However, the therapeutic options have increased exponentially over the last few years. Our as yet limited experience with novel epigenetic modulators and angiogenesis inhibitors appears to indicate, for the first time, that these novel agents can provide sustained remissions and perhaps curtail the inexorable and relentless progression of MDS. It is hoped that an increasing understanding of the molecular basis of the genetic and immunologic events driving the pathogenesis of these disorders will facilitate the design of better tolerated and more specific targeted therapies.

To this end, it is important to ascertain the role of persistent polyclonal hematopoiesis in MDS and determine the frequency and prognostic significance of point mutations in various candidate genes such as *RAS*, *AML1*, *C/EBPα*, and *PU.1*. Moreover, the role of constitutively activated tyrosine kinases, such as FLT3, must be determined; and our search to discover other constitutively active tyrosine kinases amenable for targeted therapies needs to be expanded. Identifying the genes associated with recurrent chromosomal deletions and numerical abnormalities in patients with MDS, including studies and tests for haplo-insufficiency are also important directions to pursue. As a result of these efforts, novel therapies will be generated that will likely include the use of gene therapy strategies to overcome acquired genomic defects involved in the pathogenesis of the disease, more selective hypomethylating agents and HDAC inhibitors capable of restoring the disrupted transcriptional cellular machinery, thereby facilitating the maturation of hematopoietic progenitors, and more refined immunotherapeutic approaches to target specific antigens selectively expressed by malignant MDS stem cells. Undoubtedly, a key element for the furtherance of our knowledge of the molecular underpinnings of MDS will be the development of appropriate animal models that allow us to understand MDS progression and in which to test novel therapeutic agents. The pace with which MDS therapy has evolved during the last decade appears to herald a much brighter future for patients with this condition.

REFERENCES

1. Aul C, Giagounidis A, Germing U. Epidemiological features of myelodysplastic syndromes: results from regional cancer surveys and hospital-based statistics. Int J Hematol 2001;73:405–10.
2. Ma X, Does M, Raza, A, et al. Myelodysplastic syndromes: incidence and survival in the United States. Cancer 2007;109:1536–42.
3. Cazzola M, Malcovati L. Myelodysplastic syndromes—coping with ineffective hematopoiesis. N Engl J Med 2005;352:536–8.
4. Bennett JM, Catovsky D, Daniel MT, et al. Proposals for the classification of the myelodysplastic syndromes. Br J Haematol 1982;51:189–99.
5. Vardiman JW, Harris NL, Brunning RD. The World Health Organization (WHO) classification of the myeloid neoplasms. Blood 2002;100:2292–302.
6. Greenberg P, Cox C, LeBeau MM, et al. International scoring system for evaluating prognosis in myelodysplastic syndromes. Blood 1997;89:2079–88.
7. Olney HJ, Le Beau MM. The cytogenetics of myelodysplastic syndromes. Best Pract Res Clin Haematol 2001;14:479–95.
8. Bianchi E, Rogge L. Dissecting oncogenes and tyrosine kinases in AML cells. Med Gen Med 2003;5:10.
9. Russell M, List A, Greenberg P, et al. Expression of EVI1 in myelodysplastic syndromes and other hematologic malignancies without 3q26 translocations. Blood 1994;84:1243–8.
10. Dreyfus F, Bouscary D, Melle J,et al. Expression of the Evi-1 gene in myelodysplastic syndromes. Leukemia 1995;9:203–5.
11. Kelly LM, Gilliland DG. Genetics of myeloid leukemias. Annu Rev Genomics Hum Genet 2002;3:179–98.
12. Corey SJ, Minden MD, Barber DL, et al. Myelodysplastic syndromes: the complexity of stem-cell diseases. Nat Rev Cancer 2007;7:118–29.
13. Quesnel B, Guillerm G, Vereecque R, et al. Methylation of the p15(INK4b) gene in myelodysplastic syndromes is frequent and acquired during disease progression. Blood 1998;91:2985–90.
14. Uchida T, Kinoshita T, Nagai H, et al. Hypermethylation of the p15INK4B gene in myelodysplastic syndromes. Blood 1997;90:1403–9.
15. Nightingale KP, O'Neill LP, Turner BM. Histone modifications: signalling receptors and potential elements of a heritable epigenetic code. Curr Opin Genet Dev 2006;16:125–36.
16. Roth SY, Denu JM, Allis CD. Histone acetyltransferases. Annu Rev Biochem 2001;70:81–120.
17. Silverman LR, Demakos EP, Peterson BL, et al. Randomized controlled trial of azacitidine in patients with the myelodysplastic syndrome: a study of the cancer and leukemia group B. J Clin Oncol 2002;20:2429–40.
18. Kaminskas E, Farrell A, Abraham S, et al. Approval summary: azacitidine for treatment of myelodysplastic syndrome subtypes. Clin Cancer Res 2005;11:3604–8.
19. Gryn J, Zeigler ZR, Shadduck RK, et al. Treatment of myelodysplastic syndromes with 5-azacytidine. Leuk Res 2002;26:893–7.
20. Hellstrom-Lindberg E. Update on supportive care and new therapies: immunomodulatory drugs, growth factors and epigenetic-acting agents. Hematology (Am Soc Hematol Educ Program) 2005;161–6.
21. Momparler RL, Rossi M, Bouchard J, et al. Kinetic interaction of 5-AZA-2'-deoxycytidine-5'-monophosphate and its 5'-triphosphate with deoxycytidylate deaminase. Mol Pharmacol 1984;25:436–40.
22. Santini V, Kantarjian HM, Issa JP. Changes in DNA methylation in neoplasia: pathophysiology and therapeutic implications. Ann Intern Med 2001;134:573–86.
23. Juttermann R, Li E, Jaenisch R. Toxicity of 5-aza-2'-deoxycytidine to mammalian cells is mediated primarily by covalent trapping of DNA methyltransferase rather than DNA demethylation. Proc Natl Acad Sci U S A 1994;91:11797–801.
24. Rivard GE, Momparler RL, Demers J, et al. Phase I study on 5-aza-2'-deoxycytidine in children with acute leukemia. Leuk Res 1981;5:453–62.

25. Van Groeningen CJ, Leyva A, O'Brien AM, Gall HE, Pinedo HM. Phase I and pharmacokinetic study of 5-aza-2'-deoxycytidine (NSC 127716) in cancer patients. Cancer Res 1986; 46:4831–6.

26. Zagonel V, Lo Re G, Marotta G, et al. 5-Aza-2'-deoxycytidine (Decitabine) induces trilineage response in unfavourable myelodysplastic syndromes. Leukemia 1993;7(suppl 1):30–5.

27. Issa JP, Garcia-Manero G, Giles FJ, et al. Phase 1 study of low-dose prolonged exposure schedules of the hypomethylating agent 5-aza-2'-deoxycytidine (decitabine) in hematopoietic malignancies. Blood 2004;103:1635–40.

28. Wijermans PW, Krulder JW, Huijgens PC, et al. Continuous infusion of low-dose 5-aza-2'-deoxycytidine in elderly patients with high-risk myelodysplastic syndrome. Leukemia 1997;11(suppl 1):S19–23.

29. Wijermans P, Lubbert M, Verhoef G, et al. Low-dose 5-aza-2'-deoxycytidine, a DNA hypomethylating agent, for the treatment of high-risk myelodysplastic syndrome: a multicenter phase II study in elderly patients. J Clin Oncol 2000;18:956–62.

30. Lubbert M, Wijermans P, Kunzmann R, et al. Cytogenetic responses in high-risk myelodysplastic syndrome following low-dose treatment with the DNA methylation inhibitor 5-aza-2'-deoxycytidine. Br J Haematol 2001;114:349–57.

31. Van den Bosch J, Lubbert M, Verhoef G, et al. The effects of 5-aza-2'-deoxycytidine (Decitabine) on the platelet count in patients with intermediate and high-risk myelodysplastic syndromes. Leuk Res 2004;28:785–90.

32. Kantarjian H, Issa JP, Rosenfeld CS, et al. Decitabine improves patient outcomes in myelodysplastic syndromes: results of a phase III randomized study. Cancer 2006;106:1794–803.

33. Kantarjian H, Oki Y, Garcia-Manero G, et al. Results of a randomized study of 3 schedules of low-dose decitabine in higher-risk myelodysplastic syndrome and chronic myelomonocytic leukemia. Blood 2007;109:52–7.

34. Gao L, Cueto, MA, Asselbergs, F, et al. Cloning and functional characterization of HDAC11, a novel member of the human histone deacetylase family. J Biol Chem 2002;277:25748–55.

35. Novogrodsky A, Dvir A, Ravid A, et al. Effect of polar organic compounds on leukemic cells: butyrate-induced partial remission of acute myelogenous leukemia in a child. Cancer 1983;51:9–14.

36. Gore SD, Weng LJ, Zhai S, et al. Impact of the putative differentiating agent sodium phenylbutyrate on myelodysplastic syndromes and acute myeloid leukemia. Clin Cancer Res 2001;7:2330–9.

37. Marcucci G, Bruner, RJ, Binkley, PE, et al. Phase I trial of the histone deacetylase inhibitor depsipeptide (FR901228) in acute myeloid leukemia (AML). Blood 2002;100:86a. Abstract.

38. Byrd JC, Marcucci G, Parthun MR, et al. A phase 1 and pharmacodynamic study of depsipeptide (FK228) in chronic lymphocytic leukemia and acute myeloid leukemia. Blood 2005;105:959–67.

39. Gottlicher M, Minucci S, Zhu P, et al. Valproic acid defines a novel class of HDAC inhibitors inducing differentiation of transformed cells. EMBO J 2001;20:6969–78.

40. Kuendgen A, Strupp C, Aivado M, et al. Treatment of myelodysplastic syndromes with valproic acid alone or in combination with all-trans retinoic acid. Blood 2004;104:1266–9.

41. Pilatrino C, Cilloni D, Messa E, et al. Increase in platelet count in older, poor-risk patients with acute myeloid leukemia or myelodysplastic syndrome treated with valproic acid and all-trans retinoic acid. Cancer 2005;104:101–9.

42. Marks PA, Miller T, Richon VM. Histone deacetylases. Curr Opin Pharmacol 2003;3:344–51.

43. Kelly WK, Richon VM, O'Connor O, et al. Phase I clinical trial of histone deacetylase inhibitor: suberoylanilide hydroxamic acid administered intravenously. Clin Cancer Res 2003;9:3578–88.

44. Garcia-Manero G, Yang, H, Sanchez-Gonzalez, B, et al. Final results of a phase I study of the histone deacetylase inhibitor vorinostat (suberoyanilide hydroxamic acid, SAHA), in patients with leukemia and myelodysplastic syndrome. Blood 2005;106. Abstract 2801.

45. Garcia-Manero G, Minden, M, Estrov, Z, et al. Clinical activity and safety of the histone deacetylase inhibitor MGCD0103: results of a phase I study in patients with leukemia or myelodysplastic syndromes (MDS). J Clin Oncol 2006;24. Abstract 6500.

46. Giles F, Fischer T, Cortes J, et al. A phase I study of intravenous LBH589, a novel cinnamic hydroxamic acid analogue histone deacetylase inhibitor, in patients with refractory hematologic malignancies. Clin Cancer Res 2006;12:4628–35.

47. Plumb JA, Finn PW, Williams RJ, et al. Pharmacodynamic response and inhibition of growth of human tumor xenografts by the novel histone deacetylase inhibitor PXD101. Mol Cancer Ther 2003;2:721–8.

48. Gimsing P, Wu, F, Qian, X, et al. Activity of the histone deacetylase (HDAC) inhibitor PXD101 in preclinical studies and in a phase I study in patients with advanced haematological tumors. Blood 2005;106. Abstract 3337.

49. Gojo I, Jiemjit A, Trepel JB, et al. Phase 1 and pharmacological study of MS-275, a histone deacetylase inhibitor, in adults with refractory and relapsed acute leukemias. Blood 2007;109:2781–90.

50. Gore SD, Baylin S, Sugar E, et al. Combined DNA methyltransferase and histone deacetylase inhibition in the treatment of myeloid neoplasms. Cancer Res 2006;66:6361–9.

51. Garcia-Manero G, Kantarjian HM, Sanchez-Gonzalez B, et al. Phase 1/2 study of the combination of 5-aza-2'-deoxycytidine with valproic acid in patients with leukemia. Blood 2006;108:3271–9.

52. Gore S, Jiemjit, A, Silverman, LB, et al. Combined methyltransferase/histone deacetylase inhibition with 5-azacitidine and MS-275 in patients with MDS, CMMoL and AML: clinical response, histone acetylation and DNA damage. Blood 2006;108. Abstract 517.

53. Sanchez-Gonzalez B, Yang H, Bueso-Ramos C, et al. Antileukemia activity of the combination of an anthracycline with a histone deacetylase inhibitor. Blood 2006;108:1174–82.

54. Aguayo A, Kantarjian, H, Manshouri, T, et al. Angiogenesis in acute and chronic leukemias and myelodysplastic syndromes. Blood 2000;96:2240–5.

55. Albitar M. Angiogenesis in acute myeloid leukemia and myelodysplastic syndrome. Acta Haematol 2001;106:170–6.

56. Bellamy WT, Richter L, Sirjani D, et al. Vascular endothelial cell growth factor is an autocrine promoter of abnormal localized immature myeloid precursors and leukemia progenitor formation in myelodysplastic syndromes. Blood 2001;97:1427–34.

57. Aguayo A, Kantarjian, H, Estey, EH, et al. Plasma vascular endothelial growth factor levels have prognostic significance in patients with acute myeloid leukemia but not in patients with myelodysplastic syndromes. Cancer 2002;95:1923–30.

58. Schafer PH, Gandhi AK, Loveland MA, et al. Enhancement of cytokine production and AP-1 transcriptional activity in T cells by thalidomide-related immunomodulatory drugs. J Pharmacol Exp Ther 2003;305:1222–32.

59. Raza A, Meyer P, Dutt D, et al. Thalidomide produces transfusion independence in long-standing refractory anemias of patients with myelodysplastic syndromes. Blood 2001;98:958–65.

60. Strupp C, Germing U, Aivado M, et al. Thalidomide for the treatment of patients with myelodysplastic syndromes. Leukemia 2002;16:1–6.

61. Musto P, Falcone A, Sanpaolo G, et al. Thalidomide abolishes transfusion-dependence in selected patients with myelodysplastic syndromes. Haematologica 2002;87:884–6.

62. Moreno-Aspitia A, Colon-Otero G, Hoering A, et al. Thalidomide therapy in adult patients with myelodysplastic syndrome: a North Central Cancer Treatment Group phase II trial. Cancer 2006;107:767–72.

63. Bouscary D, Legros L, Tulliez M, et al. A non-randomised dose-escalating phase II study of thalidomide for the treatment of patients with low-risk myelodysplastic syndromes: the Thal-SMD-2000 trial of the Groupe Francais des Myelodysplasies. Br J Haematol 2005;131:609–18.

64. Musto P, Falcone A, Sanpaolo G, et al. Combination of erythropoietin and thalidomide for the treatment of anemia in patients with myelodysplastic syndromes. Leuk Res 2006;30:385–8.

65. Raza A, Lisak L, Billmeier J, et al. Phase II study of topotecan and thalidomide in patients with high-risk myelodysplastic syndromes. Leuk Lymphoma 2006;47:433–40.

66. Muller GW, Chen R, Huang SY, et al. Amino-substituted thalidomide analogs: potent inhibitors of TNF-alpha production. Bioorg Med Chem Lett 1999;9:1625–30.

67. Dredge K, Horsfall R, Robinson SP, et al. Orally administered lenalidomide (CC-5013) is anti-angiogenic in vivo and inhibits endothelial cell migration and Akt phosphorylation in vitro. Microvasc Res 2005;69:56–63.

68. Bartlett JB, Dredge K, Dalgleish AG. The evolution of thalidomide and its IMiD derivatives as anticancer agents. Nat Rev Cancer 2004;4:314–22.

69. Sole F, Espinet B, Sanz GF, et al. Incidence, characterization and prognostic significance of chromosomal abnormalities in 640 patients with primary myelodysplastic syndromes: Grupo Cooperativo Espanol de Citogenetica Hematologica. Br J Haematol 2000;108:346–56.

70. Van den Berghe H, Vermaelen K, Mecucci C, et al. The 5q-anomaly. Cancer Genet Cytogenet 1985;17:189–255.

71. Gandhi AK, Kang J, Naziruddin S, et al. Lenalidomide inhibits proliferation of Namalwa CSN.70 cells and interferes with Gab1 phosphorylation and adaptor protein complex assembly. Leuk Res 2006;30:849–58.

72. List A, Kurtin S, Roe DJ, et al. Efficacy of lenalidomide in myelodysplastic syndromes. N Engl J Med 2005;352:549–57.

73. List A, Dewald G, Bennett J, et al. Lenalidomide in the myelodysplastic syndrome with chromosome 5q deletion. N Engl J Med 2006;355:1456–65.

74. List A, Dewald, GW, Bennettt, JM, et al. Long-term clinical benefit of lenalidomide (Revlimid) treatment in patients with myelodysplastic syndrome and chromosome deletion 5q. Blood 2006;108. Abstract 251.

75. Raza A, Reeves, J, Feldman, EJ, et al. Long term clinical benefit of lenalidomide (Revlimid) treatment in patients with myelodysplastic syndrome without Del 5q cytogenetic abnormalities. Blood 2006;108. Abstract 250.

76. Ferrara N. VEGF as a therapeutic target in cancer. Oncology 2005;69(suppl 3):11–6.

77. Gotlib J, Jamieson CHM, List A, et al. Phase II study of bevacizumab (anti-VEGF humanized monoclonal antibody) in patients with myelodysplastic syndrome (MDS): preliminary results. Blood 2003;102. Abstract 1545.

78. Giles FJ, Stopeck AT, Silverman LR, et al. SU5416, a small molecule tyrosine kinase receptor inhibitor, has biologic activity in patients with refractory acute myeloid leukemia or myelodysplastic syndromes. Blood 2003;102:795–801.

79. Foran J, Paquette, R, Copper, M, et al. A phase I study of repeated oral dosing with SU11248 for the treatment of patients with acute myeloid leukemia who have failed or are not eligible for conventional chemotherapy. Blood 2002;100:558a. Abstract.

80. Roboz GJ, Giles FJ, List AF, et al. Phase 1 study of PTK787/ZK 222584, a small molecule tyrosine kinase receptor inhibitor, for the treatment of acute myeloid leukemia and myelodysplastic syndrome. Leukemia 2006;20:952–7.

81. Giles FJ, Bellamy WT, Estrov Z, et al. The anti-angiogenesis agent, AG-013736, has minimal activity in elderly patients with poor prognosis acute myeloid leukemia (AML) or myelodysplastic syndrome (MDS). Leuk Res 2006;30:801–11.

82. John AM, Thomas NS, Mufti GJ, et al. Targeted therapies in myeloid leukemia. Semin Cancer Biol 2004;14:41–62.

83. Beaupre DM, Kurzrock R. RAS and leukemia: from basic mechanisms to gene-directed therapy. J Clin Oncol 1999;17:1071–9.

84. Downward J. Targeting RAS signalling pathways in cancer therapy. Nat Rev Cancer 2003;3:11–22.

85. Rowinsky EK, Windle JJ, Von Hoff DD. Ras protein farnesyltransferase: a strategic target for anticancer therapeutic development. J Clin Oncol 1999;17:3631–52.

86. Lackner MR, Kindt RM, Carroll PM, et al. Chemical genetics identifies Rab geranylgeranyl transferase as an apoptotic target of farnesyl transferase inhibitors. Cancer Cell 2005;7:325–36.

87. Ashar HR, James L, Gray K, et al. Farnesyl transferase inhibitors block the farnesylation of CENP-E and CENP-F and alter the association of CENP-E with the microtubules. J Biol Chem 2000;275:30451–7.

88. Kurzrock R, Kantarjian, HM, Cortes, JE, et al. Farnesyltrasnferase inhibitor R115777 in myelodysplastic syndrome: clinical and biologic activities in the phase I setting. Blood 2003;102:4527–34.

89. Kurzrock R, Albitar M, Cortes JE, et al. Phase II study of R115777, a farnesyl transferase inhibitor, in myelodysplastic syndrome. J Clin Oncol 2004;22:1287–92.

90. Feldman E, Cortes, J, Holyoake, TL, et al. Continuous oral lonafarnib (Sarasar) for the treatment of patients with myelodysplastic syndrome. Blood 2003;102:421a. Abstract.

91. Cortes J, Faderl S, Estey E, et al. Phase I study of BMS-214662, a farnesyl transferase inhibitor in patients with acute leukemias and high-risk myelodysplastic syndromes. J Clin Oncol 2005;23:2805–12.

92. Heidel F, Cortes J, Rucker FG, et al. Results of a multicenter phase II trial for older patients with c-Kit-positive acute myeloid leukemia (AML) and high-risk myelodysplastic syndrome (HR-MDS) using low-dose Ara-C and Imatinib. Cancer 2007;109:907–14.

93. Golub TR, Barker GF, Lovett M, et al. Fusion of PDGF receptor beta to a novel ets-like gene, tel, in chronic myelomonocytic leukemia with t(5;12) chromosomal translocation. Cell 1994;77:307–16.

94. Ross TS, Bernard OA, Berger R, et al. Fusion of Huntingtin interacting protein 1 to platelet-derived growth factor beta receptor (PDGFbetaR) in chronic myelomonocytic leukemia with t(5;7)(q33;q11.2). Blood 1998;91:4419–26.

95. Drechsler M, Hildebrandt B, Kundgen A, et al. Fusion of H4/D10S170 to PDGFRbeta in a patient with chronic myelomonocytic leukemia and long-term responsiveness to imatinib. Ann Hematol 2007;86:353–4.

96. Apperley JF, Gardembas M, Melo JV, et al. Response to imatinib mesylate in patients with chronic myeloproliferative diseases with rearrangements of the platelet-derived growth factor receptor beta. N Engl J Med 2002;347:481–7.

97. David M, Cross NC, Burgstaller S, et al. Durable responses to imatinib in patients with PDGFRB fusion gene-positive and BCR-ABL-negative chronic myeloproliferative disorders. Blood 2007;109:61–4.

98. Griffin JD. FLT3 tyrosine kinase as a target in acute leukemias. Hematol J 2004;5(suppl 3):S188–90.

99. Smith BD, Levis M, Beran M, et al. Single-agent CEP-701, a novel FLT3 inhibitor, shows biologic and clinical activity in patients with relapsed or refractory acute myeloid leukemia. Blood 2004;103:3669–76.

100. Stone RM, DeAngelo DJ, Klimek V, et al. Patients with acute myeloid leukemia and activating mutations in FLT3 respond to small-molecule FLT3 tyrosine kinase inhibitor, PKC412. Blood 2005;105(1):54–60.

101. Braun T, Carvalho G, Coquelle A, et al. NF-kappaB constitutes a potential therapeutic target in high-risk myelodysplastic syndrome. Blood 2006;107:1156–65.

102. Shetty V, Verspoor, F, Nguyen, H, et al. Effect of proteasome inhibition by bortezomib on tumor necrosis factor alpha (TNF-alpha) and apoptosis in patients with myelodysplastic syndromes (MDS). Blood 2003;102:1534. Abstract.

103. Raza A, Buonamici S, Lisak L, et al. Arsenic trioxide and thalidomide combination produces multi-lineage hematological responses in myelodysplastic syndromes patients, particularly in those with high pre-therapy EVI1 expression. Leuk Res 2004;28:791–803.

104. Schiller GJ, Slack J, Hainsworth JD, et al. Phase II multicenter study of arsenic trioxide in patients with myelodysplastic syndromes. J Clin Oncol 2006;24:2456–64.

105. Molldrem JJ, Lee PP, Wang C, et al. Evidence that specific T lymphocytes may participate in the elimination of chronic myelogenous leukemia. Nat Med 2000;6:1018–23.

106. Molldrem JJ, Lee PP, Kant S, et al. Chronic myelogenous leukemia shapes host immunity by selective deletion of high-avidity leukemia-specific T cells. J Clin Invest 2003;111:639–47.

107. Qazilbash M, Wieder, E, Rios, R, et al. Vaccination with the PR1 leukemia-associated antigen can induce complete remission in patients with myeloid leukemia. Blood 2004;104. Abstract 259.

108. Cilloni D, Saglio G. WT1 as a universal marker for minimal residual disease detection and quantification in myeloid leukemias and in myelodysplastic syndrome. Acta Haematol 2004;112:79–84.

109. Bellantuono I, Gao L, Parry S, et al. Two distinct HLA-A0201-presented epitopes of the Wilms tumor antigen 1 can function as targets for leukemia-reactive CTL. Blood 2002;100:3835–7.

110. Mailander V, Scheibenbogen C, Thiel E, et al. Complete remission in a patient with recurrent acute myeloid leukemia induced by vaccination with WT1 peptide in the absence of hematological or renal toxicity. Leukemia 2004;18:165–6.

111. Oka Y, Tsuboi A, Murakami M, et al. Wilms tumor gene peptide-based immunotherapy for patients with overt leukemia from myelodysplastic syndrome (MDS) or MDS with myelofibrosis. Int J Hematol 2003;78:56–61.

12 Targeted Therapy in Epithelial Ovarian Cancer

Maurie Markman, MD

ABSTRACT

Despite the high objective response rate (70%–80%) of ovarian cancer to standard cytotoxic chemotherapeutic agents, most patients ultimately experience a recurrence of their disease. Thus, there is a critical need to find novel agents that might favorably influence the course of the malignancy. A number of molecular abnormalities have been identified in ovarian cancer that might be rational candidates for a "targeted" therapeutic approach. Unfortunately, to date, there has been limited evidence of the effectiveness of a variety of "targeted" strategies in ovarian cancer. However, recent data revealing the surprisingly high objective response rate (approximately 15%) of recurrent and platinum-resistant disease to single-agent bevacizumab has stimulated considerable interest in employing antiangiogenic agents for the malignancy. Phase III trials are currently underway to define a possible role for use of this approach in routine management of ovarian cancer as a component of the primary treatment.

Key Words: Ovarian cancer, Cisplatin, Carboplatin, Antiangiogenic agents, Bevacizumab, Targeted therapy

1. EPIDEMIOLOGY AND NATURAL HISTORY OF OVARIAN CANCER

There are approximately 25,000 new cases of epithelial ovarian cancer diagnosed in the United States each year, with 70%–80% documented to have spread beyond the confines of the ovary at the time of initial presentation *(1)*. In approximately two-thirds of cases,

From: *Current Clinical Oncology: Targeted Cancer Therapy*
Edited by: R. Kurzrock and M. Markman © Humana Press, Totowa, NJ

the ovarian malignancy is considered to be high grade (grade 3). Although the morphologic description of epithelial ovarian cancer currently does not influence the choice of management, there is increasing evidence that mucinous ovarian cancers respond poorly to standard platinum-based chemotherapy (2). The only well established risk factor for ovarian cancer is a strong family history of the malignancy (approximately 5% of all cases), now known to be related to BRCA-1 and BRCA-2 abnormalities in most patients with a genetic component to their illness. Of note, patients with BRCA-1-related ovarian cancer appear to have a superior prognosis compared to non-BRCA-1-related cancers, which has been speculated to be due to an inherent inability within the cancer cell to repair platinum-induced damage.

A somewhat unique feature of ovarian cancer is its propensity to remain principally confined to the peritoneal cavity in most patients for the greater part of its natural history, despite the presence of extensive disease at diagnosis (3). Knowledge of this fact led investigators to examine regional antineoplastic drug delivery as a therapeutic strategy for the malignancy (discussed below).

2. MANAGEMENT OF ADVANCED OVARIAN CANCER

Most patients with ovarian cancer undergo an initial attempt at maximal surgical cytoreduction prior to the administration of cytotoxic chemotherapy (4). The principle justification for this rather unique oncologic management approach is the extensive retrospective data indicating superior survival for women with the malignancy who initiate systemic therapy with the smallest volume of residual cancer. It remains uncertain to this day whether the favorable outcome results principally from the successful surgery, the inherent biology of the cancers that are able to be "cytoreduced" effectively, or a combination of these factors. Although an appropriate definition of "optimal residual" advanced disease remains a controversial issue, the Gynecologic Oncology Group (GOG) currently considers patients with stage 3 ovarian cancer (malignancy confined to the peritoneal cavity) to be "optimally cytoreduced" (small-volume residual disease) if the largest remaining mass is < 1 cm in maximum diameter (5). Patients whose largest residual malignant lesion is > 1 cm or when stage 4 is documented are stated to have "suboptimal residual" advanced disease.

Over the past several decades a series of well designed and conducted randomized Phase III trials have defined the standard primary chemotherapy approach for advanced ovarian cancer (1). The platinum agents cisplatin and carboplatin remain the cornerstone of treatment, with carboplatin generally preferred because of its more favorable toxicity profile (5–7). Individual randomized trials and several meta-analyses have confirmed the major impact of this class of agents in ovarian cancer (8). Based on existing data, it is highly unlikely that future trials in ovarian cancer (including studies of "targeted therapy") will attempt to replace a platinum agent; rather, the efforts will be to enhance the effectiveness of this cytotoxic drug.

Either paclitaxel or docetaxel is routinely employed with a platinum agent in the primary chemotherapy setting (5–7,9). There is no evidence for the superiority of one of these taxanes in ovarian cancer, although in combination with carboplatin the drugs have quite different toxicity profiles, with the paclitaxel-containing program being associated with more peripheral neuropathy, in contrast to the significant neutropenia observed with docetaxel. The anticipated objective response rate to a primary platinum/taxane combination regimen is approximately 70% to 80%. Unfortunately, most of the responding patients ultimately experience recurrence of the cancer and are candidates for a second-line treatment approach (discussed below). The median survivals for patients with "small-volume residual" and "large-volume residual" advanced ovarian cancer are currently approximately 5 years and 3 years, respectively. Despite multiple attempts to examine the issue in Phase III trials, there is currently no evidence that adding a third cytotoxic drug to a platinum/taxane program or increasing the dose intensity of a platinum agent improves outcome with this malignancy *(10–12)*.

As previously noted, the known natural history of ovarian cancer led a number of investigators to explore the therapeutic potential of regional antineoplastic drug delivery *(13)*. Three randomized multiinstitutional Phase III trials comparing an intravenous to an intraperitoneal cisplatin-based strategy as primary therapy of small-volume residual advanced ovarian cancer have demonstrated that the regional approach improves overall survival in this clinical setting *(14–16)*. These results led the National Cancer Institute to issue a "Clinical Announcement" in early 2006 to inform physicians, patients, and the public of the benefits of this innovative strategy *(17)*.

Although the concept of "maintenance" or "consolidation" chemotherapy has not been shown to be an effective management approach in solid tumor oncology *(18)*, including several platinum-based trials for advanced ovarian cancer, a somewhat controversial Phase III study has revealed that the continuation of single-agent paclitaxel for 12-months in women with advanced ovarian cancer who had achieved a clinically defined complete response to a platinum/paclitaxel primary chemotherapy regimen substantially improves progression-free survival *(19)*. This outcome led to a decision by the study's Data Safely and Monitoring Committee to close the trial with only one-half of the initial planned accrual having been entered. As a result, the sample size was insufficient to make a definitive statement regarding an impact of 12 months of single-agent paclitaxel maintenance therapy on overall survival in women with ovarian cancer. However, at a minimum, this study serves as a critically important "proof of principle" that a maintenance strategy can exert a clinically relevant effect on the natural history of advanced ovarian cancer.

Despite the high objective response rate (70%–80%) of advanced ovarian cancer to platinum-based chemotherapy, most patients experience a recurrence of the disease process. A relatively large number of antineoplastic agents as well as some combination chemotherapy regimens may be employed in this clinical setting, including retreatment with previously employed drugs *(20)*. It is interesting to note that although current primary chemotherapy of advanced ovarian cancer is based on a series of impressive evidence-based clinical trials, there has been a distressing paucity of such studies to define optimal disease management in the "second-line" setting.

3. UNIQUE ASPECTS OF OVARIAN CANCER PERMITTING STUDY OF NOVEL MANAGEMENT STRATEGIES

It has been recognized for several decades that epithelial ovarian cancer is highly responsive to cytotoxic chemotherapy, being appropriately considered the most "chemosensitive" solid tumor (excluding germ cell cancers). Multiple antineoplastic agents have been shown to produce at least a modest objective regression rate (> 10%) in the platinum-resistant setting, and retreatment with a platinum-based program has been recognized as a rational approach, often associated with apparent considerable extension of survival, in patients who have responded to initial therapy but who experience subsequent recurrence of the cancer *(20)*. However, there is currently no evidence that any second-line regimen in ovarian cancer has a legitimate curative potential. Despite this fact, women with ovarian cancer may live for many years with an excellent quality of life following evidence the initial treatment program has failed to control the disease process. It is of note that the extended survival and lack of curative options in this setting have led some investigators to argue it is reasonable to approach the malignancy as a "serious chronic illness."*(21,22)*

One gynecologic cancer investigative group noted that although ovarian cancer patients may respond two, three, or more times to a platinum-based regimen, the duration of each subsequent response is shorter than the prior response, assuming the same agents (or class of agents) are employed in the treatment regimen *(23)*. This observation has the potential to be useful in the preliminary examination of the utility of a novel antineoplastic agent in the management of ovarian cancer. For example, if such a drug is added to a second-line carboplatin/paclitaxel regimen and the duration of a documented secondary response in a particular patient is longer than that of the initial response, although the measured "objective tumor shrinkage" may have been due solely to the two established cytotoxic drugs it would be reasonable to suggest that it was the new drug that was largely responsible for the extended duration of that response. By permitting each patient to act as her "own control," the percentage of "secondary responses" that are longer in duration than the "initial response" (e.g., none, 20%, 70%) may provide an important preliminary "window" into how this drug will perform when subsequently subjected to a rigorous analysis in a Phase III randomized trial.

Finally, an evaluation of the status of ovarian cancer and of the activity of antineoplastic therapy in this malignancy is assisted by the availability of a remarkably useful serum tumor marker, CA-125. Although CA-125 is not specific for ovarian cancer and is frequently not elevated in early-stage disease (thus being of limited value as a "screening test"), in the presence of known malignancy either a documented (and subsequently confirmed) rise or fall in this marker is a highly reliable indicator of progression or regression of the cancer, respectively *(24–26)*. It is currently unknown if treating a patient solely on the basis of an elevation in the CA-125 level or if altering therapy based on that change exerts a favorable impact on the patient's ultimate outcome. However, in the context of a clinical trial, use of the tumor marker may be extremely helpful for evaluating the biologic activity of treatment, including novel agents whose activity is presumed to be cytostatic, rather then cytotoxic. In this setting, the benefits of the drug may be measured solely by a delay in the time to disease progression, rather than on the objective response rate.

4. POTENTIAL FOR "TARGETED THERAPY" OF OVARIAN CANCER

Owing to the previously noted inherent sensitivity of ovarian cancer to cytotoxic chemotherapy and the favorable history of early drug development for this malignancy (e.g., cisplatin, carboplatin, paclitaxel, topotecan, liposomal doxorubicin), there has been a natural desire on the part of both investigators and the pharmaceutical/biotech industry to explore a possible role for "targeted" therapy in this clinical setting. As with multiple other tumor types, there have been considerable efforts in both the laboratory and clinical settings to predict which target may be relevant for ovarian cancer.

On the basis of preclinical evaluation, ovarian cancer appears to be an excellent tumor model in which to explore such agents, with studies demonstrating overexpression or unique expression of several recognized molecular targets present on the malignant cell population or in the serum of patients with ovarian cancer. Of note, these molecular abnormalities have been successful "targets" of drugs in other malignancies. However, as will become evident, the clinical data available to date with delivery of these agents in the treatment of ovarian cancer reveals the complexity of translating preclinical evaluation into a beneficial management strategy in this malignancy.

5. EXPERIENCE WITH "TARGETED THERAPY" OF OVARIAN CANCER

5.1. HER2 Overexpression

One of the earliest experiences with targeted therapy of ovarian cancer was an attempt to duplicate the highly favorable results associated with the administration of trastuzumab in the management of breast cancer. Initial reports had suggested that approximately 30% of epithelial ovarian cancers overexpress the HER2 receptor (a rate similar to that noted in breast cancer), and that such overexpression was associated with an unfavorable clinical outcome (27–29). However, in a study conducted by the GOG, a far lower incidence of HER2 overexpression in ovarian cancer was demonstrated (11%); and among the patient population with this particular biologic feature (HER2 overexpression) who received trastuzumab, a disappointingly low objective response rate of only 7% was observed (30).

Of interest, preliminary reported data employing pertuzumab, a HER dimerization inhibitor, suggests that this agent may be more active in the malignancy than trastuzumab, potentially in particular subsets of patients with ovarian cancer (31). Further investigation of this agent seems indicated.

5.2. Epidermal Growth Factor Receptor Overexpression

Preclinical data had revealed that overexpression of epidermal growth factor receptor (EGFR) was common in ovarian cancer (70% incidence), with this molecular marker being associated with an unfavorable clinical outcome (32,33). Unfortunately, similar to the previously noted experience with therapy directed to HER2 overexpression in ovarian cancer, single-agent trials of several commercially available or investigative EGFR inhibitors (erlotinib, gefitinib, matuzumab) failed to reveal significant clinical activity (objective response rates < 10%) (34–37). Of interest, in the GOG trial of gefitinib, the cancer in the single patient who achieved a partial response following treatment with this agent contained an activating mutation of EGFR (36). It remains to be shown if it will be worthwhile to examine the molecular profile of the individual tumors of women with advanced ovarian cancer to determine if treatment with an EGFR inhibitor is a reasonable management strategy. The relevance of such a strategy can certainly be questioned if the chances of finding such an abnormality are limited (< 10% of ovarian malignancies). Furthermore, as recently demonstrated for lung cancer (38), even cancers responding to EGFR inhibition are quite capable of developing strategies to overcome this biologic effect. Thus, in addition to the issue of the percentage of individuals who are likely to respond to EGFR agents, it will also be important to understand the legitimate opportunity for extended responses (e.g., > 6–12 months) versus short-term responses (e.g., < 3–4 months).

5.3. Tyrosine Kinase Inhibition

The established and rather dramatic effectiveness of imatinib in the management of chronic myelocytic leukemia and gastrointestinal stromal tumors (GISTs) (39,40), along with preclinical data in ovarian cancer revealing the relatively common expression of several molecular markers (c-ABL, c-KIT, PDGFRβ) that might be favorably influenced following inhibition by this agent, led several groups to initiate clinical trials exploring a possible role for imatinib in the second-line treatment of ovarian cancer *(41–43)*. Unfortunately, limited biologic activity has been observed, again demonstrating the major difficulty with attempting to translate the beneficial results of treatment in one cancer to another based solely on the apparent presence of a particular molecular "target" *(44,45)*.

5.4. *Antiangiogenesis Agents*

Ovarian cancer is an important tumor in which to evaluate antiangiogenic agents. Vascular endothelial growth factor (VEGF) expression has been shown to correlate with both the presence of the malignant ovarian phenotype and the poor prognosis in the cancer *(46)*. In addition, studies have revealed high VEGF serum levels in ovarian cancer to be associated with the presence of ascites and inferior survival.

Although the clinical relevance of these biologic markers has been unclear, the previously noted favorable results observed in the randomized trial of "maintenance paclitaxel" may be considered a possible "proof of principle" of the concept of inhibition of angiogenesis in ovarian cancer *(19)*. Existing preclinical data have suggested that relatively low concentrations of paclitaxel can produce an antiangiogenic effect *(47)*. Thus, it is conceivable that the favorable impact on outcome documented in this Phase III study may have been at least partially related to the impact of this agent on the tumor vasculature.

Several Phase II trials of single-agent bevacizumab have demonstrated a somewhat surprising level of biologic activity of the drug, with approximately 15% of patients with recurrent and platinum-resistant ovarian cancer achieving an objective response of measurable tumor masses *(48,49)*. Investigators have also explored a possible role for combining cytotoxic chemotherapy with bevacizumab *(50,51)*. Although responses have been reported in several series, it is important to note that there currently exist no randomized trial data to demonstrate if the level of biologic activity observed, and clinical benefit achieved, by adding this antiangiogenic agent to second-line ovarian cancer chemotherapy is superior to either bevacizumab or chemotherapy delivered alone. Ongoing Phase III randomized trials are examining the role of adding bevacizumab to primary chemotherapy in the management of advanced ovarian cancer. Based on the favorable experience with bevacizumab, it is likely that other agents with known antiangiogenic properties will be explored for possible use in advanced ovarian cancer.

Of particular clinical relevance is the fact that in several reports on the use of bevacizumab in ovarian cancer bowel perforation was observed as a particular side effect, an event uncommonly seen with other antineoplastic agents employed in this setting or associated with the natural history of the malignancy *(49)*. This unfortunate effect is likely to be related to the property of antiangiogenic agents to inhibit specific repair mechanisms (e.g., wound healing), a normal biologic process that may be quite important in preventing such events in individuals with significant intraabdominal tumor volumes. It is currently recommended by many investigators that this drug not be given to ovarian cancer patients with large-volume intraperitoneal disease or women who have "recently" (i.e., within the past few weeks) undergone major surgical cytoreductive procedures.

A second antiangiogenic agent, VEGF-Trap, has also been examined in a large Phase II trial in recurrent heavily pretreated ovarian cancer *(52)*. A response rate of approximately 10% has been reported in a preliminary analysis of the ongoing trial.

6. CONCLUSION

Despite the obvious attraction for both testing and subsequently routinely employing "targeted therapy" in the management of advanced ovarian cancer—it is a highly chemosensitive malignancy; there is an opportunity for extended survival with good quality of life despite documented disease recurrence; there exists a highly reliable tumor maker (CA-125)—progress in this arena has been surprisingly slower and more limited than in the setting of other malignancies. It is hoped that the provocative, but nonrandomized data regarding the biological activity of antiangiogenic agents in the second-line setting will subsequently be translated into a documented favorable impact on clinically relevant outcomes in ovarian cancer (e.g., improvement in symptom-free or overall survival, delay in cancer progression).

REFERENCES

1. Cannistra SA. Cancer of the ovary. N Engl J Med 2004;351:2519–9.
2. Hess V, A'Hern R, Nasiri N, et al. Mucinous epithelial ovarian cancer: a separate entity requiring specific treatment. J Clin Oncol 2004;22(6):1040–4.
3. Bergman F. Carcinoma of the ovary: a clinicopathological study of 86 autopsied cases with special reference to mode of spread. Acta Obstet Gynecol Scand 1966;45:211–31.
4. Covens AL. A critique of surgical cytoreduction in advanced ovarian cancer. Gynecol Oncol 2000;78(3 Pt 1):269–74.
5. Ozols RF, Bundy BN, Greer BE, et al. Phase III trial of carboplatin and paclitaxel compared with cisplatin and paclitaxel in patients with optimally resected stage III ovarian cancer: a Gynecologic Oncology Group study. J Clin Oncol 2003;21(17):3194–200.
6. Covens A, Carey M, Bryson P, et al. Systematic review of first-line chemotherapy for newly diagnosed postoperative patients with stage II, III, or IV epithelial ovarian cancer. Gynecol Oncol 2002;85(1):71–80.
7. McGuire WP, Hoskins WJ, Brady MF, et al. Cyclophosphamide and cisplatin compared with paclitaxel and cisplatin in patients with stage III and stage IV ovarian cancer. N Engl J Med 1996;334(1):1–6.
8. Advanced Ovarian Cancer Trialists Group. Chemotherapy in advanced ovarian cancer: four systematic meta-analyses of individual patient data from 37 randomized trials. Br J Cancer 1998;78(11):1479–87.
9. Vasey PA, Jayson GC, Gordon A, et al. Phase III randomized trial of docetaxel-carboplatin versus paclitaxel-carboplatin as first-line chemotherapy for ovarian carcinoma. J Natl Cancer Inst 2004;96(22):1682–91.
10. McGuire WP, Hoskins WJ, Brady MF, et al. Assessment of dose-intensive therapy in suboptimally debulked ovarian cancer: a Gynecologic Oncology Group study. J Clin Oncol 1995;13(7):1589–99.
11. Gore M, Mainwaring P, A'Hern R, et al. Randomized trial of dose-intensity with single-agent carboplatin in patients with epithelial ovarian cancer: London Gynaecological Oncology Group. J Clin Oncol 1998;16(7):2426–34.
12. Conte PF, Bruzzone M, Carnino F, et al. High-dose versus low-dose cisplatin in combination with cyclophosphamide and epidoxorubicin in suboptimal ovarian cancer: a randomized study of the Gruppo Oncologico Nord-Ovest. J Clin Oncol 1996;14(2):351–6.
13. Dedrick RL, Myers CE, Bungay PM, et al. Pharmacokinetic rationale for peritoneal drug administration in the treatment of ovarian cancer. Cancer Treat Rep 1978;62:1–9.
14. Alberts DS, Liu PY, Hannigan EV, et al. Intraperitoneal cisplatin plus intravenous cyclophosphamide versus intravenous cisplatin plus intravenous cyclophosphamide for stage III ovarian cancer. N Engl J Med 1996;335(26):1950–5.
15. Markman M, Bundy BN, Alberts DS, et al. Phase III trial of standard-dose intravenous cisplatin plus paclitaxel versus moderately high-dose carboplatin followed by intravenous paclitaxel and intraperitoneal cisplatin in small-volume stage III ovarian carcinoma: an Intergroup study of the Gynecologic Oncology Group, Southwestern Oncology Group, and Eastern Cooperative Oncology Group. J Clin Oncol 2001;19(4):1001–7.
16. Armstrong DK, Bundy B, Wenzel L, et al. Intraperitoneal cisplatin and paclitaxel in ovarian cancer. N Engl J Med 2006;354(1):34–43.
17. Trimble EL, Alvarez RD. Intraperitoneal chemotherapy and the NCI clinical announcement. Gynecol Oncol 2006;103(suppl 1):S18–9.
18. Hakes TB, Chalas E, Hoskins WJ, et al. Randomized prospective trial of 5 versus 10 cycles of cyclophosphamide, doxorubicin, and cisplatin in advanced ovarian carcinoma. Gynecol Oncol 1992;45(3):284–9.

19. Markman M, Liu PY, Wilczynski S, et al. Phase III randomized trial of 12 versus 3 months of maintenance paclitaxel in patients with advanced ovarian cancer after complete response to platinum and paclitaxel-based chemotherapy: a Southwest Oncology Group and Gynecologic Oncology Group trial. J Clin Oncol 2003;21(13):2460–5.

20. Markman M, Bookman MA. Second-line treatment of ovarian cancer. Oncologist 2000;5(1):26–35.

21. Markman M. Why study third-, fourth-, fifth-, ...line chemotherapy of ovarian cancer? Gynecol Oncol 2001;83(3):449–50.

22. Markman M. Viewing ovarian cancer as a "chronic disease": what exactly does this mean? Gynecol Oncol 2006;100(2):229–30.

23. Markman M, Markman J, Webster K, et al. Duration of response to second-line, platinum-based chemotherapy for ovarian cancer: implications for patient management and clinical trial design. J Clin Oncol 2004;22(15):3120–5.

24. Bridgewater JA, Nelstrop AE, Rustin GJ, et al. Comparison of standard and CA-125 response criteria in patients with epithelial ovarian cancer treated with platinum or paclitaxel. J Clin Oncol 1999;17(2):501–8.

25. Rustin GJ, Marples M, Nelstrop AE, et al. Use of CA-125 to define progression of ovarian cancer in patients with persistently elevated levels. J Clin Oncol 2001;19(20):4054–7.

26. Rustin GJ, Timmers P, Nelstrop A, et al. Comparison of CA-125 and standard definitions of progression of ovarian cancer in the intergroup trial of cisplatin and paclitaxel versus cisplatin and cyclophosphamide. J Clin Oncol 2006;24(1):45–51.

27. Berchuck A, Kamel A, Whitaker R, et al. Overexpression of HER-2/neu is associated with poor survival in advanced epithelial ovarian cancer. Cancer Res 1990;50(13):4087–91.

28. Felip E, del Campo JM, Rubio D, et al. Overexpression of c-erbB-2 in epithelial ovarian cancer: prognostic value and relationship with response to chemotherapy. Cancer 1995;75(8):2147–52.

29. Meden H, Marx D, Roegglen T, et al. Overexpression of the oncogene c-erbB-2 (HER2/neu) and response to chemotherapy in patients with ovarian cancer. Int J Gynecol Pathol 1998;17(1):61–5.

30. Bookman MA, Darcy KM, Clarke-Pearson D, et al. Evaluation of monoclonal humanized anti-HER2 antibody, trastuzumab, in patients with recurrent or refractory ovarian or primary peritoneal carcinoma with overexpression of HER2: a phase II trial of the Gynecologic Oncology Group. J Clin Oncol 2003;21(2): 283–90.

31. Makhija S, Glenn D, Ueland F, et al. Results from a phase II randomized, placebo-controlled, double-blind trial suggest improved PFS with the addition of pertuzumab to gemcitabine in patients with platinum-resistant ovarian, fallopian tube, or primary peritoneal cancer. J Clin Oncol 2007;25(18s):275s. Abstract 5507.

32. Kohler M, Janz I, Wintzer HO, et al. The expression of EGF receptors, EGF-like factors and c-myc in ovarian and cervical carcinomas and their potential clinical significance. Anticancer Res 1989;9(6):1537–47.

33. Berchuck A, Rodriguez GC, Kamel A, et al. Epidermal growth factor receptor expression in normal ovarian epithelium and ovarian cancer. I. Correlation of receptor expression with prognostic factors in patients with ovarian cancer. Am J Obstet Gynecol 1991;164(2):669–74.

34. Wagner U, duBois A, Pfisterer J, et al. Gefitinib in combination with tamoxifen in patients with ovarian cancer refractory or resistant to platinum-taxane based therapy—a phase II trial of the AGO Ovarian Cancer Study Group (AGO-OVAR 2.6). Gynecol Oncol 2007;105(1):132–7.

35. Seiden MV, Burris HA, Matulonis U, et al. A phase II trial of EMD72000 (matuzumab), a humanized anti-EGFR monoclonal antibody, in patients with platinum-resistant ovarian and primary peritoneal malignancies. Gynecol Oncol 2007;104(3):727–31.

36. Schilder RJ, Sill MW, Chen X, et al. Phase II study of gefitinib in patients with relapsed or persistent ovarian or primary peritoneal carcinoma and evaluation of epidermal growth factor receptor mutations and immuno-histochemical expression: a Gynecologic Oncology Group Study. Clin Cancer Res 2005;11(15):5539–48.

37. Posadas EM, Liel MS, Kwitkowski V, et al. A phase II and pharmacodynamic study of gefitinib in patients with refractory or recurrent epithelial ovarian cancer. Cancer 2007;109:1323–30.

38. Engelman JA, Zejnullahu K, Mitsudomi T, et al. MET amplification leads to gefitinib resistance in lung cancer by activating ERBB3 signaling. Science 2007;316:1039–43.

39. Goldman JM, Melo JV. Targeting the BCR-ABL tyrosine kinase in chronic myeloid leukemia. N Engl J Med 2001;344(14):1084–6.

40. Demetri GD, von MM, Blanke CD, et al. Efficacy and safety of imatinib mesylate in advanced gastrointestinal stromal tumors. N Engl J Med 2002;347(7):472–80.

41. Schmandt RE, Broaddus R, Lu KH, et al. Expression of c-ABL, c-KIT, and platelet-derived growth factor receptor-beta in ovarian serous carcinoma and normal ovarian surface epithelium. Cancer 2003;98(4): 758–64.

42. Apte SM, Fan D, Killion JJ, et al. Targeting the platelet-derived growth factor receptor in antivascular therapy for human ovarian carcinoma. Clin Cancer Res 2004;10:897–908.

43. Matei D, Chang DD, Jeng MH. Imatinib mesylate (Gleevec) inhibits ovarian cancer cell growth through a mechanism dependent on platelet-derived growth factor receptor alpha and Akt inactivation. Clin Cancer Res 2004;10:681–90

44. Coleman RL, Broaddus RR, Bodurka DC, et al. Phase II trial of imatinib mesylate in patients with recurrent platinum- and taxane-resistant epithelial ovarian and primary peritoneal cancer. Gynecol Oncol 2006;101:126–31.

45. Alberts DS, Liu PY, Wilczynski SP, et al. Phase II trial of imatinib mesylate in recurrent, biomarker positive, ovarian cancer. Int J Gynecol Cancer 2007;17:784–8.

46. Frumovitz M, Sood AK. Vascular endothelial growth factor (VEGF) pathway as a therapeutic target in gynecologic malignancies. Gynecol Oncol 2007;104(3):768–78.

47. Bocci G, Nicolaou KC, Kerbel RS. Protracted low-dose effects on human endothelial cell proliferation and survival in vitro reveal a selective antiangiogenic window for various chemotherapeutic drugs. Cancer Res 2002;62:6938–43.

48. Burger RA, Sill M, Monk BJ, et al. Phase II trial of bevacizumab in persistent or recurrent epithelial ovarian cancer or primary peritoneal cancer: a Gynecologic Oncology Group study. J Clin Oncol 2005;23 (suppl 1):457s. Abstract 5009.

49. Cannistra SA, Matulonis U, Person R, et al. Bevacizumab in patients with advanced platinum-resistant ovarian cancer. J Clin Oncol 2006;34(18S):257s. Abstract 5006.

50. Garcia AA, Oza AM, Hirte H, et al. Interim report of a phase II clinical trial of bevacizumab and low dose metronomic oral cyclophosphamide in recurrent ovarian and primary peritoneal carcinoma: a California Cancer Consortium Trial. J Clin Oncol 2005;23(suppl 1):455s. Abstract 5000.

51. Wright JD, Hagemann A, Rader JS, et al. Bevacizumab combination therapy in recurrent, platinum-refractory epithelial ovarian carcinoma. Cancer 2006;107:83–9.

52. Tew WP, Colombo N, Ray-Coquard I, et al. VEGF-Trap for patients with recurrent platinum-resistant epithelial ovarian cancer: preliminary results of a randomized multi-center phase II study. J Clin Oncol 2007;25(18s):276s. Abstract 5008.

13 Targeted Drug Therapy in Pancreatic Cancer

Don L. Gibbons, MD, PhD, Robert A. Wolff, MD, and Gauri Varadhachary, MD

Contents

Abstract

Only modest progress has been made in improving the overall survival of pancreatic cancer patients during the past 20 years with standard cytotoxic chemotherapy drugs. More work needs to be done to address the key biologic characteristics of pancreatic cancer that make it so aggressive, metastasizing at an early stage, and more refractory to standard treatments than most other solid tumor types. Here, we discuss the emerging role of targeted therapy in pancreatic cancer and the status of currently available and tested agents. We also point out the potential pitfalls in current trial designs and recommend new methods for testing novel compounds in this heterogeneous and difficult-to-treat group of patients.

Key Words: Targeted therapy, Pancreatic cancer, Chemotherapy, Clinical trials

From: *Current Clinical Oncology: Targeted Cancer Therapy*
Edited by: R. Kurzrock and M. Markman © Humana Press, Totowa, NJ

1. INTRODUCTION

Pancreatic adenocarcinoma is a challenging disease to treat owing to its late stage of detection, with a disproportionate number of patients presenting with locally advanced or metastatic disease, and its resistance to conventional cytotoxic chemotherapy drugs. As a result, approximately 33,000 of the estimated 37,000 patients diagnosed with pancreatic adenocarcinoma in the United States in 2007 will die of the disease (1). Only 20% of newly diagnosed patients will have early-stage, potentially resectable disease. However, 75% of these will have computed tomography (CT)-occult extrapancreatic disease that eventually leads to recurrence. The 1-year overall survival rate of the remaining 80% of newly diagnosed patients with locally advanced or metastatic pancreatic adenocarcinoma is a dismal 18%.

Historically, chemotherapy for advanced pancreatic adenocarcinoma centered on the use of fluorouracil (5-FU), either alone or in combination with other cytotoxic agents, with significantly variable response rates (2). However, improvements in cross-sectional imaging techniques revealed that in many early studies the benefits of 5-FU treatment were likely overestimated (2,3).

More recent studies have consistently demonstrated that single-agent gemcitabine, a ribonucleotide reductase inhibitor, is modestly effective against pancreatic adenocarcinoma (4). Burris et al. (5) performed the landmark trial comparing gemcitabine and 5-FU that led to gemcitabine's approval by the U.S. Food and Drug Administration (FDA) and established it as the standard of care for patients with advanced pancreatic cancer. The authors demonstrated both a clinical benefit response (as measured by pain medication need, weight gain, and improvement in performance status) of 23.8% in patients treated with gemcitabine compared to 4.8% for patients treated with 5-FU. The study also revealed a 1-year overall survival rate of 18% with gemcitabine and 2% with 5-FU. Median overall survival durations of 5.6 and 4.4 months were found for patients treated with gemcitabine and 5-FU, respectively ($p = 0.0025$). However, the objective response rates were only 5.4% with gemcitabine and 0% with 5-FU. In other trials, objective response rates of approximately 10% have been found for gemcitabine. Because gemcitabine is associated with relatively mild toxicity, it has become the standard of care for palliative treatment of patients with advanced pancreatic cancer.

Researchers have attempted to optimize the effectiveness of gemcitabine by adjusting the method of delivery to match the mechanism of cellular uptake and activation. On the basis of the results of preclinical and pharmacokinetic studies, an alternative infusion method was devised, termed fixed dose rate (FDR). With FDR infusion, gemcitabine is given at 10 mg/m/hr, rather than the standard 30-minute infusion. The plasma concentration using FDR infusion results in maximal intracellular levels of the active gemcitabine triphosphate moiety. In a multicenter Phase II trial of 92 patients (6), a statistically significant longer median survival duration was found among patients in the FDR arm than in the standard dose schedule arm (5 vs. 8 months). Similarly, the 1- and 2-year overall survival rates in the standard dose versus FDR arms were 9.0% vs. 28.8% and 2.2% vs.18.3%, respectively. Unfortunately, the preliminary results of a recent randomized Phase III trial (ECOG 6201) of 833 patients (7) demonstrated no significant difference in response rate or overall survival between standard-dose gemcitabine, FDR gemcitabine, and standard-dose gemcitabine combined with oxaliplatin.

Recent data from a randomized Phase III trial (8) revealed that gemcitabine combined with oxaliplatin resulted in a higher response rate (26.8% vs. 17.3%), clinical benefit rate (38.2% vs. 26.9%), and progression-free survival (PFS) duration (5.8 vs. 3.7 months) than single-agent gemcitabine; however, the combination resulted in only nonsignificant improvement in the median overall survival duration (9.0 vs. 7.1 months; p = NS). Similar but slightly less robust results have also been shown for the combination of gemcitabine and cisplatin (9). To our knowledge, no combination of cytotoxic chemotherapy drugs has clearly demonstrated superiority to gemcitabine alone in a randomized trial; thus, more effective agents are needed for this intransigent disease.

2. BIOLOGY OF THE DISEASE

We discuss here various pathways that have been implicated in pancreatic cancer oncogenesis and review clinical trials of agents that target these pathways. Of note, several of the most promising trials rely on a combination of treatments, such as standard cytotoxic therapy plus a targeted agent or two different targeted agents.

A substantial number of studies have been conducted in recent years to understand better the biologic characteristics of pancreatic adenocarcinoma and thus improve treatment with cytotoxic agents and develop agents that target specific molecular and cellular defects, such as is being done in breast and colon cancer treatment. Three main biologic characteristics of pancreatic adenocarcinoma still need to be clarified: the role of particular genes in each step of oncogenesis, the molecular mechanisms by which the tumor becomes locally invasive at an early stage and metastasizes, and the cellular or molecular basis for pancreatic cancer cells' resistance to chemotherapy.

The results of studies of the biologic characteristics of pancreatic adenocarcinoma in both animal models and human pathologic specimens suggest that normal tissue progresses through multiple stages of dysplasia characterized by small-caliber ductal changes in the type of epithelium, distortion of the cellular architecture, and increasing numbers of atypical nuclei (termed PanIN, for pancreatic intraepithelial neoplasia), eventually developing into invasive adenocarcinoma (10). This progression is caused by the accumulation of mutations in multiple cellular pathways and the development of substantial genetic instability. Studies of surgical pancreatic cancer specimens have revealed focal areas of adenocarcinoma on a background of dysplastic changes throughout the tissue, with genetic heterogeneity seen in both adjacent and distant nonmalignant tissue (10,11). These pathologic changes do not appear to follow a strict timeline, as multiple initiating molecular events can substitute for one another, but this overall model of cumulative genetic and histologic changes is well supported in preclinical studies, revealing that particular pathways are prominent in pancreatic cancer oncogenesis. This linear evolution model is similar to those proposed for other malignancies, such as colon cancer.

Understanding the mechanisms of pancreatic adenocarcinoma oncogenesis is critical to treating the disease because patients' disease characteristics may vary, producing significant variability in their response to treatment. Several molecules have been identified as being commonly involved in the development of pancreatic cancer; these molecules are either involved in early carcinogenic events or in the development of genomic instability and thus an invasive and metastatic phenotype (Table 1) (10,12). In most cases, an activating event, such as a gain-of-function mutation, loss of regulatory interaction, or overexpression, allows one or several mitogenic pathways to be engaged, resulting in cells receiving stimuli for unregulated growth and proliferation. Often, these stimuli are concomitant with dysregulation of the normal apoptotic pathways.

It is argued that tumor xenografts and cell-based assays are not the most optimal method for evaluating the efficacy of a new agent as they do not simulate the histology or genetic

Table 1
Molecules Commonly Involved in the Development of Pancreatic Cancer

Gene	Event	Percent of cases	Stage of progression
KRAS (30–32)	Activating mutation	~100	Early
p53 (83,84)	Inactivating mutation	> 50	Late
EGFR (21,22)	Over-expression Ligand over-expression	90	Early
INK4A (83,84)	Mutation Deletion Hypermethylation	80–95	Middle to late
SMAD4 (83,85)	Homozygous deletion Inactivating mutation	50	Late

mutations seen in human pancreatic cancer. Development of targeted mouse models is showing promise and may prove to be a better model for predicting therapeutic efficacy in pancreatic cancer. A number of mouse models have been developed during the past few years. The "KPC" mouse model is of particular interest because it develops advanced pancreatic cancer with 100% penetrance at an early age and mimics many features of human pancreatic cancer, including histology, metastasis to relevant sites, cachexia, activation of biochemical pathways, and evidence of genomic instability (13).

Figure 1 iillustrates several pathways that have been implicated in the oncogenic transformation and phenotypic perpetuation of pancreatic adenocarcinoma. In the following paragraphs we discuss various pathways involved and agents tested to target these pathways.

3. AGENTS TARGETING EPIDERMAL GROWTH FACTOR RECEPTOR

Epidermal growth factor receptor (EGFR), or ErbB-1/HER1, is a receptor tyrosine kinase (TK) that belongs to the ErbB family, which has four members: EGFR, ErbB-2/HER2 (neu), ErbB-3/HER3, and ErbB-4/HER4 (14,15). The basic structure of this receptor family includes an extracellular ligand-binding domain, a membrane-spanning domain, and an intracellular TK domain (16). Multiple ligands for these receptors have been identified, including epidermal growth factor (EGF) and the EGF-like growth factors transforming growth factor-α (TGFα), epiregulin, amphiregulin, and members of the neuregulin family (14,15,17,18). EGFR is an inactive monomer; and after binding of the extracellular domain of the receptor to a ligand, it forms homodimers or heterodimers with another monomer from the ErbB family. This dimerization step activates the autophosphorylation of the TK domain at multiple sites (19). Three major (Tyr1068, Tyr1148, Tyr1173) and two minor (Tyr992, Tyr1086) sites of phosphorylation have been identified in the TK domain (14,15). Phosphorylation of any of these sites induces structural changes in the protein, allowing it to interact with several intracellular proteins and resulting in the activation of at least two major signal transduction pathways: the mitogen-activated protein kinase (MAPK) and AKT pathways (Fig. 1). Both of these pathways are involved in cell proliferation, apoptosis, angiogenesis promotion, and metastasis (20). As EGF is the upstream activator of these pathways, specific inhibition of EGFR or EGFR-TK activity should be effective against tumors with aberrant expression or activation of EGFR.

Two available strategies to target these pathways are (1) monoclonal antibodies that specifically bind the extracellular portion of EGFR (the antibody studied in pancreatic

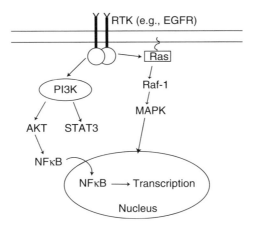

Fig. 1. Activated pathways involved in oncogenesis of pancreatic adenocarcinoma. A simplified schema illustrates general receptor tyrosine kinase activation, with downstream signaling pathway activation. Activation of the mitogen-activated protein kinase (MAPK) pathway and the phosphoinositol-3-kinase (PI3K) pathways, with their downstream effectors, have been demonstrated to be involved in cellular activation and transformation.

adenocarcinoma is cetuximab); and (2) small molecules with TK inhibitory activity (EGFR-TK inhibitors). The latter compounds reversibly or irreversibly compete with ATP molecules by directly or indirectly blocking the ATP binding site in the TK domain of EGFR, thereby interrupting downstream signaling. The most widely studied members of this drug class are erlotinib and gefitinib.

Several studies have evaluated the role of EGFR activation in the development and progression of pancreatic cancer. An immunohistochemical analysis of pancreatic cancer specimens revealed that EGFR was overexpressed in up to 90% of samples, as were the activating ligands EGF and TGFα; thus, it is possible that pancreatic adenocarcinoma cells are driven to proliferate by the activation of a paracrine loop (21,22). In fact, expression of the receptor and its ligands was correlated with the clinical aggressiveness of the cancer and patient survival (23). This overexpression has also been found in premalignant lesions and chronic pancreatitis tissue specimens, suggesting that it plays a role in the earliest stages of tumor development (24). Of interest, activating EGFR mutations, similar to those identified for non-small-cell lung cancer, have been found in a few clinical pancreatic cancer specimens after laser-capture microdissection (25). The results of these studies suggest that multiple mechanisms exist by which EGFR is aberrantly activated in pancreatic cancer. The difficulty of applying this information to the development of new treatments lies in understanding by what specific mechanism EGFR mutation or overexpression results in unregulated cell growth, especially given the likely coexistence of other mutational events in the same or interacting pathways (e.g., activation of the downstream KRAS molecule in a large percentage of tumors) (see further discussion below).

Cetuximab is a human-mouse chimeric monoclonal antibody with high affinity and specificity for EGFR, which acts to block EGF binding. It was approved by the U.S. Food and Drug Administration (FDA) for the treatment of colorectal carcinoma and squamous cell carcinoma of the head and neck. Xiong and colleagues reported their Phase II data with cetuximab and gemcitabine in 41 patients with locally advanced (15%) or metastatic (85%) pancreatic carcinoma, all of whom had positive staining for EGFR on immunohistochemical analysis of either the primary or metastatic tissue (26). In total, 5 patients (12%) experienced a partial response and 26 had stable disease (SD) (63%), with a median time to progression of 3.8 months and median overall survival duration of 7.1 months. The 1-year overall survival rate was 31.7%, which was better than that for gemcitabine alone (18%) and justified further study. The results of this study also highlight an emerging theme in clinical trials of targeted agents: Many of these agents have cytostatic rather than cytotoxic effects, making it difficult to compare the two types of agent directly or to assess the effectiveness of the new agents.

Based on the Phase II data with cetuximab and gemcitabine, the Southwest Oncology Group closed enrollment in April 2006 for an open-label Phase III trial (SWOG 0205) of > 700 patients who have been randomly assigned to receive either gemcitabine alone or gemcitabine and cetuximab for advanced pancreatic adenocarcinoma. Preliminary analysis of data from this trial show disappointing results with no survival benefit after the addition of cetuximab to gemcitabine *(27)*.

Other researchers are evaluating the effectiveness of cetuximab in combination with doublet chemotherapy. Cetuximab plus gemcitabine and oxaliplatin is currently being tested as a first-line treatment for metastatic pancreatic cancer in a Phase II study of 64 patients *(28)*. A similar combination is being studied at The University of Texas M. D. Anderson Cancer Center for locally advanced pancreatic cancer (C. Crane, NCT338039). The patients are treated with gemcitabine, oxaliplatin, and cetuximab for 2 months, followed by concomitant cetuximab and capecitabine plus radiation therapy and then maintenance doses of gemcitabine and cetuximab. The goal of these and other ongoing studies is to determine the optimal method of combining monoclonal antibody-mediated inhibition of the EGFR pathway and cytotoxic therapy. Ultimately, Phase III studies are needed to determine whether these combination regimens are more effective than standard treatment.

Small-molecule EGFR-TK inhibitors bind the C-terminal domain of the protein and compete for ATP binding, thereby inhibiting phosphorylation. These inhibitors have been effective in specific subsets of patients with metastatic non-small-cell lung cancer and gained their first FDA-approved indication in that setting. In a recent Phase III trial conducted by the National Cancer Institute of Canada *(29)*, 569 patients with pancreatic cancer were randomly assigned to receive either gemcitabine alone or gemcitabine and erlotinib. Patients were treated with 100 mg or 150 mg daily of erlotinib, an orally bioavailable TK inhibitor, and gemcitabine 1000 mg/m^2/week for 7 of 8 weeks. Patients in the erlotinib group had higher overall survival [hazard ratio (HR) 0.81] and progression-free survival (PFS) (HR 0.76) rates than patients in the gemcitabine alone arm. The median survival durations were 6.37 and 5.91 months, respectively ($p = 0.025$), and the 1-year survival rates were 24% and 17%, respectively. This study was the first to demonstrate in a Phase III trial that a combination regimen results in a significantly greater survival benefit than gemcitabine alone. On the basis of these data, erlotinib in combination with gemcitabine was approved by the FDA for the treatment of advanced pancreatic cancer. An immunohistochemical analysis of the tumor specimens from this trial revealed that 53% were EGFR-positive (> 10% of tumor cells with membrane staining for EGFR) and 47% were EGFR-negative ($\leq$ 10% stained). No apparent correlation was found between overall survival and receptor expression, as determined by immunohistochemical analysis. No tests are currently available to identify which patients would benefit from the addition of this agent to their chemotherapy regimen(s). This problem is further complicated by the coexistence of EGFR-independent mechanisms of cellular activation, the mutation or overexpression of which could nullify or bypass the effect of EGFR inhibition.

4. AGENTS TARGETING THE *KRAS* PROTO-ONCOGENE

The *KRAS* proto-oncogene contains a mutated codon 12 in 75% to 90% of pancreatic adenocarcinoma cases. The mutation appears to occur early in the oncogenic process *(30–32)* and is also found in some patients with chronic pancreatitis *(33)*. The mutated *KRAS* proto-oncogene releases Ras from regulation by the small GTPase-activating proteins, resulting in constitutive activation of Ras and the multiple downstream pathways that drive proliferation, growth, and antiapoptosis (Fig. 1); it thus allows the transformed phenotype to be maintained *(34)*.

Because the *KRAS* mutation stabilizes the ATP-bound form of Ras protein and makes it resistant to the activating effects of GTPase-activating proteins, pharmacologic inhibition of Ras activity has been difficult to achieve. Consequently, efforts to inhibit the Ras signaling pathway have centered on targeting the isoprenylation reaction performed by farnesyltransferase, the enzyme responsible for the addition of a 15-carbon farnesyl lipid moiety to the carboxyl-terminal cysteine *(35,36)*. Farnesylation is the posttranslational modification responsible for the targeting and partial anchoring of the Ras protein to the plasma membrane, where it is anchored to the internal leaflet of the cell membrane and is an intermediary in regulated signaling pathways (Fig. 1).

Several Phase II studies showed that the farnesyltransferase inhibitor tipifarnib (R115777), when used as a single agent, was not effective against locally advanced or metastatic pancreatic cancer, despite positive preclinical findings *(37,38)*. In a large multicenter, Phase III trial, 688 patients with metastatic or locally advanced disease were randomly assigned to receive either gemcitabine plus tipifarnib or gemcitabine alone *(39)*. The combination therapy was well tolerated but provided no clinical benefit or survival advantage over gemcitabine alone.

Tipifarnib may not be effective against pancreatic cancer cells because these cells have other prenyltransferase enzymes, such as geranylgeranyltransferase I and II, that produce similar posttranslational modifications and thus allow the inhibited farnesyltransferase pathway to be bypassed *(35,36)*. In addition, prenylation does not permanently anchor the protein to the membrane; and depending on the Ras isoform, additional protein modification occurs by palmitoylation or acylation. The overall outcome of peripheral membrane association is influenced by the additional complexities of regulated membrane protein association, including interaction with membrane lipid microdomains and protein polybasic motifs that mediate protein-lipid head binding, along with protein–protein interactions.

5. AGENTS TARGETING VASCULAR ENDOTHELIAL GROWTH FACTOR

Tumors are extremely vascular structures, although the vasculature of new tumors is immature and poorly functional *(40,41)*. Vascular endothelial growth factor (VEGF) is critical to this process *(42)*. The VEGF gene family includes VEGF-A, VEGF-B, VEGF-C, VEGF-D, VEGF-E, and placental growth factor, which are processed by undergoing splice variation into multiple isoforms with variable biologic functions *(43)*. The protein ligands homodimerize or heterodimerize and then bind to a related set of receptor TKs, the VEGF receptor (VEGFR) family, which includes *fms*-like TK-1 (FLT1, VEGFR-1), the kinase insert domain-containing receptor (KDR, VEGFR-2), and *fms*-like TK-4 (FLT4, VEGFR-3), all of which have been found on vascular or lymphatic endothelial cells. VEGF overexpression in malignant cells disrupts the careful homeostatic balance of angiogenesis or lymphangiogenesis, allowing malignant cells to produce a change in the surrounding environment by effecting an overabundance of immature and leaky vasculature.

Pancreatic cancer tumor samples have been found to have higher VEGF expression levels than normal pancreatic tissue, which are correlated with microvasculature density, liver metastasis, and overall survival (44–46). As with EGFR, VEGFR activity can be inhibited using one of several agents—antibodies against VEGF, soluble decoy receptors (so-called VEGF Trap), VEGFR antibodies, or small-molecule inhibitors that target the TK activity of the receptor (some of which are multikinase inhibitors). One of the most studied of these agents is bevacizumab, a humanized monoclonal antibody that recognizes VEGF.

Researchers initially believed that targeting the angiogenic process would disrupt the vasculature of extremely sensitive tumors, cutting off the blood supply and causing cell death. However, it is now believed that the antiangiogenic effects have preferential activity on small, immature vessels in the tumor, causing a "pruning" effect that leads to pseudonormalization of the remaining large vasculature (41,47). This streamlining of vascular architecture is believed to enhance the delivery of cytotoxic agents given in combination. In addition, the use of two compounds more effectively targets the two cell types—rapidly proliferating tumor cells and vascular endothelial cells. The use of antivascular agents such as bevacizumab with cytotoxic chemotherapy has resulted in significant clinical benefits in trials of other tumor types, including lung, colon, and breast tumors (48).

In a Phase II trial (49) of 52 patients with metastatic pancreatic adenocarcinoma (83% of whom had liver metastases), the combination of gemcitabine and bevacizumab resulted in partial responses (PRs) in 11 patients (21%) and stabilized disease (SD) in 24 patients (46%), with a median survival duration of 8.8 months. On the basis of these findings, the Cancer and Leukemia Group B conducted a randomized, placebo-controlled Phase III trial (CALGB 80303) of single-agent gemcitabine versus gemcitabine with bevacizumab in 602 patients with pancreatic adenocarcinoma (50). The overall disease control [combined complete responses (CR), PR, and SD] rates were 54% for gemcitabine plus bevacizumab and 47% for gemcitabine alone; this difference was not statistically significant. The median overall survival and PFS durations were also similar (6.0 vs. 4.5 months, respectively). These results are disappointing given the effectiveness of bevacizumab in combination with cytotoxic agents in other tumor types. However, the different outcomes in these two trials may be attributable to differences in patient selection, with more patients having a performance status of 0 in the Phase II trial and more with a performance status of 2 in the Phase III trial.

Several studies are evaluating multidrug combinations that simultaneously target angiogenesis and EGFR, in addition to the general cytotoxic effects of gemcitabine. Moreover, a Phase III trial in Europe is being conducted to determine the effectiveness of adding bevacizumab to gemcitabine and erlotinib. A randomized Phase II trial is being conducted of gemcitabine, bevacizumab, and cetuximab or erlotinib by the University of Chicago (Chicago, IL, USA) in 126 patients (NCI 6590).

6. AGENTS TARGETING MATRIX METALLOPROTEINASES

The early stages of cancer growth and metastasis involve invasion into surrounding tissues and cellular migration from the site of origin into vascular or lymphatic structures. For this process to occur, the extracellular matrix must be degraded. The large family of zinc-dependent proteases, termed matrix metalloproteinases (MMPs) are capable of degrading the extracellular matrix *(51)*. MMPs are normally activated during physiologic events such as wound healing and embryogenesis, and their activity is regulated by tissue-specific inhibitors. An imbalance between MMP activation and tissue-specific inhibition occurs in many malignant states, which may be partially caused by up-regulated expression levels secondary to activation of the mitogen-activated kinase pathway *(52–54)*. MMP-2 and MMP-9 are two enzymes that are overexpressed in pancreatic cancer, and their overexpression is correlated with the invasion and metastasis of the primary tumor. Resected tumor specimens from patients with pancreatic cancer had elevated MMP-2 expression that was not found in normal pancreatic tissue from transplant donor patients *(55)*. MMP inhibitors demonstrate efficacy in vitro and decrease the size and number of metastatic lesions in orthotopic animal models *(56,57)* but the results of clinical trials have been less dramatic.

Several MMP inhibitors have been tested in Phase I and II trials, including marimastat and BAY 12-9566 (Bayer, West Haven, CT, USA). In a randomized Phase II study *(58)* of 414 patients with locally advanced or metastatic disease, patients receiving the highest dose of marimastat had the same median and overall 1-year survival rates as patients receiving gemcitabine alone. The toxicities were primarily musculoskeletal in nature, reversible, and considered acceptable. The National Cancer Institute of Canada *(59)* conducted a Phase II trial of BAY 12-9566 in 277 patients with advanced pancreatic cancer (68% with metastatic disease to the liver, 14% with metastases in the lungs, and 18% with locally advanced pancreatic cancer). Patients were randomly assigned to receive either oral BAY 12-9566 (800 mg twice daily) or intravenous gemcitabine (1000 mg/m^2 weekly) for 7 of 8 weeks. The trial was stopped after the second interim analysis because longer PFS (3.54 vs. 1.77 months) and median overall survival (6.4 vs. 3.2 months) durations were found among patients treated with gemcitabine than patients in the BAY 12-9566 arm.

Unfortunately, the trial designs used in the above studies may not have been optimal. Mechanistically, these drugs are expected to be most effective at preventing the metastatic spread of locally advanced disease or controlling the spread of micrometastatic disease. However, 60% to 70% of patients in these trials *(51,52)* had gross metastatic disease at the start of the studies. Rather than comparing the clinical response of patients receiving a cytotoxic drug such as gemcitabine with that of patients receiving a cytostatic drug, one could compare gemcitabine alone with gemcitabine and an oral MMP compound. Alternatively, given the high rate of disease recurrence after curative-intent surgery (suggesting a high rate of CT occult micrometastases), these cytostatic MMP drugs could be studied as adjuvant therapy.

7. AGENTS INHIBITING PHOSPHOINOSITOL-3-KINASE

Activation of the phosphoinsitol-3-kinase (PI3K) signal transduction pathway, with downstream activation of AKT and nuclear factor-kB (NFkB), has demonstrated several important roles in oncogenesis. Its two most prominent roles are cell activation and apoptosis inhibition. Increased constitutive activity of this pathway has been found in pancreatic cancer cell lines and tumor samples *(60)*. Additionally, in vitro studies have shown that treating cells with gemcitabine or cisplatin alone activates AKT and NFkB, causing the oncogenic cells to become resistant to cytotoxic agents. This chemotherapy-induced resistance is enhanced under hypoxic conditions *(61)*. PI3K inhibition has thus been studied as a way to block cellular activation and resensitize cells to chemotherapeutic agents *(62,63)*.

Genistein is a soy isoflavone that inhibits PI3K activity. It has been evaluated, in combination with erlotinib or gemcitabine, in multiple studies of pancreatic cancer cell lines to determine the relative roles of the components involved *(64)*. These in vitro experiments have demonstrated that in human pancreatic cancer cells, the combination of genistein and gemcitabine or cisplatin results in 60% to 80% growth inhibition, whereas gemcitabine alone results in only 30% inhibition. In studies of genistein in orthotopic mice, treatment with genistein decreased the size of the pancreatic mass irrespective of the metastatic potential of the tumor *(62,65)*. The inhibition of tumor cell growth by genistein appears to work by dephosphorylation of AKT, abrogating NFkB DNA-binding activity, with subsequent down-regulation of Bcl-2 and Bcl-xL, thus allowing apoptotic cell death. In vitro and in vivo studies of genistein in combination with cisplatin demonstrated that NFkB is down-regulated, resulting in enhanced cell killing by cisplatin, likely because of reduced chemoresistance *(65)*. However, these relatively short experiments in mice did not determine whether this combined regimen suppresses metastases. Taken together, the results of these studies demonstrate that the addition of genistein to chemotherapy results in enhanced growth inhibition and apoptosis.

Similar results of enhanced growth inhibition and apoptosis were found in an in vitro study comparing erlotinib with erlotinib plus genistein due to inhibition of NFkB-induced EGFR expression *(64)*. In addition, genistein appears to block the up-regulation of EGFR expression that occurs with the use of TK inhibitors alone, providing a second possible mechanism for its inhibitory effect *(66)*. Another important finding in these studies was the diversity in cell lines that accounts for their growth activation; in some cases AKT activation is EGFR–dependent, and in other cases it is partially or not dependent. These differences appear to mimic those observed clinically and should be factored into both preclinical and clinical study designs.

On the basis of the preclinical data on genistein, a multicenter Phase II trial (NCT00376948) in 40 patients is being conducted to determine whether genistein enhances the effects of gemcitabine and erlotinib regimens.

8. AGENTS TARGETING SIGNAL TRANSDUCER AND ACTIVATOR OF TRANSCRIPTION 3

Signal transducer and activator of transcription 3 (STAT3) is a cytosolic transcription factor that forms homodimers in response to Janus kinase phosphorylation, translocates to the cell nucleus, binds to STAT3-specific DNA-binding elements, and transcriptionally activates genes involved in cell cycle progression, angiogenesis, and apoptosis, such as Bcl-xL, MMP2, and VEGF. STAT3 is overexpressed in pancreatic cancer cell lines and human tumor samples, with concomitant high levels of the activated phosphoprotein *(67,68)*. Its expression level appears to increase in response to chemotherapeutic agents, such as gemcitabine, thus leading to apoptosis resistance. The results of several studies indicate that inhibition of the Janus kinase/STAT pathway modulates the invasive and metastatic phenotype of pancreatic cancer cells *(67,69)*.

When screening for molecules that could prevent or reverse the development of chemoresistance in malignant cells, a previously developed pharmaceutical was identified: bromovinyldeoxyuridine (BVDU) [(E)-5-(2-bromovinyl)-2´-deoxyuridine] *(70)*, which is being developed under the name RP101 for chemotherapeutic uses. BVDU was originally developed and marketed in Europe as an antiviral compound for herpesvirus infections (primarily herpes simplex virus-1 and varicella zoster virus) *(71)*. It acts as a substrate for the virus-encoded thymidine kinase, and this initial phosphorylation event allows further cellular phosphorylation, producing an adduct that inhibits the viral DNA polymerase. In addition, BVDU has a broad range of effects on cancer cells, including the suppression of chemotherapy-induced up-regulation of multidrug resistance genes and the pro-prosurvival and antiapoptotic pathways, as well as repression of the DNA repair machinery *(72)*. Because it prevents the development of chemoresistance, RP101 has synergistic effects with cytotoxic agents such as gemcitabine, cisplatin, doxorubicin, and methotrexate. Multiple tumor types, both in vitro and in vivo, have demonstrated an enhanced response to chemotherapy treatment with RP101.

Surprising results have been found in Phase I and II trials of patients with metastatic pancreatic cancer treated with combinations of RP101 and gemcitabine or gemcitabine and cisplatin *(73)*. In a study of 13 patients (9 with stage IV disease, 4 with stage III) treated with RP101, gemcitabine, and cisplatin, the median survival duration was 447 days, with a median time to progression of 280 days. Of the 13 patients, 10 lived longer than 1 year, and 3 lived for longer than 2 years. These results were significant when compared with those of a randomly selected group of patients in a separate study. Another small study of gemcitabine plus RP101 showed similar results. Markers of activity were not directly assayed in patient samples in these studies; but based on in vitro and animal model data, the authors of these studies believed that the compound's activity was at least partially attributable to the prevention of STAT3 activation, thereby allowing chemotherapy-induced apoptosis. However, several other mechanisms have been reported to be involved in the effects of this drug *(72)*. The results of these small trials need to be corroborated in large randomized trials.

9. AGENTS TARGETING TRANSCRIPTION FACTOR NUCLEAR FACTOR-κ B

Nuclear factor-κ B (NFkB) plays a major role in the proliferation, survival, angiogenesis, and chemoresistance of pancreatic cancer and is constitutively active in pancreatic cancer cells. Agents that block NFkB activation could reduce chemoresistance to gemcitabine. One such agent tested is curcumin (diferuloylmethane), a plant-derived dietary ingredient derivative of the spice turmeric *Curcuma longa*). Curcumin has shown to suppress NFkB and in one recently published in vitro study, curcumin inhibited the proliferation of various pancreatic cancer cell lines, potentiated the apoptosis induced by gemcitabine, and inhibited constitutive NFkB activation in the cells *(74)*. Tumor xenografts injected with pancreatic cancer cells and treated with a combination of curcumin and gemcitabine showed significant reductions in tumor volume, the Ki-67 proliferation index, NFkB activation, suppressing angiogenesis as well as reducing the expression of NFkB-regulated gene products—cyclin D1, c-myc, Bcl-2, Bcl-xL, cellular inhibitor of apoptosis protein-1, cyclooxygenase-2 (COX-2), MMP, VEGF—compared with tumors from control mice treated with olive oil only.

A recent completed Phase II clinical trial with curcumin (8 g daily) for advanced pancreatic cancer evaluated its safety, benefit, and impact on biologic correlates *(75)*. Among the 21 evaluable patients, low circulating curcumin was detected, suggesting poor oral bioavailability. Two patients showed prolonged SD (8 and 12+ months). Curcumin down-regulated expression of NFkB, COX-2, and phosphorylated STAT3 in peripheral blood mononuclear cells (PBMCs) from patients, although the decrease did not reach statistical significance for p65. At present, studies with liposomal curcumin, which has better bioavailability, are being designed.

10. AGENTS TARGETING BCL-2/ADENOVIRUS E1B 19-KDA PROTEIN-INTERACTING PROTEIN

Bcl-2/adenovirus E1B 19-kDa protein-interacting protein (BNIP3) is a member of the Bcl-2 family, which forms heterodimers with Bcl-2 and Bcl-xL, antagonizing their prosurvival activity. BNIP3 localizes to mitochondrial membranes and facilitates apoptosis by activating the permeability transition pore *(76)*. Down-regulation of this proapoptotic gene in pancreatic cancer specimens and cell lines has been found to be correlated with gemcitabine resistance and prognosis, whereas its expression levels in cell lines are not appropriately induced by hypoxia *(77,78)*. In addition, the attenuated expression levels have been demonstrated to result from epigenetic methylation of the BNIP3 promoter site *(79)*.

This epigenetic regulation has prompted investigation of the use of the demethylating agent 5-aza-2′-deoxycytidine (5-azacytidine), a compound that was approved during the past several years for the treatment of myelodysplasia syndrome and is being studied in several other cancer types. In a study in pancreatic cancer cell lines, 5-azacytidine reversed the hypermethylation of BNIP3, resensitizing the cells to hypoxia- or chemotherapy-induced cell apoptosis *(79,80)*. Currently, this drug is in Phase I development for solid tumors; its efficacy in pancreatic cancer has not been reported.

11. PATIENT SELECTION AND TRIAL DESIGN FOR STUDIES WITH TARGETED AGENTS

11.1. Patient Population Heterogeneity

An important consideration when designing trials of emerging compounds and new drug combinations is the heterogeneity of the pancreatic carcinoma patient population in terms of disease spread and overall performance status (taking into account co-morbidities). Patients with locally advanced disease but no evidence of metastasis have a median survival of 6 to 10 months, whereas those with distant metastases have a median survival duration of 3 to 6 months, depending on their overall tumor burden and performance status *(81)*. Approximately 25% of patients with advanced pancreatic cancer treated in clinical trials die within 2 months of the start of treatment, regardless of treatment type, and there are clear differences in the response rates between patients with locally advanced disease and patients with metastatic disease *(81)*. Indeed, the disparate results of the Phase II and III trials of gemcitabine versus gemcitabine plus bevacizumab demonstrate how the outcomes can be substantially affected by differences in patient selection methods *(49,50)*. Thus, it is possible that drugs useful in a subset of patients are being discounted because they are being studied in an unselected patient sample.

The heterogeneity of the pancreatic cancer patient population suggests that these patients should be stratified into homogeneous categories for clinical protocols—at a minimum into locally advanced disease and metastatic disease groups. A scoring system (as is commonly used for hematologic malignancies) may be a useful starting point, with baseline treatment matched for different scoring groups (e.g., doublet therapy such as gemcitabine plus oxaliplatin for patients with good performance status versus gemcitabine alone in those with poor performance status). The results of a recent retrospective analysis of gemcitabine versus gemcitabine and cisplatin support the use of the Karnofsky performance score to predict response to treatment and may therefore be useful for trial design *(82)*.

11.2. Appropriate Endpoints to Assess Drug Activity

Appropriate endpoints are needed in studies of cytostatic agents to assess the drug effectiveness and roles in treatment. These agents may yield substantial clinical benefits, such as control of tumor growth, prevention of new lesions, or improvements in patient symptoms but may not meet the Response Evaluation Criteria in Solid Tumors or World Health Organization criteria for tumor shrinkage and response. Any agent that allows patients to live longer with their disease under control, even without evidence of tumor shrinkage, is of benefit and should not be dismissed in early trials as a result of misplaced expectations. Therefore, as was initially developed for the evaluation of gemcitabine, appropriate standardized measures must be applied to assess clinical benefits. Overall survival of 6 months or 1 year and PFS rates are often used as the primary objectives in Phase III studies; the disease control rate and clinical benefits are reasonable secondary endpoints.

11.3. Changes in Trial Design

The standard design of clinical trials has been relatively effective in studies of drugs in other tumor types but has been less useful in studies of pancreatic cancer drugs. Several compounds have appeared promising in preclinical, Phase I, and single-arm Phase II trials that produced disappointing results in randomized Phase III trials. In addition, in these trials, little is learned about the tumor's biologic characteristics or what mechanisms are involved in the compound's effectiveness. Pancreatic cancer researchers should consider designing trials that can yield more useful information about the disease and the characteristics of patients who do and do not respond for future trials and drug development. For example, the use of randomized Phase II trials instead of single-arm trials would provide an appropriate comparator for evaluating results; such a change is further justified by the inaccuracy of historical control group comparisons, especially given the variability of outcomes found in pancreatic cancer trials. In addition, randomized Phase II trials would make it easier to determine the efficacy of compounds at an earlier point in drug development.

Rebiopsy of tumors and identifying other surrogate biomarkers may be useful for evaluating the effects of new drugs. These effects could include whether the drugs reach their target, what other pathways are activated that abrogates the drug's effectiveness, and whether the primary tumor and metastases respond differently to the drugs. In addition, a better understanding of patient characteristics is needed as aggregate analyses of large groups of patients may not be revealing enough in a heterogeneous group of pancreatic cancer patients.

12. CONCLUSION

The prognosis of patients with pancreatic cancer is bleak, and little progress in the treatment of this disease has been made during the past two decades. However, we are now gaining insight into the underlying biologic characteristics of this cancer. Development of targeted mouse models shows promise and may prove to be a better model for predicting therapeutic efficacy in pancreatic cancer compared to the use of tumor xenografts and cell-based assays. Extrapolated findings for other tumor types and empiric data from clinical trials suggest that targeting the correct effector pathways could help us improve survival outcomes. More work is needed to address the key characteristics of pancreatic cancer that make it so aggressive, metastasizing at an early stage, and more refractory to standard treatments than most other solid tumor types. By using our knowledge of pancreatic cancer's biologic characteristics and improving our patient selection methods, we will be able to make advances in pancreatic cancer clinical trials and personalize our treatment recommendations in daily practice.

REFERENCES

1. Jemal A, Siegel R, Ward E, et al. Cancer statistics, 2007. CA Cancer J Clin 2007;57(1):43–66.
2. Carter SK, Comis RL. The integration of chemotherapy into a combined modality approach for cancer treatment. VI. Pancreatic adenocarcinoma. Cancer Treat Rev 1975;2(3):193–214.
3. Freeny PC. Radiology of the pancreas: two decades of progress in imaging and intervention. AJR Am J Roentgenol 1988;150(5):975–81.
4. Eckel F, Schneider G, Schmid RM. Pancreatic cancer: a review of recent advances. Expert Opin Invest Drugs 2006;15(11):1395–410.
5. Burris HA 3rd, Moore MJ, Andersen J, et al. Improvements in survival and clinical benefit with gemcitabine as first-line therapy for patients with advanced pancreas cancer: a randomized trial. J Clin Oncol 1997;15(6):2403–13.
6. Tempero M, Plunkett W, Ruiz Van Haperen V, et al. Randomized phase II comparison of dose-intense gemcitabine: thirty-minute infusion and fixed dose rate infusion in patients with pancreatic adenocarcinoma. J Clin Oncol 2003;21(18):3402–8.
7. Saif MW. Pancreatic cancer: highlights from the 42nd annual meeting of the American Society of Clinical Oncology, 2006. JOP J Pancreas (Online) 2006;7(4):337–48.
8. Louvet C, Labianca R, Hammel P, et al. Gemcitabine in combination with oxaliplatin compared with gemcitabine alone in locally advanced or metastatic pancreatic cancer: results of a GERCOR and GISCAD phase III trial. J Clin Oncol 2005;23(15):3509–16.
9. Heinemann V, Quietzsch D, Gieseler F, et al. Randomized phase III trial of gemcitabine plus cisplatin compared with gemcitabine alone in advanced pancreatic cancer. J Clin Oncol 2006;24(24):3946–52.
10. Hezel AF, Kimmelman AC, Stanger BZ,et al. Genetics and biology of pancreatic ductal adenocarcinoma. Genes Dev 2006;20(10):1218–49.
11. Yamano M, Fujii H, Takagaki T, et al. Genetic progression and divergence in pancreatic carcinoma. Am J Pathol 2000;156(6):2123–33.
12. Bardeesy N, DePinho RA. Pancreatic cancer biology and genetics. Nat Rev Cancer 2002;2(12):897–909.
13. Olive KP, Tuveson DA. The use of targeted mouse models for preclinical testing of novel cancer therapeutics. Clin Cancer Res 2006;12(18):5277–87.
14. Schlessinger J. Cell signaling by receptor tyrosine kinases. Cell 2000;103(2):211–25.
15. Yarden Y. The EGFR family and its ligands in human cancer. signalling mechanisms and therapeutic opportunities. Eur J Cancer 2001;37(suppl 4):S3–8.
16. Wells A. EGF receptor. Int J Biochem Cell Biol 1999;31(6):637–43.
17. Salomon DS, Brandt R, Ciardiello F, et al. Epidermal growth factor-related peptides and their receptors in human malignancies. Crit Rev Oncol Hematol 1995;19(3):183–232.
18. Woodburn JR. The epidermal growth factor receptor and its inhibition in cancer therapy. Pharmacol Ther 1999;82(2–3):241–50.
19. Yarden Y, Sliwkowski MX. Untangling the ErbB signalling network. Nat Rev Mol Cell Biol 2001;2(2):127–37.
20. Hanahan D, Weinberg RA. The hallmarks of cancer. Cell 2000;100(1):57–70.
21. Korc M, Chandrasekar B, Yamanaka Y, et al. Overexpression of the epidermal growth factor receptor in human pancreatic cancer is associated with concomitant increases in the levels of epidermal growth factor and transforming growth factor alpha. J Clin Invest 1992;90(4):1352–60.
22. Lemoine NR, Hughes CM, Barton CM, et al. The epidermal growth factor receptor in human pancreatic cancer. J Pathol 1992;166(1):7–12.
23. Yamanaka Y, Friess H, Kobrin MS, et al. Coexpression of epidermal growth factor receptor and ligands in human pancreatic cancer is associated with enhanced tumor aggressiveness. Anticancer Res 1993;13(3):565–9.
24. Korc M, Friess H, Yamanaka Y, et al. Chronic pancreatitis is associated with increased concentrations of epidermal growth factor receptor, transforming growth factor alpha, and phospholipase C gamma. Gut 1994;35(10):1468–73.
25. Kwak EL, Jankowski J, Thayer SP, et al. Epidermal growth factor receptor kinase domain mutations in esophageal and pancreatic adenocarcinomas. Clin Cancer Res 2006;12(14 Pt 1):4283–7.
26. Xiong HQ, Rosenberg A, LoBuglio A, et al. Cetuximab, a monoclonal antibody targeting the epidermal growth factor receptor, in combination with gemcitabine for advanced pancreatic cancer: a multicenter phase II trial. J Clin Oncol 2004;22(13):2610–6.

27. Philip PA, Benedetti J, Fenoglio-Preiser C, et al. Phase III study of gemcitabine [G] plus cetuximab [C] versus gemcitabine in patients [pts] with locally advanced or metastatic pancreatic adenocarcinoma [PC]: SWOG S0205 study. J Clin Oncol 2007;25(18S):LBA4509.

28. Kullmann F, Hollerbach S, Dollinger M, et al. Cetuximab plus gemcitabine/oxaliplatin (GEMOXCET) in 1st line metastatic pancreatic cancer: first results from a multicenter phase II study. Presented at the American Society of Clinical Oncology, Gastrointestinal Cancers Symposium, 2007.

29. Moore MJ. Brief communication: a new combination in the treatment of advanced pancreatic cancer. Semin Oncol 2005;32(suppl 8):5–6.

30. Grunewald K, Lyons J, Frohlich A, et al. High frequency of Ki-ras codon 12 mutations in pancreatic adenocarcinomas. Int J Cancer 1989;43(6):1037–41.

31. Klimstra DS, Longnecker DS. K-ras mutations in pancreatic ductal proliferative lesions. Am J Pathol 1994;145(6):1547–50.

32. Lemoine NR, Jain S, Hughes CM, et al. Ki-ras oncogene activation in preinvasive pancreatic cancer. Gastroenterology 1992;102(1):230–6.

33. Lohr M, Kloppel G, Maisonneuve P, et al. Frequency of K-ras mutations in pancreatic intraductal neoplasias associated with pancreatic ductal adenocarcinoma and chronic pancreatitis: a meta-analysis. Neoplasia 2005;7(1):17–23.

34. Fleming JB, Shen GL, Holloway SE, et al. Molecular consequences of silencing mutant K-ras in pancreatic cancer cells: justification for K-ras-directed therapy. Mol Cancer Res 2005;3(7):413–23.

35. Pechlivanis M, Kuhlmann J. Hydrophobic modifications of Ras proteins by isoprenoid groups and fatty acids—more than just membrane anchoring. Biochim Biophys Acta 2006;1764(12):1914–31.

36. Resh MD. Trafficking and signaling by fatty-acylated and prenylated proteins. Nat Chem Biol 2006;2(11):584–90.

37. Cohen SJ, Ho L, Ranganathan S, et al. Phase II and pharmacodynamic study of the farnesyltransferase inhibitor R115777 as initial therapy in patients with metastatic pancreatic adenocarcinoma. J Clin Oncol 2003;21(7):1301–6.

38. Macdonald JS, McCoy S, Whitehead RP, et al. A phase II study of farnesyl transferase inhibitor R115777 in pancreatic cancer: a Southwest Oncology Group (SWOG 9924) study. Invest New Drugs 2005;23(5):485–7.

39. Van Cutsem E, van de Velde H, Karasek P, et al. Phase III trial of gemcitabine plus tipifarnib compared with gemcitabine plus placebo in advanced pancreatic cancer. J Clin Oncol 2004;22(8):1430–8.

40. Folkman J. Tumor angiogenesis: therapeutic implications. N Engl J Med 1971;285(21):1182–6.

41. Kerbel RS. Antiangiogenic therapy: a universal chemosensitization strategy for cancer? Science 2006;312(5777):1171–5.

42. Ferrara N, Leung DW, Cachianes G, et al. Purification and cloning of vascular endothelial growth factor secreted by pituitary folliculostellate cells. Methods Enzymol 1991;198:391–405.

43. Kiselyov A, Balakin KV, Tkachenko SE. VEGF/VEGFR signalling as a target for inhibiting angiogenesis. Expert Opin Invest Drugs 2007;16(1):83–107.

44. Itakura J, Ishiwata T, Friess H, et al. Enhanced expression of vascular endothelial growth factor in human pancreatic cancer correlates with local disease progression. Clin Cancer Res 1997;3(8):1309–16.

45. Itakura J, Ishiwata T, Shen B, et al. Concomitant over-expression of vascular endothelial growth factor and its receptors in pancreatic cancer. Int J Cancer 2000;85(1):27–34.

46. Seo Y, Baba H, Fukuda T, et al. High expression of vascular endothelial growth factor is associated with liver metastasis and a poor prognosis for patients with ductal pancreatic adenocarcinoma. Cancer 2000;88(10):2239–45.

47. Jain RK. Normalization of tumor vasculature: an emerging concept in antiangiogenic therapy. Science 2005;307:58–62.

48. Shih T, Lindley C. Bevacizumab: an angiogenesis inhibitor for the treatment of solid malignancies. Clin Ther 2006;28(11):1779–802.

49. Kindler HL, Friberg G, Singh DA, et al. Phase II trial of bevacizumab plus gemcitabine in patients with advanced pancreatic cancer. J Clin Oncol 2005;23(31):8033–40.

50. Kindler H, Niedzwiecki D, Hollis E, et al. A double-blind, placebo-controlled, randomized phase III trial of gemcitabine (G) plus bevacizumab (B) versus gemcitabine plus placebo (P) in patients (pts) with advanced pancreatic cancer (PC): a preliminary analysis of Cancer and Leukemia Group B (CALGB) 80303. Presented at the American Society of Clinical Oncology, Gastrointestinal Cancers Symposium, 2007.

51. Bloomston M, Zervos EE, Rosemurgy AS 2nd. Matrix metalloproteinases and their role in pancreatic cancer: a review of preclinical studies and clinical trials. Ann Surg Oncol 2002;9(7):668–74.

52. Lee KH, Hyun MS, Kim JR. Growth factor-dependent activation of the MAPK pathway in human pancreatic cancer: MEK/ERK and p38 MAP kinase interaction in uPA synthesis. Clin Exp Metastasis 2003;20(6): 499–505.

53. Okada Y, Eibl G, Guha S, et al. Nerve growth factor stimulates MMP-2 expression and activity and increases invasion by human pancreatic cancer cells. Clin Exp Metastasis 2004;21(4):285–92.
54. Tan X, Egami H, Abe M, et al. Involvement of MMP-7 in invasion of pancreatic cancer cells through activation of the EGFR mediated MEK-ERK signal transduction pathway. J Clin Pathol 2005;58(12):1242–8.
55. Bramhall SR, Neoptolemos JP, Stamp GW, et al. Imbalance of expression of matrix metalloproteinases (MMPs) and tissue inhibitors of the matrix metalloproteinases (TIMPs) in human pancreatic carcinoma. J Pathol 1997;182(3):347–55.
56. Haq M, Shafii A, Zervos EE, et al. Addition of matrix metalloproteinase inhibition to conventional cytotoxic therapy reduces tumor implantation and prolongs survival in a murine model of human pancreatic cancer. Cancer Res 2000;60(12):3207–11.
57. Zervos EE, Norman JG, Gower WR, et al. Matrix metalloproteinase inhibition attenuates human pancreatic cancer growth in vitro and decreases mortality and tumorigenesis in vivo. J Surg Res 1997;69(2):367–71.
58. Bramhall SR, Rosemurgy A, Brown PD, et al. Marimastat as first-line therapy for patients with unresectable pancreatic cancer: a randomized trial. J Clin Oncol 2001;19(15):3447–55.
59. Moore MJ, Hamm J, Dancey J, et al. Comparison of gemcitabine versus the matrix metalloproteinase inhibitor BAY 12–9566 in patients with advanced or metastatic adenocarcinoma of the pancreas: a phase III trial of the National Cancer Institute of Canada Clinical Trials Group. J Clin Oncol 2003;21(17):3296–302.
60. Wang W, Abbruzzese JL, Evans DB, et al. The nuclear factor-kappa B RelA transcription factor is constitutively activated in human pancreatic adenocarcinoma cells. Clin Cancer Res 1999;5(1):119–27.
61. Yokoi K, Fidler IJ. Hypoxia increases resistance of human pancreatic cancer cells to apoptosis induced by gemcitabine. Clin Cancer Res 2004;10(7):2299–306.
62. Banerjee S, Zhang Y, Ali S, et al. Molecular evidence for increased antitumor activity of gemcitabine by genistein in vitro and in vivo using an orthotopic model of pancreatic cancer. Cancer Res 2005;65(19): 9064–72.
63. Mohammad RM, Banerjee S, Li Y, et al. Cisplatin-induced antitumor activity is potentiated by the soy isoflavone genistein in BxPC-3 pancreatic tumor xenografts. Cancer 2006;106(6):1260–8.
64. El-Rayes BF, Ali S, Ali IF, et al. Potentiation of the effect of erlotinib by genistein in pancreatic cancer: the role of Akt and nuclear factor-kappaB. Cancer Res 2006;66(21):10553–9.
65. Banerjee S, Zhang Y, Wang Z, et al. In vitro and in vivo molecular evidence of genistein action in augmenting the efficacy of cisplatin in pancreatic cancer. Int J Cancer 2007;120(4):906–17.
66. Jimeno A, Rubio-Viqueira B, Amador ML, et al. Epidermal growth factor receptor dynamics influences response to epidermal growth factor receptor targeted agents. Cancer Res 2005;65(8):3003–10.
67. Huang C, Cao J, Huang KJ, et al. Inhibition of STAT3 activity with AG490 decreases the invasion of human pancreatic cancer cells in vitro. Cancer Sci 2006;97(12):1417–23.
68. Scholz A, Heinze S, Detjen KM, et al. Activated signal transducer and activator of transcription 3 (STAT3) supports the malignant phenotype of human pancreatic cancer. Gastroenterology 2003;125(3):891–905.
69. Toyonaga T, Nakano K, Nagano M, et al. Blockade of constitutively activated Janus kinase/signal transducer and activator of transcription-3 pathway inhibits growth of human pancreatic cancer. Cancer Lett 2003;201(1):107–16.
70. Fahrig R, Steinkamp-Zucht A, Schaefer A. Prevention of adriamycin-induced mdr1 gene amplification and expression in mouse leukemia cells by simultaneous treatment with the anti-recombinogen bromovinyldeoxyuridine. Anticancer Drug Des 2000;15(5):307–12.
71. De Clercq E. Discovery and development of BVDU (brivudin) as a therapeutic for the treatment of herpes zoster. Biochem Pharmacol 2004;68(12):2301–15.
72. Fahrig R, Heinrich JC, Nickel B, et al. Inhibition of induced chemoresistance by cotreatment with (E)-5-(2-bromovinyl)-2'-deoxyuridine (RP101). Cancer Res 2003;63(18):5745–53.
73. Fahrig R, Quietzsch D, Heinrich JC, et al. RP101 improves the efficacy of chemotherapy in pancreas carcinoma cell lines and pancreatic cancer patients. Anticancer Drugs 2006;17(9):1045–56.
74. Kunnumakkara AB, Guha S, Krishnan S, et al. Curcumin potentiates antitumor activity of gemcitabine in an orthotopic model of pancreatic cancer through suppression of proliferation, angiogenesis, and inhibition of nuclear factor-kappaB-regulated gene products. Cancer Res 2007;67(8):3853–61.
75. Dhillon N, Wolff RA, Abbruzzese JL, et al. Phase II clinical trial of curcumin in patients with advanced pancreatic cancer. J Clin Oncol 2007;24(18S):14151.
76. Vande Velde C, Cizeau J, Dubik D, et al. BNIP3 and genetic control of necrosis-like cell death through the mitochondrial permeability transition pore. Mol Cell Biol 2000;20(15):5454–68.
77. Akada M, Crnogorac-Jurcevic T, Lattimore S, et al. Intrinsic chemoresistance to gemcitabine is associated with decreased expression of BNIP3 in pancreatic cancer. Clin Cancer Res 2005;11(8):3094–101.
78. Erkan M, Kleeff J, Esposito I, et al. Loss of BNIP3 expression is a late event in pancreatic cancer contributing to chemoresistance and worsened prognosis. Oncogene 2005;24(27):4421–32.

79. Abe T, Toyota M, Suzuki H, et al. Upregulation of BNIP3 by 5-aza-2'-deoxycytidine sensitizes pancreatic cancer cells to hypoxia-mediated cell death. J Gastroenterol 2005;40(5):504–10.
80. Kanda T, Tada M, Imazeki F, et al. 5-Aza-2'-deoxycytidine sensitizes hepatoma and pancreatic cancer cell lines. Oncol Rep 2005;14(4):975–9.
81. Hochster HS, Haller DG, de Gramont A, et al. Consensus report of the International Society of Gastrointestinal Oncology on therapeutic progress in advanced pancreatic cancer. Cancer 2006;107(4):676–85.
82. Boeck S, Hinke A, Wilkowski R, et al. Importance of performance status for treatment outcome in advanced pancreatic cancer. World J Gastroenterol 2007;13(2):224–7.
83. Maitra A, Adsay NV, Argani P, et al. Multicomponent analysis of the pancreatic adenocarcinoma progression model using a pancreatic intraepithelial neoplasia tissue microarray. Mod Pathol 2003;16(9):902–12.
84. Rozenblum E, Schutte M, Goggins M, et al. Tumor-suppressive pathways in pancreatic carcinoma. Cancer Res 1997;57(9):1731–4.
85. Hahn SA, Schutte M, Hoque AT, et al. DPC4, a candidate tumor suppressor gene at human chromosome 18q21.1. Science 1996;271:350–3.

14 Targeted Therapy in Prostate Cancer

Amado J. Zurita, MD, John F. Ward, MD, and Jeri Kim, MD

CONTENTS

ABSTRACT

New therapeutic advances in Phase I to III clinical trials against castration-resistant prostate cancer strive to manipulate the androgen receptor, a growth and survival mediator; reduce circulating androgen concentrations; combat antiapoptotic proteins; and target pathways related to angiogenesis. Immunotherapeutic studies are based on a better understanding of the prostate's testosterone-dependent organogenesis and functional differentiation at puberty. Bone, because it is the site of first relapse in more than 80% of cases and is the tissue most frequently involved in hormone-refractory cases, remains of prominent interest for interventions.

Key Words: Prostate cancer, Prostatic neoplasms, Castration-resistant prostate cancer, Androgen receptors, Ansamycins, mTOR (mammalian target of rapamycin) inhibitors, Angiogenesis, Immunotherapy

1. INTRODUCTION

New targeted therapeutic strategies currently undergoing clinical development for prostate cancer create novel frontline treatments for castration-resistant prostate cancer.

From: *Current Clinical Oncology: Targeted Cancer Therapy*
Edited by: R. Kurzrock and M. Markman © Humana Press, Totowa, NJ

2. TARGETING THE ANDROGEN RECEPTOR

The androgen receptor (AR) is a central mediator of growth and survival in prostate cancer *(1,2)* and as such is considered by many to be the dominant oncogene in the disease (by gain of function mutations) *(1–8)*. Signaling by the AR is critical in all phases of prostate cancer progression, including castration-resistant prostate cancer (CRPC), where androgen responsiveness is still present and partial reactivation of AR-regulated genes—including those governing prostate-specific antigen (PSA)—occurs *(9,10)*. Many cases progressing after castration demonstrate these characteristics by displaying a rising PSA level and by responding to additional hormonal manipulation. However, these responses may reflect changes affecting only a subset of tumor cells, considering the high degree of heterogeneity in AR expression existing among tissue sites and even within the same tissue in individual prostate cancer patients *(11)*. As the disease progresses, AR-mediated gene expression becomes hypersensitive to androgens by various mechanisms, including increased AR levels (by gene amplification, mRNA expression, or receptor stabilization) *(6,12–15)* and/or function (through cross-talk with other signaling pathways or changes in expression of co-regulatory molecules) *(16,17)*, AR gain-of-function mutations (found in a relatively small group of cases) *(18)*, or other mechanisms such as alterations in chromatin at AR target-specific loci (e.g., PSA) *(19)*.

It has also become clear that surgical or chemical castration and treatment with currently available anti-AR antagonists do not result in an intratumoral environment that is completely depleted of androgens *(20,21)*. In such a context, prostate cancer cells increase their own production of androgens from weak adrenal androgens or synthesize androgens de novo. Molecular profiling studies have shown an increased expression of genes mediating testosterone/dihydrotestosterone (DHT) synthesis in CRPC *(9,22)*. These results demonstrate that novel strategies targeting androgens (ligands) and AR signaling mechanisms hold great potential in prostate cancer treatment. Some possibilities include:

- Targeting hormone ligands of the AR (e.g., by reducing their concentrations or antagonizing receptor binding)
- Modulating AR levels or function directly
- Disrupting nongenomic mechanisms of AR activation by signaling cross-talk

New therapeutics targeting these mechanisms are discussed below (Table 1).

2.1. Reducing Circulating Androgen Concentrations

Patients with blood testosterone concentrations in the castrate range (< 50 ng/mL) whose disease is progressing despite therapy on a combination of a gonadotropin-releasing hormone agonist and a nonsteroidal antiandrogen (e.g., flutamide) are typically treated, after discontinuation of the latter, with another antiandrogen (e.g., bicalutamide or nilutamide), an estrogen (diethylstilbestrol), a progestin (megestrol acetate), or an inhibitor of adrenal androgen synthesis (e.g., aminoglutethimide or ketoconazole with hydrocortisone). Ketoconazole, which is frequently used in this setting, is a weak inhibitor of several adrenal cytochrome P450 enzymes. A much more specific inhibitor of androgen synthesis pathways in the adrenal glands known as abiraterone acetate is being developed.

Abiraterone is a potent inhibitor of 17α-hydroxylase/C17, 20-lyase (P450 17, CYP450 C17), which is a critical enzyme in the biosynthesis of androgens *(23)*. Recently presented preliminary results of a Phase I/II trial of abiraterone in chemotherapy-naive patients with progressive CRPC have demonstrated the ability of this agent to inhibit levels of circulating

Table 1
Selected New Agents Under Investigation for the Treatment of CRPC

Target	Agent	Phase
17α-Hydroxylase/C17,20-lyase	Abiraterone acetate	I/II
Heat shock protein 90 (Hsp90)	17-Allylamino-geldanamycin (17-AAG)	II
	17-Dimethylaminoethylamino-demethoxygeldanamycin (17-DMAG)	I
Histone deacetylase (HDAC)	Suberoylanilide hydroxamic acid (SAHA) (vorinostat)	II
	FK228 (depsipeptide)	II
Androgen receptor	BMS-641988	I
	MDV-3100	I
Mammalian target of rapamycin (mTOR)	Rapamycin (sirolimus)	II
	CCI-779 (temsirolimus)	II
	RAD001 (everolimus)	II
	AP23573	II
AKT	Perifosine	II
Insulin-like growth factor-1 receptor (IGF-1R)	CP-751871	II
	IMC-A12	I
Src kinase	BMS-354825 (dasatinib)	I/II
	AZD0530	I
Clusterin	OGX-011	II/III
Survivin	YM155	II
Vascular endothelial growth factor (VEGF)	Bevacizumab	II/III
VEGF receptor	SU011248 (sunitinib malate)	II
	Sorafenib	II
	AZD2171	II
Endothelin-A receptor	ABT-627 (atrasentan)	III
	ZD4054	I/II
Receptor activator of nuclear factor B ligand (RANKL)	AMG162 (denosumab)	III
Anti-CTLA-4 monoclonal antibodies	MDX-010-01 (ipilimumab)	I
Dendritic cells	Sipuleucel-T (Provenge)	III

Abbreviations are supplied when it is the more familiar name of the target or agent

testosterone significantly *(24)*. Given continuously as an oral daily formulation, various doses of this agent induced PSA responses ($\geq$ 50% over baseline) in 18 of 30 patients (60%); and the disease was measurably regressed in bone and lymph nodes in several cases. All doses were well tolerated.

Interestingly, more than half of the patients continued on treatment for longer than 6 months (responses to ketoconazole after progression on antiandrogens are typically short-lived). Because CYP 17 inhibition results in increased concentrations of upstream C21 steroids (including pregnenolone, corticosterone, and deoxycorticosterone, which could potentially activate a mutated AR), low daily doses of dexamethasone (0.5 mg) are being added to regimens when disease progression is detected.

2.2. Modulating Protein Levels and Activation of the AR

Targeting the receptor itself can also inhibit AR-mediated signaling. Recent publication of the crystal structure of the ligand-binding domain of the AR bound to bicalutamide *(25)*, DHT *(26)*, and cyproterone acetate *(27)* and a better understanding of ligand-independent mechanisms of receptor activation, posttranslational modifications, and changes in co-regulatory molecules are facilitating the development of new agents targeting the AR.

One approach to inducing the degradation of the AR includes interfering with heat shock protein-90 (Hsp90) binding, thus affecting AR structure and stability *(28)*. The ansamycins (natural antibiotics), of which the first in clinical testing was 17-allylamino-geldanamycin (17-AAG), cause the proteosomal degradation of a number of steroid hormone receptors, including AR, as well as key oncogenic "client" proteins such as ErbB2, met, and phosphoAKT. Phase I trials have been completed, demonstrating schedule-dependent maximum-tolerated doses *(29–31)* and Hsp90 inhibition. However, the development of ansamycins has been challenged by their poor solubility and potential for hepatotoxicity. New formulations of 17-AAG as well as novel ansamycins, including the oral compound 17-DMAG, are being tested in Phase I trials.

Histone deacetylase (HDAC) inhibitors have also been shown to affect the binding of client proteins (e.g., AR to Hsp90) *(32–34)*. Additionally, these agents can directly reactivate silenced genes by inhibiting the increased HDAC activity characteristic of prostate cancer *(35)*. HDAC inhibitors enhance histone acetylation and thus reactivate transcription of repressed tumor suppressor genes by destabilizing the interactions between histones and DNA *(36)*. Several HDAC inhibitors, alone or in combination, are in clinical trials against various solid tumors, including prostate cancer. Suberoylanilide hydroxamic acid (SAHA; or vorinostat) and FK228 (depsipeptide) are the most advanced HDAC inhibitors in clinical testing against this disease *(37)*.

Another approach is to modulate AR activation. A new generation of potent AR antagonists/antiandrogens, including MDV3100 and BMS-641988, are now entering clinical trials. AR activity is directly modulated by cofactors that increase (co-activators) or decrease (co-repressors) transcription (forming co-regulatory complexes) in a tissue-specific manner *(1,2,38,39)*. AR co-activators contribute to prostate cancer progression by directly enhancing AR activity in the presence of very low levels of androgen (possibly influenced by histone modifications) through AR binding promiscuity to nonnative or alternative ligands or by facilitating cross-talk with signal transduction pathways *(40–42)*. Several in vitro studies consistently demonstrated a functionally relevant increase in levels of co-activator expression patterns related to androgen deprivation *(42–44)* and presented the possible utility of pharmacologically inducing the recruitment of AR-inhibiting co-repressors *(45)*. Thus, selective AR modulators targeting co-regulatory complexes have great potential as targets for prostate cancer therapy.

2.3. Targeting Nongenomic Mechanisms of AR Activation by Signaling Cross-Talk

Co-activator proteins facilitate ligand-independent activation of the AR through signaling cross-talk with growth factor signaling pathways *(2)*. Several classes of agents that target dysregulated pathways in prostate cancer are being tested in clinical trials.

Functional inactivation of the tumor suppressor gene phosphatase and tensin homologue deleted in chromosome 10 (*PTEN*) by loss of heterozygosity or mutational silencing is one of the most common molecular alterations in CRPC *(46)*. *PTEN* is involved in cell proliferation, adhesion, and apoptosis; and its reduction or loss can lead to increased accumulation of phosphoinositol-(3,4,5)-triphosphate via phosphoinositide-3-kinase (PI3K) and constitutive activation of AKT kinase and mammalian target of rapamycin (mTOR) *(47)*, which is a critical sensor of survival signals in cancer cells. Such activity can enhance AR stabilization and association of the AR with active transcriptional co-regulatory complexes *(2)*. Not surprisingly, active AKT not only correlates with a high Gleason score and predicts a poor prognosis, its up-regulation is also associated with progression to CRPC *(48–50)*. The PI3K/AKT/mTOR pathway is therefore an attractive therapeutic target in this disease.

The development and application of mTOR inhibitors has provided clinical proof of the feasibility of targeting the PI3K pathway in cancer. Analogues of the immunosuppressant compound rapamycin (sirolimus)—including CCI-779 (temsirolimus), RAD001 (everolimus), AP23573—and rapamycin itself have mTOR-inhibitory properties and are being studied in Phase II trials in prostate cancer as single agents and in combination. Concerns about the safety profile of mTOR inhibitors, the possibility of negative feedback with activation of upstream targets such as insulin-like growth factor-1 receptor (IGF-1R), and activation of AKT by feedback mechanisms suggest that an improved understanding of the complexities of this signaling network in prostate-specific models is required *(50,51)*. Carefully designed clinical trials emphasizing pharmacokinetics and correlations with biologic readouts are also critical. Accordingly, CCI-779, RAD001, and rapamycin are being tested in neoadjuvant preoperative pharmacodynamic and dose-determining studies in patients with disease who are at high risk for recurrence. Because these agents appear to be primarily cytostatic in prostate cancer, rational combinations with other targeted agents (e.g., RAD001 with gefitinib) or chemotherapy are being developed *(2)*. However, combining these agents with docetaxel may be challenging because of potential metabolic and myelosuppressive interactions. Regarding immunosuppression, no clear evidence of clinically significant effects has been observed with intermittent schedules, but long-term safety in prostate cancer patients has yet to be tested.

Few direct PI3K/AKT inhibitors are available, and so study results with them are rare in regard to prostate cancer. One such agent is the alkylphosphocholine perifosine, which inhibits AKT membrane localization and signaling in preclinical models of prostate cancer *(52,53)*. Two Phase II studies in patients with biochemically recurrent, hormone-sensitive, and metastatic CRPC have been reported: perifosine demonstrated little activity as a single agent in these settings *(54,55)*. A placebo-controlled, double-blind Phase II trial of perifosine in combination with docetaxel and prednisone in metastatic CRPC is currently accruing patients. Clinical testing and results with a newer generation of inhibitors of PI3K/AKT with higher selectivity are anticipated.

There is sufficient evidence to suggest that AR activity can be enhanced by harnessing cell signaling pathways used by growth factors and their receptors—including epidermal growth factor (EGF), HER-2/*neu*, and IGF-1R—as well as cytokines (interleukin-6) and neuropeptides, thereby minimizing the requirement for androgen ligand binding and promoting androgen-independent progression *(56–59)*. This has provided a rationale for targeting growth factor-mediated signaling in CRPC. Among the most interesting and best characterized in prostate cancer are the IGF/IGF-1R and the HER-kinase pathways. The IGF signaling axis consists of an intricate network of IGFs, IGF-binding proteins (IGFBPs), IGFBP proteases, and IGF tyrosine kinase receptors (RTKs) that results in activation of PI3K/AKT and Ras/mitogen-activated protein kinase (MAPK). In experimental models of prostate cancer, autocrine IGF-1R activation has been linked to castration-resistant progression *(60)*. Furthermore, levels of IGFBP change after castration to increase IGF-1R signal transduction *(61,62)*, and serum IGFBP-2 has been implicated as a biomarker for *PTEN* status and PI3K/AKT pathway activation *(63)*. The monoclonal antibody CP-751871 targeting IGF-1R is being tested in combination with docetaxel and prednisone in CRPC. A second monoclonal antibody, IMC-A12, is in Phase I testing.

Also relevant to prostate cancer progression are pathways initiated by HER kinases. In contrast to other targets, Phase II data are available for multiple agents targeting the EGF receptor (EGFR). These include the monoclonal antibodies cetuximab (EGFR/ HER-1) *(64)*, trastuzumab (HER-2) *(65–67)*, and pertuzumab (dimers of HER-2 and HER-3) *(68,69)*, and the small-molecule RTK inhibitors gefitinib *(70)*, erlotinib *(71,72)*, and lapatinib *(73)*. Unfortunately, most, if not all, of these agents have failed to demonstrate significant single-agent activity in prostate cancer despite the strong evidence provided by studies in laboratory model systems showing the importance of the HER-kinase pathways in the progression of this disease *(74)*. Clearly, future efforts targeting these pathways are needed to link molecular profiling of tumors with preclinical efficacy before the studies can proceed.

Other growth factors, cytokines, and neuropeptides are likely to be involved in activating signaling pathways that influence the AR in a manner similar to IGF and HER-kinase family members *(75)*. Those pathways exhibit cross-talk and often utilize common effectors that result in phosphorylation of the AR or its co-regulators. Protein kinases, including protein kinase C (PKC), casein kinases 1 and 2, and possibly AKT and MAPK, phosphorylate specific serine or threonine residues in the AR or co-activators, thus modulating its transcriptional activity *(16,58)*. Likewise, the AR can also be activated by non-RTKs. AR tyrosine phosphorylation sites have been recently identified by mass spectrometry analysis *(76)*, and phosphorylation of residue 534 has been linked to Src kinase activity *(76)*. Y534 phosphorylation of AR by nonsteroid peptide growth factors results in nuclear translocation of the receptor and an increase in AR transcriptional activity under androgen-depleted conditions *(76)*. Src transduces signals from upstream transcription factors (e.g., EGF, IGF-1R, hepatocyte growth factor, IL-8, neurotensin) to the AR, acting as a functional node of signaling convergence. Such convergence is likely related to disease progression to a state of hormone refractoriness, so it is rational that new therapeutics targeting Src are being tested in prostate cancer. Two small-molecule Src inhibitors (BMS-354825, or dasatinib, and AZD0530) are in Phase I/II testing in patients with prostate cancer.

3. TARGETING ANTIAPOPTOTIC PROTEINS

Prostate cancer cells activate a bypass pathway independent of AR to escape the apoptotic response induced by androgen deprivation. Bcl-2, which exerts its antiapoptotic function by heterodimerizing with proapoptotic regulators such as Bax is a critical mediator of such a response in prostate cancer. The mechanistic basis for the overexpression of this protein in CRPC is unclear but could be related to loss of *PTEN* and/or activation of AKT *(77,78)*. Oblimersen (G3139), an antisense molecule directed against Bcl-2, has been tested in patients with CRPC *(79,80)*. In prostate cancer models, this agent inhibited the expression of Bcl-2 while synergizing with chemotherapy and delaying progression to a castrate-resistant state *(81)*. Despite initial Phase II data suggesting improved efficacy *(79)*, the first results of a randomized Phase II study of oblimersen in combination with docetaxel versus docetaxel alone in CRPC have just been presented; and unfortunately the benefits of this regimen in a CRPC patient population are not clear *(80)*.

Clusterin, another antiapoptotic protein associated with prostate cancer progression, inhibits activated Bax and endoplasmic reticulum vacuolation and protein degradation under stress conditions such as androgen deprivation and chemotherapy *(82,83)*. In a neoadjuvant Phase I study of OGX-011, a second-generation antisense oligonucleotide targeting clusterin, dose-dependent increasing concentrations of the drug in prostate tissue and downregulation of the target were observed *(84)*. A Phase II randomized trial of docetaxel with or without OGX-011 in patients with CRPC has recently completed accrual. A Phase III randomized double-blind placebo-controlled trial of OGX-011 in combination with second-line mitoxantrone-based chemotherapy in CRPC is expected to begin enrolling patients in 2007.

Agents targeting survivin, a member of the inhibitor of apoptosis (IAP) family that has been implicated in resistance to antiandrogen therapy *(85)*, have entered clinical trials recently. YM155, a survivin inhibitor, has shown the ability to induce PSA responses as a single agent in CRPC patients treated in a Phase II study *(86)*.

4. TARGETING PATHWAYS RELATED TO ANGIOGENESIS

A number of cell signaling pathways critical to tumor angiogenesis are dysregulated in prostate cancer. Mediators of new blood vessel formation and stability, such as vascular endothelial growth factor (VEGF) and platelet-derived growth factor (PDGF), are implicated in metastatic spread in addition to their role in angiogenesis. VEGF is produced by tumor cells to facilitate nesting of metastatic cells in bone and to promote osteoblast differentiation *(87)*. Similarly, PDGF produced by prostate cancer cells in the bone microenvironment induces expression of the PDGF receptor (PDGFR) and its activation in tumor-associated endothelial cells *(88)*.

Bevacizumab, a monoclonal antibody that binds to and inactivates VEGF, has demonstrated no significant single-agent activity in prostate cancer *(89)*; however, because of its favorable toxicity profile and promising experience in many other tumors, such as colorectal, breast, and non-small-cell lung cancer, bevacizumab is being tested in combination with other therapies, including taxane-based chemotherapy and immunotherapy. Preliminary results from a Phase II study of combined docetaxel, estramustine, and bevacizumab conducted by the Cancer and Leukemia Group B (CALGB) showed that 81% of patients treated had an overall survival of 21 months and $\geq$ 50% decrease in PSA levels *(90)*. Based on these data from CALGB 90006, a Phase III randomized, double-blind study of docetaxel and prednisone with and without bevacizumab was launched (CALGB 90401) to determine if the addition of bevacizumab improves overall survival. Results from a Phase II study of the combination of bevacizumab plus prostatic acid phosphatase pulsed antigen-presenting cells (sipuleucel-T, or Provenge) in patients with biochemical relapse have demonstrated preliminary therapy-induced PSA modulation *(91)*.

Thalidomide, an antiangiogenic and immunomodulatory agent that attenuates the activity of VEGF, IL-6, and the hedgehog signaling pathway in prostate cancer *(92)*, has demonstrated modest single-agent activity *(93,94)* and therapeutic potential in combination with taxanes *(95)* and bevacizumab *(96)*. However, the use of thalidomide has been plagued by thromboembolic events necessitating anticoagulation. A thalidomide analogue, lenalidomide, is being tested in combinations with docetaxel and granulocyte-macrophage colony-stimulating factor (GM-CSF).

Multiple small-molecule inhibitors of the RTKs of PDGFR and/or VEGF receptors (VEGFR) are being developed in clinical trials. Based on promising preclinical data showing antivascular properties for the PDGFR inhibitor imatinib mesylate (STI571) in models of prostate cancer bone metastasis *(88)*, a modular Phase I trial was conducted in patients with CRPC. A total of 28 men, most of whom had been previously treated with chemotherapy, underwent 30-day lead-in treatment with imatinib alone followed by its combination with weekly docetaxel *(97)*. Interestingly, only 7% of the patients had a decline in PSA level of < 50%, and most experienced a median 1.8-fold increase. A similar effect has been described with sorafenib (BAY43-9006), a Raf-kinase, VEGFR, and PDGFR inhibitor *(98)*. A randomized multiinstitutional Phase II trial of docetaxel with or without imatinib in patients with CRPC and bone metastases was subsequently launched. Unfortunately, this study had to be terminated early because of excess gastrointestinal toxicity. Preliminary results suggest that imatinib does not detectably modulate docetaxel activity *(99)*.

Other multitargeted RTK inhibitors, such as sunitinib malate (SU011248), sorafenib, and AZD2171, are undergoing Phase II testing as single agents and in combination with docetaxel.

5. TARGETING PATHWAYS IN BONE METASTASIS

Bone is the first site of relapse in more than 80% of patients with prostate cancer *(100)* and is the most frequently involved tissue in men dying of hormone-refractory disease *(11)*. Once in bone, prostate cancer is a major source of morbidity in patients, typically producing pain and affecting normal hematopoiesis and bone structure. Even though the typical response to prostate cancer cells in the skeleton is bone formation, which is mediated by osteoblasts, this phenomenon is usually accompanied by a concomitant process of increased bone destruction that may be important in supporting tumor growth *(101)*.

One of the first efforts to target the osteoblastic compartment in bone therapeutically was inspired by evidence involving endothelin-1 (a powerful vasoconstrictor) in osteoblast activation and prostate cancer cell proliferation via the endothelin-A receptor *(102,103)*. Atrasentan (ABT-627), a selective endothelin-A receptor antagonist, has been shown to control markers of bone turnover while delaying progression of CRPC in some patients *(104,105)*. Two Phase III, placebo-controlled clinical trials of single-agent atrasentan in CRPC have been completed and the preliminary results presented. The first trial reported was designed to evaluate the role of atrasentan in men with metastatic CRPC *(106)*. This study was closed early because of an unexpectedly large number of early adverse events in both treatment arms. In an intent-to-treat analysis, atrasentan failed to distinguish itself as statistically significantly different from placebo in terms of time to disease progression and time to PSA progression *(106)*. However, a subset analysis of patients with bone metastases suggested that those treated with atrasentan experienced delayed disease progression *(107)*. The second trial, in which patients with nonmetastatic CRPC were enrolled, did not find that atrasentan produced a statistically significant effect on time to disease progression, probably because of a high rate of discontinuation related to PSA changes *(108)*. Both atrasentan and ZD4054, another endothelin-A receptor antagonist, are being investigated in combination with docetaxel in CRPC metastatic to bone.

Much earlier in the development process are strategies targeting the receptor activator of nuclear factor B (RANK) signaling pathway. This pathway, which consists of RANK ligand (RANKL), its receptor (RANKR), and a decoy receptor (osteoprotegerin), regulates activation and differentiation of osteoclasts, the cells primarily related to bone resorption *(109)*. Hormones and other factors stimulating bone resorption induce the expression of

RANKL by osteoblasts and stromal cells in bone. Denosumab (AMG162) is a human monoclonal antibody that binds to and neutralizes RANKL. Preliminary results of a Phase II randomized, open-label, active-controlled trial of denosumab and zoledronic acid in 24 patients with bone metastases and elevated levels of markers of bone turnover show a similar efficacy for both agents in reducing those markers *(110)*. In addition to targeting bone metastasis, denosumab is under development for the prevention and treatment of castration-induced osteoporosis in men with prostate cancer.

6. HARNESSING IMMUNOTHERAPEUTIC AGENTS

Immunotherapy for prostate cancer has evolved from an understanding of the development of the prostate. Testosterone-dependent organogenesis of the human prostate occurs at 10 to 12 weeks of gestation. Beyond that point and until the onset of puberty, the human prostate remains functionally and immunogically quiescent. Functional differentiation of the human prostate occurs only after the onset of puberty, curiously coinciding with the onset of androgen–mediated regression of both thymic and bone marrow tissues *(111)*. Despite this relatively late intrusion of epithelial cells elaborating prostate-specific proteins, the male immune system remains relatively unaware of the prostate's presence. However, a return to a low testosterone state through androgen ablative therapy results in a mononuclear cell infiltration prominent in CD4+ T cells *(112)*. The mechanism by which testosterone prevents immune surveillance of the prostate during and following puberty remains under investigation, but this observation highlights the precarious balance existing between the prostate and the host's immune system.

Inflammatory diseases of the prostate, which are frequently unassociated with an identifiable pathogen, may represent a form of chronic autoimmune disorder, as is seen in the thyroid, kidney, and intestine, where the balance between activation and inhibitory signals has been lost *(113,114)*. Additionally, both animals and humans are capable of generating robust and measurable antigen-specific cellular and humoral immune responses when exposed to both benign and cancerous prostate antigens *(115–120)*. This rather permissive immune tolerance, possibly T-cell anergy or T-cell ignorance, has become the focus of an array of novel investigations to exploit this permissiveness for therapeutic benefit in prostate cancer treatment. These inquests can broadly be considered to fall into one of two categories: (1) strategies that modify T-cell co-stimulatory pathways or (2) strategies that boost host antigen presentation.

6.1. Modifying T-Cell Co-stimulatory Pathways

The immune system seems to be programmed to avoid autoimmunity. It is now well understood that foreign or abnormal antigens alone are not enough to stimulate and expand an immune response. Thymically derived CD4 cells that co-express the IL-2 receptor α chain (CD25) appear crucial for control of autoreactive T cells (Tregs, CD3+CD4+CD25+) in vivo *(121)*. These Tregs, now identified by intracellular expression of FOXP3+ (forkhead box P3), inhibit the proliferation of CD25-effector T cells. The level of Tregs has been associated with cancer-specific outcomes. Elevated numbers of Tregs in the ascitic fluid of women with ovarian carcinoma and the peripheral blood/lymph nodes of patients with melanoma and lung cancer have been associated with poor cancer-specific survival *(122–124)*. Similarly, in the setting of prostate cancer, a low density of tumor-infiltrating lymphocytes has a demonstrated association with poor disease-specific outcome *(125)*. The mechanism of this suppression is being investigated, but the expression of cytotoxic T-lymphocyte antigen 4 (CTLA4) by Treg cells, interacting with CD80/CD86 on the surface of dendritic cells (DCs), appears to provide a negative signal for CD25-effector T-cell activation. Depleting CTLA4-expressing Tregs prior to immunization has been found to enhance the T-cell response to DC vaccine in humans *(126)*.

Two drugs in development— ipilimumab (MDX-010) (Bristol Meyers Squibb/Medarex, Princeton, NJ, USA) and ticilimumab (CP-675206) (Pfizer/Amgen, New York, NY, USA)— are antibodies directed at blocking the inhibitory CTLA-4 receptor on Treg cells, thereby releasing regulatory control. Both agents are human immunoglobulin G1 (IgG1) anti-CTLA-4 monoclonal antibodies (mAbs) that actively inhibit CTLA-4 interactions with B7.1 and B7.2 and do not show any cross-reactivity with human B7.1/B7.2-negative cell lines or cross-reactivity in normal human tissues. Ipilimumab has been administered in single and multiple doses as single-agent therapy and in combination with vaccine, chemotherapy, or IL-2 to more than 1000 patients to date. Although most studies have focused on patients with metastatic melanoma, some have included patients with prostate cancer, lymphoma, renal cell cancer, breast cancer, ovarian cancer, and human immunodeficiency virus (HIV).

A Phase I trial of ipilimumab (MDX-010-01) in patients with progressive, metastatic CRPC ($n = 14$) has been completed. Of the 14 patients treated in the study, 5 (36%) experienced one or more adverse events considered by the investigator to be related to treatment. Most patients experienced adverse events of grade 1 severity (2 patients, 14%) or grade 2 severity (2 patients, 14%). The most common adverse events reported were rash and pruritus, reported in two patients (14%). A > 50% decrease in the PSA level from baseline was observed in two patients.

Immune-mediated events, termed immune breakthrough events (IBEs), are adverse events associated with drug exposure that are consistent with an immune-based mechanism of action. In terms of organ system involvement, these events have primarily involved the gastrointestinal tract (diarrhea, colitis), the skin (rash, pruritus), or endocrine organs (thyroid, adrenals). Cancer responses across all studied malignancies are more common in patients who develop IBEs. Investigators reported no gastrointestinal perforations or colectomies in patients with breast or prostate cancer; however, trials in melanoma and renal cancer patients recorded such events associated with occasionally catastrophic results.

6.2. Boosting Host Antigen Presentation

Dendritic cells regulate cellular and humoral immunity and are considered natural adjuvants. Immunogenicity of antigens delivered on DCs has been demonstrated in patients with cancer. Thus, ex vivo generation of DCs with subsequent administration to patients has been suggested as a new immunotherapeutic approach to treating various cancers, including prostate cancer.

Immature DCs are highly efficient at endocytosis and phagocytosis followed by antigen processing and presentation to lymphocytes in secondary lymphoid tissues. They serve as the critical decision-making cells in the immune response and are therefore attractive targets for therapeutic manipulation to enhance an otherwise insufficient immune response to tumor antigens. Loading DCs with total antigen preparations and allowing "natural" processing and eptitope selection generates a diverse immune response involving many clones of CD4+ T cells and CTLs. Another approach involves exploiting the capacity of DCs to cross-prime and generate tumor-specific T lymphocytes. This approach elicits immunity against multiple antigens, regardless of the patient's human leukocyte antigen (HLA) type.

Strategic use of DCs to treat patients with CRPC have progressed beyond Phase II testing. Sipuleucel-T (Provenge) (Dendreon, Seattle, WA, USA) is the product of proprietary processing of autologous DCs obtained through patient leukopheresis and DC stimulation ex vivo with a prostate acid phosphatase GM-CSF protein (PAP-GMCSF). These activated DCs are then reintroduced intravenously to the donating patient. Initial results from small Phase III trials ($n = 225$) of men with asyptomatic metastatic CRPC did not meet the study primary endpoints—the time to disease or pain progression. Although not originally powered to measure improvements in survival, a retrospective analysis balanced for prognostic factors and use of chemotherapy after vaccination revealed an average 4-month improvement in survival for patients receiving the product. Based on these findings and the lack of other efficacious treatment options for these men, Dendreon submitted a Biologics License Application to the U.S. Food and Drug Administration (FDA). The FDA's Cellular, Tissue, and Gene Therapies Advisory Committee was scheduled to consider the application in open session March 29 and 30, 2007. Unfortunately, approval of the drug was denied by the FDA pending additional data.

Prostate GVAX (Cell Genesys, San Francisco, CA, USA) is an off-the-shelf immunotherapeutic agent that is also being evaluated for CRPC. Phase II trials are complete, and investigators are now enrolling patients in a Phase III trial. This product uses prostate cancer cell lines (PC-3, LnCaP) that have been virally transduced to express GM-CSF and then lethally irradiated. GVAX is subsequently administered intradermally, where a high concentration of antigen-presenting cells reside. A Phase II study of prostate GVAX in 34 patients with metastatic CRPC resulted in a favorable median survival of 26 months *(127)*. Further evaluation of 80 patients with metastatic CRPC treated at higher doses demonstrated one partial PSA response with improvement in bone turnover markers *(128)*. Survival analysis in this trial is ongoing. Prostate GVAX is now being directly compared with the new chemotherapeutic standard for symptomatic metastatic CRPC, docetaxel. In the VITAL-1 trial, men will be randomized to receive either prostate GVAX or docetaxel. In the VITAL-2 trial, all men with CRPC will receive docetaxel with or without the GVAX product.

7. CONCLUSION

Investigators have undertaken studies of a broad range of targeted therapeutic agents in efforts to control CRPC, including agents meant to affect androgens and AR signaling mechanisms. Among them are agents that affect binding of the AR to Hsp90, reactivate transcription of repressed tumor suppressor genes, and act in dysregulated prostate cancer pathways. Others are designed (1) to affect growth factor-mediated signaling, (2) to have antiapoptotic and antiangiogenesis effects, and (3) to function as endothelin-A receptor antagonists to affect bone turnover and thereby disease progression. With equal enthusiasm, investigators have sought to use a new understanding of the combination of the introduction of prostate-specific antigens at puberty and their androgen dependence to place prostate cancer at the forefront of cancer immunotherapeutics. Like new knowledge of the AR, apoptosis, and angiogenesis, unraveling and harnessing the power and complexity of the human immune system is beginning to lead to new pathways for treating CRPC.

REFERENCES

1. Feldman BJ, Feldman D. The development of androgen-independent prostate cancer. Nat Rev Cancer 2001;1(1):34–45.
2. Scher HI, Sawyers CL. Biology of progressive, castration-resistant prostate cancer: directed therapies targeting the androgen-receptor signaling axis. J Clin Oncol 2005;23(32):8253–61.

3. Berger R, Febbo PG, Majumder PK, et al. Androgen-induced differentiation and tumorigenicity of human prostate epithelial cells. Cancer Res 2004;64(24):8867–75.

4. Litvinov IV, De Marzo AM, Isaacs JT. Is the Achilles' heel for prostate cancer therapy a gain of function in androgen receptor signaling? J Clin Endocrinol Metab 2003;88(7):2972–82.

5. Grossmann ME, Huang H, Tindall DJ. Androgen receptor signaling in androgen-refractory prostate cancer. J Natl Cancer Inst 2001;93(22):1687–97.

6. Chen CD, Welsbie DS, Tran C, et al. Molecular determinants of resistance to antiandrogen therapy. Nat Med 2004;10(1):33–9.

7. Han G, Buchanan G, Ittmann M, et al. Mutation of the androgen receptor causes oncogenic transformation of the prostate. Proc Natl Acad Sci U S A 2005;102(4):1151–6.

8. Zegarra-Moro OL, Schmidt LJ, Huang H, et al. Disruption of androgen receptor function inhibits proliferation of androgen-refractory prostate cancer cells. Cancer Res 2002;62(4):1008–13.

9. Holzbeierlein J, Lal P, LaTulippe E, et al. Gene expression analysis of human prostate carcinoma during hormonal therapy identifies androgen-responsive genes and mechanisms of therapy resistance. Am J Pathol 2004;164(1):217–27.

10. Mousses S, Wagner U, Chen Y, et al. Failure of hormone therapy in prostate cancer involves systematic restoration of androgen responsive genes and activation of rapamycin sensitive signaling. Oncogene 2001;20(46):6718–23.

11. Shah RB, Mehra R, Chinnaiyan AM, et al. Androgen-independent prostate cancer is a heterogeneous group of diseases: lessons from a rapid autopsy program. Cancer Res 2004;64(24):9209–16.

12. Edwards J, Krishna NS, Grigor KM, et al. Androgen receptor gene amplification and protein expression in hormone refractory prostate cancer. Br J Cancer 2003;89(3):552–6.

13. Gregory CW, Johnson RT Jr, Mohler JL, et al. Androgen receptor stabilization in recurrent prostate cancer is associated with hypersensitivity to low androgen. Cancer Res 2001;61(7):2892–8.

14. Linja MJ, Savinainen KJ, Saramaki OR, et al. Amplification and overexpression of androgen receptor gene in hormone-refractory prostate cancer. Cancer Res 2001;61(9):3550–5.

15. Chen S, Xu Y, Yuan X, et al. Androgen receptor phosphorylation and stabilization in prostate cancer by cyclin-dependent kinase 1. Proc Natl Acad Sci U S A 2006;103(43):15969–74.

16. Gioeli D. Signal transduction in prostate cancer progression. Clin Sci (Lond) 2005;108(4):293–308.

17. Agoulnik IU, Weigel NL. Androgen receptor action in hormone-dependent and recurrent prostate cancer. J Cell Biochem 2006;99(2):362–72.

18. Gelmann EP. Molecular biology of the androgen receptor. J Clin Oncol 2002;20(13):3001–15.

19. Jia Li, Shen HC, Wantroba M, et al. Locus wide chromatin remodeling and enhanced androgen receptor-mediated transcription in recurrent prostate tumor cells. Mol Cell Biol 2006;26(19):7331–41.

20. Mohler JL, Gregory CW, Ford OH 3rd, et al. The androgen axis in recurrent prostate cancer. Clin Cancer Res 2004;10(2):440–8.

21. Titus MA, Schell MJ, Lih FB, et al. Testosterone and dihydrotestosterone tissue levels in recurrent prostate cancer. Clin Cancer Res 2005;11(13):4653–7.

22. Stanbrough M, Bubley GJ, Ross K, et al. Increased expression of genes converting adrenal androgens to testosterone in androgen-independent prostate cancer. Cancer Res 2006;66(5):2815–25.

23. Leroux F. Inhibition of p450 17 as a new strategy for the treatment of prostate cancer. Curr Med Chem 2005;12(14):1623–9.

24. Attard G, Yap TA, Reid AH, et al. Activity, toxicity, and effect on steroid precursor levels of abiraterone (A), an oral irreversible inhibitor of CYP17 (17α hydroxylase/17,20 lyase), in castrate men with castration refractory prostate cancer (CRPC). Presented at the Prostate Cancer Symposium, 2007. Abstract 264.

25. Bohl CE, Gao W, Miller DD, et al. Structural basis for antagonism and resistance of bicalutamide in prostate cancer. Proc Natl Acad Sci U S A 2005;102(17):6201–6.

26. Sack JS, Kish KF, Wang C, et al. Crystallographic structures of the ligand-binding domains of the androgen receptor and its T877A mutant complexed with the natural agonist dihydrotestosterone. Proc Natl Acad Sci U S A 2001;98(9):4904–9.

27. Bohl CE, Wu Z, Miller DD, et al. Crystal structure of the T877A human androgen receptor ligand-binding domain complexed to cyproterone acetate provides insight for ligand-induced conformational changes and structure-based drug design. J Biol Chem 2007;282:13648–55.

28. Solit DB, Scher HI, Rosen N. Hsp90 as a therapeutic target in prostate cancer. Semin Oncol 2003;30(5): 709–16.

29. Banerji U, O'Donnell A, Scurr M, et al. Phase I pharmacokinetic and pharmacodynamic study of 17-allylamino, 17-demethoxygeldanamycin in patients with advanced malignancies. J Clin Oncol 2005;23(18):4152–61.

30. Goetz MP, Toft D, Reid J, et al. Phase I trial of 17-allylamino-17-demethoxygeldanamycin in patients with advanced cancer. J Clin Oncol 2005;23(6):1078–87.

31. Grem JL, Morrison G, Guo XD, et al. Phase I and pharmacologic study of 17-(allylamino)-17-demethoxygeldanamycin in adult patients with solid tumors. J Clin Oncol 2005;23(9):1885–93.

32. Butler LM, Agus DB, Scher HI, et al. Suberoylanilide hydroxamic acid, an inhibitor of histone deacetylase, suppresses the growth of prostate cancer cells in vitro and in vivo. Cancer Res 2000;60(18):5165–70.

33. Chen L, Meng S, Wang H, et al. Chemical ablation of androgen receptor in prostate cancer cells by the histone deacetylase inhibitor LAQ824. Mol Cancer Ther 2005;4(9):1311–9.

34. Scroggins BT, Robzyk K, Wang D, et al. An acetylation site in the middle domain of Hsp90 regulates chaperone function. Mol Cell 2007;25(1):151–9.

35. Seligson DB, Horvath S, Shi T, et al. Global histone modification patterns predict risk of prostate cancer recurrence. Nature 2005;435(7046):1262–6.

36. Li LC, Carroll PR, Dahiya R. Epigenetic changes in prostate cancer: implication for diagnosis and treatment. J Natl Cancer Inst 2005;97(2):103–15.

37. Molife R, Patterson S, Riggs C, et al. Phase II study of FK228 in patients with hormone refractory prostate cancer (HRPC). J Clin Oncol 2006;24(18S):14554.

38. Burd CJ, Morey LM, Knudsen KE. Androgen receptor corepressors and prostate cancer. Endocr Relat Cancer 2006;13(4):979–94.

39. Bebermeier JH, Brooks JD, Deprimo SE, et al. Cell-line and tissue-specific signatures of androgen receptor-coregulator transcription. J Mol Med 2006;84(11):919–31.

40. Kang Z, Janne OA, Palvimo JJ. Coregulator recruitment and histone modifications in transcriptional regulation by the androgen receptor. Mol Endocrinol 2004;18(11):2633–48.

41. Yan J, Yu CT, Ozen M, et al. Steroid receptor coactivator-3 and activator protein-1 coordinately regulate the transcription of components of the insulin-like growth factor/AKT signaling pathway. Cancer Res 2006;66(22):11039–46.

42. Debes JD, Schmidt LJ, Huang H, et al. p300 mediates androgen-independent transactivation of the androgen receptor by interleukin 6. Cancer Res 2002;62(20):5632–6.

43. Gregory CW, Hamil KG, Kim D, et al. Androgen receptor expression in androgen-independent prostate cancer is associated with increased expression of androgen-regulated genes. Cancer Res 1998;58(24):5718–24.

44. Hong H, Kao C, Jeng MH, et al. Aberrant expression of CARM1, a transcriptional coactivator of androgen receptor, in the development of prostate carcinoma and androgen-independent status. Cancer 2004;101(1):83–9.

45. Hodgson MC, Astapova I, Cheng S, et al. The androgen receptor recruits nuclear receptor CoRepressor (N-CoR) in the presence of mifepristone via its N and C termini revealing a novel molecular mechanism for androgen receptor antagonists. J Biol Chem 2005;280:6511–9.

46. Mulholland DJ, Dedhar S, Wu H, et al. PTEN and GSK3beta: key regulators of progression to androgen-independent prostate cancer. Oncogene 2006;25(3):329–37.

47. Vivanco I, Sawyers CL. The phosphatidylinositol 3-Kinase AKT pathway in human cancer. Nat Rev Cancer 2002;2(7):489–501.

48. Kreisberg JI, Malik SN, Prihoda TJ, et al. Phosphorylation of Akt (Ser473) is an excellent predictor of poor clinical outcome in prostate cancer. Cancer Res 2004;64(15):5232–6.

49. Ayala G, Thompson T, Yang G, et al. High levels of phosphorylated form of Akt-1 in prostate cancer and non-neoplastic prostate tissues are strong predictors of biochemical recurrence. Clin Cancer Res 2004;10(19):6572–8.

50. Li B, Sun A, Youn H, et al. Conditional Akt activation promotes androgen-independent progression of prostate cancer. Carcinogenesis 2007;28(3):572–83.

51. Easton JB, Kurmasheva RT, Houghton PJ. IRS-1: auditing the effectiveness of mTOR inhibitors. Cancer Cell 2006;9(3):153–5.

52. Ruiter GA, Zerp SF, Bartelink H, et al. Anti-cancer alkyl-lysophospholipids inhibit the phosphatidylinositol 3-kinase-Akt/PKB survival pathway. Anticancer Drugs 2003;14(2):167–73.

53. Kondapaka SB, Singh SS, Dasmahapatra GP, et al. Perifosine, a novel alkylphospholipid, inhibits protein kinase B activation. Mol Cancer Ther 2003;2(11):1093–103.

54. Chee KG, Lara PN, Longmate J, et al. The AKT inhibitor perifosine in biochemically recurrent, hormone-sensitive prostate cancer (HSPC): a phase II California Cancer Consortium Trial. J Clin Oncol 2005;23(16S):4642.

55. Posadas EM, Gulley J, Arlen PM, et al. A phase II study of perifosine in androgen independent prostate cancer. Cancer Biol Ther 2005;4(10):1133–7.

56. Craft N, Shostak Y, Carey M, et al. A mechanism for hormone-independent prostate cancer through modulation of androgen receptor signaling by the HER-2/neu tyrosine kinase. Nat Med 1999;5(3):280–5.

57. Culig Z, Hobisch A, Cronauer MV, et al. Androgen receptor activation in prostatic tumor cell lines by insulin-like growth factor-I, keratinocyte growth factor, and epidermal growth factor. Cancer Res 1994;54(20): 5474–8.

58. Gregory CW, Fei X, Ponguta LA, et al. Epidermal growth factor increases coactivation of the androgen receptor in recurrent prostate cancer. J Biol Chem 2004;279(8):7119–30.

59. Fan W, Yanase T, Morinaga H, et al. Insulin-like growth factor 1/insulin signaling activates androgen signaling through direct interactions of Foxo1 with androgen receptor. J Biol Chem 2007;282(10):7329–38.

60. Nickerson T, Chang F, Lorimer D, et al. In vivo progression of LAPC-9 and LNCaP prostate cancer models to androgen independence is associated with increased expression of insulin-like growth factor I (IGF-I) and IGF-I receptor (IGF-IR). Cancer Res 2001;61(16):6276–80.

61. Miyake H, Pollak M, Gleave ME. Castration-induced up-regulation of insulin-like growth factor binding protein-5 potentiates insulin-like growth factor-I activity and accelerates progression to androgen independence in prostate cancer models. Cancer Res 2000;60(11):3058–64.

62. Kiyama S, Morrison K, Zellweger T, et al. Castration-induced increases in insulin-like growth factor-binding protein 2 promotes proliferation of androgen-independent human prostate LNCaP tumors. Cancer Res 2003;63(13):3575–84.

63. Mehrian-Shai R, Chen CD, Shi T, et al. Insulin growth factor-binding protein 2 is a candidate biomarker for PTEN status and PI3K/Akt pathway activation in glioblastoma and prostate cancer. Proc Natl Acad Sci U S A 2007;104(13):5563–8.

64. Slovin SF, Kelly WK, Cohen R, et al. Epidermal growth factor receptor (EGFr) monoclonal antibody (MoAb) C225 and doxorubicin (DOC) in androgen-independent (AI) prostate cancer (PC): results of a phase Ib/IIa study. Proc Am Soc Clin Oncol 1997;16:311a.

65. Ziada A, Barqawi A, Glode LM, et al. The use of trastuzumab in the treatment of hormone refractory prostate cancer; phase II trial. Prostate 2004;60(4):332–7.

66. Lara PN Jr, Chee KG, Longmate J, et al. Trastuzumab plus docetaxel in HER-2/neu-positive prostate carcinoma: final results from the California Cancer Consortium Screening and Phase II Trial. Cancer 2004;100(10):2125–31.

67. Morris MJ, Reuter VE, Kelly WK, et al. HER-2 profiling and targeting in prostate carcinoma. Cancer 2002;94(4):980–6.

68. De Bono JS, Bellmunt J, Attard G, et al. Open-label phase II study evaluating the efficacy and safety of two doses of pertuzumab in castrate chemotherapy-naive patients with hormone-refractory prostate cancer. J Clin Oncol 2007;25(3):257–62.

69. Agus DB, Sweeney CJ, Morris MJ, et al. Efficacy and safety of single-agent pertuzumab (rhuMAb 2C4), a human epidermal growth factor receptor dimerization inhibitor, in castration-resistant prostate cancer after progression from taxane-based therapy. J Clin Oncol 2007;25(6):675–81.

70. Canil CM, Moore MJ, Winquist E, et al. Randomized phase II study of two doses of gefitinib in hormone-refractory prostate cancer: a trial of the National Cancer Institute of Canada-Clinical Trials Group. J Clin Oncol 2005;23(3):455–60.

71. Gravis G, Goncalves A, Bladou F, et al. A phase II study of erlotinib in advanced prostate cancer. Presented at the Prostate Cancer Symposium, 2006. Abstract 245.

72. Nabhan C, Tolzien K, Newman S, et al. Phase II trial investigating the efficacy and toxicity of single agent erlotinib in chemotherapy-naïve androgen-independent metastatic prostate cancer. Presented at the Prostate Cancer Symposium, 2007. Abstract 240.

73. Sridhar SS, Hotte SJ, Chin JL, et al. A multicenter phase II study of lapatinib in hormone sensitive prostate cancer (HSPC). Presente at the Prostate Cancer Symposium, 2007. Abstract 261.

74. Solit DB, Rosen N. Targeting HER2 in prostate cancer: where to next? J Clin Oncol 2007;25(3):241–3.

75. Nelson EC, Cambio AJ, Yang JC, et al. Biologic agents as adjunctive therapy for prostate cancer: a rationale for use with androgen deprivation. Nat Clin Pract Urol 2007;4(2):82–94.

76. Guo Z, Dai B, Jiang T, et al. Regulation of androgen receptor activity by tyrosine phosphorylation. Cancer Cell 2006;10(4):309–19.

77. McDonnell TJ, Troncoso P, Brisbay SM, et al. Expression of the protooncogene bcl-2 in the prostate and its association with emergence of androgen-independent prostate cancer. Cancer Res 1992;52(24):6940–4.

78. Majumder PK, Febbo PG, Bikoff R, et al. mTOR inhibition reverses Akt-dependent prostate intraepithelial neoplasia through regulation of apoptotic and HIF-1-dependent pathways. Nat Med 2004;10(6):594–601.

79. Tolcher AW, Chi K, Kuhn J, et al. A phase II, pharmacokinetic, and biological correlative study of oblimersen sodium and docetaxel in patients with hormone-refractory prostate cancer. Clin Cancer Res 2005;11(10):3854–61.

80. Sternberg CN, Dumez H, Van Poppel H, et al. Multicenter randomized EORTC trial 30021 of docetaxel + oblimersen and docetaxel in patients (pts) with hormone refractory prostate cancer (HRPC). Presented at the Prostate Cancer Symposium, 2007. Abstract 144.

81. Miayake H, Tolcher A, Gleave ME. Chemosensitization and delayed androgen-independent recurrence of prostate cancer with the use of antisense Bcl-2 oligodeoxynucleotides. J Natl Cancer Inst 2000;92(1):34–41.

82. Zhang H, Kim JK, Edwards CA, et al. Clusterin inhibits apoptosis by interacting with activated Bax. Nat Cell Biol 2005;7(9):909–15.

83. Miyake H, Nelson C, Rennie PS, et al. Acquisition of chemoresistant phenotype by overexpression of the antiapoptotic gene testosterone-repressed prostate message-2 in prostate cancer xenograft models. Cancer Res 2000;60(9):2547–54.

84. Chi KN, Eisenhauer E, Fazli L, et al. A phase I pharmacokinetic and pharmacodynamic study of OGX-011, a 2'-methoxyethyl antisense oligonucleotide to clusterin, in patients with localized prostate cancer. J Natl Cancer Inst 2005;97(17):1287–96.

85. Zhang M, Latham DE, Delaney MA, et al. Survivin mediates resistance to antiandrogen therapy in prostate cancer. Oncogene 2005;24(15):2474–82.

86. Tolcher AW, Karavasilis V, Hudes G, et al. YM155, a novel survivin suppressant, demonstrates activity in subjects with hormone refractory prostate cancer (HRPC) previously treated with taxane chemotherapy. Presented at the International Symposium on Targeted Anticancer Therapies, 2007. Abstract 404.

87. Dai J, Kitagawa Y, Zhang J, et al. Vascular endothelial growth factor contributes to the prostate cancer-induced osteoblast differentiation mediated by bone morphogenetic protein. Cancer Res 2004;64(3):994–9.

88. Kim SJ, Uehara H, Yazici S, et al. Targeting platelet-derived growth factor receptor on endothelial cells of multidrug-resistant prostate cancer. J Natl Cancer Inst 2006;98(11):783–93.

89. Reese DM, Fratesi P, Corry M, et al. A phase II trial of humanized anti-vascular endothelial growth factor antibody for the treatment of androgen-independent prostate cancer. Prostate J 2001;3:65–70.

90. Picus J, Halabi S, Rini B, et al. The use of bevacizumab (B) with docetaxel (D) and estramustine (E) in hormone refractory prostate cancer (HRPC): initial results of CALGB 90006. Proc Am Soc Clin Oncol 2003;22. Abstract 1578.

91. Rini BI, Weinberg V, Fong L, et al. Combination immunotherapy with prostatic acid phosphatase pulsed antigen-presenting cells (provenge) plus bevacizumab in patients with serologic progression of prostate cancer after definitive local therapy. Cancer 2006;107(1):67–74.

92. Efstathiou E, Troncoso P, Wen S, et al. Initial modulation of the tumor microenvironment accounts for thalidomide activity in prostate cancer. Clin Cancer Res 2007;13(4):1224–31.

93. Figg WD, Dahut W, Duray P, et al. A randomized phase II trial of thalidomide, an angiogenesis inhibitor, in patients with androgen-independent prostate cancer. Clin Cancer Res 2001;7(7):1888–93.

94. Drake MJ, Robson W, Mehta P, et al. An open-label phase II study of low-dose thalidomide in androgen-independent prostate cancer. Br J Cancer 2003;88(6):822–7.

95. Dahut WL, Gulley JL, Arlen PM, et al. Randomized phase II trial of docetaxel plus thalidomide in androgen-independent prostate cancer. J Clin Oncol 2004;22(13):2532–9.

96. Ning YM, Gulley J, Arlen P, et al. Phase II trial of thalidomide, bevacizumab, and docetaxel in patients (pts) with metastatic androgen-independent prostate cancer (AIPC). Presented at the Prostate Cancer Symposium, 2007. Abstract 228.

97. Mathew P, Thall PF, Jones D, et al. Platelet-derived growth factor receptor inhibitor imatinib mesylate and docetaxel: a modular phase I trial in androgen-independent prostate cancer. J Clin Oncol 2004;22(16):3323–9.

98. Dahut WL, Scripture CD, Posadas EM, et al. Bony metastatic disease responses to sorafenib (BAY 43–9006) independent of PSA in patients with metastatic androgen independent prostate cancer. J Clin Oncol 2006;24:4506.

99. Mathew P, Thall PF, Johnson MM, et al. Preliminary results of a randomized placebo-controlled double-blind trial of weekly docetaxel combined with imatinib in men with metastatic androgen-independent prostate cancer (AIPC) and bone metastases (BM). J Clin Oncol 2006;24:4562.

100. Scher HI. Prostate carcinoma: defining therapeutic objectives and improving overall outcomes. Cancer 2003;97(suppl):758–71.

101. Jung K, Lein M, Stephan C, et al. Comparison of 10 serum bone turnover markers in prostate carcinoma patients with bone metastatic spread: diagnostic and prognostic implications. Int J Cancer 2004;111(5):783–91.

102. Nelson JB, Hedican SP, George DJ, et al. Identification of endothelin-1 in the pathophysiology of metastatic adenocarcinoma of the prostate. Nat Med 1995;1(9):944–9.

103. Yin JJ, Mohammad KS, Kakonen SM, et al. A causal role for endothelin-1 in the pathogenesis of osteoblastic bone metastases. Proc Natl Acad Sci U S A 2003;100(19):10954–9.

104. Nelson JB, Nabulsi AA, Vogelzang NJ, et al. Suppression of prostate cancer induced bone remodeling by the endothelin receptor A antagonist atrasentan. J Urol 2003;169(3):1143–9.
105. Carducci MA, Padley RJ, Breul J, et al. Effect of endothelin-A receptor blockade with atrasentan on tumor progression in men with hormone-refractory prostate cancer: a randomized, phase II, placebo-controlled trial. J Clin Oncol 2003;21(4):679–89.
106. Carducci M, Nelson JB, Saad F, et al. Effects of atrasentan on disease progression and biological markers in men with metastatic hormone-refractory prostate cancer: phase 3 study. J Clin Oncol 2004;22(14S):4508.
107. Sleep DJ, Nelson JB, Petrylak DP, et al. Clinical benefit of atrasentan for men with metastatic hormone-refractory prostate cancer metastatic to bone. J Clin Oncol 2006;24(18S):4630.
108. Nelson JB, Chin JL, Love W, et al. Results of a phase 3 randomized controlled trial of the safety and efficacy of atrasentan in men with nonmetastatic hormone-refractory prostate cancer (HRPC). Presented at the Prostate Cancer Symposium, 2007. Abstract 146.
109. Boyle WJ, Simonet WS, Lacey DL. Osteoclast differentiation and activation. Nature 2003;423(6937): 337–42.
110. Fizazi K, Bosserman L, Lipton A, et al. Phase II randomized trial of denosumab in patients with bone metastases from prostate cancer and elevated urine N- telopeptide levels after receiving zoledronic acid. Presented at the Prostate Cancer Symposium, 2007. Abstract 272.
111. Marker PC, Donjacour AA, Dahiya R, et al. Hormonal, cellular, and molecular control of prostatic development. Dev Biol 2003;253(2):165–74.
112. Mercader M, Bodner BK, Moser MT, et al. T cell infiltration of the prostate induced by androgen withdrawal in patients with prostate cancer. Proc Natl Acad Sci U S A 2001;98(25):14565–70.
113. Alexander RB, Brady F, Ponniah S. Autoimmune prostatitis: evidence of T cell reactivity with normal prostatic proteins. Urology 1997;50(6):893–9.
114. Ponniah S, Arah I, Alexander RB. PSA is a candidate self-antigen in autoimmune chronic prostatitis/chronic pelvic pain syndrome. Prostate 2000;44(1):49–54.
115. Simons JW, Mikhak B, Chang JF, et al. Induction of immunity to prostate cancer antigens: results of a clinical trial of vaccination with irradiated autologous prostate tumor cells engineered to secrete granulocyte-macrophage colony-stimulating factor using ex vivo gene transfer. Cancer Res 1999;59(20):5160–8.
116. Hurwitz AA, Foster BA, Kwon ED, et al. Combination immunotherapy of primary prostate cancer in a transgenic mouse model using CTLA-4 blockade. Cancer Res 2000;60(9):2444–8.
117. Kwon ED, Foster BA, Hurwitz AA, et al. Elimination of residual metastatic prostate cancer after surgery and adjunctive cytotoxic T lymphocyte-associated antigen 4 (CTLA-4) blockade immunotherapy. Proc Natl Acad Sci U S A 1999;96(26):15074–9.
118. Kwon ED, Hurwitz AA, Foster BA, et al. Manipulation of T cell costimulatory and inhibitory signals for immunotherapy of prostate cancer. Proc Natl Acad Sci U S A 1997;94(15):8099–103.
119. Fong L, Ruegg CL, Brockstedt D, et al. Induction of tissue-specific autoimmune prostatitis with prostatic acid phosphatase immunization: implications for immunotherapy of prostate cancer. J Immunol 1997;159(7):3113–7.
120. Vieweg J, Rosenthal FM, Bannerji R, et al. Immunotherapy of prostate cancer in the Dunning rat model: use of cytokine gene modified tumor vaccines. Cancer Res 1994;54(7):1760–5.
121. Shimizu J, Yamazaki S, Sakaguchi S. Induction of tumor immunity by removing CD25+CD4+ T cells: a common basis between tumor immunity and autoimmunity. J Immunol 1999;163(10):5211–8.
122. Woo EY, Yeh H, Chu CS, et al. Cutting edge: regulatory T cells from lung cancer patients directly inhibit autologous T cell proliferation. J Immunol 2002;168(9):4272–6.
123. Viguier M, Lemaitre F, Verola O, et al. Foxp3 expressing CD4+CD25(high) regulatory T cells are overrepresented in human metastatic melanoma lymph nodes and inhibit the function of infiltrating T cells. J Immunol 2004;173(2):1444–53.
124. Wolf AM, Wolf D, Steurer M, et al. Increase of regulatory T cells in the peripheral blood of cancer patients. Clin Cancer Res 2003;9(2):606–12.
125. Vesalainen S, Lipponen P, Talja M, et al. Histological grade, perineural infiltration, tumour-infiltrating lymphocytes and apoptosis as determinants of long-term prognosis in prostatic adenocarcinoma. Eur J Cancer 1994;30A(12):1797–803.
126. Dannull J, Su Z, Rizzieri D, et al. Enhancement of vaccine-mediated antitumor immunity in cancer patients after depletion of regulatory T cells. J Clin Invest 2005;115(12):3623–33.
127. Simons JW, Sacks N. Granulocyte-macrophage colony-stimulating factor-transduced allogeneic cancer cellular immunotherapy: the GVAX vaccine for prostate cancer. Urol Oncol 2006;24(5):419–24.
128. Small E, Higano C, Corman J. A phase 2 study of an allogeneic GM-CSF gene-transduced prostate cancer cell line vaccine in patients with metastatic hormone-refractory prostate cancer (HRPC). Proc Am Soc Clin Oncol 2004;22(14s). Abstract 4565

15 Targeted Therapy in Renal Cell Carcinoma

Eric Jonasch, MD and Nizar Tannir, MD

CONTENTS

ABSTRACT

Renal cell carcinoma affects close to 40,000 people per year in the United States; and once it is metastatic, treatment options have historically been limited. With our emerging understanding of the molecular biology of renal cell carcinoma, we have recently acquired an expanding armamentarium of agents that target vascular and intracellular pathways involved in renal carcinogenesis. This chapter describes the key agents and the clinical data supporting their use. The chapter concludes with several of the key dilemmas we will face over the next decade when approaching the treatment of renal cell carcinoma.

Key Words: Renal cell carcinoma, VHL mutation, Antivascular therapy, Targeted therapy, Combination therapy, Sequential therapy

1. EPIDEMIOLOGY

In 2006, renal cell carcinoma (RCC) was estimated to occur in 39,000 people in the United States, and almost 13,000 people were projected to die from their disease *(1)*. RCC represents 2% of all malignancies. Worldwide, the mortality from RCC has been estimated to exceed 100,000 per year and may be as high as 170,000 *(2)*.

The incidence of RCC is increasing *(3)*. Since 1950, there has been a 126% increase in the incidence and a 37% increase in annual mortality *(1,4)*. The 5-year survival rate of patients diagnosed with RCC has improved from 34% for those diagnosed in 1954 to 62% for those diagnosed in 1996 *(4)*. Reasons for the improved outcome include earlier detection through computed tomography (CT) imaging and advances in surgical technique. Incidental discovery of RCC increased from approximately 10% during the 1970s to 60% in 1998 *(4)*.

From: *Current Clinical Oncology: Targeted Cancer Therapy*
Edited by: R. Kurzrock and M. Markman © Humana Press, Totowa, NJ

2. PATHOLOGY AND GENETICS

Renal cell carcinomas are divided into four major categories: clear cell (conventional), papillary, chromophobe, and collecting duct tumors. Rarer subtypes exist, including medullary, mucinous tubular, and spindle cell cancers and Xp11 translocation tumors of the kidney.

Clear cell or conventional RCC, which comprises 75% to 85% of the tumors, is characterized by a deletion or functional inactivation in one or both copies of chromosome 3p *(5)*. A higher nuclear grade (Fuhrman classification) or the presence of a sarcomatoid pattern correlates with a poorer prognosis *(6,7)*.

Papillary carcinomas make up approximately 10% of RCCs. In the hereditary setting, papillary carcinomas are multifocal and bilateral and commonly present as small tumors *(8)*. These lesions are both morphologically and genetically distinct from clear cell carcinomas and have multiple genetic abnormalities, including monosomy Y, trisomy 7, and trisomy 17 *(9)* but no abnormalities in 3p *(10)*. Although these tumors often present at a low stage and are thus assigned a more favorable prognosis *(8,11)*, in advanced stages their prognosis is equivalent to that of clear cell RCC *(12)*.

Chromophobe histology (cells do not take up colored dye readily) is found in approximately 4% of all RCCs. Chromophobe tumors have a hypodiploid number of chromosomes and no 3p loss *(13–15)*. Patients with chromophobe RCC generally have an excellent prognosis. Once they metastasize, chromophobe carcinomas are generally refractory to immunotherapy and chemotherapy but are nevertheless associated with better prognosis than clear cell carcinomas, with median overall survivals (OSs) of 29 and 13 months, respectively *(12)*.

Carcinomas of the collecting ducts (Bellini duct tumors) are also rare and are frequently extremely aggressive *(16)*. Collecting duct tumors have not been associated with a consistent pattern of genetic abnormalities.

Medullary RCC is a rare aggressive variant usually seen in individuals with sickle cell trait *(17)*. This entity was called the "seventh sickle cell nephropathy."*(17)* Little is known about the cytogenetics of this tumor. Monosomy of chromosome 11 *(18)* and BCR-ABL translocation *(19)* have been described. Other authors have described up-regulation of the *ABL* gene without BCR-ABL translocation *(20)*.

The Xp11.2 translocation carcinoma was first described in 1991 by Tomlinson et al. *(21)*. This translocation results in the fusion of RCC17 on chromosome 17q25 with the transcription factor TFE3 located on the Xp11 chromosomal region *(22)*. The resulting tumors usually occur in children and young adults. Although relatively indolent, they are refractory to systemic therapy.

3. MOLECULAR BIOLOGY

Much of our current knowledge of the molecular biology of clear cell RCC is derived from the discovery of the von Hippel-Lindau gene mutation in 1993 *(23)*. Von Hippel-Lindau (VHL) disease is an autosomal dominant hereditary illness that induces clear cell RCC, renal cysts, retinal angiomas, spinal and cerebellar hemangioblastomas, pheochromocytomas, pancreatic neuroendocrine tumors, and pancreatic cysts *(24)*. Clear cell RCC develops in 40% to 70% of patients with VHL and is a major cause of death. Tumor development in this setting is linked to somatic inactivation of the remaining wild-type allele. Biallelic VHL inactivation due to somatic mutations and/or hypermethylation is observed in more than

50% of patients with sporadic clear cell RCC, demonstrating a unique similarity between inherited and somatic disorders.

The von Hippel-Lindau protein (pVHL) is an E3 ubiquitin ligase that has several key functions, including regulation of hypoxia inducible factor (HIF) *(25)*. HIF is a heterodimer composed of HIFα and HIFβ subunits *(26)*. HIFβ is constitutively expressed, and HIFα is normally degraded in the normoxic state *(27,28)*. A 200-amino-acid oxygen-dependent degradation domain lies within the central region of HIF1α *(29,30)*. This region permits recognition by pVHL and subsequent degradation *(30,31)*. The interaction of pVHL with HIF is regulated by a prolyl hydroxylase acting on residue 564 of HIF1α or residue 531 of HIF2α *(27,29–31)*. In the presence of oxygen, HIFα becomes hydroxylated, is recognized by pVHL, and is degraded. In the hypoxic state, the prolyl hydroxylase remains inactivated, and HIF heterodimerization and transcriptional activation occur. Mutated or functionally inactivated HIF replicates the hypoxic state. The downstream consequences of unbridled HIF-related transcription include increased production of vascular endothelial growth factor (VEGF), platelet-derived growth factor (PDGF), transforming growth factor-α (TGFα), erythropoietin, glucose transport (GLUT1), carbonic anhydrase IX, and several dozen other HIF-responsive genes. Low carbonic anhydrase IX, which is associated with the absence of VHL mutation and with aggressive tumor characteristics, is a significant predictor of poor prognosis in patients with clear cell RCC. Clear cell RCC was considered an ideal disease in which to evaluate the efficacy of antivascular therapy because of the relation between the VHL mutation and the production of proangiogenic factors.

The hereditary papillary RCC (*PRC*) gene was identified on chromosome 7q31.1-34 and codes for the c-*Met* proto-oncogene. Germline missense mutations in the tyrosine kinase domain of the c-*Met* proto-oncogene were detected in several hereditary PRC families *(32)*. These mutations result in a constitutively active form of c-Met. The ligand for c-Met is hepatocyte growth factor (HGF) *(33)*. HGF-Met signaling has been shown to regulate growth, invasion, tumor metastasis, angiogenesis, wound healing, and tissue regeneration *(34,35)*. Individuals with germline mutations of c-Met develop multifocal bilateral papillary RCC. Tumors from individuals who develop sporadic papillary RCC carry c-*Met* mutations approximately 15% of the time.

Several disorders are associated with fumarate hydratase (*FH*) gene mutations, including autosomal dominant multiple cutaneous and uterine leiomyomas (MCUL or MCL) and hereditary leiomyomatosis and RCC syndrome (HLRCC). An autosomal recessive condition, fumarate deficiency is associated with progressive encephalopathy, cerebral atrophy, seizures, hypotonia, and renal developmental delay. Carriers of FH are rarely shown to exhibit leiomyomas *(36)*. HLRCC is characterized by cutaneous leiomyomas, uterine fibroids, and RCCs, which are predominantly solitary *(37,38)*. The renal tumors are aggressive, and they may metastasize and lead to death in patients in their thirties. Although originally classified as hereditary papillary type 2 RCC, the unique cytomorphologic features of the renal tumors, as well as the finding of mutations in the *FH* gene in affected families suggest that it is a distinct entity *(39,40)*. The *FH* gene product is a component of the Krebs cycle and catalyzes the conversion of fumarate to malate. It also exists in a cytosolic form, thought to be involved in amino acid metabolism *(36)*. It is not known why this mutation results in the development of RCC.

The dominantly inherited Birt-Hogg-Dube (BHD) syndrome is characterized by cutaneous lesions (fibrofolliculomas); lung cysts, which may result in spontaneous pneumothoraces; and a predisposition to kidney neoplasms. The renal lesions include chromophobe RCC, oncocytomas, or lesions that have features of both (termed mixed oncocytic tumors) *(41–43)*. The affected gene, folliculin (*FLCN*), was described in 2002 *(44)*. The folliculin gene is localized on chromosome 17p and functions as a tumor suppressor gene *(44)*. How folliculin mutations induce RCC is not understood.

Tuberous sclerosis is an autosomal dominant condition associated with mutations in the tuberous sclerosis complex genes (*TSC1* or *TSC2*) *(45,46)*. Affected individuals typically manifest facial angiofibromas and cognitive impairment, and they develop renal angiomyolipomas *(47)*. The incidence of RCC is slightly increased in patients with *TSC* mutations.

The molecular biology of medullary carcinoma is poorly understood. No mutation or genetic disorder is associated with this disease, although it is found with increased frequency in individuals with sickle cell trait. Gene expression profiling in medullary renal carcinoma shows close clustering with urothelial (transitional cell) carcinoma of the renal pelvis *(48)*. Further work is needed to determine if unique genetic lesions exist in this disease.

4. TARGETING AGENTS FOR RENAL CELL CARCINOMA

The use of targeting agents has been most successful in diseases with well defined genetic lesions that drive tumor biology, against which agents have been developed to "drug" the abnormal pathway or molecule implicated in carcinogenesis. Key examples include HER2/Neu and trastuzumab for breast carcinoma and BCR-ABL and imatinib for chronic myelogenous leukemia. RCC may become another example of such a paradigm. The tumor biology of clear cell RCC appears to be driven by VHL mutations and that of papillary RCC by c-*MET* mutations. Most of the molecules tested so far have been designed to down-regulate HIF target genes. This model is intuitively attractive, but there are clearly some problems associated with it. As has recently been shown, objective responses are more likely to occur in patients with a mutated *VHL* gene, but lack of the mutation in the tumor specimen does not preclude a response to VEGF-targeted therapy *(49)*. In addition, emerging research implicates the disruption of non-HIF VHL functions in the development of clear cell RCC. Most importantly, these agents are failing to cure most individuals who receive them.

The following section outlines the key agents approved for, or studied in, RCC. With the exception of temsirolimus, these agents have been almost exclusively investigated in patients with clear cell histology. To date, no trials have been published specifically assessing the role of targeted agents in the treatment of patients with non-clear-cell histology.

4.1. Bevacizumab (Avastin)

Phase I studies using bevacizumab, a recombinant humanized anti-VEGF monoclonal antibody, demonstrated several responses in patients with metastatic RCC (mRCC). A subsequent Phase II study of 116 patients was reported in 2003. This study randomized patients who had progressive disease or were ineligible to receive interleukin-2 (IL-2) immunotherapy, comparing placebo with bevacizumab at doses of 3 or 10 mg/kg *(50)*. Progression-free survival (PFS) for patients on the high-dose arm was 4.8 months versus 2.5 months for the patients on placebo ($p < 0.001$). The study was stopped early on the basis of an interim analysis showing a significant difference in favorable outcome for the high-dose bevacizumab arm. Two large randomized, Phase III trials comparing frontline administration of bevacizumab plus subcutaneous interferon-α (IFNα) to IFNα alone or IFNα plus placebo completed accrual. The AVOREN study, sponsored by Roche, showed superiority of the combination of bevacizumab plus IFNα over IFNα plus placebo, with a median PFS of 10.2 months versus 5.4 months [hazard ratio (HR) = 0.63; $p < 0.0001$] and a response rate of 30.6% versus 12.4% ($p < 0.0001$) *(51)*. Studies looking at the role of erlotinib in combination with bevacizumab were completed and ultimately failed to show improved outcome compared to bevacizumab alone *(52,53)*. These studies are described in more detail below in the section on epidermal growth factor blocking agents.

4.2. Sorafenib (Bay 43-9006)

Sorafenib is a bis-aryl urea multikinase inhibitor originally developed as a potent inhibitor of wild-type and mutant (V599E) B-Raf and c-Raf proteins. It was also found to have inhibitory activity against VEGF receptor (VEGFR), PDGF receptor (PDGFR), c-Kit, and FLT3. A Phase II randomized discontinuation study accrued 202 patients with metastatic RCC *(54)*. All patients in this study received a lead-in of 12 weeks of treatment with sorafenib. Patients who had more than 25% tumor shrinkage or growth continued or discontinued therapy, respectively. Individuals with less than 25% change in tumor dimensions were randomized between sorafenib and placebo. PFS for patients on sorafenib was 24 weeks versus 6 weeks in the placebo group ($p < 0.0001$).

A large-scale Phase III clinical trial was subsequently performed in patients with mRCC who had failed one prior therapy. Patients were randomized between sorafenib and placebo. The median PFS was 5.5 months in the treatment arm and 2.8 months in the placebo arm ($p < 0.0001$). A subsequent survival analysis showed a difference in survival favoring the sorafenib arm ($p = 018$), which did not reach the predetermined threshold of 0.0005 required for early study termination. Tumor responses, all partial, were reported in 10% of the sorafenib-treated patients, although more than 70% of sorafenib-treated patients exhibited some degree of tumor shrinkage *(55)*. Largely on the basis of these data, sorafenib received approval by the FDA in late 2005 for use in patients with advanced RCC.

A randomized Phase II trial of sorafenib versus IFN in the first-line setting in mRCC showed no significant difference in median PFS between sorafenib and IFN (5.7 vs. 5.6 months, respectively). The overall response rate (ORR) was 5% with sorafenib and 9% with IFN *(56)*. In a recent Phase II trial of intrapatient dose-escalated sorafenib for mRCC, 91% of patients received 1200 or 1600 mg daily; 52% of the patients treated achieved a complete response (CR) or partial response (PR), with the median PFS 8.8 months *(57)*.

4.3. Sunitinib (Sutent)

Sunitinib is a small-molecule inhibitor of VEGFR, PDGFR, c-Kit, and FLT3. Two Phase II studies were performed in cytokine-refractory patients with mRCC. The first trial enrolled 63 patients, most of whom had tumors with clear cell histology and had undergone prior nephrectomy. The ORR was 40% with no complete responders, and the median PFS was 8.1 months *(58)*. A subsequent 106 patient study, in which 105 individuals had clear cell carcinoma (one patient had transitional cell carcinoma of the renal pelvis and was ineligible), had undergone prior nephrectomy, and had failed cytokine therapy, showed a 25% ORR after independent review. On the basis of these Phase II data, sunitinib was approved for use in patients with advanced RCC in January 2006.

A subsequent large-scale, frontline Phase III trial randomizing patients between sunitinib and IFNα resulted in an ORR of 31% and a median PFS of 11 months for sunitinib-treated patients versus a 6% ORR and 5 months median PFS for patients treated with IFN (both $p < 0.0001$). No significant difference in OS was observed *(59)*. A recent update of the Phase III trial shows the benefit of sunitinib extending to all Memorial Sloan-Kettering Cancer Center prognostic subgroups. The updated ORR by investigator assessment was 44% for sunitinib versus 11% for IFN, including 4 patients achieving a CR with sunitinib and 2 patients achieving a CR with IFN *(60)*. A Phase II trial of sunitinib in bevacizumab-refractory mRCC yielded an ORR of 23% and a median PFS of 30 weeks *(61)*.

4.4. Axitinib (AG-013736)

Axitinib is a potent inhibitor of VEGFR 1, 2, and 3 and showed substantial efficacy in a Phase II trial in patients with cytokine-refractory RCC, with a 46% ORR and median PFS close to 8 months *(62)*. A recent Phase II trial of this agent in patients with sorafenib-refractory mRCC showed a PR of 14%. Preliminary analysis indicates a median PFS of > 7.1 months *(63)*.

4.5. Temsirolimus (CCI-779)

Temsirolimus is a rapamycin analogue that inhibits mammalian target of rapamycin (mTOR) downstream of AKT and results in cell cycle arrest. Temsirolimus was approved for poor-risk mRCC in May 2007. Atkins et al. *(64)*. reported results of a randomized, double-blind, Phase II trial examining weekly intravenous doses of 25, 75, or 250 mg of temsirolimus in RCC patients who were either refractory to or were thought to be poor candidates for cytokine-based therapy *(64)*. A total of 29 patients (26%) showed a PR or a minor response, with a median time to progression (TTP) of 6 months. OS in this pretreated, predominantly poor prognosis group was 15 months. No obvious dose–response curve was seen, and the 25 mg dose was chosen for subsequent studies in RCCs. A reanalysis of the trial suggested that patients with intermediate and poor prognostic features appeared to benefit most compared to individuals with similar prognostic features receiving cytokine therapy.

A Phase III study randomized 625 patients with mRCC and poor prognostic features between temsirolimus 25 mg IV weekly, IFNα 9 MU three times a week, and temsirolimus 15 mg IV weekly plus IFNα 6 MU units three times a week. Results showed that the OS of patients receiving temsirolimus alone was significantly longer than those receiving IFN alone (10.9 vs. 7.3 months, $p = 0.0069$). The OS of patients receiving both agents was 8.4 months and was not significantly different from the temsirolimus-only arm *(65)*. In addition to clear cell RCC (approximately 80% of patients treated in the study), the benefit of temsirolimus extended to tumors with non-clear-cell RCC histology. This study established a survival benefit for temsirolimus in patients with mRCC and poor prognostic features, as defined by Motzer and colleagues, but its value in patients with better prognostic features remains to be established *(66)*.

4.6. Epidermal Growth Factor Blocking Agents

The epidermal growth factor (EGF) receptor antagonists, despite the presence of encouraging preclinical data, have not yet lived up to their promise. A high rate of EGF receptor expression on renal cell tumors coupled with loss of VHL, resulting in increased expression of TGFα, supports the presence of an autocrine loop in many RCCs. Inhibition of this autocrine loop by blocking the cell surface receptor (EGFR) or the ligand would be expected to result in growth inhibition and clinical response. As described below, blockade of the EGFR pathway has failed to show consistent clinical benefit.

4.6.1. CETUXIMAB (ERBITUX)

Cetuximab is a humanized (murine) inactivating anti-EGFR antibody first described in 1995. Results from a Phase II clinical trial evaluating cetuximab in 55 patients with mRCC were published in 2003. Patients received single-agent cetuximab administered by intravenous infusion at a loading dose of 400 or 500 mg/m^2 followed by weekly maintenance doses at 250 mg/m^2. No patient experienced a CR or PR. The median TTP was 57 days *(67)*.

4.6.2. PANITUMUMAB (ABX-EGF)

Panitumumab is a fully humanized anti-EGFR antibody. Phase II study results after evaluating panitumumab in patients with mRCC were reported in 2004. Panitumumab was administered to 88 previously treated patients at doses of 1.0, 1.5, 2.0, or 2.5 mg/kg weekly for 8 weeks. The study resulted in three PRs and two minor responses, and disease stabilization occurred in 44 patients at the 8-week time point *(68)*. The median PFS was 100 days.

4.6.3. GEFITINIB (IRESSA, ZD1839)

Gefitinib is a small-molecule inhibitor of EGFR. Druker et al. treated 18 mRCC patients with gefitinib at a dose of 500 mg daily. Of 12 evaluable tumor specimens, 11 stained positive for the EGF receptor. No CRs or PRs were seen. Thirteen patients (81%) progressed within 4 months of initiating therapy. VEGF and basic fibroblast growth factor (bFGF) serum levels were tested before starting therapy and every 3 months on therapy, but there was no correlation between pretreatment level and TTP *(69)*.

In late 2004, Dawson et al. published their experience with gefitinib in 21 patients with RCC. Patients had received a median of one prior therapy. The best response was stable disease in 8 patients (38%). The median PFS was 2.7 months, and the median OS was 8.3 months *(70)*. EGF receptor analysis and corresponding best response were assessed. There was no correlation between the intensity of EGF receptor staining (0 or 1 vs. 2 or 3) and having stable versus progressive disease.

Jermann et al. published a Phase II trial of open-label gefitinib 500 mg daily in 28 patients with locally advanced, metastatic, or relapsed RCC. Stable disease was reported in 14 patients (53.8%). The median TTP was 110 days, and the median OS was 303 days. In total, 91% of pretreatment tumor biopsies demonstrated that at least 70% of tumor cells expressed membrane EGF receptor *(71)*.

4.6.4. ERLOTINIB (TARCEVA)

Erlotinib is another small-molecule inhibitor of EGFR. Results from combining bevacizumab and erlotinib were reported in by Hainsworth et al. in November 2005. A group of 63 patients with metastatic clear cell RCC were treated with bevacizumab 10 mg/kg intravenously every 2 weeks and erlotinib 150 mg orally daily. Most of these individuals had not received prior systemic therapy. Of 59 assessable patients. 15 (25%) had objective responses to treatment, and an additional 36 patients (61%) had stable disease after 8 weeks of treatment; the disease had progressed in only 8 patients (14%) at that time point. The median and 1-year PFSs were 11% and 43%, respectively. After a median follow-up of 15 months, median survival had not been reached; survival at 18 months was 60% *(52)*.

A 104-patient follow-up study randomized patients with untreated metastatic RCC between bevacizumab plus placebo versus bevacizumab plus erlotinib. All patients received bevacizumab with either erlotinib 150 mg by mouth daily or placebo until disease progression or unacceptable toxicity. Patients who received bevacizumab alone had a median PFS of

8.5 months, and those who received both agents had a median PFS of 9.9 months. The difference was not statistically different, and there was no survival difference between the two arms *(53)*. The conclusion from these two studies is that erlotinib did not add a significant PFS or OS benefit to bevacizumab therapy.

4.6.5. LAPATINIB (TYKERB)

Lapatinib is a small-molecule dual HER1 and HER2 inhibitor. A Phase III study of 417 patients with advanced RCC of any histology who failed first-line cytokine therapy randomized patients between oral lapatinib 1250 mg OD or hormonal therapy with megestrol acetate. The primary efficacy endpoint was TTP, with a secondary endpoint of OS. At the time of analysis, median TTP did not differ between arms, with 15.3 weeks for lapatinib and 15.4 weeks for medroxyprogesterone; the median OS was 46.9 weeks for lapatinib versus 43.1 weeks for medroxyprogesterone (HR = 0.88; p = 0.29) *(72)*.

All tumors were assessed for EGFR expression by immunohistochemistry. For the 241 patients whose tumors had a high level of EGFR expression (3+ by immunohistochemistry), the median TTP was 15.1 weeks for lapatinib versus 10.9 weeks for medroxyprogesterone (HR = 0.76; p = 0.06); the median OS was 46.0 weeks for lapatinib versus 37.9 weeks for medroxyprogesterone (HR = 0.69; p = 0.02) *(73)*. This is the first study of RCCs that demonstrated an association between a biomarker and improved survival with a therapy targeting that specific biomarker. Unfortunately, the differences between arms were numerically small, suggesting either inadequate blockade of the target, acquisition of early resistance, or the possibility that EGFR signaling plays only a minor role in the pathogenesis of RCC.

5. SUMMARY AND FUTURE DIRECTIONS

Much has been learned about the molecular biology of RCC during the past decade, and we now have access to targeted agents that have a consistent, albeit modest, effect on tumor progression. Unfortunately, we still cure only a small number of individuals, and most patients with mRCC still die of their disease.

There are a number of potential explanations for our failure to achieve a significant cure fraction with these agents. Pharmacodynamic and pharmacokinetic factors must be considered as well as alternate signaling pathways or cellular processes. Finally, acquired versus inherent resistance to therapy is a possibility.

5.1. Pharmacokinetics and Pharmacodynamics

It is possible we are hitting the appropriate target but with an insufficient dose. If this is the case, either a dose escalation of the same agent or a "vertical" blockade of the same pathway might improve inhibition. Efforts to combine antivascular agents and to escalate dosages of single agents are underway in an attempt to resolve this possible difficulty.

5.2. Necessity Versus Sufficiency of Pathway Inhibition

It is possible that hitting our target is necessary but insufficient to achieve maximal antitumor activity and that alternate pathways must also be inhibited. The multikinase inhibitors sorafenib and sunitinib and the combination of bevacizumab with erlotinib are examples of multitarget inhibition. Nevertheless, as discussed above, studies have demonstrated the inability of these agents or combinations of these agents to achieve consistent tumor eradication in most patients. It is possible that other signaling pathways or cellular processes need to be targeted to achieve consistent tumor eradication. To date, we do not have an efficient screen that permits us to determine which pathways are central to tumorigenesis. Creating in vivo or in vitro screens may allow us to accelerate this process.

5.3. Inherent or Acquired Resistance to Therapy

The presence or acquisition of mutations that impart resistance to the agents being utilized is another obstacle to the use of targeted therapies. The example of imatinib in gastrointestinal stromal tumors is instructive. Specific mutations in the c-Kit receptor tyrosine kinase are predictive for inherent or acquired resistance to imatinib *(73)*. It is possible that the same processes are operative in RCC. We need to evaluate treated RCC tissue at the genetic and proteomic levels to understand better the determinants of response and resistance to therapy.

As we gain a better understanding of RCC tumor biology, and as we gain access to an ever-increasing number of agents targeting specific pathways, the chance of making progress increases. Fundamental to our success are tissue-rich clinical trials and validated preclinical models that accelerate the pace of discovery. We have to move beyond an empirical approach and ensure that future treatments paradigms are based on validated targets.

REFERENCES

1. Jemal A, Siegel R, Ward E, et al. Cancer statistics, 2006. CA Cancer J Clin 2006;56(2):106–30.
2. Patel PH, Chaganti RS, Motzer RJ. Targeted therapy for metastatic renal cell carcinoma. Br J Cancer 2006;94(5):614–9.
3. Chow WH, Devesa SS, Warren JL, et al. Rising incidence of renal cell cancer in the United States. JAMA 1999;281(17):1628–31.
4. Pantuck AJ, Zisman A, Belldegrun AS. The changing natural history of renal cell carcinoma. J Urol 2001;166(5):1611–23.
5. Presti JC Jr, Rao PH, Chen Q, et al. Histopathological, cytogenetic, and molecular characterization of renal cortical tumors. Cancer Res 1991;51(5):1544–52.
6. Weiss GR, Margolin KA, Sznol M, et al. A phase II study of the continuous intravenous infusion of interleukin-6 for metastatic renal cell carcinoma. J Immunother Emphasis Tumor Immunol 1995;18(1):52–6.
7. Fuhrman SA, Lasky LC, Limas C. Prognostic significance of morphologic parameters in renal cell carcinoma. Am J Surg Pathol 1982;6(7):655–63.
8. Mancilla-Jimenez R, Stanley RJ, Blath RA. Papillary renal cell carcinoma: a clinical, radiologic, and pathologic study of 34 cases. Cancer 1976;38(6):2469–80.
9. Kovacs G, Wilkens L, Papp T, et al. Differentiation between papillary and nonpapillary renal cell carcinomas by DNA analysis. J Natl Cancer Inst 1989;81(7):527–30.
10. Kovacs G, Fuzesi L, Emanual A, et al. Cytogenetics of papillary renal cell tumors. Genes Chromosomes Cancer 1991;3(4):249–55.
11. Sene AP, Hunt L, McMahon RF, et al. Renal carcinoma in patients undergoing nephrectomy: analysis of survival and prognostic factors. Br J Urol 1992;70(2):125–34.
12. Motzer RJ, Bacik J, Mariani T, et al. Treatment outcome and survival associated with metastatic renal cell carcinoma of non-clear-cell histology. J Clin Oncol 2002;20(9):2376–81.
13. Akhtar M, Kardar H, Linjawi T, et al. Chromophobe cell carcinoma of the kidney: a clinicopathologic study of 21 cases. Am J Surg Pathol 1995;19(11):1245–56.
14. Speicher MR, Schoell B, du Manoir S, et al. Specific loss of chromosomes 1, 2, 6, 10, 13, 17, and 21 in chromophobe renal cell carcinomas revealed by comparative genomic hybridization. Am J Pathol 1994;145(2):356–64.
15. Kovacs A, Kovacs G. Low chromosome number in chromophobe renal cell carcinomas. Genes Chromosomes Cancer 1992;4(3):267–8.
16. Kennedy SM, Merino MJ, Linehan WM, et al. Collecting duct carcinoma of the kidney. Hum Pathol 1990;21(4):449–56.

17. Davis CJ Jr, Mostofi FK, Sesterhenn IA. Renal medullary carcinoma: the seventh sickle cell nephropathy. Am J Surg Pathol 1995;19(1):1–11.
18. Laissy JP, Menegazzo D, Debray MP, et al. Renal carcinoma: diagnosis of venous invasion with Gd-enhanced MR venography. Eur Radiol 2000;10(7):1138–43.
19. Stahlschmidt J, Cullinane C, Roberts P, et al. Renal medullary carcinoma: prolonged remission with chemotherapy, immunohistochemical characterisation and evidence of bcr/abl rearrangement. Med Pediatr Oncol 1999;33(6):551–7.
20. Simpson L, He X, Pins M, et al. Renal medullary carcinoma and ABL gene amplification. J Urol 2005;173(6):1883–8.
21. Tomlinson GE, Nisen PD, Timmons CF, et al. Cytogenetics of a renal cell carcinoma in a 17-month-old child: evidence for Xp11.2 as a recurring breakpoint. Cancer Genet Cytogenet 1991;57(1):11–7.
22. Heimann P, El Housni H, Ogur G, et al. Fusion of a novel gene, RCC17, to the TFE3 gene in t(X;17)(p11.2;q25.3)-bearing papillary renal cell carcinomas. Cancer Res 2001;61(10):4130–5.
23. Gnarra JR, Glenn GM, Latif F, et al. Molecular genetic studies of sporadic and familial renal cell carcinoma. Urol Clin North Am 1993;20(2):207–16.
24. Lonser RR, Glenn GM, Walther M, et al. von Hippel-Lindau disease. Lancet 2003;361(9374):2059–67.
25. Kaelin WG Jr. Molecular basis of the VHL hereditary cancer syndrome. Nat Rev Cancer 2002;2(9):673–82.
26. Semenza GL. HIF-1 and human disease: one highly involved factor. Genes Dev 2000;14(16):1983–91.
27. Masson N, William C, Maxwell PH, et al. Independent function of two destruction domains in hypoxia-inducible factor-alpha chains activated by prolyl hydroxylation. EMBO J 2001;20:5197–206.
28. Lonergan KM, Iliopoulos O, Ohh M, et al. Regulation of hypoxia-inducible mRNAs by the von Hippel-Lindau tumor suppressor protein requires binding to complexes containing elongins B/C and Cul2. Mol Cell Biol 1998;18(2):732–41.
29. Jaakkola P, Mole DR, Tian Y-M, et al. Targeting of HIF-alpha to the von Hippel-Lindau ubiquitylation complex by O_2-regulated prolyl hydroxylation. Science 2001;292(5516):468–72.
30. Yu F, White SB, Zhao Q, et al. HIF-1alpha binding to VHL is regulated by stimulus-sensitive proline hydroxylation. Proc Natl Acad Sci U S A 2001;98(17):9630–5.
31. Bruick RK, McKnight SL. A conserved family of prolyl-4-hydroxylases that modify HIF. Science 2001;294(5545):1337–40.
32. Schmidt L, Duh FM, Chen F, et al. Germline and somatic mutations in the tyrosine kinase domain of the MET proto-oncogene in papillary renal carcinomas. Nat Genet 1997;16(1):68–73.
33. Comoglio PM, Tamagnone L, Boccaccio C. Plasminogen-related growth factor and semaphorin receptors: a gene superfamily controlling invasive growth. Exp Cell Res 1999;253(1):88–99.
34. Stella MC, Comoglio PM. HGF: a multifunctional growth factor controlling cell scattering. Int J Biochem Cell Biol 1999;31(12):1357–62.
35. Van der Voort R, Taher T, Derksen P, et al. The hepatocyte growth factor/MET pathway in development, tumorigenesis, and B-cell differentiation. Adv Cancer Res 2000;79:39–90.
36. Alam NA, Rowan AJ, Wortham NC, et al. Genetic and functional analyses of FH mutations in multiple cutaneous and uterine leiomyomatosis, hereditary leiomyomatosis and renal cancer, and fumarate hydratase deficiency. Hum Mol Genet 2003;12(11):1241–52.
37. Kiuru M, Launonen V, Hietala M, et al. Familial cutaneous leiomyomatosis is a two-hit condition associated with renal cell cancer of characteristic histopathology. Am J Pathol 2001;159(3):825–9.
38. Launonen V, Vierimaa O, Kiuru M, et al. Inherited susceptibility to uterine leiomyomas and renal cell cancer. Proc Natl Acad Sci U S A 2001;98(6):3387–92.
39. Tomlinson IP, Alam NA, Rowan AJ, et al. Germline mutations in FH predispose to dominantly inherited uterine fibroids, skin leiomyomata and papillary renal cell cancer. Nat Genet 2002;30(4):406–10.
40. Toro JR, Nickerson ML, Wei MH, et al. Mutations in the fumarate hydratase gene cause hereditary leiomyomatosis and renal cell cancer in families in North America. Am J Hum Genet 2003;73(1):95–106.
41. Pavlovich CP, Walther MM, Eyler RA, et al. Renal tumors in the Birt-Hogg-Dube syndrome. Am J Surg Pathol 2002;26(12):1542–52.
42. Zbar B, Alvord WG, Glenn G, et al. Risk of renal and colonic neoplasms and spontaneous pneumothorax in the Birt-Hogg-Dube syndrome. Cancer Epidemiol Biomarkers Prev 2002;11(4):393–400.
43. Pavlovich CP, Grubb RL 3rd, Hurley K, et al. Evaluation and management of renal tumors in the Birt-Hogg-Dube syndrome. J Urol 2005;173(5):1482–6.
44. Nickerson M, Warren M, Toro J, et al. Mutations in a novel gene lead to kidney tumors, lung wall defects, and benign tumors of the hair follicle in patients with the Birt-Hogg-Dube syndrome. Cancer Cell 2002;2(2):157.
45. Van Slegtenhorst M, de Hoogt R, Hermans C, et al. Identification of the tuberous sclerosis gene TSC1 on chromosome 9q34. Science 1997;277(5327):805–8.

46. Dabora SL, Jozwiak S, Franz DN, et al. Mutational analysis in a cohort of 224 tuberous sclerosis patients indicates increased severity of TSC2, compared with TSC1, disease in multiple organs. Am J Hum Genet 2001;68(1):64–80.
47. Roach ES, Gomez MR, Northrup H. Tuberous sclerosis complex consensus conference: revised clinical diagnostic criteria. J Child Neurol 1998;13(12):624–8.
48. Yang XJ, Sugimura J, Tretiakova MS, et al. Gene expression profiling of renal medullary carcinoma: potential clinical relevance. Cancer 2004;100(5):976–85.
49. Rini BI, Jaeger E, Weinberg V, et al. Clinical response to therapy targeted at vascular endothelial growth factor in metastatic renal cell carcinoma: impact of patient characteristics and Von Hippel-Lindau gene status. BJU Int 2006;98(4):756–62.
50. Yang JC, Haworth S, Steinberg SM, et al. A randomized double-blind placebo-controlled trial of bevacizumab (anti-VEGF antibody) demonstrating a prolongation in time to progression in patients with metastatic renal cancer. Proc Am Soc Clin Oncol 2002;21(1):15.
51. Escudier B, Koralewski P, Pluzanska A, et al. A randomized, controlled, double-blind phase III study (AVOREN) of bevacizumab/interferon-α2a vs placebo/interferon- α2a as first-line therapy in metastatic renal cell carcinoma. J Clin Oncol 2007;25(18S):3.
52. Hainsworth JD, Sosman JA, Spigel DR, et al. Treatment of metastatic renal cell carcinoma with a combination of bevacizumab and erlotinib. J Clin Oncol 2005;23(31):7889–96.
53. Bukowski RM, Kabbinavar F, Figlin RA, et al. Bevacizumab with or without erlotinib in metastatic renal cell carcinoma (RCC). In: ASCO, 2006, p 4523.
54. Ratain MJ, Eisen T, Stadler WM, et al. Phase II placebo-controlled randomized discontinuation trial of sorafenib in patients with metastatic renal cell carcinoma. J Clin Oncol 2006;24(16):2505–12.
55. Escudier B, Eisen T, Stadler WM, et al. Sorafenib in advanced clear-cell renal-cell carcinoma. N Engl J Med 2007;356(2):125–34.
56. Szcylik C, Dermkow T, Staehler M, et al. Randomized phase II trial of first-line treatment with sorafenib versus interferon in patients with advanced renal cell carcinoma: final results. J Clin Oncol 2007;25(18S):241s.
57. Amato RJ, Harris P, Dalton M, et al. A phase II trial of intra-patient dose-esclated sorafenib in patients(pts) with metastatic renal cell cancer (MRCC). J Clin Oncol 2007;25(18S):241s.
58. Motzer RJ, Michaelson MD, Redman BG, et al. Activity of SU11248, a multitargeted inhibitor of vascular endothelial growth factor receptor and platelet-derived growth factor receptor, in patients with metastatic renal cell carcinoma. J Clin Oncol 2006;24(1):16–24.
59. Motzer RJ, Hutson TE, Tomczak P, et al. Sunitinib versus interferon alfa in metastatic renal-cell carcinoma. N Engl J Med 2007;356(2):115–24.
60. Motzer RJ, Figlin R, Hutson TE, et al. Sunitinib versus interferon alfa as first-line treatment of metastatic renal cell carcinoma (mRCC): updated results and analysis of prognostic factors. In: ASCO, 2007, p 5024.
61. George DJ, Michaelson D, Rosenberg SA, et al. Phase II trial of sunitinib in bevacizumab-refractory metastatic renal cell carcinoama (mRCC): updated results and analysis of circulating biomarkers. In: ASCO, 2007, p 5035.
62. Rini B, Rixe O, Bukowski R, et al. AG-013736, a multi-target tyrosine kinase receptor inhibitor, demonstrates anti-tumor activity in a Phase 2 study of cytokine-refractory, metastatic renal cell cancer (RCC). In: 2005; 2005. p. 4509.
63. Rini BI, Wilding GT, Hudes G, et al. Axitinib (AG-013736; AG) in patients (pts) with metastatic renal cell cancer (RCC) refractory to sorafenib. J Clin Oncol 2007;25(18s):242s.
64. Atkins MB, Hidalgo M, Stadler WM, et al. A randomized double-blind phase 2 study of intravenous CCI-779 administered weekly to patients with advanced renal cell carcinoma. In: Proc Am Soc Clin Oncol; 2002; 2002. p. 36.
65. Hudes G, Carducci M, Tomczak P, et al. Temsirolimus, interferon alfa, or both for advanced renal-cell carcinoma. N Engl J Med 2007;356(22):2271–81.
66. Motzer RJ, Bacik J, Murphy BA, et al. Interferon-alfa as a comparative treatment for clinical trials of new therapies against advanced renal cell carcinoma. J Clin Oncol, 2002; 20:289.
67. Motzer RJ, Amato R, Todd M, et al. Phase II trial of antiepidermal growth factor receptor antibody C225 in patients with advanced renal cell carcinoma. Invest New Drugs 2003;21(1):99–101.
68. Rowinsky EK, Schwartz GH, Gollob JA, et al. Safety, pharmacokinetics, and activity of ABX-EGF, a fully human anti-epidermal growth factor receptor monoclonal antibody in patients with metastatic renal cell cancer. J Clin Oncol 2004;22(15):3003–15.
69. Druker BJ, Schwartz L, Marion S, et al. Phase II trial of ZD 1839 (Iressa), and EGF receptor inhibitor, in patients with renal cell carcinoma. Proc Am Soc Clin Oncol 2002;720. No. 150.

70. Dawson NA, Guo C, Zak R, et al. A phase II trial of gefitinib (Iressa, ZD1839) in stage IV and recurrent renal cell carcinoma. Clin Cancer Res 2004;10(23):7812–9.
71. Jermann M, Stahel RA, Salzberg M, et al. A phase II, open-label study of gefitinib (IRESSA) in patients with locally advanced, metastatic, or relapsed renal-cell carcinoma. Cancer Chemother Pharmacol 2005;1–7.
72. Ravaud A, Gardner J, Hawkins R, et al. Efficacy of lapatinib in patients with high tumor EGFR expression: results of a phase III trial in advanced renal cell carcinoma (RCC). In: ASCO 2006;4502.
73. Heinrich MC, Corless CL, Demetri GD, et al. Kinase mutations and imatinib response in patients with metastatic gastrointestinal stromal tumor. J Clin Oncol 2003;21(23):4342–9.

16 Targeted Therapy of Sarcoma

Joseph Ludwig, MD
and Jonathan C. Trent, MD, PhD

CONTENTS

INTRODUCTION
TARGETED THERAPIES
CONCLUSIONS
REFERENCES

ABSTRACT

Sarcomas represent a heterogeneous group of tumors that are composed of a wide range of tumor types with different natural histories and therapeutic approaches. Recent discoveries have identified specific molecular alterations in the pathogenesis of many of these tumors. These specific molecular alterations acquired during sarcomagenesis lead to the phenotypic changes of malignancy, namely proliferation, survival, invasion, metastasis, and angiogenesis. Inhibition of these molecular alterations by targeted therapy represents an opportunity to reverse the biologic basis of tumor formation in soft tissue sarcomas (STSs) and bone tumors (BTs). In this chapter we discuss a general overview of sarcomas and give specific examples of successful and proposed approaches to targeted therapy for this disease.

Key Words: Sarcoma, Molecular, Targeted, Personalized therapy

1. INTRODUCTION

1.1. Overview of Soft Tissue Sarcomas and Bone Tumors

In the United States there are an estimated 15,000 new cases of tumors arising from connective tissues leading to approximately 5000 deaths per year *(1)*. These tumors are heterogeneous and rare, making this entity a diagnostic challenge for pathologists. For instance, some sarcomas have been misclassified as "benign" despite well recognized risks of local recurrence, invasion, or metastasis. Thus, variations in pathologic definitions have made it difficult to obtain the exact number of patients with sarcomas. Despite the low incidence, sarcomas are within the same order of magnitude as myeloma, cervical carcinomas, gliomas, and carcinomas of the esophagus; and it occurs more frequently than testicular carcinomas

From: *Current Clinical Oncology: Targeted Cancer Therapy*
Edited by: R. Kurzrock and M. Markman © Humana Press, Totowa, NJ

or Hodgkin's disease. Most patients with sarcoma are in the younger years of their lives; thus, the disease is a significant public health problem despite its low incidence.

Progress in the treatment of STS and BTs from 1970 to 1990 included improvements in histopathologic classification, staging, use of radiotherapy as an adjunct to other modalities, surgical advances in functional preservation, and identification of doxorubicin and ifosfamide as active systemic therapy. Doxorubicin and ifosfamide are the two most widely used agents for the treatment of advanced STSs, giving an overall response rate of 64%(2) when used in combination at full therapeutic doses. A more recent regimen with activity in STS is the combination of gemcitabine with docetaxel, resulting in an overall response rate of 50% (3). BTs are treated with regimens including doxorubicin, ifosfamide, cisplatin, and methotrexate (4,5). After failure of these agents, the therapeutic options are limited. Although efficacious, some of these therapies are not commonly used by community oncologists and may be best administered at a tertiary referral center.

Given the rarity of STS, most clinical trials have grouped all tumor subtypes together when evaluating both existing and experimental drugs. Yet, progress in translational research over the last two decades has identified a number of cytogenetic and immunohistochemical properties that enables STS to be diagnosed more precisely. Similar to the gradual transition from a morphology-based to a genetic-based system that has occurred for lymphomas, better delineation of STS subtypes has allowed improved understanding of their unique prognosis, response to chemotherapy, and mechanisms of resistance. That information is critically important, as it helps avoid treating certain tumor types—e.g., alveolar soft-parts sarcoma, conventional skeletal chondrosarcoma, gastrointestinal stromal tumor (GIST) and clear cell sarcoma—with standard sarcoma chemotherapy regimens to which they are unlikely to respond and opens the door to future drug development targeted to the unique molecular aberrations responsible for their malignant behavior. Therefore, improved treatment of these chemotherapy-resistant sarcomas will require the novel discovery of drug that are both more effective and safer to administer.

Research has begun to unravel the molecular etiology of these tumors by identifying specific molecular alterations that are acquired during sarcomagenesis. Several act directly to induce features typical of malignant transformation, including growth factor independence, resistance to apoptosis, angiogenesis, cell cycle dysregulation, loss of genomic integrity, and the ability to invade and metastasize (6). The ability to inhibit these molecular perturbations represents a therapeutic opportunity to counteract the driving factors that promote growth and metastasis of STSs and BTs (Table 1). In this chapter we give an overview of the targeted therapy of sarcoma in the context of tumor cell characteristics as they apply to specific sarcoma histologic subtypes.

1.2. Molecular Alterations in Soft Tissue Sarcomas and Bone Tumors

1.2.1. GENERAL INFORMATION

As used for other more homogeneous solid tumors, sarcomas have traditionally been staged using AJCC criteria incorporating tumor size, depth, nodal status, grade, and extent of disease. The prognostic and clinical relevance of this 'one size fits all' staging approach to STS is less than ideal, however, as it fails to incorporate equally important factors such as STS subtype or location. This process of grouping of STS by name rather than by their diverse tissue of origin, seems to have hampered studies of biology, prognostic markers, and targeted therapy. For example, low response rates to conventional or experimental therapies in studies combining sarcoma histologic subtypes may have obscured higher

Table 1
Soft Tissue Sarcoma Chromosomal Translocations

Tumor type	Cytogenetics	Genes
Ewing's sarcoma/PNET	t(11;22)(q24;q12)	EWSR1, FLI1
	t(21;22)(q22;q12)	EWSR1, ERG
	t(7;22)(p22;q12)	EWSR1, ETV1
	t(2;22)(q33;q12)	EWSR1, FEV
	t(17;22)(q12;q12)	EWSR1, E1AF
	inv(22)	EWSR1, ZSG
Desmoplastic small round cell tumor	t(11;22)(p13;q12)	EWSR1, WT1
Extraskeletal myxoid chondrosarcoma	t(9;22)(q22;q12)	EWSR1, CHN
	t(9;17)(q22;q11)	RBP56, CHN
	t(9;15)(q22;q21)	CHN, TCF12
Clear cell sarcoma	t(12;22)(q13;q12)	EWSR1, ATF1
	t(2;22)(q32;q12)	EWSR1, CREB1
Alveolar rhabdomyosarcoma	t(2;13)(q35;q14)	PAX3, FKHR
	t(1;13)(p36;q14)	PAX7, FKHR
Myxoid liposarcoma	t(12;16)(q13;p11)	CHOP, TLS (FUS)
	t(12;22)(q13;q12)	EWSR1, CHOP
Synovial sarcoma	t(X;18)(p11;q11)	SSX1/2, SYT
Alveolar soft part sarcoma	t(X;17)(p11.2;q25)	ASPL, TFE3
Dermatofibrosarcoma protuberans (and Giant cell fibroblastoma)	t(17;22)(q22;q13) ring form of 17 & 22	COL1A1, PDGFB COL1A1, PDGFB
Low grade fibromyxoid sarcoma	t(7;16)(q32-34;p11)	FUS, CREB3L2 FUS, CREB3L1
Angiomatoid fibrous histiocytoma	t(12;16)(q13;p11)	FUS, ATF1
	t(12;22)(q13;q12)	EWSR1, ATF1
	t(2;22)(q32;q12)	EWSR1, CREB1
Congenital fibrosarcoma (and mesoblastic nephroma)	t(12;15)(p13;q25)	ETV6, NTRK3
Endometrial stromal sarcoma	t(7;17)(p15;q21)	JAZF1, JJAZ1
Inflammatory myofibroblastic tumor	translocations at 2p23	ALK, multiple fusion partners

response rates in individual unrecognized subtypes. Some sarcomas, such as osteosarcoma, pleomorphic sarcoma, angiosarcoma, leiomyosarcoma, adult fibrosarcoma, and conventional skeletal chondrosarcoma, are cytogenetically complex, and others have well recognized reciprocal translocations [e.g., *Col1A1-PDGF-B* in dermatofibrosarcoma protuberans (DFSP)] or activating mutations (e.g., *KIT* mutations in GISTs).

Interestingly, inactivation of the p53 pathway appears to be a key differentiating factor between sarcomas with simple genetic alterations and those with karyotypic complexity. In sarcomas with specific reciprocal translocations such as DFSP, p53 pathway alteration is a rare event, but when present it has been a strong prognostic factor, associated with significantly decreased survival in synovial sarcoma, myxoid liposarcoma, and Ewing's sarcoma/primitive neuroectodermal tumor (PNET). In contrast, in sarcomas with complex molecular alterations, p53 pathway inactivation [through point mutations or deletions, homozygous deletion of *CDKN2A* (which that encodes both p14ARF and p16), or *MDM2* amplification] may be a common early event needed to overcome checkpoints triggered by senescence, telomere erosion, or double-strand breaks in these sarcomas as they progress molecularly toward a cancer with multiple, complicated molecular abnormalities.

Table 2
Classification of Sarcomas by Potential Target

Targeted approach and histology	Target	Potential agent
Antivascular		
Angiosarcoma	VEGF	
Hemangioendothelioma	VEGF	
Hemangiopericytoma	PDGFR	
Growth factor pathway inhibitor		
Gastrointestinal stromal tumor	Kit	Imatinib, sunitinib
Dermatofibrosarcoma protuberans	PDGFR	Imatinib, sunitinib
Inflammatory myofibroblastic tumor	ALK	ALK inhibitor
Neurogenic sarcoma	NGFR	NGFR kinase inhibitor
Congenital fibrosarcoma	NTRK-3	NGFR kinase inhibtor
Desmoid tumor	Estrogen receptor-beta	Tamoxifen, aromatase inhibitor
Chondrosarcoma	AKT, MAPK	Perifosine
Dedifferentiated liposarcoma and atypical lipomatous tumor	MDM-2	Nutlin-3
Dedifferentiated liposarcoma, and atypical lipomatous tumor	CDK-4	CDK inhibitor
Tenosynovial giant cell tumor, pigmented villonodular synovitis	CSF-1	Imatinib, sunitinib
Proapoptotic		
Chondrosarcoma	DR3, DR4	Apo2L/TRAIL
Osteosarcoma	DR3, DR4	Apo2L/TRAIL
Transcription factor effector gencs		
Ewing's sarcoma	IGFR-1	IGFR-1 inhibitor
Rhabdomyosarcoma	CXCR-4	CXCR-4 inhibitor
Clear cell sarcoma	Met	Met inhibitor
Differentiation agents		
Dedifferentiated chondrosarcoma	DNA methylation	SAHA, decitabine
Dedifferentiated liposarcoma	DNA methylation	SAHA, decitabine

VEGF, vascular endothelial growth factor; PDGFR, platelet-derived growth factor receptor; ALK, anaplastic lymphoma kinase; NGFR, nerve growth factor receptor; MAPK, mitogen-activated protein kinase; MDM, murine double minute; CDK, cyclin-dependent kinase; CSF, colony-stiulating factor; DR3, death receptor-3; IGFR, insulin-like growth factor receptor; CXCR, chemokine receptor-4; TRAIL, tumor-necrosis factor apoptosis-inducing ligand; SAHA, suberoylanilide hydroxamic acid

Chromosomal translocations constitute most of the specific genetic alterations associated with sarcomas and are apparent in approximately one-third of histologic subtypes. Most of the common chromosomal translocations have been cloned, and many of the resulting fusion genes have been identified (Table 2). Surprisingly, the *EWS* gene or *EWS* family members (*TLS, TAF2N*) occur in a variety of sarcomas. In addition to providing a powerful diagnostic marker, fusion genes resulting from these translocations encode chimeric proteins that are important to the biology of the tumors, acting as abnormal transcription factors that dysregulate multiple downstream genes and pathways. The key role of these fusion proteins in pathogenesis is supported by the observation that they are required for sarcoma cell line proliferation and downregulation with antisense or RNAi inhibits cell proliferation and survival. Furthermore, specific translocations are associated with unique sarcoma histologies, presumably by inducing differential gene expression. This strong translocation-subtype relationship also implies the possibility of targeted therapy against either the fusion proteins themselves or the downstream effects induced by their binding. In those sarcomas that express aberrant transcriptional proteins, they appear to be important for maintenance of the malignant phenotype and determines the behavior of the sarcoma after initiation. The causative effects of proteomic alterations are exemplified by the limited spectrum of abnormalities that occur in the *kit* gene in GISTs and the translocation involving the collagen *1A-1* and *PDGF* genes in DFSP. These mechanisms, among others, are discussed in the following sections.

2. TARGETED THERAPIES

2.1. Targeting Growth Factor Pathways

Aberrant signal transduction pathways represent potential targets for anticancer drug designs, as pathways with mutated or overexpressed tyrosine kinases are frequently associated with tumor growth. Dysregulated signal transduction has been described in a wide variety of solid human cancers, including soft tissue and bone sarcomas *(7)*. They have often been associated with features of advanced disease and poor prognosis. Proliferation and differentiation of mesenchyme-derived cells are coordinated by factors that activate corresponding receptors expressing tyrosine kinase activity *(8)*. Growth factors may be produced by the tumor cell, the stromal cell (e.g., fibroblasts, endothelial cells), or circulating cells such as platelets or leukocytes. Once bound to their respective receptors located in the plasma membrane of both malignant and adjacent stromal cells, a complex network of autocrine/paracrine growth stimulation exists. Although the complexity of this tumor–stroma relationship remains poorly understood, some pathways are increasingly well defined. Generically, growth factor receptors remain in their inactivated state unless bound to their respective ligand or growth factor. In the case of tyrosine kinases, for example, the receptor–ligand interaction leads to receptor dimerization, kinase activation, and autophosphorylation. This, in turn, leads to the promotes phosphorylation and activation of downstream intermediary signaling molecules, such as MAP kinase, AKT, and the STAT molecules, which ultimately promotes transcriptional changes in gene expression affecting cell cycle progression, cell division, and tumor growth (Fig. 1a).

For other, more prevalent cancers, new therapies have been developed that interrupt tumor cell growth factor autonomy. Examples include the use of trastuzamab to target Her-2/neu in breast cancer, C-225 or gefitinib in colon and head and neck cancers, and imatinib for the treatment of GISTs. Other sarcomas that appear to rely on the activation of growth factor signaling are inflammatory myofibroblastic tumor (IMFT) and DFSP.

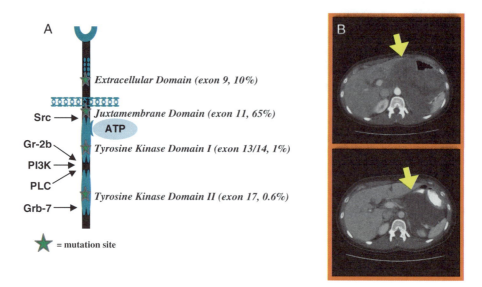

Fig. 1. a Structure of the KIT receptor tyrosine kinase displaying common sites of mutation observed in gastrointestinal stromal tumors (GISTs) tested for *kit* mutation at our institution, sites of imatinib interaction, and docking sites of downstream molecules. b Computed tomography (CT) displaying a baseline image of a gastric GIST (upper panel) and an image obtained from the same patient after 8 weeks of therapy with imatinib. The yellow arrow denotes a large, heterogeneous GIST that becomes cystic in response to imatinib therapy.

2.2. KIT Receptor Tyrosine Kinase in Gastrointestinal Stromal Tumors

Once thought to be relatively rare, the need to accurately distinguish GISTs from other STSs when considering imatinib-based therapy has led to a dramatic increase in the recognition and reporting of this tumor type. As discussed earlier, many sarcomas including GISTs were previously misdiagnosed as smooth muscle tumors of the gastrointestinal (GI) tract (GI leiomyosarcoma, leiomyoblastoma, leiomyoma), schwannoma, or desmoid tumor *(9)*. With better histologic and molecular techniques to distinguish them from tumors of similar morphologic appearance, GISTs are now recognized as the most common mesenchymal tumor of the GI tract *(10)*. They account for approximately 2% of all stomach cancers, 14% of all small intestinal tumors, and 0.1% of colon cancers, with an annual incidence of approximately 20 cases/million inhabitants *(11)*. The median age of patients at diagnosis is around 58 years and there is an equal distribution between men and women *(10)*. Recent advances in molecular and histopathologic approaches have aided in preventing misclassification *(9)*.

Given the remarkable efficacy of imatinib in treatment of GIST tumors, this tumor type now serves as the paradigm for the development of targeted therapy for sarcoma. Initially used for the treatment of chronic myelogenous leukemia (CML), imatinib mesylate (Gleevec, Glivec; Novartis, Basel, Switzerland) was later discovered to bind the Kit receptor (stem cell factor receptor, CD117) ubiquitously expressed by GISTs *(10)*. Whereas GISTs had previously been found to be resistant to all standard and experimental chemotherapeutic agents (response rate < 5%), the response rate of GIST tumors to imatinib now exceeds 90%.

The proposed major target of imatinib mesylate in GIST cells is the KIT tyrosine kinase receptor, which is composed of extracellular and intracellular domains (Fig. 1a). The extracellular domains correspond with exons 2 to 9 on the *kit* gene and the intracellular domain corresponds with exons 11 to 19 on the *kit* gene. Exon 11, the intracellular juxtamembrane domain plays a critical role in autoinhibiting KIT *(13)*. Mutations in exon 11, often in-frame deletions, confer constitutive activation of KIT by loss of autoinhibition. The effectiveness of imatinib has been demonstrated with receptors containing exon 11 mutations as well as exon 13 (tyrosine kinase domain 1). Exons 12 to 14 encode the ATP binding site (and the site of imatinib binding), the kinase insert is exon 15, and the phosphotransferase activity domain is exons 16 to 19. Mutations in the KIT receptor seen in GISTs are most commonly found on exons 9, 11, 13, and 17 *(14)*. It should be noted that patients with low Kit-expressing or Kit-negative GISTs have not been specifically studied prospectively but still may benefit from imatinib therapy in our experience *(15,16)*.

Imatinib has been studied in a number of clinical trials and is now the standard therapy for GIST. Responses to therapy can be dramatic, as seen in Figure 1b. The two largest Phase III studies conducted to date were undertaken nearly simultaneously by two independent consortia. The primary aim of these studies was to assess the impact of imatinib mesylate dose (400 vs. 800 mg daily) on survival; secondary aims were to evaluate response rates and confirm the tolerability of imatinib mesylate therapy in patients with GISTs. Patients initially randomized to receive the 400 mg daily dose were allowed to cross over to the 800 mg daily dose if they had progressive disease. At a median follow-up of 760 days ($\sim$25 months), 56% of patients on the once-daily arm had progressed compared with only 50% of patients on the twice-daily arm [estimated hazard ratio (HR) 0.82, 95% confidence interval (95% CI) 0.69–0.98; $p = 0.026$]. Although response rates were similar, the benefit in terms of median progression-free survival was an extra 5 months for patients on the arm receiving the higher dose (400 mg twice daily). At 2 years, overall survival estimates were 69% and 74% for the once-daily and twice-daily arms, respectively *(17)*. Both were substantially superior to the historical control (doxorubicin).

The toxicity results were reported at a median follow-up of 760 days ($\sim$25 months) *(17)*. The most common hematologic event was anemia (879 patients, 93%) and the most common nonhematologic side effects were edema (748, 80%), fatigue (693, 74%), nausea (515, 55%), diarrhea (494, 52%), and rash (345, 37%). Patients randomized to receive imatinib 400 mg twice daily as their initial dose were more likely to experience edema, anemia, rash, nausea, bleeding, and diarrhea compared to patients on the arm receiving 400 mg once daily The patients on high-dose imatinib were also more likely to have dose reductions [282 (60%) vs. 77 (16%); $p < 0.0001$] or treatment interruptions [302 (64%) vs. 189 (40%); $p < 0.0001$] than those receiving 400 mg daily. These toxicities were more generally nonhematologic, falling into the categories of edema and fatigue. Interestingly, these toxicities tended to resolve after first 4 weeks of therapy. The crossover arms reported lower rates of dose reduction or dose interruption when the dose was escalated from 400 mg to 800 mg than in the patients who started at the 800 mg dose.

In summary, the two largest of the two indicate the clinical trials to date imatinib mesylate is safe and generally well tolerated at doses up to 800 mg daily, particularly if given a 4 week lead-in at 400 mg daily. Patients enrolled in either of the large Phase III trials of imatinib were found to benefit from dose escalation after progression on imatinib 400 mg daily. Patients who crossed over to the higher dose arm (800 mg daily) had confirmed partial responses (2% in the EORTC study, 6% in the North American study) and stable disease (31%) *(18,19)*.

U.S. Food and Drug Adminstration (FDA)-approved therapeutic options for patients with imatinib-refractory GIST are limited. Sunitinib malate was approved on the basis of a median time-to-progression endpoint of 6 months that was superior to placebo *(20)*. However, the appropriate management of metastatic GIST that has not responded or has become resistant to imatinib mesylate and sunitinib malate is not known. To answer that question, a number of trials are planned or ongoing, including clinical trials combining imatinib mesylate with perifosine (Keryx, New York, NY, USA), single-agent Amgen 706 (Amgen, Thousand Oaks, CA, USA), and nilotinib (AMN107, Tasigna; Novartis Pharmaceuticals, Cambridge, MA, USA). Physicians should be encouraged to refer patients with GIST to centers that have access to these clinical trials.

Patients with localized sites of progression despite continuation of imatinib have been treated with percutaneous radiofrequency ablation (RFA) *(21)* as well as hepatic arterial embolization. Our experience with 110 GIST patients treated with hepatic arterial embolization (or chemoembolization) provided a response rate of 14%, with stabilization of disease in an additional 50% of patients. In selected patients with liver dominant disease, this approach appears to be a safe and effective treatment for those with localized progression. For patients whose disease becomes refractory to imatinib mesylate and who are not eligible for a clinical trial, palliative therapy—hepatic artery embolization, surgical debulking, intraperitoneal chemotherapy—should be considered.

In conclusion, imatinib mesylate has quickly become the most active targeted, small-molecule therapy used in patients with solid tumors. Imatinib mesylate is the frontline agent for metastatic GIST and is currently being evaluated for other tumor types. To address the important issues of efficacy of adjuvant therapy, efficacy of neoadjuvant therapy, duration of therapy, safety during the perioperative period, and molecular response measured by positron emission tomography (PET) imaging, several studies of imatinib mesylate in GIST are ongoing. The use of imatinib mesylate for treating patients with GIST will ultimately be tailored by the final results of these neoadjuvant, adjuvant, and metastatic clinical trials and their associated correlative studies. The identification of imatinib mesylate as an agent to target specifically the critical pathogenetic mechanisms of GIST represents a major advance in the treatment of this disease. The information gained from the success of imatinib mesylate in GIST will enhance drug development for oncology in general, although many challenges lie ahead in the applications of these strategies to other human cancers.

On the basis of studies published in abstract form, it appears that few patients with metastatic GIST exhibit complete responses to imatinib mesylate therapy, perhaps owing to relatively slow responses or imatinib mesylate's failure to induce cell death in some cases. Tumors from some patients whose disease relapses after an initial response to imatinib mesylate therapy appear to be undergoing clonal selection for tumor cells encoding a *KIT* mutation in an imatinib mesylate-resistant domain, such as the ATP binding site. Alternatively, resistance may develop through the activation of pathways located downstream or in parallel to KIT and therefore not sensitive to inhibition by imatinib mesylate. Whatever the outcome, this is an amazing opportunity to understand the biologic basis of resistance to one of the most successful therapeutic advances in oncology. Therefore, identification of molecular abnormalities that are essential for tumorigenesis will lead to the development of new anticancer therapies. Understanding diseases such as GIST may lay the foundation for understanding the more complex types of human cancer.

2.3. Platelet-Derived Growth Factor in Dermatofibrosarcoma Protuberans

PDGF/PDGFR autocrine and paracrine-driven proliferation are well described in sarcoma. Fibrosarcomas, osteosarcomas, and glioblastomas have all been shown to produce PDGF or PDGF-like substances *(22–27)*. Binding of PDGF to the PDGFR results in autophosphorylation and oligomerization *(28–30)*. The intrinsic kinase activity of the PDGFR leads to activation of downstream signaling cascades and ultimately induction of RNA synthesis and production of specific proteins *(31)*. These proteins, in turn, regulate tumor cell functions such as proliferation, evasion of apoptosis, angiogenesis, and cell–cell inter-actions *(32)*. The oncogene product of the simian sarcoma virus (v-sis) is transforming and is homologous to the human PDGF molecule c-sis. Moreover, treatment of fibroblasts with PDGF-BB results in the phenotypic transformation of the fibroblasts *(28)*.

With respect to sarcomas in particular, dysregulated PDGF is an important etiologic factor for DFSP. DFSP is thought to develop in cells expressing the fusion protein of Col1A1 and PDGF-B (Fig. 2a), the genes of which are located on chromosomes 17 and 22, respectively *(33)*. This leads to constitutive production of PDGF-B, activation of the PDGFR, and subsequent activation of downstream signaling pathways. The tyrosine kinase inhibitor imatinib blocks PDGFR signaling and DFSP cell growth in vitro *(34)*. Imatinib has been recently shown to prevent tumor growth in patients with DFSP and should be considered a therapeutic option for patients with this disease *(35)*. Figure 2b depicts a patient with multiply recurrent DFSP requiring increasingly large and complex resections for his scalp DFSP (Fig. 2b, baseline upper panel). He was enrolled in a clinical trial studying imatinib in DFSP and was found to have a dramatic response 2 weeks after initiation of therapy with this agent (Fig. 2b, lower panel). This patient has continued adjuvant imatinib postoperatively. Because DFSP is primarily managed surgically and local recurrence is more common than distant metastases, this is an entity for which patients with locally advanced

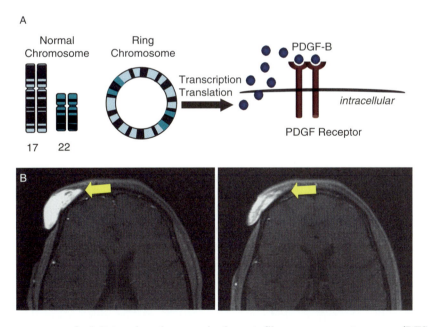

Fig. 2. a Common type of adult translocation seen in dermatofibrosarcoma protumerans (DFSP): a super-numerary ring chromosome derived from chromosome 22, containing sequences from 17q22-qter and 22q10-q13.1 in addition to the normal chromosome 17 and 22 pairs. Translocation of the collagen 1A gene on chromosome 17 with the platelet-derived growth factor-B (PDGF-B) gene on chromosome 22 leads to formation of the col1A-PDGFB fusion protein and constitutive expression of PDGFB in cells that also express the PDGFR. **b** Patient with DFSP treated with imatinib showed a marked response (arrows) after only 2 weeks of therapy.

disease may be able to be treated preoperatively with the goal of down-staging the surgical procedure or making an unresectable tumor respectable. Now, with imatinib targeted therapy against the PDGFR, it is less likely that patients with DFSP will require the morbid surgical procedures.

2.4. ALK Kinase in Inflammatory Myofibroblastic Tumors

Similar to DFSP, the inflammatory myofibroblastic tumor (IMFT) is a locally recurring tumor that is usually managed surgically. IMFT is synonymous with inflammatory, plasma cell, or xanthomatous pseudotumors (36). Histologically, IMFTs are composed of inflammatory and myofibroblastic cells. Clinically, they often present as an incidentally discovered mass in the chest or abdomen, although they may appear anywhere in the body. Less often they present as a syndrome of unexplained fever, weight loss, microcytic hypochromic anemia, thrombocytosis, polyclonal hyperglobulinemia, and elevated erythrocyte sedimentation rate (36). Resection of the IMFT leads to resolution of constitutional symptoms and laboratory abnormalities within a few days to weeks. Reappearance of the clinical syndrome often heralds an IMFT recurrence. Patients with extrapulmonary IMFTs usually are in their first and second decades, whereas patients with the pulmonary form tend to be in middle adulthood (36). The overall average age is 10 years (37). The exact etiology and pathogenesis of IMFTs remain to be elucidated, although both Epstein-Barr virus (38) and human herpesvirus-8 (39) may play a role. In recent years, some of the clinical and pathologic aspects of IMFT began to suggest the possibility that these lesions are more similar to neoplasms than a postinflammatory process (40). Some of the first strong evidence that IMFT was actually neoplastic, rather than being a pseudotumor, was the presence of clonal chromosomal abnormalities in several cases of IMFT (41,42). More recently, it has been suggested that the chromosomal abnormality in IMFT involves 2p23 and that, specifically, alterations near or within the ALK (anaplastic lymphoma kinase) gene are consistently involved in this neoplasm (43). The ALK gene at 2p23 was initially discovered when the breakpoint of the t(2;5)(p23;q35) translocation was cloned (44). Further study of the ALK gene has revealed that a recurrent oncogenic mechanism that occurs in IMFTs is the fusion of tropomyosin (TPM) N-terminal coiled-coil domains to the ALK C-terminal kinase domain, leading to ALK activation. Two ALK fusion genes have been cloned: TPM4-ALK and TPM3-ALK. Fusion of ALK to either TPM3 or TPM4 results in ALK activation (45). Of interest, the same TPM3-ALK oncogenic fusion proteins have been reported in a subset of anaplastic large-cell lymphomas (46). Abnormalities of ALK and evidence of chromosomal rearrangements of 2p23 occur most often in abdominal and pulmonary IMFTs during the first decade of life and are also associated with a higher frequency of recurrence. This suggests that patients with IMFT who have ALK abnormalities experience a more aggressive clinical course (37).

In the past, it was generally agreed that treatment of IMFTs required complete surgical removal of the main tumor mass and any surrounding individual nodules. The role of chemotherapy and radiation therapy in those with tumor recurrence has been controversial and associated with treatment-related morbidity (40). New therapies for locally recurrent and the rare metastatic IMFT are needed. A relatively high frequency (> 60%) of ALK staining has been found in IMFT, which suggest that ALK dysregulation is an important mechanism in the tumorigenesis of IMFT. Moreover, there are inhibitors in development that target intermediary signaling molecules downstream of ALK. NPM/ALK has been shown to induce continuous activation of STAT3 in T/null-cell lymphoma (TCL). It has been proposed that activated STAT3, which is known to display oncogenic properties, may be a promising target for novel therapies in ALK+ TCL*(47)* and, in turn, maybe also in ALK+ IMFT. UCN-01, a novel inhibitor that targets protein kinase C and CHK kinases, has been used with success in the treatment of a patient with an ALK+ anaplastic large-cell lymphoma *(48)*. Thus, until a specific ALK inhibitor is available, therapeutically targeting downstream molecules in the ALK receptor pathway may be an effective strategy for treating IMFTs *(37)*.

2.5. *Desmoid Tumor–ERβ Inhibition*

Extraabdominal fibromatosis (desmoid tumor) is a sarcoma arising in the soft tissue of the shoulder, trunk, abdominal wall, buttock, arm, or leg. Desmoid tumors almost never metastasize but have a propensity for local recurrence. Because these tumors can be quite large, patients with desmoid tumors often suffer from disfiguration, unrelenting pain, and limited mobility. Once surgical and radiotherapeutic options are exhausted, these patients are offered systemic therapy.

During the development of systemic therapy for this disease, investigators astutely observed that these tumors occur more commonly in women, especially during pregnancy. Early histopathologic studies reported the presence of the estrogen receptor (ER) on desmoid tumor tissue by a ligand-binding assay, raising the suspicion that the pathobiology of this disease involved ER signaling similar to invasive ductal breast carcinoma (Fig. 3a). Thus, antiestrogens such as tamoxifen have been used for many years by sarcoma medical oncologists as an effective systemic therapy for desmoid tumors. Figure 3b depicts a patient with an intraabdominal desmoid tumor that had been treated for 6 months with tamoxifen and exhibited a favorable response to therapy (Fig. 3b, lower panel). A series of confounding contemporary clinicopathologic studies reported that there was no correlation between expression of the estrogen receptor and the clinical benefit from tamoxifen. Moreover, the estrogen receptor was reported to be rarely expressed on desmoid tumors when analyzed by immunohistochemistry. Deyrup et al. made the observation that the older ligand-binding assay detected both ER-alpha and ER-beta, whereas the more recent

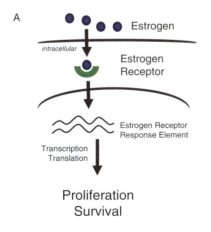
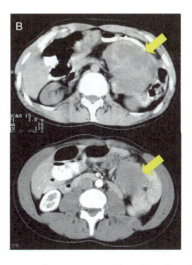

Fig. 3. a Mechanism of antiestrogen therapy in desmoid tumors that appears to involve signaling through the estrogen receptor-β. **b** CT was performed as part of the initial evaluation of a patient with a desmoid tumor (upper panel). The patient was treated for 6 months with tamoxifen, resulting in a substantial decrease (arrows) in tumor size (lower panel).

immunohistochemical studies for breast cancer employed antibodies that were raised specifically against the ER-alpha. In this elegant study the authors found that all desmoid tumors expressed detectable ER-beta while none expressed ER-alpha by using antibodies specific to each receptor isoform. Altogether, 33 (83%) of the patients' tumors had more than 50% of cells with nuclear staining, whereas the remaining 7 (17%) patients had fewer cells exhibiting nuclear staining of ERβ. Although a larger study should be performed to validate these findings, it seems that the therapeutic effectiveness of tamoxifen in desmoid tumors may be due to expression of the ERβ.

The efficacy of tamoxifen and antiestrogen therapy for this aggressive disease of the connective tissue is another compelling example of targeted therapy for sarcomas. It is interesting to hypothesize whether the importance of ERs is due to an activating genetic event such as mutation or whether the ER is a downstream activator of the APC/β-catenin pathway. Additional investigation may help determine the discrete biologic importance of primary mutation effectors and downstream molecules. Determination of ERβ expression and the APC/β-catenin/Wnt signaling pathway in a large number of desmoid tumors is an initial step. Perhaps eventual comparison of ER-responsive desmoid tumors with resistant ones could include comprehensive immunohistochemical studies, genomic microarray analysis, cytogenetic studies, and cytogenetic genomic hybridization.

2.6. Inducing Apoptosis

Tumor growth is determined by the rate of cell proliferation and the rate of cell death. Cells die by two major mechanisms: apoptosis and necrosis. Recent evidence suggests that acquired resistance to apoptosis is a important mechanism in tumor growth and resistance to chemotherapy (49). In 1972, Kerr et al. described apoptosis in rapidly growing cells after hormone withdrawal (50).

In vitro, induction of apoptosis can result from withdrawal of necessary support (growth factors, oxygen, nutrients), by activation of death receptors (tumor necrosis factor or FAS receptors), or by intracellular sensors (DNA damage, oncogene signaling imbalance) (51). Members of the Bcl-2 family of proteins exert either proapoptotic (Bax, Bak, Bid, Bim) or antiapoptotic (Bcl-2, Bcl-XL, Bcl-W) functions (52). These molecules regulate mitochondrial release of cytochrome C, a catalyst leading to the induction of apoptosis (53). The p53 tumor suppressor protein can induce apoptosis by up-regulating the expression of proapoptotic Bax in response to DNA damage (and subsequent mitochondrial release of cytochrome C). Cytochrome C then activates a cascade of molecules known caspases, beginning with caspase-8 and caspase-9 (54). Caspases are also activated by the death receptors in the tumor necrosis factor (TNF) family of receptors (54). The downstream effectors of caspases then execute the destruction of DNA (55).

These apoptotic pathways hold important implications for the development of novel types of antitumor therapy as many tumor cells already express the machinery necessary to undergo apoptosis. It is likely that new drugs will be able to block apoptosis inhibitors or activate apoptotic signaling pathways, resulting in substantial therapeutic benefit.

2.7. Apo2 Ligand/TRAIL and Bone Tumors

Recently, a new member of the TNF-cytokine family has been discovered (Fig. 4a). Apolipoprotein (Apo2) ligand, also known as TRAIL (TNF-related apoptosis-inducing ligand), is a type II transmembrane protein that transduces the apoptotic signal in association and interaction with DR4 and DR5 death domain receptors (56). There are also three known

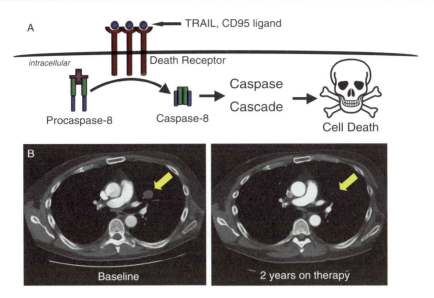

Fig. 4. a Apolipoprotein-2 (Apo2)-L/TRAIL is a ligand that binds and activates death receptors resulting in cell death. **b** Patient with a left perihilar lung metastasis (left panel) was treated with Apo2-L/TRAIL and has sustained a near-complete response (arrows) for more than 2 years (right panel).

decoy receptors for Apo2L/TRAIL. DcR1 and DcR2 both bind Apo2L/TRAIL but do not have active death domains; therefore, apoptosis does not occur *(57,58)*. It has been shown that Apo2L/TRAIL death receptors and decoy receptors are located in different locations along the cell membrane, and there is redistribution of the receptor locations after treatment with Apo2L/TRAIL *(59)*. Decoy receptors may be responsible for some Apo2L/TRAIL-induced apoptosis resistance; however, it appears that the mechanism of resistance is complex and may be multifactorial. Melanoma cell lines resistant to Apo2L/TRAIL-induced apoptosis have been shown to express high levels of FLIP, which is an intracellular protein that blocks the proapoptotic activity of caspase-8 and caspase-10, which in turn inhibits Apo2L/TRAIL-induced apoptosis *(60)*. In melanoma cell lines that were sensitive to Apo2L/TRAIL, the levels of FLIP protein were much lower or absent, suggesting that resistance to Apo2L/TRAIL is mediated by several factors. Apo2L/TRAIL may still be a novel agent for therapy despite possible resistance mechanisms.

Apo2L/TRAIL has been shown to induce apoptosis in multiple cancer cell lines; however, when tested in normal tissues it has been found to be nontoxic and safe *(57,61)*. There has been evidence that some preparations of Apo2L/TRAIL induced apoptosis in cultured human hepatocytes *(62)*; however, recent studies with a clinical grade of Apo2L/TRAIL continued to have minimal toxicity to normal human tissues *(63)*. Apo2L/TRAIL has been shown to be active in tumor cell lines as a single agent. When used in combination with various chemotherapeutic agents, Apo2L/TRAIL was found to have a synergistic effect in sensitive cells *(57,64,65)*. There is also evidence that the combination of Apo2L/TRAIL and chemotherapeutic agents can induce apoptosis in Apo2L/TRAIL-resistant cell lines *(57,64,65)*.

Evdokiou et al. *(57)* studied the effects of Apo2L/TRAIL alone and in combination with several chemotherapeutic agents in osteosarcoma cell lines. They found that Apo2L/TRAIL alone or in combination had no effect on primary normal human bone cells; however, in a Apo2L/TRAIL-sensitive BT cell line, the investigators found an 80% apoptosis rate. In five other cell lines tested, which were found to be Apo2L/TRAIL-resistant, apoptosis rates were elevated with Apo2L/TRAIL when combined with doxorubicin, cisplatin, or etoposide but not when combined with methotrexate or cyclophosphamide. This enhanced efficacy may have been mediated through up-regulation of the DR4 and DR5 death receptors when the chemotherapeutic agents were added. They also evaluated the mechanisms of cell death induced by Apo2L/TRAIL and found that apoptosis was mediated through caspase-8 and caspase-3 pathways as specific inhibition of these pathways led to loss of the proapoptotic effect. In view of the increase in apoptosis, the enhanced effects with doxorubicin and cisplatinum combination, and the minimal toxicity seen, the use of Apo2L/TRAIL may have implications for the treatment of osteosarcoma.

Several Phase I and II clinical trials are underway to study these drugs in patients with BTs as well as other cancer types. Encouraging results have been observed in the therapy of patients with chondrosarcoma. One such patient chondrosarcoma with metastatic resistant to several conventional chemotherapeutic agents (Fig. 4b, upper panel). Apo2L had a durable and dramatic response to TRAIL therapy (Fig. 4b, lower panel). A Phase II study of this agent is underway for patients with sarcoma.

2.8. Rhabdomyosarcoma and Potential Therapeutic Targets

Rhabdomyosarcoma (RMS) is a rare tumor in adults, representing < 0.1% of all malignancies in the adult U.S. population (1). Despite its low prevalence, RMS is of interest and concern because it is a typically aggressive neoplasm as evidenced by the 5-year median survival of 20% to 40% in adults with primary disease (66–68). Moreover, RMS is a public health concern with respect to the predominance of the disease in younger individuals (66–68). Despite advances in chemotherapeutic and surgical techniques, the 5-year median survival rate for adults with primary RMS remains between 20% and 40%; patients with metastatic disease have a 5-year survival rate of < 5% (66–68).

Receptor tyrosine kinases have been extensively investigated in both preclinical and clinical trials in a wide variety of carcinoma and sarcoma histologies, yet their role in adult RMS is unknown. EGFR inhibitors are used in the therapy of lung, colorectal, and head and neck cancers, and the potential for using them exists for RMS (69–71). Overexpression and amplification of c-erb-b2 (HER2/neu) in breast cancer correlates with poor overall survival and benefit from trastuzumab (72).

Even less is known about the role of Bcl-2 and Bax expression in soft tissue tumors. Understanding the frequency of expression and clinical correlations of these markers may lead to biologic observations and identification of potential therapeutic targets. To address this issue we recently analyzed tumor specimens from a cohort of 105 RMS patients treated at a single institution for the expression of EGFR, c-erb-b2, PDGFRα, PDGFRβ, KIT, Bcl-2, and Bax (manuscript in review).

RMS rarely expresses KIT (2%), and only 9% of the tested samples showed any c-erb-B2 expression. We found that 57% of our embryonal RMS tumors expressed EGFR. We also found that patients whose tumors expressed PDGFRα had a significantly shorter median overall survival than patients whose tumors did not express this marker. In our study, a combination of PDGFRα absence and PDGFR-β presence conferred a trend toward long-term overall survival. This result is intriguing given the possibility of the different actions of each PDGFR isoform. Although these observations are drawn from a small sample, further investigation into the relation between PDGFRα and PDGFRβ and the development of

PDGFRα-specific inhibitors is of interest and may lead to targeted therapy of PDGFR or EGFR in this sarcoma histology.

3. CONCLUSIONS

Sarcomas are a heterogeneous group of diseases that are often defined by precise molecular alterations, as in the examples described above. These diseases may not follow the conventional hypothesis of multistep tumorigenesis but may obtain the tumor phenotype via the acquisition of single molecular defects. For example, an isolated missense mutation, deletion, or translocation might result in aberrant expression of a gene and be sufficient to promote tumor proliferation, survival, invasion, metastasis, and angiogenesis. One could speculate that this is the reason we have observed such great success with imatinib in GISTs and DFSP, as well as in chronic myelogenous leukemia. Continued progress in the molecular understanding of sarcomas will help in the identification of specific genetic abnormalities that may be therapeutically targeted.

The success of imatinib in the treatment of GISTs and DFSP provides hope to patients suffering from intractable cancers that novel therapeutics can dramatically alter their prognosis. Targeting the AKT pathway with perifosine against imatinib-refractory GIST is a novel second-line targeted approach. Furthermore, therapy with Apo2L/TRAIL in osteosarcomas is appealing as it may be synergistic with cytotoxic chemotherapy. RMS appears to express PDGFRs and EGFR frequently, suggesting a target for new therapeutic approaches.

While laboratory investigations continue to unravel the molecular pathology that is important in sarcomagenesis, drugs targeting those pathways will almost certainly coevolve. Tyrosine kinase inhibitors (TKIs) such as imatinib provide just an initial example of what may someday be the paradigm for successful targeted therapy have proven successful for the leukemias, sarcomas, and recently renal cell cancers. Continued success will require a concerted effort by academia and the pharmaceutical industry to extend the therapeutic options to include inhibiting non-TKI targets such as transcription factors. The goal of a more personalized therapy for subtypes of sarcoma is within reach; the discovery and application of future biologic therapies can make that goal a reality.

REFERENCES

1. Jemal A, Siegel R, Ward E, et al. Cancer statistics, 2006. CA Cancer J Clin 2006;56(2):106–30.
2. Patel S, Vadhan-Raj S, Burgess M, et al. Results of two consecutive trials of dose-intensive chemotherapy with doxorubicin and ifosfamide in patients with sarcomas. Am J Clin Oncol 1998;21(3):317–21.
3. Hensley ML, Maki R, Venkatraman E, et al. Gemcitabine and docetaxel in patients with unresectable leiomyosarcoma: results of a phase II trial. J Clin Oncol 2002;20(12):2824–31.
4. Patel S, Vadhan-Raj S, Papadopoulos N, et al. High-dose Ifosfamide in bone and soft-tissue sarcomas: results of phase II and pilot studies—dose response and schedule dependence. J Clin Oncol 1997;15:2378–84.
5. Picci P, Bohling T, Bacci G, et al. Chemotherapy-induced tumor necrosis as a prognostic factor in localized Ewing's sarcoma of the extremities. J Clin Oncol 1997;15(4):1553–9.
6. Hanahan D, Weinberg RA. The hallmarks of cancer. Cell 2000;100(1):57–70.
7. Slominski A, Wortsman J, Carlson A, et al. Molecular pathology of soft tissue and bone tumors: a review. Arch Pathol Lab Med 1999;123(12):1246–59.
8. Schlessinger J. Cell signaling by receptor tyrosine kinases. Cell 2000;103(2):211–25.
9. Price N, Trent J, El-Naggar A, et al. Highly accurate two-gene classifier for differentiating gastrointestinal stromal tumors and leiomyosarcomas. Proc Natl Acad Sci USA 2007;104(9):3414–9.
10. Clary BM, DeMatteo RP, Lewis JJ, et al. Gastrointestinal stromal tumors and leiomyosarcoma of the abdomen and retroperitoneum: a clinical comparison. Ann Surg Oncol 2001;8(4):290–9.

11. Andersson J, Sjèogren H, Meis-Kindblom JM, et al. The complexity of KIT gene mutations and chromosome rearrangements and their clinical correlation in gastrointestinal stromal (pacemaker cell) tumors. Am J Pathol 2002;160(1):15–22.

12. Trent JC, Beach J, Burgess MA, et al. A two-arm phase II study of temozolomide in patients with advanced gastrointestinal stromal tumors and other soft tissue sarcomas. Cancer 2003;98(12):2693–9.

13. Mol CD, Dougan DR, Schneider TR, et al. Structural basis for the autoinhibition and STI-571 inhibition of c-Kit tyrosine kinase. J Biol Chem 2004;279(30):31655–63.

14. Mechtersheimer G, Egerer G, Hensel M, et al. Gastrointestinal stromal tumours and their response to treatment with the tyrosine kinase inhibitor imatinib. Virchows Arch 2004;444(2):108–18.

15. Chirieac L, Trent J, Steinert DM, et al. Correlation of immunophenotype with clinical outcome of GIST patients treated with imatinib mesylate. Presented to the Connective Tissue Oncology Society, Barcelona, 2003.

16. Medeiros F, Corless CL, Duensing A, et al. KIT-negative gastrointestinal stromal tumors: proof of concept and therapeutic implications. Am J Surg Pathol 2004;28(7):889–94.

17. Verweij J, Casali PG, Zalcberg J, et al. Progression-free survival in gastrointestinal stromal tumours with high-dose imatinib: randomised trial. Lancet 2004;364(9440):1127–34.

18. Zalcberg A, Verweij J, Casali PG, et al. Outcome of patients with advanced gastro-intestinal stromal tumors (GIST) crossing over to a daily imatinib dose of 800 mg (HD) after progression on 400 mg (LD)—an international, intergroup study of the EORTC, ISG and AGITG. Presented to the American Society of Clinical Oncology, New Orleans; 2004. p 815. Abstract 9004.

19. Rankin C, von Mehren M, Blanke C, et al. Dose effect of imatinib in patients with metastatic GIST: a phase III sarcoma group study S0033. Presented to the American Society of Clinical Oncology, New Orleans, 2004, p 815.

20. Demetri GD, von Oosterom AT, Blackstein M, et al. Phase 3, multicenter, randomized, double-blind, placebo-controlled trial of SU11248 in patients (pts) following failure of imatinib for metastatic GIST. Presented to the American Society of Clinical Oncology, Orlando, 2005. Abstract 4000.

21. Dileo P, Randhawa R, Vansonnenberg E. Safety and efficacy of percutaneous radio-frequency ablation (RFA) in patients (pts) with metastatic gastrointestinal stromal tumor (GIST) with clonal evolution of lesions refractory to imatinib mesylate (IM). Presented to the American Society of Clinical Oncology, New Orleans, 2004, p 820. Abstract 9024.

22. Allam M, Martinet N, Martinet Y. Differential migratory response of U-2 OS osteosarcoma cell to the various forms of platelet-derived growth factor. Biochimie 1992;74(2):183–6.

23. Badache A, De Vries GH. Neurofibrosarcoma-derived Schwann cells overexpress platelet-derived growth factor (PDGF) receptors and are induced to proliferate by PDGF BB. J Cell Physiol 1998;177(2):334–42.

24. Fahrer C, Brachmann R, von der Helm K. Expression of c-sis and other cellular proto-oncogenes in human sarcoma cell lines and biopsies. Int J Cancer 1989;44(4):652–7.

25. Gisselsson D, Hoglund M, O'Brien KP, et al. A case of dermatofibrosarcoma protuberans with a ring chromosome 5 and a rearranged chromosome 22 containing amplified COL1A1 and PDGFB sequences. Cancer Lett 1998;133(2):129–34.

26. Benito M, Lorenzo M. Platelet derived growth factor/tyrosine kinase receptor mediated proliferation. Growth Regul 1993;3(3):172–9.

27. Werner S, Hofschneider PH, Heldin CH, et al. Cultured Kaposi's sarcoma-derived cells express functional PDGF A-type and B-type receptors. Exp Cell Res 1990;187(1):98–103.

28. Clarke MF, Westin E, Schmidt D, et al. Transformation of NIH 3T3 cells by a human c-sis cDNA clone. Nature 1984;308(5958):464–7.

29. Betsholtz C, Westermark B, Ek B, et al.Coexpression of a PDGF-like growth factor and PDGF receptors in a human osteosarcoma cell line: implications for autocrine receptor activation. Cell 1984;39(3 Pt 2):447–57.

30. Kazlauskas A, Bowen-Pope D, Seifert R, et al. Different effects of homo- and heterodimers of platelet-derived growth factor A and B chains on human and mouse fibroblasts. EMBO J 1988;7(12):3727–35.

31. Callahan M, Cochran BH, Stiles CD. The PDGF-inducible 'competence genes': intracellular mediators of the mitogenic response. Ciba Found Symp 1985;116:87–97.

32. Heldin CH, Westermark B. Mechanism of action and in vivo role of platelet-derived growth factor. Physiol Rev 1999;79(4):1283–316.

33. O'Brien KP, Seroussi E, Dal Cin P, et al. Various regions within the alpha-helical domain of the COL1A1 gene are fused to the second exon of the PDGFB gene in dermatofibrosarcomas and giant-cell fibroblastomas. Genes Chromosomes Cancer 1998;23(2):187–93.

34. Sjoblom T, Shimizu A, O'Brien K, et al. Growth inhibition of dermatofibrosarcoma protuberans tumors by the platelet-derived growth factor receptor antagonist STI571 through induction of apoptosis. Cancer Res 2001;61(15):5778–83.

35. Maki RG, Awan RA, Dixon RH, et al. Differential sensitivity to imatinib of 2 patients with metastatic sarcoma arising from dermatofibrosarcoma protuberans. Int J Cancer 2002;100(6):623–6.

36. Coffin CM, Watterson J, Priest JR, et al. Extrapulmonary inflammatory myofibroblastic tumor (inflammatory pseudotumor): a clinicopathologic and immunohistochemical study of 84 cases. Am J Surg Pathol 1995;19(8):859–72.

37. Cook JR, Dehner LP, Collins MH, et al. Anaplastic lymphoma kinase (ALK) expression in the inflammatory myofibroblastic tumor: a comparative immunohistochemical study. Am J Surg Pathol 2001;25(11):1364–71.

38. Arber DA, Weiss LM, Chang KL. Detection of Epstein-Barr Virus in inflammatory pseudotumor. Semin Diagn Pathol 1998;15(2):155–60.

39. Gomez-Roman JJ, Sanchez-Velasco P, Ocejo-Vinyals G, et al. Human herpesvirus-8 genes are expressed in pulmonary inflammatory myofibroblastic tumor (inflammatory pseudotumor). Am J Surg Pathol 2001;25(5):624–9.

40. Coffin CM, Dehner LP, Meis-Kindblom JM. Inflammatory myofibroblastic tumor, inflammatory fibrosarcoma, and related lesions: an historical review with differential diagnostic considerations. Semin Diagn Pathol 1998;15(2):102–10.

41. Su LD, Atayde-Perez A, Sheldon S, et al. Inflammatory myofibroblastic tumor: cytogenetic evidence supporting clonal origin. Mod Pathol 1998;11(4):364–8.

42. Snyder CS, Dell'Aquila M, Haghighi P, et al. Clonal changes in inflammatory pseudotumor of the lung: a case report. Cancer 1995;76(9):1545–9.

43. Griffin CA, Hawkins AL, Dvorak C, et al. Recurrent involvement of 2p23 in inflammatory myofibroblastic tumors. Cancer Res 1999;59(12):2776–80.

44. Morris SW, Kirstein MN, Valentine MB, et al. Fusion of a kinase gene, ALK, to a nucleolar protein gene, NPM, in non-Hodgkin's lymphoma. Science 1994;263(5151):1281–4. Erratum: Science 1995;20;267(5196):316–7.

45. Lawrence B, Perez-Atayde A, Hibbard MK, et al. TPM3-ALK and TPM4-ALK oncogenes in inflammatory myofibroblastic tumors. Am J Pathol 2000;157(2):377–84.

46. Lamant L, Dastugue N, Pulford K, et al. A new fusion gene TPM3-ALK in anaplastic large cell lymphoma created by a (1;2)(q25;p23) translocation. Blood 1999;93(9):3088–95.

47. Zhang Q, Raghunath PN, Xue L, et al. Multilevel dysregulation of STAT3 activation in anaplastic lymphoma kinase-positive T/null-cell lymphoma. J Immunol 2002;168(1):466–74.

48. Sausville EA, Arbuck SG, Messmann R, et al. Phase I trial of 72-hour continuous infusion UCN-01 in patients with refractory neoplasms. J Clin Oncol 2001;19(8):2319–33.

49. Shmitt C, Fridman J, Yang M, et al. A Senescence program controlled by p53 and p16(INK4a) contributes to the outcome of cancer therapy. Cell 2002;109:335–46.

50. Kerr JF, Wyllie AH, Currie AR. Apoptosis: a basic biological phenomenon with wide-ranging implications in tissue kinetics. Br J Cancer 1972;26(4):239–57.

51. Reed JC. Mechanisms of apoptosis avoidance in cancer. Curr Opin Oncol 1999;11(1):68–75.

52. Reed JC. Regulation of apoptosis by bcl-2 family proteins and its role in cancer and chemoresistance. Curr Opin Oncol 1995;7(6):541–6.

53. Matsuyama S, Reed JC. Mitochondria-dependent apoptosis and cellular pH regulation. Cell Death Differ 2000;7(12):1155–65.

54. Gao CF, Ren S, Zhang L, et al. Caspase-dependent cytosolic release of cytochrome c and membrane translocation of Bax in p53-induced apoptosis. Exp Cell Res 2001;265(1):145–51.

55. Thornberry NA, Lazebnik Y. Caspases: enemies within. Science 1998;281(5381):1312–6.

56. Sheridan JP, Marsters SA, Pitti RM, et al. Control of TRAIL-induced apoptosis by a family of signaling and decoy receptors. Science 1997;277(5327):818–21.

57. Evdokiou A, Bouralexis S, Atkins GJ, et al. Chemotherapeutic agents sensitize osteogenic sarcoma cells, but not normal human bone cells, to Apo2L/TRAIL-induced apoptosis. Int J Cancer 2002;99(4):491–504.

58. Marsters SA, Sheridan JP, Pitti RM, et al. A novel receptor for Apo2L/TRAIL contains a truncated death domain. Curr Biol 1997;7(12):1003–6.

59. Zhang XD, Franco AV, Nguyen T, et al. Differential localization and regulation of death and decoy receptors for TNF-related apoptosis-inducing ligand (TRAIL) in human melanoma cells. J Immunol 2000;164(8):3961–70.

60. Griffith TS, Chin WA, Jackson GC, et al. Intracellular regulation of TRAIL-induced apoptosis in human melanoma cells. J Immunol 1998;161(6):2833–40.

61. Ashkenazi A, Pai RC, Fong S, et al. Safety and antitumor activity of recombinant soluble Apo2 ligand. J Clin Invest 1999;104(2):155–62.

62. Jo M, Kim TH, Seol DW, et al. Apoptosis induced in normal human hepatocytes by tumor necrosis factor-related apoptosis-inducing ligand. NatMed2000;6(5):564–7.

63. Lawrence D, Shahrokh Z, Marsters S, et al. Differential hepatocyte toxicity of recombinant Apo2L/TRAIL versions. Nat Med 2001;7(4):383–5.
64. Lacour S, Hammann A, Wotawa A, et al. Anticancer agents sensitize tumor cells to tumor necrosis factor-related apoptosis-inducing ligand-mediated caspase-8 activation and apoptosis. Cancer Res 2001;61(4): 1645–51.
65. Mizutani Y, Nakao M, Ogawa O, et al. Enhanced sensitivity of bladder cancer cells to tumor necrosis factor related apoptosis inducing ligand mediated apoptosis by cisplatin and carboplatin. J Urol 2001;165(1): 263–70.
66. Esnaola NF, Rubin BP, Baldini EH, et al. Response to chemotherapy and predictors of survival in adult rhabdomyosarcoma. Ann Surg 2001;234(2):215–23.
67. Ferrari A, Dileo P, Casanova M, et al. Rhabdomyosarcoma in adults: a retrospective analysis of 171 patients treated at a single institution. Cancer 2003;98(3):571–80.
68. Hawkins WG, Hoos A, Antonescu CR, et al. Clinicopathologic analysis of patients with adult rhabdomyosarcoma. Cancer 2001;91(4):794–803.
69. Bonner JA, Harari PM, Giralt J, et al. Radiotherapy plus cetuximab for squamous-cell carcinoma of the head and neck. N Engl J Med 2006;354(6):567–78.
70. Cunningham D, Humblet Y, Siena S, et al. Cetuximab monotherapy and cetuximab plus irinotecan in irinotecan-refractory metastatic colorectal cancer. N Engl J Med 2004;351(4):337–45.
71. Shepherd FA, Rodrigues Pereira J, Ciuleanu T, et al. Erlotinib in previously treated non-small-cell lung cancer. N Engl J Med 2005;353(2):123–32.
72. Slamon DJ, Leyland-Jones B, Shak S, et al. Use of chemotherapy plus a monoclonal antibody against HER2 for metastatic breast cancer that overexpresses HER2. N Engl J Med 2001;344(11):783–92.

17 Targeted and Functional Imaging

Vikas Kundra, MD, PhD, Dawid Schellingerhout, MD, and Edward F. Jackson, PhD, MS

CONTENTS

ABSTRACT

The emerging field of targeted therapy is ushering in a new era of targeted/functional imaging, which compliments and sometimes improves upon traditional anatomic imaging for diagnosis, early assessment of treatment response, and estimation of durability of therapeutic success. Targeted/functional imaging has already had an impact on clinical management. With such methods, one may either measure the target directly or assess downstream effects. The former may provide greater specificity, whereas, the latter may have broader applicability. The clinical question will guide selection between the two. The primary modalities currently used clinically include nuclear medicine techniques, such as planar or single photon emission computed tomography or positron emission tomography, and MR based techniques, such as dynamic contrast enhanced MR imaging. An understanding of the physics and clinical applications of targeted/functional imaging and their requisite molecular imaging agents aides image interpretation. Combining such imaging with anatomic imaging is often advantageous. For the future, clinical trials of targeted/functional imaging are needed in addition to and in parallel with clinical trials of targeted therapeutics given the obvious synergy between the two.

From: *Current Clinical Oncology: Targeted Cancer Therapy*
Edited by: R. Kurzrock and M. Markman © Humana Press, Totowa, NJ

Key Words: Targeted imaging, Functional imaging, Molecular Imaging, SPECT, PET, MR, DCE-MR

1. INTRODUCTION

The emerging field of targeted therapy is ushering in a new era of targeted/functional imaging. Although powerful in most circumstances, meta-analyses of some tumor types found that an anatomic reduction in tumor size alone had no or only a weak correlation with patient survival *(1,2)*. Two recent Phase III trials of therapies targeting the epidermal growth factor receptor demonstrated similar small reductions in tumor size; however, one drug improved the median overall survival rate by more than 50% compared to placebo, whereas the other did not *(3,4)*. When present, anatomic changes in tumors take time to occur. Instead of waiting weeks to months to see an anatomic change in tumor size, a goal of targeted/functional imaging is to evaluate the response to a drug in a matter of days to a few weeks, before anatomic change occurs. This can be especially important for patients with short life spans such as those with advanced lung cancer who may have only months to live. In this case, selecting the appropriate therapy and gauging its efficacy in an individual patient in a timely fashion is paramount. Furthermore, some tumors, such as pancreatic cancer, can undergo a desmoplastic response, which is difficult to distinguish from residual tumor after treatment by anatomic imaging.

In such situations and if the therapy is tumoristatic instead of tumoricidal, functional imaging may prove useful. Functional imaging may also prove useful for selecting patients who are most likely to respond to a given drug. This is an important goal given the known heterogeneity of response to treatment in populations of patients thought to have the same tumor phenotype. Furthermore, within a patient, different metastases may respond variably to a given therapy, and identifying the nonresponding metastases may guide treatment alterations, including whether to institute local therapy. Thus, there are a number of situations where functional imaging may be useful for guiding patient care.

2. CLINICAL USE OF FUNCTIONAL IMAGING

Functional imaging has already had an impact on patient care. There is a great deal of experience with some imaging agents in oncology such as ^{111}In-octreotide for imaging neuroendocrine tumors that express somatostatin receptors and metaiodobenzylguanidine (MIBG), which mimics norepinephrine and accumulates in neurosecretory granules such as those of pheochromocytomas. Newer nuclear medicine imaging agents for single photon emission computed tomography (SPECT) imaging and for positron emission tomography (PET) imaging as well as functional imaging with magnetic resonance (MR) techniques are adding to the armamentarium of targeted/functional imaging methods.

Targeted therapy and targeted/functional imaging have already found synergy in the clinical setting. In addition to diagnosis and staging, imaging can be used for patient selection, for example, to select patients that have a positive or negative response to a functional imaging agent at baseline. This can then be used for comparison after a targeted therapy is delivered. For example, patients with suspected gastrointestinal stromal tumors (GISTs) may be screened for tumors positive for ^{18}F-fluoro-2-deoxyglucose (^{18}F-FDG) uptake on PET imaging prior to initiation of imatinib therapy.

Imaging can also be used for monitoring the effect of imatinib treatment. For example, dramatically decreased ^{18}F-FDG uptake by GISTs signifies that imatinib is effective (Fig. 1)

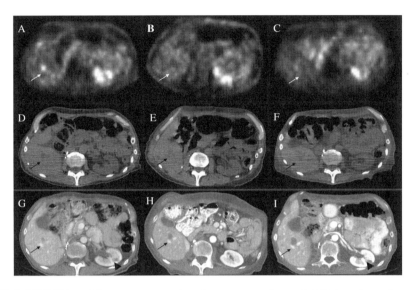

Fig. 1. ^{18}F-FDG PET-CT and intravenous and oral contrast enhanced CT imaging of a patient with a gastrointestinal stromal tumor. ^{18}F-FDG PET (A, B, C) with unenhanced CT (D, E, F) imaging was performed pre (A and D), seven days post (B and E), and three months post (C and F) therapy with imatinib of a GI stromal tumor metastasis (arrow). Intravenous and oral contrast enhanced CT was performed pre (G), one month post, (H), and two and a half months post-therapy with imatinib. Notice the rapid reduction in ^{18}F-FDG uptake at seven days post therapy (B) compared to pre-therapy (A) is maintained at the three month post-imaging time point (C), but the lesion appears to be stable 7 days post-therapy (E) or larger one month post-therapy (H) compared to pre-therapy (D and G) and larger still two and a half months (I) or three months (F) post-therapy. The timing after the contrast bolus can alter the appearance of a metastasis, and with some tumors such as GI stromal tumor metastasis, the rim of enhancement of the live tumor that can be seen at earlier phases (late arterial phase) can appear as adjacent liver tissue in the later portal venous phase, the phase of the intravenous contrast in images G, H, and I, making the tumor appear smaller. Incidental renal cysts (arrowheads).

and can be seen within 2 days of initiation of therapy *(5)*. Return of ^{18}F-FDG uptake of a nodule in a treated tumor or a new tumor suggests loss of tumor control by imatinib therapy *(6)*.

Traditional therapy can also show dramatic responses by functional imaging. For example, within one to four cycles of chemotherapy, an early response by ^{18}F-FDG PET can predict the response, progression-free survival, and overall survival. If there is treatment failure, the same imaging can predict the response to secondary treatment; and upon completion of the secondary therapy, it can predict a remission versus residual disease *(7)*. Cognizant that imaging is part of the entire clinical assessment, findings suggest that ^{18}F-FDG PET may be a general marker for lymphoma in predicting both early treatment response and durability of response after therapy. It may also have a potential role in evaluating targeted therapies for lymphoma. In a small study, Torizuka et al. found that ^{18}F-FDG PET at 1 to 2 months, but not 5 to 7 days after radioimmunotherapy with an ^{131}I-anti-B1 antibody, correlated with the response *(8)*. This small study also pointed out that the timing between therapy and imaging plays an important role in the value of a functional imaging endpoint.

3. IMAGING IN CLINICAL TRIALS

In Phase I or II drug trials, the main point is the drug(s), not the imaging. For example, Phase I trials assess the toxicity of the drug and are powered for this effect, not for the value of the imaging. In this case, the imaging is held stable, and there may or may not be efficacy of the drug. Imaging may be exploratory, but it can have value in suggesting that the functional/targeted imaging may be a predictor of response for future trials or to evaluate the mechanism of action of the new drug. When developing imaging agents or methods, the trial needs to be powered to assess the efficacy of the imaging agent or method, and the drug needs to be held stable or known to function. The trial design may be as follows: test an imaging agent/method with a drug known to function compared to the same imaging agent/method without drug.

In Phase I drug trials, imaging results may be suggestive, but often there is not enough power for a definitive assessment of the value of imaging, particularly if drug efficacy is not found or in the unlikely event that the drug has near 100% efficacy. In Phase II or III trials, there is a better chance of having enough power for assessing the value of new imaging agents/methods to assess therapeutic efficacy if the drug is effective.

Because evaluating imaging agents is not the main focus of this book, it is not be a focus of this chapter. In cases where both drug and imaging agent/method are being evaluated, imaging results may be divided as: patients who respond to the drug versus those who do not respond to the drug. Response may be measured simultaneously or subsequently by the change in tumor size using, for example, World Health Organization (WHO) or response evaluation criteria in solid tumors (RECIST) criteria, or tumor histology/signaling/target expression. Trials may also assess whether imaging predicts outcomes, such as patient survival. Eventually, trials are needed that focus on whether altering therapy, including targeted therapy, based on imaging findings improves patient outcome.

4. IMAGING AGENTS

Owing to the exquisite sensitivity and linearity of nuclear imaging cameras, most targeted/functional imaging agents are designed for imaging by either gamma cameras (planar or SPECT imaging) or by PET cameras. In terms of sensitivity for visualizing imaging agents, PET imaging is often more sensitive than SPECT imaging, both of which, however, are more sensitive than MR imaging (MRI), which is more sensitive than ultrasonography or computed tomography (CT). Each modality, however, offers its own particular benefits. For example, MRI does not use ionizing radiation and allows tissue characterization such as T1 and T2 characteristics, dynamic contrast enhancement, diffusion-weighted imaging, and spectroscopy. Currently, CT has the highest spatial resolution clinically; and unlike MRI, measurement of contrast enhancement has a linear relation with the concentration of the agent. In contrast, with MRI, contrast enhancement may be affected by the local environment and does not, in general, have a linear association with the agent. Ultrasonography does not use ionizing radiation, can demonstrate vascular flow including the direction of flow, and is a more portable modality. Combining modalities, such as PET/CT or SPECT/CT, allows simultaneous evaluation of both functional signal and anatomy, which can aid interpretation.

5. MEASURING TARGET DIRECTLY VERSUS DOWNSTREAM EFFECTS

Trials may be designed that include imaging of the target itself versus imaging of its downstream effects. Theoretically, the target itself may be imaged to determine if it is present. If the targeted is present, the drug may be effective. On the other hand, if the target is not present, the target therapy is not likely to be effective. Although target presence may be evaluated by biopsy, the following would be better or would be reasonably only evaluated by imaging: In large tumors, heterogeneity of expression within the tumor may be assessed. Without a bystander effect, areas of tumor without expression may not respond to the targeted drug. In patients with metastases, heterogeneity of expression in the various metastases may be assessed. If expression is present in some metastases but not others, there may be a mixed response to the therapy, suggesting that adding another chemotherapeutic agent or local therapy may be useful to enhance efficacy. As with other forms of imaging, imaging the target itself may be used to monitor therapeutic efficacy (9). Repetitive imaging for therapy monitoring may be used to assess change in expression over time. In patients who were responding to the targeted therapy, decreased expression in one, several, or all tumors may portend loss of tumor control and resistance to therapy.

Careful interpretation is necessary when using targeted imaging with a new targeted therapy. For example, the targeted therapy may compete with the imaging agent or vice versa. Alternatively, the imaging agent may bind to a site separate from that bound by the therapeutic agent and thus may not reflect the binding site of the agent. Imaging agents seek to visualize the target or its action; causing phenotypic change is not the goal. Therapy, on the other hand, seeks to cause phenotypic change. Thus, even if the target is visualized by imaging, it may not mean that the therapeutic agent is effective. For example, the imaging agent may bind, but not inhibit, a tyrosine kinase domain; but the therapeutic agent needs to perform both functions to be effective. In comparison, the therapeutic agent need not demonstrate favorable biodistribution in terms of signal-to-noise for imaging such as low background distribution in the organ of interest and relatively high uptake in the target. Another potential outcome is that the imaging agent images the target and the drug inhibits target function, yet the tumor grows. In other words, the drug is ineffective, which may because the primary growth/maintenance signaling pathway for the tumor was not targeted or was not adequately suppressed, or secondary/redundant pathways supported growth. As with all tests, one must also keep in mind the possibility of false positives and false negatives.

An example of receptor targeting is imaging of tumors expressing somatostatin receptors (Fig. 2). Most clinical studies focusing on the somatostatin receptor utilize the somatostatin analogue ^{111}In-labeled octreotide. Of the five receptor subtypes, this radiopharmaceutical has highest affinity for subtype 2 (SSRT2) and intermediate affinity for subtypes 3 and 5 (10–14). It is used principally to identify primary neuroendocrine tumors and their metastases for diagnosis, staging, predicting therapeutic response, and monitoring therapy. Depending on the radiopharmaceutical employed, virtually all neuroendocrine malignancies may be imaged, including islet cell tumors, carcinoids, small-cell lung cancers, pheochromocytomas, paragangliomas, and medullary thyroid cancers (15–17). These lesions often cause symptoms by secreting hormones. Fortunately, finding receptor expression by imaging predicts that therapeutic somatostatin analogues will inhibit hormone secretion by the tumor (16). With new bifunctional drugs using somatostatin analogues to deliver cytotoxic and cytostatic agents,(18–20) imaging should also become important in selecting patients whose tumors are likely to respond.

An example of a receptor-targeting agent that is still in clinical trials is ^{18}F-fluoroestradiol (FES). PET imaging with this agent correlates with estrogen receptor (ER) expression and predicts response to tamoxifen (9). In a study of 47 patients with heavily pretreated metastatic breast cancer, seminquantitative analysis of initial ^{18}F-FES uptake by imaging predicted subsequent tumor response to treatment predominantly with aromatase inhibitors (21). Using another estrogen receptor analogue, ^{123}I-labeled cis-11β-methoxy-17α-iodovinyl-estradiol

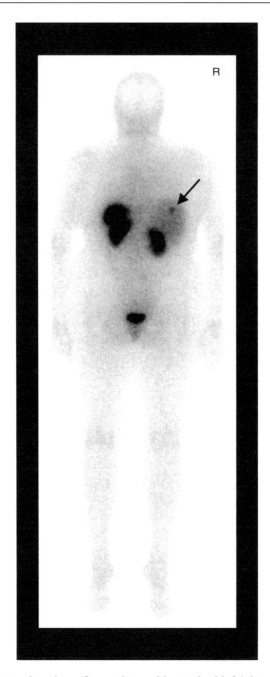

Fig. 2. Planar gamma-camera imaging of a patient with carcinoid 24 hours after injection of ^{111}In-octreotide. ^{111}In-octreotide localizes to the carcinoid metastasis in the liver (arrow) due to the expression of somatostatin receptors by the tumor. In this posterior view, the liver is on the right side. Physiologic excretion of the radiopharmaceutical is seen in the spleen, kidneys, and bladder.

(Z-^{123}I-MIVE), 21 of 23 patients had clear uptake before therapy and 2 had faint uptake. Four weeks later, 17 of 21 patients with clear uptake before therapy had clear uptake again, whereas 4 did not. Patients with faint baseline uptake or posttherapy mixed or no ER blockade after tamoxifen showed progressive disease despite antiestrogen treatment.

Moreover, patients with clear baseline uptake and complete ER blockade after tamoxifen had a significantly longer progression-free interval (PFI): 14.4 ± 1.6 vs. 1.8 ± 0.8 months. Thus, one could determine if the target was present. Mechanistically, one could determine whether the therapeutic was binding its target. Moreover, the targeted imaging predicted success of the targeted therapy.

Other examples of targeted imaging guiding targeted therapy include the use of radiolabeled antibodies aiming at cellular antigens. CD20 on non-Hodgkin's lymphoma has been successfully targeted for therapy. A ^{90}Y labeled antibody, ^{90}Y-ibritumomab tiuxetan, is a therapeutic agent. Seven to nine days before its use, the antibody labeled instead with ^{111}In may be employed to confirm the presence of the target. Imaging is performed with a gamma camera. Clearance can vary, but dosimetry does not correlate with toxicity *(22)*. It is thought that this antibody itself may have biologic activity. Another antibody to CD-20 is ^{131}I-tositumomab. At 7 to 14 days before its use, a lower dose of the same antibody may be employed to confirm the presence of the target. Imaging is performed with a gamma camera. Clearance can vary, but in this case dosimetry does appear to predict toxicity *(23)*.

Instead of the primary target, one may also study downstream effects of the drug, such as alterations in glucose metabolism by ^{18}F-FDG or changes in the function of the tumor vasculature by dynamic contrast-enhanced imaging. With downstream targets, the process being imaged may be affected by various pathways. This may be advantageous because a variety of targeted agents may be tested using a similar readout. This may be disadvantageous because the effect may be due to nonspecific mechanisms; therefore, interpreting that the process imaged is directly due to the mechanism of action of the targeting agent may be spurious.

^{18}F-FDG is an analogue of glucose. It enters cells primarily via GLUT transporters. Once inside the cell, it serves as a substrate for hexokinase. Phosphorylation of ^{18}F-FDG is a terminal event because, unlike glucose-6-phosphate, phosphorylated FDG cannot continue along the glycolytic pathway. The negative charge added upon phosphorylation prevents efflux out of the cell. Thus, phosphorylated ^{18}F-FDG accumulates in the cell. Also unlike glucose, ^{18}F-FDG does not undergo tubular reabsorption and is more readily excreted through the urine, decreasing background activity. Uptake of ^{18}F-FDG is thought to reflect the metabolic rate of the cell. Although its uptake is considered to reflect primarily GLUT transporter activity and hexokinase activity, it is a complex event. For example, ^{18}F-FDG accumulates to a greater degree in many cancers compared with normal tissues, the reasons for which may include increased transport due to overexpression of membrane GLUT transporters (primarily GLUT1) and an increased rate of glycolysis—e.g., due to increased metabolic demand, hypoxia, signaling from oncogenes, increased hexokinase expression (primarily HK-1 and HK-2) and activity, and decreased glucose-6-phosphatase activity. Blood flow to the tumor may also be a factor. Increased PET activity can be found not only in cancer but also in infections, including granulomatous disease.

Currently, ^{18}F-FDG imaging has its greatest impact in oncology for diagnosis and staging and is becoming increasingly utilized to monitor many cancers. It has also had a significant impact in cardiology, primarily for assessing ischemia and infarction. One of its major influences in neurology has been seizure focus imaging. The applications of ^{18}F-FDG PET imaging illustrate the myriad pathologic events that may be evaluated by developing a radiotracer for a central biologic event (e.g., metabolism) and at the molecular level for studying a key enzyme such as hexokinase.

6. NUCLEAR MEDICINE IMAGING

6.1. Radiopharmaceuticals

In general, radiopharmaceuticals for gamma camera imaging consist of three parts: (1) a localizing agent; (2) a linker; and (3) a radionuclide. Commonly used radionuclides include ^{99m}Tc, ^{111}In, and ^{123}I. The linker strategy has proven successful for many clinical applications as examples above illustrate. In comparison, the radionuclides used in PET most often allow direct labeling of the localization agent without need of a linker. For example, a hydroxyl group may be replaced by fluorine-18, usually with retention of biologic activity. Other radionuclides (e.g., ^{11}C, ^{15}O, ^{13}N, ^{82}Rb, ^{64}Cu, ^{68}Ga) have been used and may be more advantageous in particular situations. One advantage of ^{68}Ga is that it can be produced from a generator and thus may be more available than radionuclides that need to be produced in a cyclotron. ^{18}F is commonly used because of its chemistry and its favorable half-life of 110 minutes.

6.2. Physics

Radionuclides are unstable atoms. Atoms are made up of neutrons, protons, and electrons. The ratio of protons to neutrons and protons to electrons determines the stability and reactivity of an atom. A charge-neutral atom has the same number of protons and electrons. Electrons reside in orbital shells at different distances from the protons and neutrons, or nucleons. The closer shells have greater binding energy; and if an electron from a lower orbital shell is lost, one from a higher orbital shell usually replaces it, resulting in a release of energy in the form of an x-ray. The movement of an electron from one shell to another results in an x-ray with a characteristic amount of energy.

Similarly, nucleons in their ground state are stable, but if the ratio of neutrons to protons is not optimal or the nucleons are not in their ground state, they may release energy/particles, including gamma rays, with characteristic energy. The deexcitation may occur immediately or be delayed. If the latter, the nucleus is said to be in a metastable state. The decay of ^{99m}Tc (m for metastable) is commonly imaged in nuclear medicine. X-rays arise from electron shells and tend to have lower energy than gamma rays. They are usually delivered from outside the body, and their attenuation as they pass through the body is used for medical imaging, such as for radiography (i.e., chest x-ray) or CT. Gamma rays usually arise from nucleon energy changes and have higher energy than x-rays. They are used in nuclear medicine imaging and usually arise from radiopharmaceuticals delivered into the body. The characteristic energy signature is used to distinguish radioactive decay arising directly from the radionuclide from background/scatter reactions that result in different energies from the source of interest. Gamma cameras are used in nuclear medicine to image gamma rays from radiopharmaceuticals administered to patients. The camera may form a two-dimensional, or planar, image; or the camera may rotate around, more commonly than encircle, the patient to obtain multiple planar images in different projections that can be processed into three-dimensional images as in SPECT.

6.3. PET Physics Introduction

Unstable nucleons with too many protons or neutrons may decay to more stable states by releasing particles. PET is based on imaging radionuclides that decay by positron emission, which reduces the number of protons in the nucleus by transforming a proton to a neutron and ejecting both a positron and a neutrino from the nucleus. A positron has the same mass but opposite charge as an electron. After traveling a short distance (usually millimeters), it loses kinetic energy and collides with an electron in an annihilation reaction that transforms their combined mass into energy, releasing two gamma ray photons (each 511 keV) traveling in opposite trajectories. In nuclear medicine, gamma cameras attempt to image single gamma rays from the atom itself and distinguish them from scatter by characteristic energy windows and collimators that are designed to filter scatter. Because of the former, gamma cameras can theoretically be used for infinite magnification imaging. Because positrons travel a short distance before decay, magnification for localization is theoretically limited. Positron annihilation into gamma rays traveling in opposite trajectories allows coincidence detection, which is capitalized on in PET imaging to localize the annihilation event along a line called the line of response (LOR), which connects the two detectors that detected the two 511-keV gamma rays. In PET imaging, a ring of radiation detectors encircles the patient and detects the gamma rays on opposite sides within a specified period of time. Unlike SPECT, PET imaging does not require a collimator to help identify the source of activity; and clinically it currently has higher sensitivity.

6.3.1. PET IMAGING

In clinical trials, the workhorse for PET imaging has been ^{18}F-FDG. Its use is based on the Warburg effect, which suggests that tumors have aberrantly high rates of glycolysis. With therapy, often two types of change in ^{18}F-FDG uptake are found: early (within days) and delayed (within weeks to months). The former may reflect immediate effects on signaling pathways regulating glucose metabolism more so than cell viability. If persistent, cell viability is lost with time. If only the latter is seen, it more likely reflects loss of cell viability; less likely, it may reflect late effects of signaling pathways on glucose metabolism. Early changes may be more specific for targeted therapy predicted to effect signaling pathways involved in glucose metabolism, whereas later changes may reflect a more generalized tumor response to therapy. One must be careful with this interpretation, however, because an early decrease in ^{18}F-FDG uptake can be seen with less specific chemotherapy regimens targeting events downstream of glucose signaling. For example, Yamane et al. demonstrated a reduction in ^{18}F-FDG uptake 1 day after initiation of chemotherapy for non-Hodgkin's lymphoma. The chemotherapy used was primarily a CHOP (cyclophosphamide/doxorubicin/vincristine/prednisone) or CHOP-like regimen blocking primarily DNA replication. The authors suggested that the particular drug used may have an effect on whether decreased or potentially increased ^{18}F-FDG uptake is found. It could not be determined from this small study of 12 patients whether the decreased standard uptake value (SUV) 1 day after therapy translated into a durable tumor response *(24)*.

Early decreased uptake often persists as delayed decreased uptake compared to the baseline (pretherapy) value with effective therapy (Fig. 1). As mentioned above, an example of early decreased ^{18}F-FDG uptake with targeted therapy is treatment with imatinib *(5)*. The primary driver of the malignant phenotype of GISTs is the c-kit receptor, a tyrosine kinase inhibited by imatinib. With tyrosine kinase inhibitors, early changes in ^{18}F-FDG uptake may precede cell death,*(25)* implying that changes in cell signaling altering glucose uptake and/or metabolism precede those that affect proliferation. The low uptake in patients treated with imatinib is often maintained upon serial imaging for extended periods of time, and usually tumor necrosis is seen at later time points, consistent with cell killing. Indeed, return of ^{18}F-FDG uptake in a nodule within a treated tumor or a new tumor suggests development of resistance to imatinib therapy *(6)*. Thus, ^{18}F-FDG PET imaging appears to be a good marker of the efficacy of therapy targeting the tyrosine kinase activity of the c-kit receptor in GISTs.

In non-Hodgkin's lymphoma, decreased ^{18}F-FDG uptake can be seen 7 days after standard therapy (CHOP) with or without mitoguazone *(26)*. Even lower values were seen at day 42, and this parameter correlated better with long-term outcome in a small group of patients. In a more recent study in 12 patients with non-Hodgkin's lymphoma, reduction in SUV was seen 1 day after initiation of chemotherapy *(24)*. Larger studies of interim therapy analysis have evaluated patients after two to four cycles of therapy and found that they predict the therapeutic response in both Hodgkin's and non-Hodgkin's lymphoma *(27)*.

Figure 3 demonstrates ^{18}F-FDG PET and PET/CT imaging of a patient with non-Hodgkin's lymphoma before and 1.5 months after the first cycle of chemotherapy. On the pretherapy PET scan (Fig. 3A), increased uptake is seen in the region of the mesentery and retroperitoneum. Note the heterogeneity of the uptake on PET/CT scans (Fig. 3C), with some lymph nodes taking up significantly more ^{18}F-FDG than others, as well as the heterogeneity

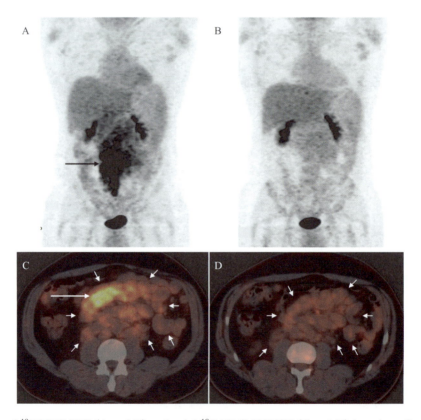

Fig. 3. Coronal ^{18}F-FDG PET (A and B) and axial ^{18}F-FDG PET/CT (C and D) imaging of a patient with non-Hodgkin's lymphoma before (A and C) and one and a half months after (B and D) the first cycle of chemotherapy (hyper-CVAD + rituximab). Increased uptake (long arrow) is seen in the retroperitoneum and the mesentery pre-therapy on both the PET scan (A) and PET/CT (B). The uptake in the enlarged lymph nodes (short arrows) is heterogeneous on the PET/CT (C). Post-therapy there is near resolution of ^{18}F-FDG uptake (B and D); however, although smaller, lymphadenopathy remains substantial (D). Thus, uptake of an imaging agent may be quite heterogeneous in one tumor and among tumors and the degree of functional signal loss may precede or be significantly greater than the change in tumor size – both of these points are better appreciated using multimodality combined PET/CT.

of the uptake in a single enlarged lymph node. Thus, uptake of an imaging agent may be quite heterogeneous in one tumor and among tumors. After therapy, the PET-only image (Fig. 3B) suggests near resolution of ^{18}F-FDG uptake. On the PET/CT image, again, near resolution of ^{18}F-FDG uptake is noted; and although smaller, lymphadenopathy remains substantial. Thus, the degree of functional signal loss may precede or be significantly greater than the change in tumor size. Multimodality imaging such as with PET/CT allows evaluation of both the distribution of the functional signal and the tumor morphology/size simultaneously.

Delayed responses can be seen in a variety of tumors, including breast cancer. In an initial study by Wahl et al.,(28) modest reduction in ^{18}F-FDG uptake was seen 8 days following chemotherapy, but a greater reduction of approximately 50% was noted at 2 months. The chemotherapy primarily used agents that inhibit DNA replication and conjugated estrogens. The importance of the chemotherapeutic agent is attested to by the study of Mortimer et al., who found that increased ^{18}F-FDG uptake 1 to 2 weeks after starting tamoxifen predicted the subsequent response and may represent an early agonist "flare" response (29). Semiquantitative analysis of ^{18}F-FDG uptake weeks to months after chemotherapy or chemoradiotherapy was prognostic of increased median survival for several tumors, including esophagus, gastric, head and neck, ovarian, and lung cancer (30).

Imaging at the end of therapy has also been used to predict eventual treatment failure. In a study of patients with breast cancer treated with high-dose chemotherapy and stem cell transplantation, patients with a negative end-of-therapy ^{18}F-FDG PET scan survived longer than those with a positive scan, but the overall survival after 4 years was similar (31). In several other tumor types, including esophagus, lung, head and neck, cervix, and soft tissue sarcomas, the median survival increased in patients demonstrating an ^{18}F-FDG PET response at the end of chemotherapy or chemoradiotherapy compared to nonresponders (30). Response is often described as lack of ^{18}F-FDG uptake in these end-of-treatment studies and may be assessed visually. In contrast, at earlier time points at the end of one to two cycles of therapy, there is commonly residual, but lower ^{18}F-FDG uptake that is often better assessed using semiquantitative evaluation.

Studies suggest that ^{18}F-FDG PET imaging at the end of therapy can be valuable in the management of lymphoma. In an analysis of seven studies with a mixed population of patients with Hodgkin's and non-Hodgkin's lymphoma, an overall sensitivity to predict treatment failure was 79%, specificity was 92%, positive predictive value (PPV) was 90%, negative predictive value (NPV) was 81%, and accuracy was 90% for ^{18}F-FDG PET at the end of treatment (7). Debate persists as to whether ^{18}F-FDG PET imaging after two to four cycles of chemotherapy is as predictive as end-of-therapy imaging. In addition, the type of lymphoma is an important factor in the use of ^{18}F-FDG PET.

In a subgroup analysis of 15 studies, 84% sensitivity and 90% sensitivity for ^{18}F-FDG PET was found for detecting residual disease at the end of treatment in Hodgkin's disease and 72% and 100%, respectively, for non-Hodgkin's lymphoma (32). ^{18}F-FDG PET has been reported to have better test characteristics than ^{67}Ga-citrate scintigraphy for predicting subsequent relapse in non-Hodgkins's lymphoma after two cycles of therapy (33). The type of lymphoma can influence whether it takes up an imaging agent at baseline. For example, Tsukamoto et al. found that only approximately 50% of cases of small lymphocytic lymphoma and splenic marginal zone lymphoma demonstrated increased ^{18}F-FDG uptake. In comparison, ^{18}F-FDG-PET identified > 97% of disease sites of Hodgkin's lymphoma and aggressive and highly aggressive non-Hodgkin's lymphoma; and for indolent lymphoma, the detection rate was 91% for follicular lymphoma (FL) and 82% for extranodal marginal zone B-cell lymphoma of mucosa-associated lymphoid tissue, irrespective of plasmacytic differentiation *(34)*.

Although there have been encouraging results, trials to demonstrate that PET-response-adapted therapy improves outcome in patients with lymphoma are needed. One possible methodology for incorporating PET into criteria for assessing the therapeutic response of lymphoma is provided by the international Harmonization Project initiated by the German Competence Network Malignant Lymphoma. Unlike many clinical studies, this group suggests that visual inspection, instead of quantitative or semiquantitative measures, is adequate for evaluating whether a PET scan is positive. The consensus statement from the Cancer Imaging Program of the National Cancer Institute (NCI) in the United States recommended quantitative or semiquantitative assessment of PET Images *(35)*.

Among the methods for quantitative analysis of PET imaging, SUV is most commonly employed. SUV measurements can be affected by various factors*(36)* and which SUV (e.g., SUV_{mean}, $SUV_{maximum}$, SUV_{peak}) has been debated. Various derivations of SUV have been proposed based on equations for quantifying the glucose utilization rate. A simplified SUV calculation is as follows.

$$SUV = \frac{\text{tissue } ^{18}F - FDG \text{ uptake derived from region of interest analysis of the image}}{\text{injected dose/patient weight}}$$

Once an SUV is obtained, one must decide whether absolute values or percent change from baseline implies the response. In the United States, a consensus has not yet been established about which absolute SUV amount or percent decrease in SUV constitutes a response, and it will likely vary depending on the tumor type, the duration of time between therapy and imaging, and the therapy itself. Of course, the method of PET imaging needs to be held constant, particularly in clinical trials; and having a pretherapy scan for comparison is ideal.

Tumors change size on and off of therapy. SUV alone is limited in accounting for the size and morphology of the underlying tumor. Portions of a tumor may be necrotic and therefore would not contribute to a signal generated by living cells. Modern anatomic imaging techniques have higher resolution than functional imaging techniques. Combining anatomic imaging with functional imaging can be used to normalize the functional signal to the underlying tumor morphology and size or weight so the degree of signal per gram tissue may be obtained *(37)*. With appropriate use of phantoms for calibration, the percent injected dose per gram of tumor (akin to ex vivo tissue biodistribution studies used in general tracer studies) may be derived. This should be applicable to a variety of functional imaging agents, such as those for light-based imaging or for nuclear medicine. Fusion systems such as PET/CT or SPECT/CT should ease such evaluation.

Combined-modality imaging can improve test characteristics of either test alone. For example, Antoch et al *(38)*. found heterogeneous ^{18}F-FDG uptake in GISTs by PET and noted that CT detected a larger number of lesions, but combined PET/CT detected the most lesions overall. Discerning pathologic uptake of radiopharmaceuticals is limited in small lesions, particularly those near the spatial resolution of the camera, and can be confounded by normal physiologic uptake. A study of esophageal cancer *(39)* found that mean ^{18}F-FDG uptake did not distinguish 10% viable tumor cells from no residual disease after chemoradiotherapy, underlining the fact that small, residual disease may not be distinguishable by ^{18}F-FDG PET. As with all imaging studies, tumor size matters. Image resolution is a limitation, and microscopic disease can be missed. In this context, waiting too long in the course of therapy may decrease the residual tumor volume enough that residual signal in responding and eventually nonresponding tumors may become difficult to distinguish.

6.3.2. NEWER PET AGENTS

6.3.2.1. Nucleosides. Nucleoside analogues are being evaluated for PET, such as ^{18}F-FLT (3'-deoxy-3'-[^{18}F]fluorothymidine) and ^{18}F-FMAU [1-(2'-deoxy-2'-fluoro-β-D-arabinofuranosyl)thymine], which mimic thymidine. More clinical trial literature is available for ^{18}F-FLT, which has so far demonstrated variable correlation with DNA synthesis and variable imaging of lymph node metastases. In patients with breast cancer, although 13 of 14 primary and 7 of 8 lymph node metastases were identified, ^{18}F-FLT uptake did not correlate with the Ki-67 marker of proliferation *(40)*. A correlation was also not seen in a study of 10 patients with esophageal cancer, and 8 of 10 cancers were detected by ^{18}F-FLT compared to 10 of 10 with ^{18}F-FDG *(41)*. In patients with lung tumors, a study involving 26 patients found that ^{18}F-FLT did not perform as well as ^{18}F-FDG in identifying tumors, but ^{18}F-FLT did correlate with the proliferation marker *(42)*. A more recent study in thoracic tumors also found a correlation between ^{18}F-FLT uptake and Ki-67 *(43)*. In another study of 16 patients, 36 of 38 primarily thoracic malignancies were detected, but there was a weak correlation with Ki-67 *(44)*. Muzi et al. suggested that instead of static measures, such as SUV, dynamically measuring the flux constant of ^{18}F-FLT may better correlate with proliferation *(45)*.

^{18}F-FLT could not differentiate reactive from malignant lymph nodes in 10 patients with head and neck tumors owing to low specificity *(46)*, whereas in studies of patients with lung cancer *(43,47)* low sensitivity (53%) for mediastinal lymph node involvement was noted. The different findings for specificity and sensitivity may be due to the degree of proliferative/thymidine metabolism activity of the metastases from different tumor types and to the reactive nature of the lymph nodes (lymph nodes in the neck usually are exposed to more infectious organisms). The studies pointed out that before using new markers in clinical trials of targeted therapies, it is important to validate the mechanism of action of new imaging agents and confirm that these mechanisms are relevant in the model system to be employed for the chemotherapeutic agent.

6.3.2.2. Amino Acids. Several agents for imaging amino acid metabolism are being developed. In a recent study, ^{11}C-methionine, an amino acid analogue, was used to evaluate the effects of temozolomide therapy in gliomas (primarily grade III or IV tumors) *(48)*. ^{11}C-methionine uptake by tumor was compared to uptake in normal brain and was evaluated prior to and after three cycles of chemotherapy. Responders (9 of 15 patients with reduced or persistent "normal low" ^{11}C-methionine after therapy) had a mean time to progression of 23 months versus 3.5 months for nonresponders. Thus, ^{11}C-methionine PET could predict relatively early in this chemotherapeutic setting which patients were likely to do well on temozolomide by assessing its effects on amino acid metabolism. ^{18}F-FDG-PET was much less successful in this setting, likely due to the relatively high rate of background glucose metabolism of the brain *(49)*.

6.3.2.3. Hypoxia. Several agents for imaging hypoxia are under development. One, ^{18}F-misonidazole (^{18}F-FMISO), was recently used in 40 patients with advanced head and neck cancer ($n = 26$) or non-small-cell lung cancer ($n = 14$). ^{18}F-FMISO PET imaging was performed before curative radiotherapy *(50)*. For patients with head and neck cancer, but not for patients with lung cancer, SUV > 2 separated patients with or without disease-free survival. However, tumor/muscle (> 2.0) or tumor/mediastinum (> 1.6) ratios separated patients with or without disease-free survival with both tumor types. This suggests that ^{18}F-FMISO PET imaging can select patients more likely to respond to radiation therapy and that those patients with increased ^{18}F-FMISO uptake may benefit from treatment targeting regions of hypoxia. It also illustrates the fact that the method used for semiquantitative analysis can affect the study outcome.

In a clinical trial (51) of patients with head and neck tumors, patients were randomly assigned to conventional chemoradiation (irradiation, cisplatin/5-fluorouracil) versus chemoradiation (cisplatin) plus tirapazamide (tirapazamide is a hypoxia-activated prodrug). PET imaging using ^{18}F-FMISO was performed before and during therapy to detect tumor hypoxia. Of 45 patients, 32 (71%) had detectable hypoxia in either the primary cancer or neck nodes at baseline on ^{18}F-FMISO PET imaging, and these patients on either regimen were subsequently found to have a greater rate of locoregional treatment failure than nonhypoxic cases. Furthermore, the locoregional failure rate was less in patients with hypoxia treated with the regimen that included the hypoxia-activated agent tirapazamine. This study suggests that ^{18}F-FMISO imaging may be used to select patients for hypoxia-specific therapies.

7. MAGNETIC RESONANCE

7.1. Physics

7.1.1. T$_1$-WEIGHTED AND T$_2$-WEIGHTED IMAGES

The wide range of contrast mechanisms in MRI frequently makes it the modality of choice for soft tissue imaging. Although several nuclei can be used in MR applications, the near 100% natural abundance and highest relative sensitivity makes hydrogen (proton) the most commonly used for in vivo studies. When a collection of nuclei with nonzero spin (odd number of protons, neutrons, or both) is placed in a strong static magnetic field, a small net excess of them preferentially align with the magnetic field. In clinical MRI, it is this net excess of protons (roughly 10 out of a million in a 1.5-T MR scanner) that ultimately gives rise to the detected signal. Along with the strong static magnetic field that creates the net magnetization, additional time-varying magnetic fields are applied to convert the net magnetization to a measurable form (the radiofrequency, or B$_1$, field) and to encode positional information in the detected signals (the magnetic field gradients applied in each orthogonal direction). The signals created by the application of these magnetic fields are then used to create the MR image.

Undoubtedly, two of the most common types of clinical MR images are T$_1$-weighted and T$_2$-weighted spin-echo images. In spin-echo images, a pair of radiofrequency pulses (a 90° pulse and a 180° pulse) are applied repeatedly to excite the protons. The separation of the 90^0 and 180^0 pulses in time determines the echo time (TE), and the time between repeated applications of these pulse pairs determines the repetition time (TR). The choices of echo time (TE) and repetition time (TR) determine whether one achieves T1 or T2 weighting. In the case of T$_1$-weighted images, the image contrast depends primarily on the T1 (spin-lattice) relaxation times, with substances with short T1 relaxation times (e.g., lipids) being hyperintense (brighter) and substances with long T1 relaxation times (e.g., as low-viscosity fluids) being hypointense (darker). In addition, the most commonly utilized MR contrast agents, based on the gadolinium atom (which has seven unpaired electrons), cause shortening of T1 relaxation times of water protons in the local vicinity of the contrast agent. Therefore tissues that take up such contrast agents become hyperintense on T$_1$-weighted images. In the case of T$_2$-weighted images, the image contrast depends primarily on the T2 (spin-spin) relaxation times, with substances with long T2 relaxation times, such as fluids (e.g., cerebrospinal fluid, cysts, vitreous humor), being hyperintense. Iron-based contrast agents decrease T2 relaxation times of adjacent water molecules resulting in a hypointense signal on such T_2-weighted images. Because tissue injury is frequently associated with edema, T_2-weighted images are ubiquitously used for clinical MR imaging.

7.1.2. FLAIR

In neuroimaging applications, FLAIR (fluid attenuated inversion recovery) sequences are also commonly used. Basically, FLAIR images are T_2-weighted images in which signals from low viscosity, nonproteinacious fluids are purposely suppressed. Because these fluids represent the brightest components of a T_2-weighted image, their suppression improves visibility of edema, infarcts, multiple sclerosis plaques, and other lesions or tissue responses that have associated hyperintense signal levels on T_2-weighted images but not as hyperintense as "pure" fluids such as cerebrospinal fluid (CSF). With the signal from CSF suppressed, periventricular lesions and cortical infarcts, for example, are much more conspicuous and less susceptible to being masked by partial volume averaging of brain tissue or small lesions with CSF. In addition, FLAIR images have been used to assess response of therapy as reflected in decreased peritumoral edema *(52,53)*. T_1-weighted, T_2-weighted, and intravascular contrast (commonly gadolinium-based) enhanced images are commonly used in clinical practice to characterize lesions and assess therapeutic response.

7.1.3. DIFFUSION-WEIGHTED IMAGING

The "apparent diffusion coefficient" of water protons may be quantitatively measured by MRI. All water protons undergo random thermal motion due to diffusion. Modern MR systems with high speed imaging capabilities can produce images in which the signal intensity is proportional to the rate of water proton diffusion. This is accomplished by applying a matched pair of strong diffusion sensitizing gradient pulses symmetrically about the spin-echo (180°) pulse in a spin-echo imaging study. If protons being imaged with such a technique are stationary, the combined effects of the two diffusion sensitizing gradient pulses cancel. If protons are moving, however, the effect of the first gradient pulse is not completely canceled by the second gradient pulse. In this case, the signal is attenuated exponentially with a rate constant that depends on the product of two measures: the apparent diffusion coefficient (ADC) and a quantity known as the "*b* value." The ADC value is a measure of the proton diffusion (in mm^2/s). The value of *b* (in s/mm^2) depends on the amplitude, width, and spacing of the diffusion sensitizing gradient pulses; and as *b* is increased, the diffusion sensitization increases.

Diffusion sensitized images are displayed as "diffusion weighted (DWI) images," where low signal intensity implies increased diffusion and high signal intensity implies restricted (decreased) diffusion, or as "apparent diffusion coefficient (ADC) images," in which high signal implies increased diffusion and low signal implies restricted (decreased) diffusion. The ADC images, although computationally more demanding, have the advantage that they decrease the amount of T2 "shine through" that can occur in DWI images owing to the inherently high T2 weighting of DWI images. In such DWI images, areas of edema, for example, can appear artificially bright rather than dark (as would be expected in areas of increased diffusion) due to the long T2 relaxation times for fluids.

Because the rate of proton diffusion is not necessarily isotropic (the same in all directions) (e.g., water protons diffuse more rapidly along white matter fiber tracts) diffusion sensitizing gradients are usually applied in at least three orthogonal directions to create an average, or "trace," diffusion image that avoids the effects of anisotropic diffusion. One may also exploit anisotropic diffusion to generate diffusion tensor images (e.g., to image the white matter tracts and the effect of lesions or interventions on the tracts).

The power of diffusion imaging is its ability to assess changes in intracellular versus extracellular water. For example, in the acute stages of an ischemic event, cell swelling results in a decrease in the apparent diffusion coefficient owing to the increase in intracellular volume (with more restricted water diffusion due to the presence of intracellular structures that decrease the mean free path of water molecules) relative to the extracellular volume (where water diffusion is more rapid). In terms of assessing novel therapeutics, diffusion MRI techniques have been proposed as a means of noninvasively assessing changes in cell density and/or changes in the intracellular to extracellular volume fractions.

7.1.4. FLAIR in Clinical Trials

In general, a reduction in T2 (FLAIR)-bright signal and enhancement signifies a favorable treatment response. In neuroimaging, this corresponds to a reduction in edema and blood-brain barrier breakdown and a likely reduction in tumor cell burden. Traditional tumor response measures have been based on the measurement of enhancing volume.

The relation between imaging findings and tumor recurrence does not always hold and may break down in the setting of radiation necrosis, a treatment effect that can lead to increased enhancement and T2-bright signal, but not due to tumor. Such cases often require biopsy or advanced imaging to guide therapy. Traditional MRI has been criticized too for failing to demonstrate adequately the borders of ill-defined gliomas and for not allowing fast assessment of the treatment response. Figure 4 demonstrates that FLAIR can demonstrate

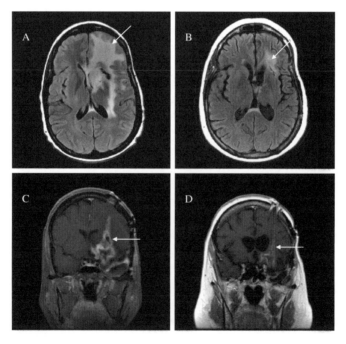

Fig. 4. Flair and intravenous contrast enhanced T_1-weighted MR imaging of a patient with a gliobastoma multiforme. Flair (A and B) and gadolinium based intravenous contrast enhanced T_1-weighted (C and D) imaging of the brain demonstrates increased T_2-weighted signal on FLAIR (arrow) and increased enhancement on T_1-weighted MR images (arrow) primarily in the frontal lobe pre-therapy (A and C), with marked decrease three weeks (one cycle, B and D) after CPT-11 and bevacizumab therapy. Images coutesy of Dr. A. J. Kumar.

the response to treatment with a chemotherapeutic agent and an antibody to the vascular epithelial growth factor (VEGF), bevacizumab, within 3 weeks of starting therapy.

FLAIR imaging can also be used to monitor treatment of complications of cancer therapy, such as radiation necrosis of the brain. In a recent study of eight patients with biopsy-proven radiation necrosis,[54] bevacizumab was used to block the effects of VEGF. The reasoning for this was that an excess of VEGF was likely a critical event in the pathogenesis of radionecrosis, with ischemia causing excess VEGF secretion, resulting in blood-brain barrier breakdown and edema. Imaging findings changed markedly at 6 to 8 weeks after therapy with either bevacizumab or a bevacizumab combination (with temozolamide, carboplatin, or irinotecan). The areas of FLAIR abnormalities decreased in area by 60% ($\pm$ 18% SD), and gadolinium-enhanced T_1-weighted images decreasing in size by 48% ($\pm$ 22% SD). Dexamethasone requirements also decreased by 8.6 mg daily, suggesting reduced edema. This pilot study showed that bevacizumab has a marked effect on radiation necrosis, as measured by imaging findings.

7.1.5. DWI in Clinical Trials

For brain tumors, there have been conflicting reports as to the usefulness of DWI imaging in assessing tumor edema versus infiltration or treatment effect versus recurrence. In the setting of brain tumors, DWI imaging was found useful for distinguishing edema from tumor infiltration by some authors (54,55) but not by others (56–58). It is likely that there is overlap in ADC values for infiltrating tumor and edema; thus, it is unlikely that ADC alone can make this distinction in individual patients (59). In the setting of glioma, DWI imaging showed significantly higher ADC values in patients with recurrent tumor (mean 1.23×10^{-3} mm^2/s) than in those with treatment effects (mean 1.07×10^{-3} mm^2/s) in a study of 19 patients; (60) however, there have been conflicting reports as to whether ADC should be lower in recurrence or necrosis (61–64).

It has been suggested that DWI imaging may predict treatment effect. Changes in the functional diffusion map in 20 glioma patients predicted the response at 3 weeks from the initiation of therapy (irradiation, chemotherapy, or a combination of irradiation and chemotherapy) (65). In addition, ADC and FLAIR imaging has been used to demonstrate decreased vasogenic edema associated with primary brain gliomas upon treatment with an oral tyrosine kinase inhibitor of VEGF receptors (see below) (53).

8. DCE-MRI

Gadolinium-based intravenous contrast-enhanced imaging has been used for some time to characterize lesions. Solid lesions enhance, whereas cysts do not. With faster scanners, temporal resolution has allowed evaluation of the dynamics of contrast enhancement. For liver imaging, differences in enhancement time and morphology during the early arterial, portal venous, and delayed phases help distinguish neoplasms. Early techniques looking at the rate of wash-in and washout have proven useful for characterizing some tumors. For example, rapid wash-in and slow washout is used clinically to differentiate breast cancer from nonmalignant pathology, such as fibroadenomas. Increased temporal resolution and mathematic modeling have enabled quantitative assessment of vascular parameters; however, methodology has not been standardized.

8.1. DCE-MR Physics

In recent years, the image acquisition rates for state-of-the-art MR systems have improved dramatically, enabling improved imaging of moving organs as well as enabling dynamic imaging of MR contrast agent uptake. Two such dynamic contrast imaging techniques are commonly used.

The first technique, and the one currently most commonly used in clinical trials, is dynamic contrast agent-enhanced MRI (DCE-MRI). With DCE-MRI techniques, heavily T_1-weighted images are obtained rapidly ($\sim$ 0.5–1.0 s/image) before, during, and following a rapid injection of gadolinium-based contrast agent. The dynamic enhancement (enhancement over time) in a region of interest can be evaluated in a variety of ways, including qualitative visual review or quantitative measures such as rate of enhancement, time to peak enhancement, washout rate, and total and/or initial area under the enhancement versus time among others. The most quantitative and physiologically relevant model is the pharmacokinetic model in which, most commonly, two compartments are considered: the vascular space and the extravascular, extracellular space (EES) *(66)*. Using the two-compartment pharmacokinetic model, physiologically relevant parameters, such as the vascular volume fraction (v_p, unitless), endothelial transfer constant (K^{trans}, min^{-1}, representing the rate of transfer from the vascular space to the EES), the reflux rate (k_{ep}, min^{-1}, representing the rate of transfer from the EES back to the vascular space), and the EES volume fraction (v_e, unitless), can be computed from a chosen region of interest or pixel by pixel throughout the imaged volume. K^{trans} measures are relatively commonly used as secondary or exploratory endpoints in the assessment of acute response to tyrosine kinase inhibitors targeting VEGFR because such inhibitors cause an acute decrease in vascular permeability. In general, the initial area under the signal intensity versus time curve (IAUC, typically integrated over the first 90–120 seconds following contrast agent administration) yields longitudinal response measures that compare favorably with those obtained with K^{trans} measures. Given the simplicity of the IAUC calculation relative to K^{trans} calculations, IAUC measures in tumor, usually normalized to an IAUC measure in blood, may be described in DCE-MRI studies of treatment response.

The second relatively commonly used dynamic MR technique is known as dynamic susceptibility change MRI (DSC-MRI). In this technique, T2- or "apparent" T_2-weighted images are obtained rapidly ($\sim$100–300 ms/image) before, during, and immediately following a rapid bolus administration of gadolinium-based MR contrast agent. The first pass of the agent bolus through the microvasculature causes a localized transient loss of signal. Analysis of the signal change over time allows estimation of the regional blood volume (rBV). If the mean transit time (MTT, arterial-to-venous) can be computed from the same data, the central volume theorem can be used to compute the regional blood flow (rBF) (i.e., rBF = rBV/MTT). Finally, if extraction of the contrast agent is computed as a function of time, an estimate of the permeability-surface area can be obtained. This DSC-MRI technique is therefore a direct analogue of the dynamic contrast agent-enhanced computed tomography (DCE-CT) technique. Unlike DCE-CT, however, the signal intensity change as a function of contrast agent concentration is not linear, and therefore DSC-MRI data modeling is more complex.

There is an important limitation of both the DSC-MRI and DCE-MRI techniques (or, in fact, the DCE-CT technique): The contrast agents approved for clinical MRI (or CT) are all low-molecular-weight agents ($\sim$500–800 daltons). As a result, all of these agents extravasate into normal tissue, with a first-pass extraction fraction as high as 40% to 50%. The resulting nonspecific uptake places limits on the interpretation of resulting quantitative measures. For example, in the case of DCE-MRI, the frequently cited K^{trans} parameter, commonly reported as a measure of "permeability," really represents the extraction–flow product unless it can be verified that the extraction is not flow-limited. When extraction is not flow-limited, transport of the imaging agent out of the vasculature is slow enough that the concentration of the imaging agent in the intravascular space is essentially not depleted over the time of imaging. Similar constraints apply to DSC-MRI and DCE-CT measures. It is only if the molecular weight of the contrast agent is substantially higher than that of current clinically available contrast agents that one can be assured that K^{trans}, for example, reflects the true permeability–surface area. However, in this case the rate of extraction is low, and measurement times are therefore long. Despite these limitations, however, DCE-MRI, DSC-MRI, and DCE-CT techniques have been, and continue to be, useful for assessing antivascular/antiangiogenic agents so long as the limitations of the resulting parameters are appreciated and the acquisition and analysis methodologies are validated and reproducible.

8.2. Clinical Trials Using DCE-MRI

Most clinical trials incorporating DCE-MRI with targeted therapy have been in the Phase I or II setting. DCE-MRI has been used successfully for assessing antiangiogenic therapy *(67)*. For example, in patients with glioblastoma, an oral tyrosine kinase inhibitor of VEGF receptors, AZD2171, had a rapid but reversible onset of action. It had greater effect on large than on small vessels, including an immediate decrease in blood volume in large vessels and decreased blood flow in both small and large vessels. Sustained decrease in K^{trans} and v_e corresponded with a decrease in brain edema. In addition, FLAIR lesion volumes and ADC decreased, again consistent with reduced vasogenic edema. The patients also demonstrated a reduced mass effect, consistent with efficacy. The DCE-MR vascular parameter changes were seen by day 1; and the FLAIR, ADC, and mass effect improvements were better visualized at the next imaging session, on day 27 of imaging.

In inflammatory breast cancer, an antibody to VEGF, bevacizumab, appeared to cause a decrease in DCE-MRI *(68)* parameters, suggesting reduced angiogenesis, including a median decrease of 34% in the inflow transfer rate constant, 15% in the backflow extravascular-extracellular rate constant, and 14% in the extravascular-extracellular volume fraction.

In Phase I or II trials evaluating the tyrosine kinase inhibitor vatalanib *(69)* (PTK787/ZK222584; Novartis, Cambridge, MA, USA), which has specificity for VEGF receptors, the bidirectional transfer constant (K_i), reflecting tumor vascular permeability and flow and proportional to K^{trans}, was associated with "nonprogressive disease" or tumor stabilization of patients with hepatic metastases from colorectal cancer. The DCE-MRI was performed before therapy and on days 2 and 28 after therapy. The changes at day 2 likely reflect effects on vascular permeability, with the later time points more reflective of morphologic changes in the vasculature. There was an inverse relation between a decrease in K_i and increasing doses and plasma levels of the drug with a plateau below the maximal tolerated dose, suggesting that biologic activity may be gleaned by DCE-MRI *(70,71)*.

Figure 5 demonstrates DCE-MR imaging of a patient treated with a tyrosine kinase inhibitor targeting VEGF. In patient 1, both intravenous contrast enhancement and K^{trans} decreased 48 hours after therapy and persisted after cycle 1, suggesting a sustained response to therapy. The effect at the end of cycle 1 suggests a sustained condition that likely altered the tumor vessels. In patient 2, both intravenous contrast enhancement and K^{trans} decreased 48

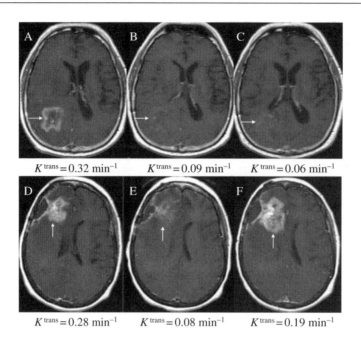

$K^{trans} = 0.32$ min^{-1} $K^{trans} = 0.09$ min^{-1} $K^{trans} = 0.06$ min^{-1}

$K^{trans} = 0.28$ min^{-1} $K^{trans} = 0.08$ min^{-1} $K^{trans} = 0.19$ min^{-1}

Fig. 5. DCE-MRI. Dynamic contrast-enhanced imaging of a patient with glioblastoma multiforme before and after treatment with a tyrosine kinase inhibitor targeting the VEGF receptor. In patient 1 (A, B, C), pre-therapy (A) enhancement (arrow) of the tumor is seen in the parietal lobe. There is a significant reduction in gadolinium-based intravenous contrast enhancement and K^{trans} 48 hours after therapy (B) that persists into the end of cycle 1 (C). In patient 2 (D, E, F), pre-therapy (D) enhancement of the tumor is seen in the frontal lobe. There is a significant reduction in gadolinium-based intravenous contrast enhancement and K^{trans} 48 hours after therapy (E); however, enhancement returns and K^{trans} increases at the end of cycle 1 (F).

hours after therapy but "rebounded" after cycle 1, suggesting an early effect on permeability but no effect on or development of resistance by tumor vessels.

Similarly, with the angiogenesis inhbitor axitinib (AG-013736; Pfizer, New York, NY, USA), a linear correlation was found. The percentage change from baseline to day 2 after therapy of DCE-MRI parameters K^{trans} and IAUC were inversely proportional to the dose and could be used to predict response (72).

With the vascular disrupting (antitubulin) agent combretastatin A4-phosphate (CA-4-P; OxiGene, Waltham, MA, USA), perfusion was decreased within hours of delivering the drug, as assessed by K^{trans} and AUC by DCE-MRI (73) and by PET using ^{15}O-labeled water (74). The imaging helped determine that the mechanistic goal of reducing blood supply to the tumor was achieved. However, the dose for biologic activity suggested by the tumor did not differ much from the dose based on toxicity data. Although this may suggest that the imaging is not helpful in selecting a biologically relevant dose, it may also simply suggest that for efficacy with this drug the dose for biologic efficacy is similar to that based on toxicity data. The PET data suggested that the reduction in tumor perfusion was approximately 49% at 30 minutes but only 13% at 24 hours. If mechanistic parameters are used, this finding suggests that dosing be performed approximately every day instead of longer dosing schedules of once a week or even longer. Of course, the frequent dosing schedule would need to be tempered by toxicity data. This example suggests the concept that functional imaging may help guide dosing schedules.

As with other downstream imaging modalities, less-targeted therapies may have an effect on tumor enhancement. For example, radiation therapy can decrease dynamic tumor enhancement, and it may correlate with the response *(75)*. When therapy is likely to be highly successful, such as radiation therapy to small cervical tumors, the value of adding a functional test is limited; however, when there is less certainty, such as radiation therapy to moderate or large cervical tumors, the functional test may help discriminate responders from nonresponders. Combining functional and anatomic data such as DCE-MRI and tumor size may be more predictive of outcome than either parameter alone. For example, an early study by Mayr et al. found that volume analysis with dynamic tumor enhancement together was more predictive of cervical cancer recurrence after radiation therapy than either test alone *(75)*.

In a study of brain gliomas by Law et al., *(76)* cerebral blood volume (CBV) measurements were made in a group of patients with low-grade gliomas. Altogether, 35 patients with a variety of treatments were followed for a mean of 4.2 years at 3-month intervals. Patients, irrespective of treatment, were divided into two groups based on a peak CBV cutoff value of 1.75. Although the pathologic grade was constant for both of these groups, Kaplan-Meier plots showed that the low-CBV group had a mean time to progression of 4620 days, in contrast to 245 days for the high-CBV group. This trial did not study a specific drug. Its result suggests a potentially fundamental significance of blood flow as a prognostic indicator in brain gliomas and highlights the role of functional imaging in studying vascular parameters. The findings suggest that DSC-MRI may be used for both patient selection and stratification, which may aid future trial designs.

9. MR SPECTROSCOPY

9.1. Physics

MR spectroscopy (MRS) techniques enable noninvasive assessment of biochemical agents by obtaining spectroscopic information from a localized region (or multiple regions) defined on an existing anatomic MR image. Although other atoms such as phosphorus may be evaluated, hydrogen is commonly interrogated because of its high natural abundance and its presence in numerous molecules. Two primary MRS techniques are used in clinical and clinical research applications for obtaining spectra. The first, known as single voxel localization, obtains a spectrum from a single volume of interest. Although this technique is relatively rapid, it does not allow assessment of heterogeneity, and the volume of interest is, in general, rather large (commonly on the order of 3.5 cm^3). The second technique is called multivoxel spectroscopic imaging. After a large volume of interest is initially localized, this volume is subsequently subdivided into smaller volumes using phase-encoding techniques similar to those utilized for routine clinical imaging such that voxels on the order of 1.5 to 0.4 cm^3 are obtained. With either technique, signals from water protons must be substantially suppressed to allow the detection of signals from metabolites of interest, which generally are present in concentrations 1000 to 10,000 times less than that of water. The output is a series of spectral peaks whose areas are proportional to the concentration of different amounts metabolites or moieties in the volume of interest.

Multivoxel spectroscopic imaging techniques take longer than single voxel localization techniques, but the spectral data are obtained from multiple smaller volumes, allowing assessment of heterogeneity and/or the comparison of spectral data from suspected abnormal tissues with spectra from nearby or contralateral normal tissue. It should be noted that the choice of echo time has a strong effect on the resulting spectra, because the T2 relaxation times vary for various metabolites. This T2 variation means that the spectral peaks from the various metabolites change in amplitude (and area) depending on the choice of echo time. Therefore, when comparisons are made between spectra obtained longitudinally or with published findings, it is critically important to take the echo times into account. An echo time in the range of 135 to 145 ms is commonly used in brain MRS applications because it results in inversion of the doublet peak due to lactate, which allows distinction between these peaks and the methylene and methyl spectral peaks that occupy the same region of the spectrum but are not inverted at this echo time. In general, more spectral peaks are seen in spectra obtained with short echo times, as the T2 relaxation times of some metabolites (such as *myo*-inositol) are quite short and the corresponding peaks are not seen if the echo times are longer than approximately 30 ms. With good water suppression and a highly homogeneous magnetic field, both critical requirements for successful proton MRS applications, the following spectral peaks can generally be detected.

- Brain: *N*-Acetylaspartate (NAA), total creatine (creatine + phosphocreatine), choline-containing compounds (e.g., phosphotidylcholine), and *myo*-inositol. In abnormal brain tissue, spectral peaks from lipids and lactate may also be present. In high-grade neoplasms, a common finding is elevated choline and decreased *N*-acetylaspartate. In regions of necrosis, elevated lipid peaks are a common finding. Lactate peaks may be seen in ischemic/hypoxic conditions such as stroke or in some higher-grade neoplasms.
- Prostate: Relatively high levels of citrate and low levels of choline. In malignant disease, citrate levels are usually markedly decreased and choline levels are elevated.
- Breast: Relatively high levels of lipids and low levels of choline. In malignant disease, choline levels are commonly elevated.
- Muscle: Relatively high levels of lipids and moderate levels of choline and creatine. Lactate can be detected in ischemic conditions.

9.2. Clinical Trials Using MR Spectroscopy

Magnetic resonance spectroscopy has been used to improve tumor detection with promising results. The most commonly studied markers in prostate cancer include choline, creatine, and citrate; but others have also been identified, such as lipids and lysine. Most commonly, prostate cancer is identified by an increase in choline, which is involved in cell membrane metabolism, and a decrease in citrate. For assessing therapeutic response, it has been suggested that "metabolic atrophy" may be assessed (Fig. 6), one definition for which is spectra containing no significant metabolite peaks, specifically spectra having peak area/noise ratios of < 5 for choline, polyamines, creatine, and citrate. After hormone ablation therapy using antiandrogens and/or leuteinizing hormone-releasing hormone (LHRH) agonists, metabolic atrophy in the tumor that signified tumor response increased with increasing duration of therapy; a greater effect was noted in patients treated for more than 16 weeks. In some patients with prostate-specific antigen (PSA) < 0.2 ng/ml, metabolic activity remained at the tumor site, suggesting residual disease *(77)*. Even with such a low PSA, prostate cancer can remain. Histologically, in patients treated with neoadjuvant hormone therapy and PSA < 0.2 ng/ml, prostate cancer can be found upon radical prostatectomy *(78)*. MR spectroscopy has also shown potential in evaluating for metabolic atrophy posttreatment and for distinguishing recurrence after external beam-radiation therapy *(79)*. In a small number of patients biopsied, MRS imaging (MRSI) and biopsy results corresponded, but the PSA results did not. In the patients biopsied, negative MRSI and negative biopsy results

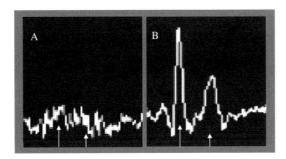

Fig. 6. Spectroscopy of the prostate. A. Spectrum of a prostate cancer treated with radiation therapy demonstrates no significant metabolite peaks. B. For comparison, spectrum of an untreated prostate cancer demonstrates an elevated choline+creatine peak (long arrow) compared to the citrate peak (short arrow).

were seen in the setting of elevated PSA; and when MRSI was positive, so was the biopsy and the PSA assay (79). These studies suggest that assessing metabolic atrophy by MR spectroscopy may aid in assessing therapeutic efficacy in prostate cancer.

Many neurologic disease processes have distinctive metabolic profiles, and measuring them with MR spectroscopy is useful when characterizing intracranial pathology. MRS has been used to distinguish tumor from tumefactive demyelinative plaque, encephalitis, or seizure effects (80–84). MRS is also useful for appropriately staging gliomatous tumors to high-grade or low-grade disease (83,84,86,87). The classic tumor signature of a gliomatous tumor is an elevated choline/creatine ratio, reduced NAA, and possibly a lactate doublet. Higher-grade gliomas tend to have higher choline/creatine ratios. *Myo*-inositol in an intra-ventricular tumor may signify a choroid plexus papilloma (88).

MR spectroscopy can distinguish cerebral radiation necrosis from gliomatous tumor recurrence (85,89,90). Tumor recurrence is characterized by the tumor signature of an elevated choline/creatine ratio, and treatment effects show a lack of metabolite peaks. As always, close radiologic supervision and interpretation is a key requirement for obtaining reliable MRS results.

MRS, MR perfusion, and ^{18}F-FDG PET (in some patients) were used in a clinical trial assessing the effects of irradiation and thalidomide on patients with brain stem gliomas. MR imaging was performed at 2-week intervals for the first 8 weeks and monthly thereafter with ^{18}F-FDG PET (91). Altogether, 13 patients with brain stem gliomas underwent radiotherapy and an escalating dose of thalidomide (12–24 mg/kg). The median duration of therapy was 5 months. Advanced imaging was not useful for predicting a response (9/13 patients progressed), but MRS, MR perfusion, and ^{18}F-FDG-PET were useful for discriminating radiation necrosis from tumor recurrence (3/13 patients).

MRS has been used with traditional MRI measures to monitor temozolomide therapy (92). Temozolomide is a DNA-chelating chemotherapeutic agent with good bioavailability behind the blood-brain barrier after oral dosing. A total of 12 patients were followed over the course of 1 year. The authors showed reduced choline levels at 12 months, in keeping with an overall tumor volume decrease of 33%. The changes in spectroscopic and volumetric appearances were gradual over the 12 months of the study and appeared to occur in parallel with volumetric changes. Thus, seems that in this study the MRS response did not add much information beyond that already available from tumor volumetric analysis.

10. BIOPSY

Unlike imaging, biopsy samples only a part of a tumor; and when multiple tumors are present, usually only one is sampled. Commonly, there is heterogeneity of functional signal within a tumor and among multiple tumors. In glioblastoma multiforme, high cerebral blood volume and K^{trans} assessed by DCE-MRI correspond with high-grade malignancy (93); therefore, many centers target such areas in a tumor at the time of biopsy. Others have noted that elevated choline/NAA levels correlate with high histologic grade and high cell density in gliomas and can be used to select a site for biopsy (94). Clinically, when there are multiple lesions, as in lymphoma, a lesion that has high ^{18}F-FDG uptake is often selected at the time of biopsy as the tumor most likely to yield diagnostic information. This suggests that when considering targeted therapy at biopsy, areas of higher functional signal before and after therapy may be informative to predict and/or assess drug efficacy.

11. FUTURE OF TARGETED IMAGING

Many new imaging agents are being developed for both nuclear medicine (95) and MR imaging. Some of these agents have moved beyond testing in animals and have been tested in clinical trials. Some examples include FLT (40,42,44,96,97) and FMAU for imaging thymidine metabolism and theoretically proliferation, ^{11}C-labeled methionine (98) for amino acid imaging, and ^{11}C-labeled choline (99) for imaging lipid precursors. Iron-based particles (SPIOs) are being developed for assessing lymph nodes for metastases by MRI. New intravascular imaging agents are also being developed. Microbubbles for vascular imaging by ultrasonography are approved for human use in Europe but not yet in the United States. Targeted microbubbles are being developed. Intravascular agents are also being developed for CT and MRI. These agents may further improve calculation of vascular parameters by CT and MR, such as K^{trans} without flow limitation and the functional vascular space in tumors as only a portion of a tumor may be perfused at a time. Quantitative in vivo imaging of gene expression (37) using reporter technology will open the way for evaluating gene therapy, for example whether, where, and what amount of gene expression occurred. It will guide dosing regimens of gene therapeutics. It will also enable imaging direct and indirect effects of pharmacologic agents on transcription and potentially imaging of protein–protein interactions.

Clinical trials of imaging agents/functional imaging are needed in addition to and in parallel with clinical trials of therapeutic agents given the obvious synergy between the two. Ideally, design of an imaging agent would begin simultaneously with that of a targeted therapy so both may be ready for clinical use. Once an imaging agent for a particular target is found, it may be amenable for use with other drugs focused on the same target. One target may be relevant for multiple cancers or other diseases. Thus, pathways for approval of new imaging agents/techniques for assessing biochemical changes, in contrast to indications that are tied solely to a particular disease type/state, are needed. Validation studies of functional imaging that can be applied to various targeted agents are also needed. The tumor type, patient population, timing of the imaging, and mode of acquisition can have a significant impact on image interpretation. Finally, studies are needed to demonstrate that the targeted imaging is predictive of outcome and change in therapy on the basis of imaging findings improves patient outcome. Thus, there is a need to develop imaging tools to perform targeted therapy assessments. This is a paradigm shift from the traditional drug-centered trials where it is assumed that imaging tools are already in place and ready to use. The development of imaging tools will require imaging trials, where the main point of the research is to assess imaging agents/techniques and imaging findings, not to investigate drugs. In the new era of targeted therapy, investment in imaging development is necessary for future drug trials and patient care.

REFERENCES

1. Ratain MJ. Clin Cancer Res 2005;11:5661–2.
2. Goffin J, Baral S, Tu D, et al. Clin Cancer Res 2005;11:5928–34.
3. Shepherd FA, Rodrigues Pereira J, et al. N Engl J Med 2005;353:123–32.
4. Thatcher N, Chang A, Parikh P, et al. Lancet 2005;366:1527–37.
5. Stroobants S, Goeminne J, Seegers M, et al. Eur J Cancer 2003;39:2012–20.
6. Shankar S, van Sonnenberg E, Desai J, et al. Radiology 2005;235:892–8.
7. Jerusalem G, Hustinx R, Beguin Y, et al. Semin Nucl Med 2005;35:186–96.
8. Torizuka T, Zasadny KR, Kison PV, et al. J Nucl Med 2000;41:999–1005.
9. Dehdashti F, Flanagan FL, Mortimer JE, et al. Eur J Nucl Med 1999;26:51–6.
10. Kluxen FW, Bruns C, Lubbert H. Proc Natl Acad Sci U S A 1992;89:4618–22.
11. Bell GI, Reisine T. Trends Neurosci 1993;16:34–8.
12. Panetta R, Greenwood MT, Warszynska A, et al. Mol Pharmacol 1994;45:417–27.
13. O'Carroll AM, Lolait SJ, Konig M, et al. Mol Pharmacol 1993;44:1278.
14. Yamada Y, Reisine T, Law SF, et al. Mol Endocrinol 1992;6:2136–42.
15. Termanini B, Gibril F, Reynolds JC, et al. Gastroenterology 1997;112:335–47.
16. Lamberts SW, Hofland LJ, Nobels FR. Front Neuroendocrinol 2001;22:309–39.
17. Kwekkeboom D, Krenning E, de Jong M. J Nucl Med 2000;41:1704–13.
18. Plonowski A, Schally AV, Nagy A, et al. Cancer Res 2000;60:2996–3001.
19. Schally AV, Nagy A. Eur J Endocrinol 1999;141:1–14.
20. Kwekkeboom DJ, Bakker WH, Kooij PP, et al. Eur J Nucl Med 2001;28:1319–25.
21. Linden HM, Stekhova SA, Link JM, et al. J Clin Oncol 2006;24:2793–9.
22. Wiseman GA, Kornmehl E, Leigh B, et al. J Nucl Med 2003;44:465–74.
23. Wahl RL. Semin Oncol 2003;30:31–8.
24. Yamane T, Daimaru O, Ito S, et al. J Nucl Med 2004;45:1838–42.
25. Su H, Bodenstein C, Dumont RA, et al. Clin Cancer Res 2006;12:5659–67.
26. Romer W, Hanauske AR, Ziegler S, et al. Blood 1998;91:4464–71.
27. Brepoels L, Stroobants S, Verhoef G. Leuk Lymphoma 2007;48:270–82.
28. Wahl RL, Zasadny K, Helvie M, et al. J Clin Oncol 1993;11:2101–11.
29. Mortimer JE, Dehdashti F, Siegel BA, et al. J Clin Oncol 2001;19:2797–803.
30. Weber WA, Wieder H. Eur J Nucl Med Mol Imaging 2006;33(suppl 1):27–37.
31. Cachin F, Prince HM, Hogg A, et al. J Clin Oncol 2006;24:3026–31.
32. Zijlstra JM, Lindauer-van der Werf G, Hoekstra OS, et al. Haematologica 2006;91:522–9.
33. Zijlstra JM, Hoekstra OS, Raijmakers PG, et al. Br J Haematol 2003;123:454–62.
34. Tsukamoto N, Kojima M, Hasegawa M, et al. Cancer 2007;110:652–9.
35. Shankar LK, Hoffman JM, Bacharach S, et al. J Nucl Med 2006;47:1059–66.
36. Huang SC. Nucl Med Biol 2000;27:643–6.
37. Yang D, Han L, Kundra V. Radiology 2005;235:950–8.
38. Antoch G, Kanja J, Bauer S, et al. J Nucl Med 2004;45:357–65.
39. Swisher SG, et al. Cancer 2004;101(8):1776–85.
40. Smyczek-Gargya B, Fersis N, Dittmann H, et al. Eur J Nucl Med Mol Imaging 2004;31:720–4.
41. Van Westreenen HL, Cobben DC, Jager PL, et al. J Nucl Med 2005;46:400–4.
42. Buck AK, Halter G, Schirrmeister H, et al. J Nucl Med 2003;44:1426–31.
43. Yap CS, Czernin J, Fishbein MC, et al. Chest 2006;129:393–401.
44. Dittmann H, Dohmen BM, Paulsen F, et al. Eur J Nucl Med Mol Imaging 2003;30:1407–12.
45. Muzi M, Vesselle H, Grierson JR, et al. J Nucl Med 2005;46:274–82.
46. Troost EG, Vogel WV, Merkx MA, et al. J Nucl Med 2007;48:726–35.
47. Buck AK, Hetzel M, Schirrmeister H, et al. N. Eur J Nucl Med Mol Imaging 2005;32:525–33.
48. Galldiks N, Kracht LW, Burghaus L, et al. Eur J Nucl Med Mol Imaging 2006;33:516–24.
49. Brock CS, Young H, O'Reilly SM, et al. Br J Cancer 2000;82:608–15.
50. Eschmann SM, Paulsen F, Reimold M, et al. J Nucl Med 2005;46:253–60.
51. Rischin D, Hicks RJ, Fisher R, et al. J Clin Oncol 2006;24:2098–104.

52. Gonzalez J, Kumar AJ, Conrad CA, et al. Int J Radiat Oncol Biol Phys 2007;67:323–6.
53. Batchelor TT, Sorensen AG, di Tomaso E, et al. Cancer Cell 2007;11:83–95.
54. Bastin ME, Sinha S, Whittle IR, et al. Neuroreport 2002;13:1335–40.
55. Sinha S, Bastin ME, Whittle IR, et al. AJNR Am J Neuroradiol 2002;23:520–7.
56. Castillo M, Smith JK, Kwock L, et al. AJNR Am J Neuroradiol 2001;22:60–4.
57. Stadnik TW, Chaskis C, Michotte A, et al. AJNR Am J Neuroradiol 2001;22:969–76.
58. Provenzale JM, McGraw P, Mhatre P, et al. Radiology 2004;232:451–60.
59. Field AS, Alexander AL. Top Magn Reson Imaging 2004;15:315–24.
60. Dong Q, Welsh RC, Chenevert TL, et al. J Magn Reson Imaging 2004;19:6–18.
61. Le Bihan D, Douek P, Argyropoulou M, et al. Top Magn Reson Imaging 1993;5:25–31.
62. Tung GA, Evangelista P, Rogg JM, et al. AJR Am J Roentgenol 2001;177:709–12.
63. Hein PA, Eskey CJ, Dunn JF, et al. AJNR Am J Neuroradiol 2004;25:201–9.
64. Biousse V, Newman NJ, Hunter SB, et al. J Neurol Neurosurg Psychiatry 2003;74:382–4.
65. Moffat BA, Chenevert TL, Lawrence TS, et al. Proc Natl Acad Sci U S A 2005;102:5524–9.
66. Tofts PS. J Magn Reson Imaging 1997;7:91–101.
67. Jackson A, O'Connor JP, Parker GJ, et al. Clin Cancer Res 2007;13:3449–59.
68. Wedam SB, Low JA, Yang SX, et al. J Clin Oncol 2006;24:769–77.
69. Morgan B, Thomas AL, Drevs J, et al. J Clin Oncol 2003;21:3955–64.
70. Thomas AL, Morgan B, Horsfield MA, et al. J Clin Oncol 2005;23:4162–71.
71. Mross K, Drevs J, Muller M, et al. Eur J Cancer 2005;41:1291–9.
72. Liu G, Rugo HS, Wilding G, et al. J Clin Oncol 2005;23:5464–73.
73. Galbraith SM, Maxwell RJ, Lodge MA, et al. J Clin Oncol 2003;21:2831–42.
74. Anderson HL, Yap JT, Miller MP, et al. J Clin Oncol 2003;21:2823–30.
75. Mayr NA. Yuh WT, Zheng J, et al. AJR Am J Roentgenol 1998;170:177–82.
76. Law M, Oh S, Johnson G, et al. Neurosurgery 2006;58:1099–107.
77. Mueller-Lisse UG, Swanson MG, Vigneron DB, et al. Magn Reson Med 2001;46:49–57.
78. Gleave ME, Goldenberg SL, Jones EC, et al. J Urol 1996;155:213–9.
79. Pickett B, Kurhanewicz J, Coakley F, et al. Int J Radiat Oncol Biol Phys 2004;60:1047–55.
80. Castillo M. AJNR Am J Neuroradiol 2001;22:597–8.
81. Kwock L, Smith JK, Castillo M, et al. Technol Cancer Res Treat 2002;1:17–28.
82. Smith JK, Castillo M, Kwock L. Magn Reson Imaging Clin N Am 2003;11:415–29, v-vi.
83. Vuori K, Kankaanranta L, Hakkinen AM, et al. Radiology 2004;230:703–8.
84. De Stefano N, Bartolozzi ML, Guidi L, et al. J Neurol Sci 2005;233:203–8.
85. Croteau D, Scarpace L, Hearshen D, et al. Neurosurgery 2001;49:823–9.
86. Butteriss DJ, Ismail A, Ellison DW, et al. Br J Radiol 2003;76:662–5.
87. Chang YW, Yoon HK, Shin HJ, et al. M. Pediatr Radiol 2003;33:836–42.
88. Krieger MD, Panigrahy A, McComb JG, et al. Neurosurg Focus 2005;18, E4.
89. Kamada K, Houkin K, Abe H, et al. Neurol Med Chir (Tokyo) 1997;37:250–6.
90. Weybright P, Sundgren PC, Maly P, et al. AJR Am J Roentgenol 2005;185:1471–6.
91. Turner CD, Chi S, Marcus KJ, et al. J Neurooncol 2007;82:95–101.
92. Murphy PS, Viviers L, Abson C, et al. Br J Cancer 2004;90:781–6.
93. Patankar TF, Haroon HA, Mills SJ, et al. AJNR Am J Neuroradiol 2005;26:2455–65.
94. McKnight TR, Lamborn KR, Love TD, et al. J Neurosurg 2007;106:660–6.
95. Wester HJ. Clin Cancer Res 2007;13:3470–81.
96. Francis DL, Visvikis D, Costa DC, et al. J. Eur J Nucl Med Mol Imaging 2003;30:988–94.
97. Sun H, Sloan A, Mangner TJ, et al. Eur J Nucl Med Mol Imaging 2005;32:15–22.
98. Nunez R, Macapinlac HA, Yeung HW, et al. J Nucl Med 2002;43:46–55.
99. Hara T, Kosaka N, Kishi H. J Nucl Med 1998;39:990–5.

18 Combining Targeted Therapies

David Hong, MD and Lakshmi Chintala, MD

CONTENTS

ABSTRACT

Many new agents have emerged in the drug development pipeline that target the mechanisms driving the development and progression of specific cancers. Ultimately, the goal is to create personalized treatment plans for each patient's tumor(s). Despite promising early preclinical data, only a handful of the targeted molecules developed thus far have shown benefit when used as single agents. The need to combine individual agents with existing therapies or in novel combinations has become increasingly important. A primary objective is to design drug combinations that can overcome drug resistance. Cross talk among signaling pathways and parallel pathways that contribute to tumor pathogenesis is thought to contribute to single-agent resistance. Combining cytostatic and cytotoxic therapies with targeted agents could help overcome resistance or prevent its development. The issues surrounding the combinatorial approach that are covered in this chapter are patient selection, toxicity profiles from additive and synergistic effects of combining chemotherapy with targeted therapy, and the importance of timing when combining targeted therapy with cytotoxic chemotherapy. The variables that need to be considered when designing effective combinations of targeted agents are discussed. Finally, the chapter looks at ways to improve preclinical models. Sophisticated technologies, including microarray technologies leading to genomic profiling through gene set enrichment analysis (GSEA) or reverse phase array (RPPA) proteomic technology, which evaluates microarry data at the level of the gene and protein, are also covered along with the experience that investigators have had with

From: Current Clinical Oncology: Targeted Cancer Therapy
Edited by: R. Kurzrock and M. Markman © Humana Press, Totowa, NJ

various targeted agents that have been tested in preclinical and clinical studies, including trastuzumab, epithelial growth factor receptor tyrosine kinase inhibitors, sorafenib and its combinations, and others.

Key Words: Targeted therapy, Combinational therapy, Personalized therapy, Signaling pathways, Drug resistance, Drug development

1. INTRODUCTION

The previous chapters have looked at the increasing role of targeted therapies in cancer therapy for specific cancers. The concept underlying the strategy of combining therapeutic modalities has evolved from the historical experience of empirically combining chemotherapy agents with known activity and toxicity profiles to what is now a more rational approach, which involves combining agents with the goal of overcoming drug resistance, targeting specific biochemical pathways, and using dose-dense combinations to overcome specific tumor kinetics. As the mechanisms underlying growth and differentiation in cancer have been increasingly elucidated, many new agents have emerged in the drug development pipeline that target the mechanisms driving the development and progression of specific cancers. Despite promising early preclinical data, only a handful of these targeted molecules have shown any benefit when used as single agents. Therefore, the need to combine individual agents with existing therapies or in novel combinations has become increasingly important. Moreover, as the number of available drugs continues to expand, the number of combinations exponentially escalates. The need for a rational and strategic approach to testing drug combinations is obviously warranted. This chapter reviews the success of combining current targeted therapies with existing modes of therapy, explores strategies for future novel combinations, and addresses some of the challenges in both the research and regulatory arenas.

2. WHY COMBINE ANTICANCER AGENTS AND SPECIFICALLY TARGETED THERAPIES?

The justification for combining targeted therapies with existing cancer therapies and other targeted therapies is fundamentally the same as the rationale for combining conventional cytotoxic chemotherapies. First is the desire for additive or synergistic combinations of drugs and molecules that increase clinical benefit over their use as single agents. With few exceptions, most effective cancer treatments are combinations of drugs. Few of these combinations have been tested critically in the preclinical setting to determine optimal scheduling and dosing, and even fewer have demonstrated clear clinical evidence of synergy, but many of these combinations have proved efficacy over single-agent administration (1).

Development of a resistant phenotype to chemotherapy is a major problem in oncology. Therefore, a second important objective is to design drug combinations that can overcome drug resistance. Tumors can be intrinsically resistant to a given therapy or can initially be responsive but develop resistance. One example is the use of imatinib mesylate to treat gastrointestinal stromal tumors (GISTs). Although this is a highly successful treatment for GISTs, in some patients disease relapse appears to be caused by clonal selection for tumor cells encoding a *KIT* mutation in an imatinib mesylate-resistant domain, such as the ATP binding site. Alternatively, resistance may develop through the activation of pathways located downstream or in parallel to KIT and that, therefore, are not sensitive to inhibition by imatinib mesylate. Multiple other factors are responsible for intrinsic or acquired resistance. Combining targeted agents that target these multiple pathways could help to overcome resistance or prevent the development of resistance.

3. TARGETED AGENTS IN COMBINATION WITH CYTOTOXIC CHEMOTHERAPEUTIC AGENTS

Thus far, combining targeted agents with standard chemotherapy has been the most successful strategy. Notable successes in cancer drug development have changed the standard of care, and some of these have been described in previous chapters in this book. However, the road to success has also been littered with many failed attempts. Our exploration of some of these successes and failures in this chapter narrates some of the lessons learned and gives directions for future success.

3.1. Experience With Trastuzumab

The humanized monoclonal antibody trastuzumab has been one of the most successful targeted agents to be combined with standard therapy. Trastuzumab in combination with a taxane has become has become the standard of care for HER2+-overexpressing metastatic breast cancer tumors and recently has shown significant survival advantage in the adjuvant setting (2,3). Several key steps in the development of trastuzumab underline important factors in targeted therapy development in combination with chemotherapy.

Trastuzumab's development is an ideal case study, highlighting the power of patient selection through biomarker development. HER2 is significantly associated with the increased expression of P-glycoprotein, a cell surface molecule with intrinsic tyrosine activity involved in a cascade of events leading to breast cancer growth and development and associated with multidrug resistance. The initial observation that the HER2 gene was amplified in 25% of lymph node-positive breast cancer patients and was correlated with a worse prognosis, shorter relapse-free survival, and overall survival set the stage for the development both of a predictive biomarker and an agent that was used as a specific targeted therapy (4,5). HER2 overexpression and its association with a more aggressive breast cancer suggested that the proto-oncogene had an important pathogenetic role in this patient subset. This finding led to the development of trastuzumab, a humanized recombinant monoclonal antibody directed at the extracellular domain of HER2 protein. The strong correlation between trastuzumab efficacy and HER2 overexpression in preclinical models led to the design of trials requiring HER2 overexpression as the predominant inclusion criterion. The trial sponsor, Genentech (South San Francisco, CA, USA), made the wise decision to limit the population to HER2+-overexpressing patients throughout all Phase I to III trials. This early incorporation of a specific assay in all stages of clinical development led to its refinement and was instrumental in the approval of trastuzumab by the U.S. Food and Drug Administration (FDA) (6).

Some important lessons from combining targeted agents with chemotherapy can be drawn from these early clinical trials with trastuzumab. One is that patient selection is a vital factor in developing a targeted therapy both for monotherapy and for combination with chemotherapy. Second, toxicity can be significantly increased when targeted agents are combined with chemotherapy. Trastuzumab monotherapy clearly showed activity in HER2+ patients. The pivotal Phase II trial of trastuzumab as monotherapy demonstrated a higher objective response in HER2+-overexpressing patients (7). Immunohistochemical

(IHC) staining revealed greater efficacy with a score of 3+ or higher (18% vs. 6%) for patients with 3+ and 2+ IHC results, respectively. The same HER2+ subpopulation was also evaluated in combination studies with chemotherapy. Preclinical evidence showed trastuzumab's additive or synergistic activity when combined with chemotherapy *(8)*. The pivotal clinical trial by Slamon et al. of paclitaxel, doxorubicin with cyclophosphamide (AC), or epirubicin plus cyclophosamide (EC) with or without trastuzumab in untreated HER2-positive metastatic breast cancer patients confirmed the preclinical data *(4,7)*. Trastuzumab increased time to tumor progression for all chemotherapy regimens (7.4 vs. 4.6 months with chemotherapy alone), had a higher response rate (50% vs. 32%) and a longer median survival (25.1 vs. 20.3 months). Moreover, no benefit was seen for HER-2-normal patients regardless of the dosing schedule in a recent CALGB study looking at different schedules of paclitaxel with traztuzumab in HER-2-positive and HER-2-normal patients *(9)*. Unfortunately, trastuzumab in combination with AC chemotherapy resulted in significant cardiac toxicity in 27% of patients treated with this combination compared to 8% in the AC alone arm and 13% in the paclitaxel with trastuzumab arm. Trastuzumab monotherapy produced cardiotoxicty in 5% of patients *(10)*. Because adding trastzumab to AC chemotherapy significantly increased cardiac toxicity, the evidence-based clinical recommendation is to avoid using this drug combination. The example of trastuzumab points out the necessity of defining a patient subpopulation that has a specific target throughout the development process from monotherapy to combination trials with chemotherapy. However, it is clear from the cardiotoxicity seen when trastuzumab is combined with an anthracycline that when choosing chemotherapy combinations the additive effect of overlapping toxicities needs to be taken into consideration.

3.2. Lessons from the Use of EGFR Tyrosine Kinase Inhibitors as Targeted Agents

The failures of the epithelial growth factor receptor (EGFR) tyrosine kinase inhibitors (TKIs) give the clinical trialist further guidance vis-à-vis developing efficacious targeted therapies. The failures of erlotinib (Tarceva) and gefitinib (Iressa), EGFR TKIs in combination trials with chemotherapy in non-small-cell lung cancer (NSCLC) also demonstrate the need to identify a specific subset of treatable patients and a valid biomarker that can be used to identify these patients. Second, the subset analysis of the combination trial results suggest that some instances of combination therapy may be more detrimental than beneficial. Gefitinib in combination studies as first-line regimens in the INTACT (Iressa NSCLC Trial Assessing Combination Treatment) 1 and INTACT 2 trials combining gefitinib with cisplatin plus gemcitibine or carboplatin plus paclitaxel failed to show benefit with the addition of gefitinib *(11,12)*. Likewise, no statistical difference in survival was noted in the two trials of erlotinib with chemotherapy regimens in the TALENT study of erlotinib with gemcitibine and cisplatin and the TRIBUTE Phase III study of erlotinib combined with carboplatin and paclitaxel *(13)*.

Unlike the experience with trastuzumab, identifying a predictive biomarker for EGFR inhibitors has been a difficult task. The failed Phase III trials of EGFR TKIs did not incorporate a patient selection biomarker such as HER2+ IHC staining as in the trastuzumab trials and therefore did not test the combinations in a specifically targeted subset of patients. In early Phase II trials in NSCLC, EGFR overexpression shown in IHC analysis did not seem to correlate with response as trastuzumab did with HER2+ breast cancer. Later, however, Paez et al. and Lynch et al. identified a predictive marker that correlated with dramatic responses to gefitinib therapy *(14,15)*. These groups discovered somatic mutations, small in-frame deletions or amino acid missense substitutions clustered around the adenosine triphosphate (ATP) binding pocket of the EGFR TK catalytic domain. These heterozygous mutations are thought to augment EGFR-induced tyrosine autophosphorylation. Interestingly, the subset of patients that harbored these mutations fit the same patient profile that appeared most likely to respond to gefitinib revealed in a subset analysis of the initial IDEAL trial. These gefitinib-responsive patients were Asian female nonsmokers with adenocarcinoma histology. These initial findings were supported by several studies showing the association between EGFR mutations and increased response, progression-free survival (PFS), and overall survival with EGFR TKI treatment *(16–21)*.

Moreover, a further detailed *EGFR* and *KRAS* mutation analysis by Eberhard et al. of a subset of 274 patient tumors from the TRIBUTE trial identified a subset of patients with wild-type (wt) *EGFR* who, when treated with the combination of chemotherapy and erlotinib, demonstrated statistically inferior results for time to progression and overall survival compared to all patient subsets, including those treated with chemotherapy alone *(22)*. Recent preclinical studies provide a rationale for these findings. These studies show that EGFR TKIs result in G_1 cell cycle arrest in cancer cell lines with wt *EGFR*, whereas EGFR TKIs induce apoptosis of cells with mutant *EGFR (23)*. Combination studies in vitro and in vivo demonstrated that these agents induced G_1 arrest and may block the effects of subsequent chemotherapy *(24)*. Finally, Eberhard et al. found that 21% of the specimens tested had no *EGFR* mutations but had mutant *KRAS*, and the patients with this mutation had poorer clinical outcomes when treated with combination erlotinib and chemotherapy *(25)*.

The understanding that can be taken from the combined results of the failed combination trials of erlotinib and gefitinib with chemotherapy demonstrates that there are subsets of patients who would benefit from combinations of chemotherapy and targeted agents, but that there are also populations who may fare more poorly when treated with combined agents than with standard chemotherapy alone. Preclinical identification of these subpopulations and their biomarkers is a difficult endeavor, but intensive early investment in biomarker development that leads to identifying these populations in early Phase I and Phase II trials will likely increase the success of future Phase III combination trials.

3.3. Importance of Timing When Combining Targeted Therapy and Cytotoxic Chemotherapy

A further consideration for combining targeted therapy with standard cytotoxic chemotherapy is the timing of administering targeted therapy in relation to chemotherapy. The proper sequencing of combining a targeted agent with standard chemotherapy has been shown to be a critical rationale for cyclin-dependent kinase (CDK) inhibitors being added to a chemotherapeutic regimen. Cell cycle inhibitors, specifically CDK inhibitors, which are important mediators of the cell cycle, have emerged as a new class of anticancer agents. Cell cycle-mediated drug resistance is a recognized mechanism of drug resistance to cytotoxic chemotherapy. A cancer cell may become insensitive to an agent due to the activation of cell cycle checkpoints that interrupt cell cycle progression, allowing time for the cell to repair itself. However, in combination regimens, the first treatment with chemotherapy may alter the cell cycle so the second chemotherapeutic agent is less effective *(26)*.

The experience with CDK inhibitors such as flavopiridol when combined with cytotoxic chemotherapy illustrates how proper sequencing is an essential consideration in rationally combining these targeted agents and avoiding cell cycle-mediated drug resistance. For example, experiments with the CDK inhibitors flavopiridol and bryostatin-1 in combination with paclitaxel showed that proper sequencing is essential for efficacy. MKN-74, a human gastric cancer cell line, and the human breast adenocarcinoma MCF-7 cell line when exposed to flavopirodol prior to paclitaxel are prevented from entering the M phase of the cell cycle. This is the cell cycle phase during which paclitaxel is most active; and thus when the cells are treated with CDK inhibitors using that schedule, paclitaxel sensitivity is significantly decreased *(25)*. Similar results have been shown with bryostatin-1 in mammary xenograft models. Bryostatin-1 given prior to paclitaxel exposure leads to a reduction of cyclin B1-cdc2 kinase and results in cells arresting in G_2, which is a necessary step in the cell cycle before they are able to enter the M phase, thus leading to paclitaxel insensitivity *(27)*. In contrast, the reverse is true when both of these CDK inhibitors are sequenced after paclitaxel, resulting in increased sensitivity to paclitaxel and induction of apoptosis *(25,28)*. Early Phase I trials of the combination of paclitaxel followed by flavopiridol showed promise in patients with esophageal cancer. Five of seven esophageal cancer patients responded to the combination, with three patients having progressed previously on paclitaxel, supporting the validity of the preclinical findings *(29)*.

Interestingly and pertinently, the importance of properly sequencing a targeted agent in relation to chemotherapy has been underestimated. Few targeted agents used in combination are subjected to a rigorous preclinical sequencing evaluation prior to entering the clinic. Several other targeted agents, including bortezimab (Velcade) and erlotinib may also require a favorable sequencing schedule with chemotherapy for maximum results *(30)*.

As the previous examples and current trials illustrate, chemotherapy and cytotoxic agents will continue to serve as a foundation for the next generation of cancer therapy. The role of the new generation of targeted therapy may well be as modulators and potentiators of chemotherapy *(31)*. Although, it is unlikely there will be a unifying approach for combining targeted agents with chemotherapy, the lessons learned from both the successes and failures of these novel combinations must be incorporated when designing future drug combinations.

4. COMBINATIONS OF MOLECULARLY TARGETED ANTICANCER AGENTS

As increasing numbers of targeted agents emerge, opportunities and challenges arise in how to combine these targeted agents. The opportunities include developing rationally targeted combinations that can overcome single-agent resistance, result in greater efficacy and clinical benefit, and lay a foundation for the continuing development of personalized cancer therapy. The challenges include narrowing the vast array of possible combinations of targeted agents into clinically relevant combinations, finding combinations with minimal toxicity, and developing reliable assays for patient selection or for determining the pharmacodynamic effect of various drug combinations.

4.1. Underlying Mechanisms of Tumorigenesis and Combination Therapies: Pertinent Considerations

The first question to bear in mind before combining targeted agents is what pathways or mechanisms of tumor pathogenesis do we want to target? The answer lies in understanding the signaling pathways involved in the pathogenesis and resistance to some of the therapies given to treat any particular tumor. Our current understanding of the signaling pathways involved is likely much less complex than the totality of components of the signaling pathways that are actually involved in the development and progression of a particular tumor. So, a second question to consider is, given our current understanding of these pathways, the following: What strategies can we employ to select rational combinations of targeted agents?

Several strategies specifically targeting the growth factor receptor kinase pathways are illustrated in Figure 1 and can be applied to other combinations targeting diverse tumor processes such as cell cycle regulation, chromatin modeling, and apoptosis among others.

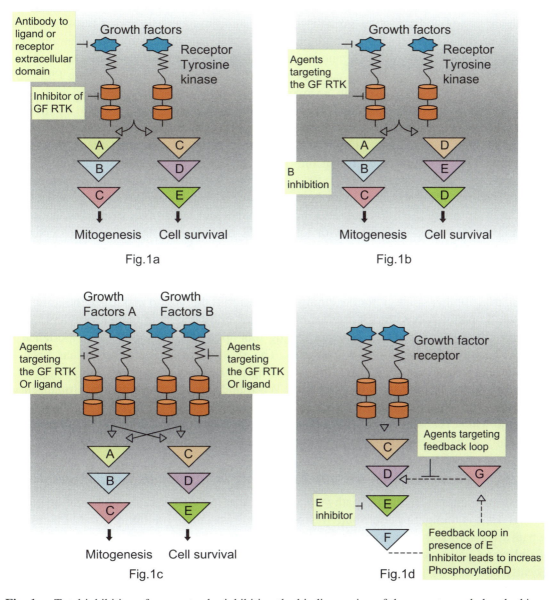

Fig. 1. a Total inhibition of a receptor by inhibiting the binding region of the receptor and also the kinase segment. **b** Dual inhibition of a specific pathway by inhibiting the receptor (antibody or tyrosine kinase inhibitor) and a downstream molecule involved in signaling. **c** Dual inhibition of parallel pathways with inhibition of the receptor at the receptor binding site or the kinase portion. **d** Targeting a feedback loop may overcome resistance of inhibition of a specific pathway. GFRTK (growth factor receptor kinase) (From Dancey and Chen, *(1)* with permission).

368 Hong and Chintala

Although, only a few trials have reported their results, several of these strategies have already been incorporated into clinical trials and have shown some evidence of proof of principle (Table 1).

4.2. Lessons Learned from Sorafenib and its Combinations

One approach involves maximizing the inhibition of receptor ligand-binding of a growth receptor and the tyrosine kinase activity of the same receptor (Fig. 1a). Several trials are utilizing this rationale to combine targeted agents. A recent combination used was sorafenib, a synthetic compound targeting growth signaling and angiogenesis and a tyrosine kinase inhibitor of the VEGF receptor, combined with bevacizumab, a humanized monoclonal antibody that binds to the VEGF ligand in renal cell cancer. The findings of that trial showed that such combinations are able to act synergistically against tumorigenesis. In a Phase I/II study of sorafenib and bevacizumab Sosman et al. recently reported partial responses in 10 of the 24 patients enrolled. Additionally, among 24 patients on the trial for 4 to 14 months, only 3 patients were taken off study due to disease progression (32).

As mentioned earlier, it is an unfortunate truth that the same combined agents that target a single pathway and increase growth inhibition can also lead to increased toxicity, as in the experience of Sosman et al. (32). Patients treated with the full dose of sorafenib (400 mg twice daily) in combination with bevacizumab had significant toxicities. Most of the toxicities were related to sorafenib and included hand-foot syndrome, stomatitis, anorexia, and weight loss (>15%). Studies with total EGFR inhibition of the EGFGR receptor by cetuximab and gefitinib or erlotinib are ongoing in both colon and lung cancer (Table 1). Future results from these studies will reveal the veracity of the observed effect of the concomitance of increased effect with increased toxicity.

Similarly, another strategy for designing combinatorial therapy to maximize the inhibition of a specific pathway is to block a series of signaling components in the pathway, as shown in Figure 1b. Several trials have begun testing this approach, including our experience in a Phase I study of tipifarnib and sorafenib. The strategy used in this study has been to block the RAS/RAF/MAPK pathway by inhibiting the farneslyation of the Ras protein with tipifarnib and the Raf kinase with sorafenib. We found that the combination is much more toxic than single-agent therapy, with a significant increase of rash, drug fever, and hand-foot syndrome. However, preliminary findings suggest that the combination may be synergistic, specifically in patients with medullary thyroid cancer (33).

4.3. Signaling Pathways and Cross Talk in Combination Therapies

Cross talk among signaling pathways and parallel pathways that contribute to tumor pathogenesis is thought to contribute to single-agent resistance. Inhibiting parallel pathways or pathways involved in such cross talk may increase the clinical response over the inhibition of only one pathway (Fig. 1c). A study that explored inhibiting parallel pathways was recently reported for the combination of sorafenib, a Raf inhibitor, and temsirolimus (CCI-779), an mTOR inhibitor, in advanced cancer patients. Patnaik showed that the combination increased mucocutaneous toxicity at the current maximum tolerated dose (MTD) of sorafenib (400 mg PO b.i.d.) and temsirolimus (15 mg IV weekly) (34). The study is ongoing; but given the high number of dose-limiting toxicities, the recommended combination doses will be much lower than the current single-agent doses of sorafenib and temsirolimus or of only one of the agents.

Table 1
Clinical Trials for Combinations of Novel Targeted Agents

Strategy and targets	Clinical trial	Cancer	Phase of the trial
Maximize inhibition of a target			
VEGFR2 + VEGF	AZD2171 + bevacizumab	Leukemia, lymphoma, small intestine	I
	Bevacizumab + sunitinib	Kidney	I
	Bevacizumab + sorafenib + temsirolimus	Kidney	II
VEGF+ (EGFRab+EGFR TKI)	Bevacizumab + sorafenib	Solid tumors, kidney	I
	Bevacizumab + cetuximab + erlotinib	Colorectal, head and neck, kidney, lung, pancreatic cancer	I
EGFRab+EGFR TKI	Cetuximab + erlotinib	Head and neck, non-small-cell lung, colorectal cancer, gastrointestinal carcinomas	II
PanHER TKI + HER2ab	Lapatinib + trastuzumab	Breast cancer	II
HER2 dimerization+HER2	Pertuzumab + trastuzumab	Breast cancer	II
Maximize inhibition of a pathway			
EGFR + VEGFR2 + FTI + mTOR	Erlotinib + sorafenib + Temsirolimus + tipifarnib	Brain and CNS tumors	I/II
PanHER + VEGF	Lapatinib + bevacizumab	Breast cancer	II
mTOR + EGFR	Erlotinib + everolimus	Breast cancer	I/II
	Erlotinib + rapamune	Kidney	II
	Erlotinib + RAD001	Non-small-cell lung cancer	I/II
mTOR+HER2	Rapamycin + trastuzumab	Breast cancer	II
	RAD001 + trastuzumab	Breast cancer	I/II
	Everolimus + lapatinib	Lymphoma, adult solid tumor	I
Inhibition of parallel pathways			
VEGF + Angiogenesis	ABT-510 + Bevacizumab	Adult Solid Tumor	I
FGFR + EGFR	BMS-582664 + erbitux	Colorectal Cancer	I
VEGF + (EGFR + mTOR)	Bevacizumab + erlotinib	Lung Cancer	II
EGFR + SRC	Erlotinib + dasatinib	Non-small-cell Lung	I

(Continued)

Table 1
(Continued)

Strategy and targets	Clinical trial	Cancer	Phase of the trial
EGFR + HER2	Cetuximab + trastuzumab	Breast Cancer	I
EGFR + VEGFR2 + (FTI + mTOR)	Erlotinib + sorafenib + Temsirolimus + tipifarnib	Brain, CNS Tumors	I/II
PDGF + mTOR	Everolimus + imatinib	Kidney Cancer	II
Inhibition of multiple tumor processes			
Hypomethylation + HDAC	Azacitidine + vorinostat	Leukemia	I/II
VE-cadherin/ß-catenin/Akt + VEGFR2	Combretastatin A4 phosphate (CA4P) + bevacizumab	Advanced solid tumors	I
VEGF + EFGR	Bevacizumab + erlotinib	Ovarian neoplasms	II
	Cetuximab + bevacizumab	Head and neck, squamous cell, adult solid tumors	II
	Bevacizumab + sunitinib	Colon, head and neck,	I/II
	Bevacizumab + cetuximab + erlotinib	Kidney, lung, pancreatic	I
		SCCHN	II
	Bevacizumab + tarceva + sulindac	Esophageal, gastric, pancreatic,cholangiocarcinoma, gallbladder, lung, hepatocellular, thymic	II
	Bevacizumab + erlotinib		
VEGFR2 + mTOR	Everolimus + sorafenib	Lymphoma, multiple myeloma	I/II
	Sorafenib + rapamycin	Plasma cell neoplasm	I
	Sorafenib + RAD001	Advanced solid tumor	I/II
	Sorafenib + temsirolimus	Kidney	I/II
	Bevacizumab + RAD001	Adult solid tumor, brain, CNS tumors, melanoma	II
	Bevacizumab + temsirolimus	Kidney cancer	II
	Sirolimus + bevacizumab	Melanoma (skin)	I
	RAD001 + sunitinib	Liver cancer	I
		Renal cell carcinoma	
VEGFR2 + EGFR	Cetuximab + sorafenib	Colon	II
	Erlotinib + sorafenib	Unspecified adult solid tumor	II

VEGF + HER2	Bevacizumab + herceptin	Breast cancer	I/II
	SU011248 ± placebo + trastuzumab	Breast cancer	II
HDAC + proteasome	Belinostat + bortezomib	Lymphoma, leukemia	I
	Bortezomib + vorinostat	Adult solid tumor	I
CD52 + CD20	Alemtuzumab + rituximab	Chronic lymphocytic leukemia	I/II
CD80 + CD20	Galiximab + rituximab vs. rituximab + placebo	Non-Hodgkin's lymphoma	III
GFR + toll-like receptor 9	Erlotinib + PF-3512676	Non-small-cell lung cancer	II
VEGF + CD20	Bevacizumab + rituximab vs. rituximab	Lymphoma	II
CDK + mTOR	Bryostatin 1 + temsirolimus	Kidney, melanoma (skin)	I
CDK + CD20	Bryostatin 1 + rituximab	Leukemia, lymphoma	II
CDK + HDAC	Flavopiridol + vorinostat	Leukemia, adult solid tumors	I
Proteasome + IL-6	CNTO 328 + bortezomib vs. bortezomib	Multiple myeloma	II
Proteasome + HER2	PS341 + trastuzumab	Breast cancer	I
Proteasome + BCL-2	Bortezomib + obatoclax	Mantle-cell lymphoma	I
Proteasome + TRAIL-R	Mapatumumab + bortezomib vs. bortezomib	Multiple myeloma	II
Proteasome + VEGFR2	Bortezomib + sorafenib	Leukemia, multiple myeloma, plasma cell neoplasm, adult solid tumors	I
	Bevacizumab + bortezomib	Lymphoma, myeloma, solid tumors, kidney	I
Proteasome + FTI	Bortezomib + tipifarnib	Multiple myeloma, plasma cell neoplasm	I/II
Proteosome + CD20	Bortezomib + dexamethasone + rituximab	Waldenström's macroglobulinemia	II
	Bortezomib + rituximab	lymphoma	II

(Continued)

Table 1
(Continued)

Strategy and targets	Clinical trial	Cancer	Phase of the trial
EGFR + VEGFR2 + FTI + mTOR	Erlotinib + sorafenib + temsirolimus + tipifarnib	Brain, CNS tumors	I/II
Retinoid + EGFR	Bexarotene + erlotinib	Lung	I
PDGF/C-KIT + mTOR	Imatinib + temsirolimus	Leukemia	I
Pan HER + VEGF	Pazopanib + lapatinib	Glioma, cervical cancer	II
Protein kinase B + VEGFR2	Perifosine + sorafenib	Kidney	I
	Perifosine + sunitinib	Renal cancer, GIST	I
Protein kinase C + EGFR	Enzastaurin + erlotinib	Non-small-cell lung cancer	I/II
CTLA-4 + VEGFR2	CP-675,206 + SU011248	Renal cell carcinoma	I

Source: http://www.ClinicalTrials.gov
Ab, antibody; TKI, tyrosine kinase inhibitor; VEGF, vascular endothelial growth factor; VEGFR2, vascular endothelial growth factor receptor 2; EGFR, epidermal growth factor receptor; HDAC, histone deacetylase; FTI, farnesyl transferase inhibitor; mTOR, mammalian target of rapamycin; HER2, human epidermal growth factor 2; FGFR, fibroblastic growth factor; PDGF, platelet-derived growth factor; CDK, cyclin-dependent kinase; TRAIL-R, tumor necrosis factor (TNF)-related apoptosis inducing agent receptor; IL-6, interleukin-6; BCL-2, B-cell lymphoma 2; CTLA-4, cytoxic lymphocyte associated protein 4

Resistance to inhibition of a particular pathway may involve positive feedback loops that strongly amplify gene expression to regulate drug resistance and overcome inhibition of a single targeted agent to that pathway. Thus, a rational strategy to overcome resistance is to block both a specific pathway and the feedback loop involved in regulating the pathway (Fig. 1d). Several preclinical models have intimated that feedback loop regulation is an underlying mechanism of resistance so rational combinations involved in such regulation may provide an ideal approach for overcoming this resistance.

4.4. Variables to Consider When Designing Effective Combinations of Targeted Agents

After determining a strategy for combinatorial inhibition, which variables should be considered when determining which targeted agents to combine clinically? The variables to consider when choosing targeted therapies for combination are similar to considerations in single-agent studies or in the combination studies involving standard therapy: mechanism of action and interaction among drugs; synergistic preclinical demonstration of putatively beneficial activity; and a strategy for testing the combination in the clinic (1). The ideal targeted agents to be combined individually should have an acceptable pharmacologic and safety profile, show evidence of hitting the target, and possibly single-agent activity in a defined patient population with biomarkers that could each predict sensitivity and resistance. In addition, the ideal combination of targeted agents would have clinical activity for the same indication as they do acting as single agents, few overlapping toxicities, strong preclinical data suggesting synergy in multiple models, and an understanding of the underlying molecular mechanisms leading to synergy or additivity that could be incorporated into the clinical setting (1). (Drug additivity occurs when the response to both drugs equals the sum of the individual responses to each drug. In drug synergism, drugs can interact to enhance or magnify the response beyond the sum of the individual response to each drug.

This list of criteria offers up an ideal set for a perfect clinical world, but realistic combinations may not need all criteria for providing rational combinations that are effective in a treatment setting. Unfortunately, few targeted agents meet all of the above criteria alone, and even fewer combinations have been rigorously tested at the preclinical level for both synergy and toxicity (1).

4.5. Multitargeted Agents and Combination Treatment Design

Multitargeted agents provide an alternative or a possible hurdle to developing rational drug combinations. Few targeted agents are truly specific to a target. The exception is monoclonal antibodies, which are highly specific; their efficacy depends on direct binding to their respective ligand or receptor. Targeted agents that bind to the ATP binding sites of a receptor kinase or signaling protein domain may be more ubiquitous and affect numerous kinases and proteins with variable specificity in addition to their target of interest. Many of these multitargeted agents were discovered through a drug screening process that targets a specific kinase(s). Often the full inhibitory profile of the agent(s) is not initially known. Not surprisingly, the additional inhibitable kinases that are discovered generally have structural similarity to the original kinase targeted.

These agents have advantages and disadvantages (1). If multitargeted agents can overcome tumor heterogeneity in a given tumor or among patients with diverse cancers, they have a greater chance of clinical success. Likewise, a multitargeting capability could allow the drug to be developed for a number of indications. Imatinib is a case in point. Its ability to inhibit Bcr/Abl led to its approval by the FDA for use in chronic myelogenous leukemia, but its ability to target c-kit led to its approval for treating (GISTs). The ability of agents to hit multiple targets can make it difficult to combine them rationally without hitting a number of perhaps unwanted targets, leading to increased toxicity, as demonstrated in previously reported trials. An added problem is that many of these toxicities—rash and hand-foot syndrome, for example—are not toxicities that have been traditionally seen with most cytotoxic chemotherapy regimens. Thus, there are few supportive care measures that can allow for increased dosing of agents that cause these problems. This dose-limiting toxicity hurdle could ultimately limit the number of future rational combinations involving multitargeted agents. Moreover, defining a specific target and a subpopulation that will respond to the multitargeted drug may be more even difficult. Although a multi-targeted agent can provide evidence of early benefit in a specific tumor type, it may be difficult to define further why a series of patients responded, given the multiple targets involved.

5. IMPROVING PRECLINICAL MODELS

Preclinical models of cancer have rarely predicted clinical outcomes. Preclinical models have inherent limitations that pose serious challenges to transitioning their findings from the bench to the bedside in clinical trials *(35)*. Nevertheless, they remain an important tool for providing crucial information for drug development. This topic is an important area for cancer research and drug development but is far too broad and complex to cover in this chapter in depth. However, some important variables and considerations in preclinical combination studies may help develop clinically relevant drug combinations.

We have already explored some of the rationales for combining targeted agents, but which variables should be considered for optimizing preclinical models so they can better predict which targeted combinations will have synergy in the clinical setting?

In an in vitro setting that is assessing synergy, the assay system used should have a dynamic range, 3 to 4 logs of cell kill; and the combinations tested should have a twofold to threefold log improvement in cytotoxicity or growth inhibition compared to individual agents *(1,36)*. Several cell lines should be tested concomitantly, including drug-resistant cell lines; and major mechanisms of resistance should be identified. The activity of the combinations should be tested using clinically achievable doses and schedules. Diverse experimental conditions should also be entertained, including hypoxic conditions, as hypoxia may alter drug activity. Similarly, various growth conditions, including in the presence of human plasma, should be considered. Sequencing of combined agents should also be explored if the individual mechanisms of action suggest the importance of timing, as in the example of CDK inhibitors. Likewise, comparable principles should be incorporated into the in vivo setting, that is, appropriate tumor models with identified tumor targets and dosing regimens and schedules that are achievable in the clinical setting. Moreover, the combination should be compared with the best standard of care regimen as an in vivo control if the combination is to be compared to standard regimens in the clinical milieu in randomized trials.

6. MOVING TOWARD PERSONALIZED COMBINATIONS

Advances in our knowledge of the proteomics and genomic signaling of cancer cells has revealed that many cancers depend on multiple pathways and that malignant signaling pathways have several feedback and feed-forward loops that are possibly interconnected within a complex network *(37,38)*. This signaling heterogeneity in individual tumors poses a challenge for future combinations, and it may well be that a deeper understanding of the specifics of these networks is necessary to provide significant clinical benefit. Although these considerations are a significant hurdle, understanding them poses an opportunity for developing personalized targeted combination therapies.

The past several years have seen technology emerge that has led to increasing sophisticated molecular profiling of diseases, notably cancer. Microarray technologies have emerged that can profile tumors at the DNA, RNA and protein levels. Molecular profiling via gene expression arrays has shown considerable potential for identifying population subsets within a cancer subtype and profiles of drug sensitivity and resistance *(39–41)*.

Genomic and proteomic profiling, with the help of mathematic analysis/bioinformatics, has the potential to map out the complex network of signaling pathways that are involved in the pathogenesis and heterogeneity of cancer and determine how novel targeted therapies can be combined to shut down these perturbed networks *(37,42)*. Genomic profiling is a powerful tool for identifying subtle subphenotypes in a variety of cancers. This is a good start in the right direction, and it will certainly one day lead to personalized targeted cancer treatment, but significant challenges remain in understanding the underlying biology of the profiles generated.

Several new analytical/bioinformatics tools, however, show promise in using these profiles to help understand the pathways involved. Gene set enrichment analysis (GSEA) evaluates microarray data at the level of the gene. For example, the technology utilizes a list of genes that have been identified from array analysis and identifies sets of genes that are differentially regulated in one direction, distinguishing, for example, two phenotypes/classes. These two entities are then compared against a large set of signaling pathway databases. GSEA then calculates an enrichment score for a set of genes and correlates them with a specific biologic pathway *(43)*. The promise of this technology is the ability to define the pathways involved in an individual patient's tumor so a combination of targeted agents can be personalized for that patient to inhibit all the pertinent dysregulated pathways that have been identified through GSEA analysis *(37)*.

Critics of this genomic approach argue that information from the level of gene transcripts has not been found to correlate accurately with protein expression, or, more importantly, with the functional (frequently phosphorylated) forms of the encoded proteins *(44)*. The argument in favor of taking this proteomic approach is that direct profiling of the proteins involved, including the functional forms, provides a more accurate picture of the proteins and signaling networks involved in cancer. However, there are several limitations in using conventional proteomic technologies, such as two-dimensional polyacrylamide gel electrophoresis, isotope affinity tagging, and multidimensional liquid chromatography or mass spectrometry platforms *(42)*. First is the need for significant amounts of phenotypic cell equivalents—many orders more than can be obtained from a standard clinical biopsy. Second is their inability to analyze native protein samples. Because any denaturing through sampling disrupts the three-dimensional conformation of the protein, these techniques are likely not able to probe adequately the state of the cellular circuitry mediated by protein–protein interactions.

Reverse protein phase array (RPPA) is one proteomic technology that has the potential to overcome some of these barriers. Proteomic profiling by RPPA constitutes a sensitive and quantitative high-throughput means for marker screening, pathophysiology studies, identification of novel treatment targets, and therapeutic monitoring. RPPAs use an advanced immunoblotting-based technology to provide a quantitative analysis of the differential expression of multiple active (usually phosphorylated or cleaved) and parental proteins in hundreds of samples simultaneously *(44–47)*. This method is complementary and similar to mRNA expression arrays, which simultaneously measure the expression of thousands of genes and identify genomic subclasses that correlate with known subclasses and that have advanced our understanding of cancer classification *(48)*. However, as noted, comprehensive analysis of the transcriptome, a collection of all the gene transcripts present in a given cell, does not capture all levels of that cancer's biologic complexity *(49,50)*. Most potential molecular markers and targets are proteins; thus, proteomic profiling is expected to yield more direct answers to functional and pharmacologic questions than transcriptional profiling *(44)*. Furthermore, protein levels and function depend not only on translation but also on posttranslational modifications, such as phosphorylation, prenylation, and glycosylation, which influence a protein's stability and activity or affects the rate of protein destruction (e.g., ubiquitination) *(51)*. Predicting appropriate therapies and potential sites for therapeutic intervention is difficult in the absence of these data. The clinical applicability and the potential benefits of RPPAs have already been demonstrated for several tumor types, including ovarian and prostate cancers and follicular lymphoma *(46,47,52,53)*.

Another advantage of RPPA technology is that it requires only a miniscule amount of protein (nanoliters of protein lysate, picograms or femtograms of protein). Protein extracted from 200 cells is sufficient for analysis with a single antibody, with the lower level of detection being approximately three cells for many antibodies, compared to 5×10^5 cells per assay needed for Western blotting. Thus, 20,000 cells would be sufficient to analyze 100 proteins quantitatively. Each antibody is validated by demonstrating a single or predominant band on Western blots and showing that changes in the target are concordant between Western blotting results and arrays. The methodology for RPPA is outlined in Figure 2.

The vast array of proteomic data garnered from RPPA can be analyzed using mathematic and computational methods to personalize therapy or to develop more effective combinations. Several mathematic and computational methods can be used for this purpose, depending on the relevant biologic problem *(54)*. For example, detailed modeling at the level of biochemical reactions to understand small signaling subnetworks using coupled ordinary differential equations have provided new mechanistic insights into the MAPK1, MAPK2, and NFκB pathways *(55)*. Bayesian networks have also been used to analyze signaling in single cells as well as network responses to epidermal growth factor (EGF) and tumor necrosis factor (TNF), and the graph theory has been used to analyze neuronal networks *(38,56,57)*.

One of the most promising uses of this mathematical and modeling approach is the means to identify molecules whose activities or levels are rate limiting, identifying critical nodes in the signaling network of a given tumor. When the activity of the nodes or groups of nodes is altered, the behavior of the signaling network is perturbed, identifying potential molecular targets for therapeutic manipulation. The models can be used to predict the effects of targeted therapeutics, thereby providing methods to combine multiple inhibitors rationally *(42)*. Ideally, this approach could be extrapolated to personalized targeted therapy. In the future, a biopsy of a patient's tumor could be analyzed by RPPA analysis; mathematical modeling could then be performed to identify the ideal pathways or nodes or group of nodes that would be best targeted; and a prescription for an individualized cocktail of targeted therapies could be prescribed.

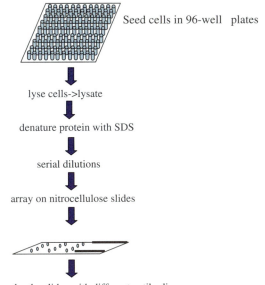

Seed cells in 96-well plates

lyse cells->lysate

denature protein with SDS

serial dilutions

array on nitrocellulose slides

probe the slides with different antibodies

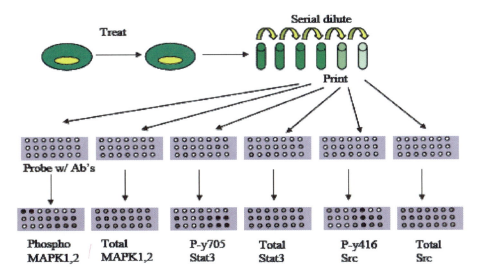

Fig. 2. Reverse phase protein array (RPPA) of cell lines seeded in a 96-well plate. Cells from tissue culture of patient samples are lysed in lysis buffer, and the detergent lysates are denatured with sodium dodecyl sulfate (SDS) sample buffer. Lysates are serially diluted with lysis buffer and spotted on nitrocellulose-coated slides, ready for probing with antibodies against total protein and their activated or phosphorylated forms (adapted from Bryan Hennessey, MD with permission).

7. BARRIERS TO COMBINATORIAL TARGETED THERAPY IN CANCER TREATMENT

We have explored some of the scientific challenges faced in developing targeted agent combinations for cancer treatment. However, among the greatest hurdles for developing these novel combinations are the regulatory and financial barriers that presently exist and that may continue to limit the ability of a therapeutic combination to move forward as a standard of care.

Two of these challenges are the regulatory time lines involved in drug development and the difficulty of the new drug application (NDA) process. Currently, the average time from initiation of clinical testing to U.S. regulatory approval for an oncology drug is 7.8 years *(58)*. Despite the fact that oncologic drug applications are often given priority review at the FDA and are reviewed 6 months faster than other drugs, this time line remains 1.5 years longer than most other classes of drugs. Even so, this prolonged developmental time line may be secondary to other deleterious factors, including difficulty recruiting patients to clinical trials and longer times needed to establish efficacy, which is problematic in and of itself in this patient population. Second, the NDA process, which is involved with the complete chemistry profile, manufacturing, toxicology, clinical pharmacology, and clinical data along with requisite complete study reports, is a rigorous process. To approve a drug combination, of two novel agents, the FDA requires that any combination of targeted agents clearly shows benefit over the single agents alone and/or standard of care (personal communication with Ramsey Dagher—Senior Official, FDA Oncology Division). This would require a registration trial that would have four stratified arms: agent A, agent B, combination of agent A and B, and possibly standard of care. Such a registration trial would likely require more patients and longer times to accrual. Ultimately, this may favor the development of multitargeted agents that may have a less difficult road to approval as a single agent than two more-specific targeted agents. However, as we have discussed, there are limitations to the development of multitargeted inhibitors, and therefore more specifically targeted combination therapies may be hindered.

Perhaps an even greater challenge in developing these targeted combinations is the increasing cost of many of these new, targeted drugs. The price tag for a combination of cytotoxic chemotherapy and a targeted agent has significantly elevated the overall cost of these regimens. For example, the cost for a colorectal patient who is 170 cm tall and 70 kg in weight and undergoes chemotherapy for 8 weeks is significantly increased with the addition of a targeted agents. The FOLFOX regimen of 5-fluorouracil, leucovorin, and oxaliplatin costs on average $11,889; but when combined with bevacizumab, the cost increases to $21,033 *(59)*. The combination of irinotecan and cetuximab for the second and third-line treatment of metastatic colorectal cancer is even more costly, with an 8-week course costing approximately $30,790. The total average calculated cost for an average metastatic colorectal patient who continues to receive treatment until median time to progression—that is, 8 months of frontline therapy and then 4.1 months of irinotecan–cetuximab therapy—would cost $161,000. In 2004, a total of 56,000 patients were diagnosed with either metastatic or recurrent metastatic disease. The estimated total cost of chemotherapy with the addition of the targeted agent would cost the health care system, based on the above patient estimate and patient numbers, $1.2 billon *(59)*.

Currently, third-party payers in the United States have continued to pay these expenses; however, other countries have questioned the cost–benefit ratio of such expensive regimens. Indeed in the United Kingdom, the National Institute for Health and Clinical Excellence (NICE) has rejected the use of cetuximab therapy as an option given the high cost/life-gained ratio *(60)*. It is conceivable that as the United States and other countries struggle with the cost of health care decisions about expensive combination targeted therapy will also be questioned by both Medicare and third-party payers unless significant gains in overall survival can be obtained with these novel combinations. Therefore, it is imperative that we continue to develop more rational and effective combination therapies.

REFERENCES

1. Dancey JE, Chen HX. Strategies for optimizing combinations of molecularly targeted anticancer agents. Nat Rev Drug Discov 2006;5(8):649–59.
2. Slamon D, Pegram M. Rationale for trastuzumab (Herceptin) in adjuvant breast cancer trials. Semin Oncol 2001;28(suppl 3):13–9.
3. Romond EH, Perez EA, Bryant J, et al. Trastuzumab plus adjuvant chemotherapy for operable HER2-positive breast cancer. N Engl J Med 2005;353(16):1673–84.
4. Slamon DJ, Godolphin W, Jones LA, et al. Studies of the HER-2/neu proto-oncogene in human breast and ovarian cancer. Science 1989;244(4905):707–12.
5. Slamon DJ, Clark GM, Wong SG, et al. Human breast cancer: correlation of relapse and survival with amplification of the HER-2/neu oncogene. Science 1987;235(4785):177–82.
6. Park JW, Kerbel RS, Kelloff GJ, et al. Rationale for biomarkers and surrogate end points in mechanism-driven oncology drug development. Clin Cancer Res 2004;10(11):3885–96.
7. Slamon DJ, Leyland-Jones B, Shak S, et al. Use of chemotherapy plus a monoclonal antibody against HER2 for metastatic breast cancer that overexpresses HER2. N Engl J Med 2001;344(11):783–92.
8. Pegram MD, Konecny GE, O'Callaghan C, et al. Rational combinations of trastuzumab with chemotherapeutic drugs used in the treatment of breast cancer. J Natl Cancer Inst 2004;96:739–49.
9. Seidman AD, Berry D, Cirrincione C, et al. CALGB 9840: phase III study of weekly (W) paclitaxel (P) via 1-hour(h) infusion versus standard (S) 3h infusion every third week in the treatment of metastatic breast cancer (MBC), with trastuzumab (T) for HER2 positive MBC and randomized for T in HER2 normal MBC. ASCO Annu Meet Proc (Post Meet Ed) 2004;22(14S):512.
10. Cobleigh MA, Vogel CL, Tripathy D, et al. Multinational study of the efficacy and safety of humanized anti-HER2 monoclonal antibody in women who have HER2-overexpressing metastatic breast cancer that has progressed after chemotherapy for metastatic disease. J Clin Oncol 1999;17(9):2639–48.
11. Giaccone G, Herbst RS, Manegold C, et al. Gefitinib in combination with gemcitabine and cisplatin in advanced non-small-cell lung cancer: a phase III trial—INTACT 1. J Clin Oncol 2004;22(5):777–84.
12. Herbst RS, Giaccone G, Schiller JH, et al. Gefitinib in combination with paclitaxel and carboplatin in advanced non-small-cell lung cancer: a phase III trial—INTACT 2. J Clin Oncol 2004;22(5):785–94.
13. Herbst RS, Prager D, Hermann R, et al. TRIBUTE: a phase III trial of erlotinib hydrochloride (OSI-774) combined with carboplatin and paclitaxel chemotherapy in advanced non-small-cell lung cancer. J Clin Oncol 2005;23(25):5892–9.
14. Paez JG, Janne PA, Lee JC, et al. EGFR mutations in lung cancer: correlation with clinical response to gefitinib therapy. Science 2004;304(5676):1497–500.
15. Lynch TJ, Bell DW, Sordella R, et al. Activating mutations in the epidermal growth factor receptor underlying responsiveness of non-small-cell lung cancer to gefitinib. N Engl J Med 2004;350(21):2129–39.
16. Han SW, Kim TY, Hwang PG, et al. Predictive and prognostic impact of epidermal growth factor receptor mutation in non-small-cell lung cancer patients treated with gefitinib. J Clin Oncol 2005;23(11):2493–501.
17. Cappuzzo F, Varella-Garcia M, Shigematsu H, et al. Increased HER2 gene copy number is associated with response to gefitinib therapy in epidermal growth factor receptor-positive non-small-cell lung cancer patients. J Clin Oncol 2005;23(22):5007–18.
18. Chou TY, Chiu CH, Li LH, et al. Mutation in the tyrosine kinase domain of epidermal growth factor receptor is a predictive and prognostic factor for gefitinib treatment in patients with non-small cell lung cancer. Clin Cancer Res 2005;11(10):3750–7.
19. Cortes-Funes H, Gomez C, Rosell R, et al. Epidermal growth factor receptor activating mutations in Spanish gefitinib-treated non-small-cell lung cancer patients. Ann Oncol 2005;16(7):1081–6.
20. Zhang GC, Lin JY, Wang Z, et al. Epidermal growth factor receptor double activating mutations involving both exons 19 and 21 exist in Chinese non-small cell lung cancer patients. Clin Oncol (R Coll Radiol) 2007;19:499–506.
21. Takano T, Ohe Y, Sakamoto H, et al. Epidermal growth factor receptor gene mutations and increased copy numbers predict gefitinib sensitivity in patients with recurrent non-small-cell lung cancer. J Clin Oncol 2005;23(28):6829–37.
22. Eberhard DA, Johnson BE, Amler LC, et al. Mutations in the epidermal growth factor receptor and in KRAS are predictive and prognostic indicators in patients with non-small-cell lung cancer treated with chemotherapy alone and in combination with erlotinib. J Clin Oncol 2005;23(25):5900–9.

23. Tracy S, Mukohara T, Hansen M, et al. Gefitinib induces apoptosis in the EGFRL858R non-small-cell lung cancer cell line H3255. Cancer Res 2004;64:7241–4.
24. Gandara DR, Gumerlock PH. Epidermal growth factor receptor tyrosine kinase inhibitors plus chemotherapy: case closed or is the jury still out? J Clin Oncol 2005;23(25):5856–8.
25. Motwani M, Delohery TM, Schwartz GK. Sequential dependent enhancement of caspase activation and apoptosis by flavopiridol on paclitaxel-treated human gastric and breast cancer cells. Clin Cancer Res 1999;5(7):1876–83.
26. Schwartz GK, Shah MA. Targeting the cell cycle: a new approach to cancer therapy. J Clin Oncol 2005;23(36):9408–21.
27. Clute P, Pines J. Temporal and spatial control of cyclin B1 destruction in metaphase. Nat Cell Biol 1999;1:82–7.
28. Wang S, Wang Z, Boise L, et al. Loss of the bcl-2 phosphorylation loop domain increases resistance of human leukemia cells (U937) to paclitaxel-mediated mitochondrial dysfunction and apoptosis. Biochem Biophys Res Commun 1999;259(1):67–72.
29. Schwartz GK, O'Reilly E, Ilson D, et al. Phase I study of the cyclin-dependent kinase inhibitor flavopiridol in combination with paclitaxel in patients with advanced solid tumors. J Clin Oncol 2002;20(8):2157–70.
30. Baselga J. Targeting of the EGFR as a modulator of cancer chemotherapy. In: Schwartz GK (ed). Combination Chemotherapy. Totowa, NJ: Humana Press Inc.; 2005:1–26.
31. Schwartz GK. Combination Cancer Therapy. Totowa, NJ: Humana; 2005.
32. Sosman JA, Puzanov I, Atkins MB. Opportunities and obstacles to combination targeted therapy in renal cell cancer. Clin Cancer Res 2007;13(2 Pt 2):764s–9s.
33. Hong D. Phase I study of tipifarnib and sorafenib in patients with bioppsable advanced cancers. ASCO Annu Meet Proc 2007;25(18S):150s.
34. Patnaik A. A phase I pharmacokinetic and pharmacodynamic study of sorafenib, a multi-targeted kinase inhibitor in combination with temsirolimus, an mTOR inhibitor in patients with advanced solid malignancies. ASCO Annu Meet Proc 2007;25(18s):141s.
35. Kamb A. What's wrong with our cancer models? Nat Rev Drug Discov 2005;4(2):161–5.
36. Gitler MS, Monks A, Sausville EA. Preclinical models for defining efficacy of drug combinations: mapping the road to the clinic. Mol Cancer Ther 2003;2(9):929–32.
37. Bild AH, Potti A, Nevins JR. Linking oncogenic pathways with therapeutic opportunities. Nat Rev Cancer 2006;6(9):735–41.
38. Ma'ayan A, Jenkins SL, Neves S, et al. Formation of regulatory patterns during signal propagation in a mammalian cellular network. Science 2005;309(5737):1078–83.
39. Baak JP, Bol MG, van Diermen B, et al. DNA cytometric features in biopsies of TaT1 urothelial cell cancer predict recurrence and stage progression more accurately than stage, grade, or treatment modality. Urology 2003;61(6):1266–72.
40. Segal E, Friedman N, Kaminski N, et al. From signatures to models: understanding cancer using microarrays. Nat Genet 2005;37(suppl):S38–45.
41. Brennan DJ, O'Brien SL, Fagan A, et al. Application of DNA microarray technology in determining breast cancer prognosis and therapeutic response. Expert Opin Biol Ther 2005;5(8):1069–83.
42. Wulfkuhle JD, Edmiston KH, Liotta LA, et al. Technology insight: pharmacoproteomics for cancer–promises of patient-tailored medicine using protein microarrays. Nat Clin Pract Oncol 2006;3(5):256–68.
43. Subramanian A, Tamayo P, Mootha VK, et al. Gene set enrichment analysis: a knowledge-based approach for interpreting genome-wide expression profiles. Proc Natl Acad Sci U S A 2005;102:15545–50.
44. Nishizuka S, Charboneau L, Young L, et al. Proteomic profiling of the NCI-60 cancer cell lines using new high-density reverse-phase lysate microarrays. Proc Natl Acad Sci U S A 2003;100:14229–34.
45. Charboneau L, Scott H, Chen T, et al. Utility of reverse phase protein arrays: applications to signalling pathways and human body arrays. Brief Funct Genomic Proteomic 2002;1(3):305–15.
46. Paweletz CP, Charboneau L, Bichsel VE, et al. Reverse phase protein microarrays which capture disease progression show activation of pro-survival pathways at the cancer invasion front. Oncogene 2001;20(16):1981–9.
47. Wulfkuhle JD, Aquino JA, Calvert VS, et al. Signal pathway profiling of ovarian cancer from human tissue specimens using reverse-phase protein microarrays. Proteomics 2003;3(11):2085–90.
48. Pusztai L, Ayers M, Stec J, et al. Gene expression profiles obtained from fine-needle aspirations of breast cancer reliably identify routine prognostic markers and reveal large-scale molecular differences between estrogen-negative and estrogen-positive tumors. Clin Cancer Res 2003;9(7):2406–15.
49. Gygi SP, Rochon Y, Franza BR, et al. Correlation between protein and mRNA abundance in yeast. Mol Cell Biol 1999;19(3):1720–30.

50. Diks SH, Peppelenbosch MP. Single cell proteomics for personalised medicine. Trends Mol Med 2004;10(12):574–7.
51. Amerik AY, Hochstrasser M. Mechanism and function of deubiquitinating enzymes. Biochim Biophys Acta 2004;1695:189–207.
52. Grubb RL, Calvert VS, Wulkuhle JD, et al. Signal pathway profiling of prostate cancer using reverse phase protein arrays. Proteomics 2003;3(11):2142–6.
53. Zha H, Raffeld M, Charboneau L, et al. Similarities of prosurvival signals in Bcl-2-positive and Bcl-2-negative follicular lymphomas identified by reverse phase protein microarray. Lab Invest 2004;84(2):235–44.
54. Ideker T. Systems biology 101—what you need to know. Nat Biotechnol 2004;22(4):473–5.
55. Bhalla US, Ram PT, Iyengar R. MAP kinase phosphatase as a locus of flexibility in a mitogen-activated protein kinase signaling network. Science 2002;297(5583):1018–23.
56. Janes KA, Albeck JG, Gaudet S, et al. A systems model of signaling identifies a molecular basis set for cytokine-induced apoptosis. Science 2005;310(5754):1646–53.
57. Sachs K, Perez O, Pe'er D, et al. Causal protein-signaling networks derived from multiparameter single-cell data. Science 2005;308(5721):523–9.
58. DiMasi JA, Grabowski HG. Economics of new oncology drug development. J Clin Oncol 2007;25(2): 209–16.
59. Schrag D. The price tag on progress—chemotherapy for colorectal cancer. N Engl J Med 2004;351:317–9.
60. Starling N, Tilden D, White J, et al. Cost-effectiveness analysis of cetuximab/irinotecan vs active/best supportive care for the treatment of metastatic colorectal cancer patients who have failed previous chemotherapy treatment. Br J Cancer 2007;96(2):206–12.

19 Drug Development in Cancer Medicine: *Challenges for Targeted Approaches*

Luis H. Camacho, MD, MPH

CONTENTS

ABSTRACT

Remarkable progress has been made in cancer medicine during the last two decades. The number of anticancer agents entering clinical trials has grown exponentially; and patients with diseases such as acute promyelocytic leukemia, chronic myelogenous leukemia, chronic lymphocytic leukemia, multiple myeloma, cutaneous T-cell lymphoma, colorectal cancer, breast cancer, GISTs, and renal cell carcinoma have already received some of the benefits from molecularly tailored strategies. Despite sustained progress, however, many patients have not yet benefited from this sophisticated approach, and cancer remains among the three most common causes of death worldwide. Carcinogenesis involves the accumulation of multiple molecular mutations responsible for deregulation of critical signaling pathways that control vital cellular functions. Targeting molecular structures on cancer cells is highly specific and can modulate vital functions such as cell growth, migration, differentiation, and survival. Targeted therapies are generally well tolerated, and the overall supportive treatments now available for cancer patients are better than in the past. Nonetheless, several challenges associated with anticancer agents, molecular targets, tumor assessment tools, clinical trial designs; and the drug development and approval process exist. Overcoming these challenges is critical to improve the early success achieved during the past two decades. It also is important to consider that the sophistication of this approach has extraordinarily increased the costs of drug development and patient care, making the application of these novel agents a privilege accorded to a small population of patients throughout the world. Some of these challenges and strategies for addressing them are summarized and discussed in this chapter.

From: *Current Clinical Oncology: Targeted Cancer Therapy*
Edited by: R. Kurzrock and M. Markman © Humana Press, Totowa, NJ

Key Words: Targeted therapy, Challenges, Obstacles, Drug development, Clinical trials, Phase I

1. INTRODUCTION

Drug development in cancer medicine has undergone dramatic progress during the last decade. In addition to conventional cytotoxic drugs targeting DNA synthesis, cell cycle elements, and structural proteins (e.g., tubulin), a new breed of rationally designed agents directed against specific molecular targets has emerged. Despite early success with differentiating agents such as retinoic acid, hormonal modulators (tamoxifen, goserelin, letrozole), and monoclonal antibodies (rituximab, myelotarg, herceptin) during the 1990s and early 2000s, the discovery of imatinib mesylate (Gleevec, Glivec; Novartis, East Hanover, NJ, USA) to treat patients with chronic myelogenous leukemia (CML) set the stage for highly successful targeted therapies in cancer medicine.

This chapter uses the example of imatinib mesylate to highlight similarities and potential pitfalls for its successors. Imatinib mesylate was synthesized and developed specifically to inhibit a mutated kinase fusion protein known as Bcr-Abl, which results from the reciprocal translocation of chromosomes 9 and 22 t(9;22), the Philadelphia chromosome, in patients with CML *(1)*. Development of this highly successful agent was not easy. Despite a complete hematologic response rate of 95% in patients with chronic-phase CML that progressed after interferon therapy and an 82% response rate in patients with accelerated-phase CML, a controlled comparison with interferon and cytarabine was requested before the new agent could be approved. A total of 1106 patients were enrolled in 177 centers over a 7-month period. The study was terminated early because of clear superiority in the imatinib arm over the combination of interferon and cytarabine in the rates of complete hematologic remission (97% vs. 69%), complete cytogenetic remission (76% vs. 14%), and drug tolerability (31% vs. 3%) *(2)*. The drug was approved by the U.S. Food and Drug Administration (FDA) in May of 2001, only 3 months after the application for approval application was filed.

Imatinib is not entirely selective for the Bcr-Abl tyrosine kinase. In vitro studies demonstrated that it also inhibits the receptor tyrosine kinases for platelet-derived growth factor (PDGF), stem cell factor (SCF), and c-Kit and inhibits PDGF- and SCF-mediated cellular events. This lack of selectivity is advantageous, as imatinib also has proven efficacious in tumor types other than CML. Van Oosterom et al. and subsequently Demetri et al. reported on the efficacy of imatinib for patients with advanced GISTs *(3,4)*; before then, GIST was a malignancy for which standard therapy consisted of surgical resection of symptomatic tumors. Imatinib is now approved to treat inoperable or metastatic GIST, and its role in the adjuvant setting is being explored. Unfortunately, several studies in other tumor types have been much less successful *(5–8)*.

The GIST experience taught us that the incomplete specificity of an agent might further serve to target molecular abnormalities common to other tumor types. Unlike in CML, GIST does not have a t(9,22) translocation. In 1998, however, Hirota et al. had described c-Kit mutations in five GIST specimens *(9)*. Subsequent investigations of tumor tissue samples of patients treated with imatinib also taught us that, in addition to c-Kit overexpression, patients with activating KIT mutations in exon 11 had partial responses in about 80% of cases, whereas patients with wild-type KIT expression without mutations had a response rate of about 18% *(10,11)*. We eventually learned that these patients likely respond because of the presence of activating mutations of PDGFRA (platelet-derived growth factor receptor, α polypeptide) in two different exons *(12)*.

Shortly after the imatinib success was celebrated by the cancer community around the world, tumor resistance to imatinib emerged as a novel challenge *(13)*. This new chapter in the history of targeted therapies reminded us of the importance of tumor resistance, prompting further research into this problem *(14)*. Once again, the mechanisms responsible for tumor progression after treatment with imatinib mesylate were identified *(13,15–17)*. Subsequently, a second targeted approach was developed to block the escape signaling mechanisms of resistant cellular clones: dasatinib (BMS-354825, Sprycel; Bristol Myers Squibb, Princeton, NJ, USA), a dual Src/Abl kinase inhibitor, was designed, developed, and approved for this indication *(18)*. The success of these continued research efforts during the past decade resulted in a substantial increase in the 5-year survival rate of patients with CML *(19)*.

Most importantly, the experience and knowledge gained from these efforts forever changed the way we see the cancer process and ramped up our hope that cancer would one day be eradicated or, at least, that we would be able modify its natural history so it would become a chronic, indolent process. This journey, however, is not uncomplicated as a number of challenges lie on the horizon requiring our immediate attention.

2. SELECTION OF TARGETS FOR CANCER THERAPEUTICS

In addition to the several molecular abnormalities identified at different levels in cancer cells, neighboring and distant structures such as blood vessels, lymphatics, stroma, and the surrounding microenvironment play a major role in human malignancy. Targeted strategies can be directed, therefore, not only against specific aberrant cellular molecules and signaling pathways but to otherwise normal physiologic mechanisms recruited by the neoplastic process. Full understanding of the role these "recruited" biologic processes play in neoplastic evolution and maintenance is pivotal. Targeting molecules critical to the functionality of these processes has resulted in substantial antitumor activity and may further refine our comprehensive approach to cancer *(20)*.

2.1. Signal Transduction Pathways

Vital cellular functions are regulated through signal transduction networks connecting the cell membrane, cytosol, and nucleus. Modulation of these signals affects cellular growth, migration, invasion, differentiation, and apoptosis. Tumor biology is largely associated with dysfunction of one or more of these pathways. Targeted therapies are primarily directed against molecular elements involved in these processes (Table 1). The following are examples of critical cellular functions and their association with particular tumor types.

2.2. Cellular Differentiation

Acute promyelocytic leukemia (APL) is a classic example of deregulation in the processes of cellular differentiation. In this neoplasm, maturation arrest at the promyelocytic stage in the myeloid lineage occurs secondary to a chromosomal translocation involving the retinoic acid receptor-α gene on chromosome 17 (*RARA*) *(21)*. In 95% of cases of APL, this gene is involved in a reciprocal translocation with the promyelocytic leukemia gene (*PML*) on chromosome 15 *(22)*.

Treatment with retinoic acid, a vitamin A analogue, results in cellular differentiation and remission in more than 80% of patients with APL *(23)*. Characterization of the molecular mechanisms involved in the leukemogenesis of APL and the subsequent identification of

Table 1
Commonly Selected Targeted Molecular Abnormalities and Their Status According
to Tumor Type

Molecule	Abnormality type	Tumor	Reference
Angiogenesis and lymphangiogenesis			
VEGF	Protein expression	GISTs (78.8%)	(104)
		Leiomyomas (60.0%)	(104)
		Schwannomas (50.0%)	(104)
	mRNA expression	Endometrial carcinoma	(105)
	Expression correlates with poor prognosis	Gastric carcinoma	(106)
	Cytoplasmic	Melanoma (84%)	(107)
VEGFR1	Protein expression	GIST (72.7%)	(104)
		Leiomyomas (80.0%)	(104)
		Schwannomas (66.7%)	(104)
		Breast cell lines	(108)
		Pancreas	(109)
VEGFR2	Protein expression	GIST (90.9%)	(104)
	Protein expression	Leiomyomas (33.3%)	(104)
	Protein expression	Schwannomas (67%)	(104)
	Amplification	Gliomas (6%–17%)	(110)
VEGFR3	mRNA expression	Glioblastoma multiforme	(111)
EGFR	Overexpression	Head and neck (80%–100%)	(112)
		Renal (50%–90%)	(112)
		Breast (14%–91%)	(112)
		Lung (40%–80%)	(112)
		Colorectal (25%–77%)	(112)
		Ovarian (35%–70%)	(112)
		Meningioma (42%)	(113)
		Pancreas (30%–50%)	(112)
		Glioma (40%–63%)	(112)
		Bladder (31%–48%)	(112)
		B-ALL (3%–31%)	(114)
	Amplification	Gliomas (0%–12%)	(110)
	Overexpression	Most Carcinomas (> 50%)	(115)
	Amplification	Breast (30%)	(115)
ERBB2	Gene amplification	Esophagus (12%; 25 tumors tested)	(116)
RAS–RAF pathway			
K-RAS	Mutation	Pancreas (90%)	(115)
		NSCLC (35%)	
		Colorectal (45%)	
		Follicular thyroid (45%)	
		Papillary thyroid (60%)	
		Seminoma (45%)	
		MDS (40%)	

N-RAS	Mutation	Follicular thyroid (55%)	*(115)*
		Papillary thyroid (60%)	
		Seminoma (45%)	
		Melanoma (15%)	
		Liver (30%)	
		MDS (40%)	
		AML (30%)	
H-RAS		Follicular thyroid (55%)	*(115)*
		Papillary thyroid (60%)	
		Kidney (10%)	
c-RAF1	Gene up-regulation after curcumin exposure	Breast Cancer cells	*(117)*
BRAF	Mutation	Melanoma (66%)	*(115,118)*
		Colorectal (12%)	
		Biliary tract (25%)	*(118)*
		Skin (44%)	*(118)*
		Ovary (16%)	
		Thyroid (26%)	
MEK1	Overexpression	Breast	
MEK2	Overexpression	Breast	*(119)*
ERK1/ERK2	ERK1 overexpression	Squamous cell carcinoma	*(120)*
	Decreased activity of ERK1/2p44/42	Squamous cell carcinoma of larynx	*(121)*
	Expression of phosphorylated ERK1/2 protein	Cholangiocarcinoma (49%)	*(122)*
	Phosphorylated ERK1/2 correlates with early stages of disease and longer relapse-free survival in women with breast carcinoma receiving tamoxifen therapy	Breast	*(123,124)*

Phosphoinosytol 3 kinase pathway

PI3K	Amplification	Ovarian (40%)	*(115)*
AKT2	Amplification	Ovarian (12%)	*(115)*
		Pancreas (10%)	*(115)*

Migration and invasion

Rac1	Overexpression	DCIS (60%–100%)	*(36)*
	Overexpression	Breast (100%)	*(36)*
	Overexpression	Squamous cell carcinoma (74%)	*(36,125)*
Rac1b	Overexpression	Breast	*(36)*
	Overexpression	Colon	*(36)*
Rac2	Overexpression	Breast	*(36)*
Rac3	Overexpression	Brain	*(36)*
	Hyperactivity	Breast	*(36)*

(Continued)

Table 1
(Continued)

Molecule	Abnormality type	Tumor	Reference
Cdc42	Overexpression	Breast	(36)
RhoA	Overexpression	Breast	(36)
		SCC	(36)
		Lung	(36)
		Colon	(36)
		Bladder	(36)
		Testicular	(36)
RhoB	Loss	Lung	(36)
RhoC	Overexpression	Lung	(36)
RhoE	Loss	Prostate	(36)
RhoG	Overexpression	Breast	(36)
RhoH	Rearrangement	Hodgkin's disease	(36)
	Deregulation	Multiple myeloma	(36)
	Point mutations	Diffuse large B-cell lymphoma	(36)
DLC-1 (RhoA and Cdc42-GAP)	Loss; methylation	Liver	(36)
DLC-2 (RhoA and Cdc42-GAP)	Loss	Liver	(36)
Vav1 (Rac-GEF)	Overexpression	Pancreas	(36)
c-Met	Overexpression	Lung (41% – 72%)	(126)
		Prostate (40%–84%)	
		Colorectal (55%–78%)	
		Breast (25%–60%)	
		Pancreas (83%–100%)	
		Ovarian (64%)	
		Head and neck (55%–68%)	
		Brain (54%–74%)	
		Renal (54%–87%)	
		Stomach (43%–69%)	
		Melanoma (17%–39%)	
		Liver (68%)	
Survival and apoptosis			
TRAIL	Cells do not express	Cholangiocarcinoma (>50%)	
	TRAIL decoy receptors lacking death domain		
	Somatic mutations of TRAIL-R1 and TRAIL-R2 genes	Non-Hodgkin's lymphoma	(127)
DR5	Loss of heterozygosity	Colorectal cancer (>50%)	(128)
	Two alterations in domain including a two-basepair insertion	Head and neck	(129)
BCL-2	Expression	Breast, metastatic (80%)	(130)

	Expression. Significant correlation with estrogen and progesterone receptors. Lack of expression in axillary lymph nodes independently correlates with disease free survival and overall survival.	Breast, invasive ductal (75%)	(131)
	Gene translocation	B cell lymphoma (80%)	(44)
	Expression	Chronic lymphocytic leukemia	(42,43)
	Low expression associated with prolonged survival	Oral squamous cell carcinoma	(132)
	Serum detection: No prognostic significance. Possible diagnostic value	Lung carcinoma (96%)	(133)
	Expression is associated with poorer outcome	Glioblastoma multiforme (33%)	(134)
	IHC expression showed longer specific survival	Hormone-refractory prostate carcinoma	(135)
Other			
IGF-IR	Ubiquitously expressed	Normal tissues	(136)
	Overexpression	Breast carcinoma (39%–93%)	(137)
		Prostate carcinoma	(138)
PDGFR	Overexpression	Uterine sarcoma (70%)	(139)
	Overexpression by immunohistochemistry	Prostate carcinoma (16%)	(140)
	PDGFR phosphory-lation/expression in the tissue of 6/6 patients	Chordoma (100%)	(141)
	Gene expression	Medulloblastoma (metastatic)	(142)
	Overexpression	Serous ovarian (13%)	(143)
	Overexpression	Lung carcinoma	(144)
	Overexpression of PDGFRA	Breast (39%)	(145)
	Expression of PDGF, PDGFR and phosphorylated PDGFR (p-PDGFR)	Colorectal	(146)
	Fusions with proteins (e.g., transcription factor Tel or rabaptin-5)	CMML	(147)
	Constitutively active PDGF α receptor fusion protein, FIPL1-PDGFRα, has been identified in patients with idiopathic hypereosinophilic syndrome	Idiopathic hypereosinophilic syndrome	(148)

(Continued)

Table 1
(Continued)

Molecule	Abnormality type	Tumor	Reference
PTEN	Loss	Glioblastoma multiforme (20%–30%)	*(115)*
		Prostate (20%)	*(115)*
		Pancreas (40%)	*(115)*

Modified from Barber et al. *(36)*. and Christensen et al. (Cancer Letters, 2005) VEGF, vascular endothelial growth factor; VEGFR1/VEGFR2, vascular endothelial growth factor receptors 1 and 2; EGFR, endothelial growth factor receptor; ERBB2, erythroblastic leukemia viral oncogene homologue 2; K-RAS, Kirsten rat sarcoma viral oncogene homologue; c-RAF1, murine leukemia viral oncogene homologue 1; BRAF, murine leukemia viral oncogene homologue 1 (A-Raf and Raf-B are two proteins with similar sequences to Raf-1); MEK1/MEK2, mitogen-activated protein kinase kinases 1 and 2; ERK1/ERK2, extracellular signal-regulated kinase 1 and 2; PI3K, phosphatidyli-nositol 3-kinase; AKT2, v-akt murine thymoma viral oncogene homologue 2; IGFR, insulin growth factor receptor; Rac1, ras-related C3 botulinum toxin substrate 1; Rac1b, a tumor associated, constitutively active Rac1 splice variant *(149)*; Cdc42, cell division cycle 42; RhoA, ras homolog gene family, member A; PDGFR, platelet-derived growth factor receptor; PTEN, Phosphatase and tensin homologue deleted on chromosome 10; TRAIL, tumor necrosis factor-related apoptosis-inducing ligand; DR4, death receptor 4; BCL-2, B-cell lymphoma-2; mRNA, messenger RNA; GIST, gastrointestinal stromal tumor; IGF, insulin growth factor

other potential targets intimately associated with this transcription complex have dramatically enhanced our understanding of this leukemia subtype, and resulted in therapeutic progress (Fig. 1). Arsenic trioxide, a poison and an ancient medicinal compound, also promotes cellular differentiation and apoptosis of APL cells, inducing remission in approximately 90% of APL patients *(24,25)*. Furthermore, the acetylation of nuclear histones is closely linked to the transcription machinery and has been associated with resistance in APL patients *(26)*. Agents that inhibit histone deacetylase may induce clinical, morphologic, and molecular remission in patients with retinoic acid-resistant APL *(27)*. In 1998, Nan et al. described methyl CpG binding protein 2 (meCP2), a linking protein between methylation and histone acetylation elements in the transcription core *(28)*. The association of these two mechanisms promptly led to clinical trials of agents directed against these biologic elements *(29–31)*. Ongoing research efforts and development of a newer generation of agents may increase the efficacy of these approaches *(32)*. To once again highlight the importance of incorporating the knowledge gained into the rational design of clinical trials, Garcia-Manero's group recently demonstrated that targeting the methylation and acetylation interactions followed by modulation of the retinoic acid receptors induces cellular differentiation and substantial clinical responses in patients with advanced non-APL AML *(33)*.

2.3. Cellular Migration/Invasion

The ability of cancer cells to detach from a primary tumor site, migrate, extravasate and invade distant tissues involves essential signaling molecules and their pathways. Several molecules have been implicated in these well organized events, and their association with particular tumor types has been confirmed. Among them, the CXCR4 (stromal cell-derived factor 1 receptor: fusin)/CXCL12 (SDF-1) pathway has been identified as critical to the migration, adhesion, and invasion of several hematologic and epithelial cancers

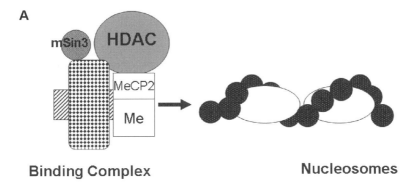

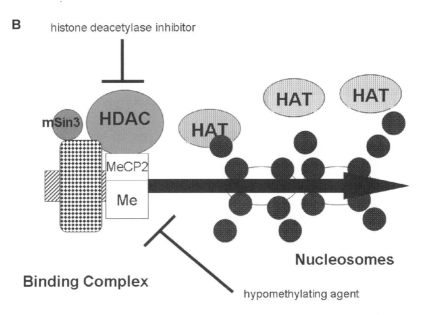

Fig. 1. Mechanisms of nuclear transcription. In an inactive transcription state, DNA is tightly coiled around the core histones of the nucleosome (**A**). Acetylation of histones by histone acetyltransferases results in conformational relaxation of the chromatin and a permissive state where transcription factors bind. Treatment with histone deacetylase inhibitors (HDACI) and hypomethylating agents may prevent the cleavage of acetyl groups from histones and induce chromatin relaxation (**B**). These configuration changes result in activation of nuclear transcription, cellular differentiation, and apoptosis.

(34). Chemokines such as CCR5, CCR6, CCR9, and CXCR6 and their ligands also play important roles in invasion and metastasis. Similarly, IL8RA and CCR3 are important contributors to cellular adhesion *(35)*. Other molecules involved in cancer cell invasion include phosphatidylinositol 3-kinase (PI3K) and the Rho family of small GTPases *(36)* and the hepatocyte growth factor and its receptor c-Met *(37)*. Targeting these pathways in humans is ongoing in early clinical trials. C-Met inhibitors are under clinical development and thus far are demonstrating clinical efficacy. Inhibition of CXCR4 was initially carried

out in patients with multiple myeloma or non-Hodgkin's lymphoma *(38)*. The agent safely induced rapid mobilization of CD34(+) cells and, in combination with granulocyte colony-stimulating factor (G-CSF), was more potent than the use of G-CSF alone *(39)*. Clinical trials evaluating its anticancer properties are underway. The investigation of this combined targeted therapy regimen through well designed clinical studies is of great interest.

2.4. Cellular Survival/Programmed Cell Death

Other mechanisms commonly affected in neoplastic cells involve the growth/programmed cell death machinery. Apoptosis or programmed cell death is complex and involves at least 11 pathways, which are subclassified as apoptotic and nonapoptotic. Whereas the former includes classic apoptotic mechanisms, the latter includes autophagic cell death, necrosis (oncosis), mitotic cell death, and caspase-independent cell death preceded by changes in the mitochondrial outer membrane *(40)*.

Chronic lymphocytic leukemia (CLL) is one of the best examples of a disease process that results from accumulation of apoptosis-resistant mature B lymphocytes. These apoptotic abnormalities result in a progressive accumulation of mature B cells that ultimately infiltrate lymph nodes, spleen, and bone marrow *(41)*. Multiple lines of evidence suggest that Bcl-2 and other antiapoptotic molecules are the driving mechanisms of CLL and other B-cell malignancies, at least in the early stages of this process *(42–46)*. Furthermore, Bcl-2 inhibition may increase sensitivity to immune-mediated tumor destruction *(47)*. The importance of targeting this mechanism in CLL has been confirmed clinically. O'Brien et al. recently reported on the activity of oblimersen, a Bcl-2 antisense molecule, among 241 CLL patients randomly assigned to receive fludarabine 25 mg/m^2/day and cyclophosphamide 250 mg/m^2/day IV for 3 days, with or without oblimersen 3 mg/kg/day given as a 7-day continuous intravenous infusion (beginning 4 days before chemotherapy), for as many as six cycles. Complete remission or nodular partial response was achieved in 20 (17%) of 120 patients in the oblimersen group and in 8 (7%) of 121 patients receiving chemotherapy only ($p = 0.025$). Therapy with oblimersen was associated with a significant survival benefit ($p = 0.05$) in this study *(48)*.

2.5. Angiogenesis

Once a nearly heretical concept, blocking the formation of new vessels to control tumor growth or to prevent its development now seems highly intuitive. As a physiologic process, angiogenesis is inherent to life. There is no growth without a proportional supply of blood, oxygen, and nutrients. In contrast, pathologic angiogenesis, which satisfies the requirement for invasive tumor growth and metastasis, is largely responsible for conditions such as cancer, psoriasis, rheumatoid arthritis, and endometriosis *(49)*. The application of the concept of antiangiogenesis was introduced nearly three decades ago by Judah Folkman. In doing so, Folkman developed one of the most controversial and successful areas of investigation and therapy in cancer medicine *(50)*.

A quarter-century later, several monoclonal antibodies—cetuximab (Erbitux), bevacizumab (Avastin)—and small molecules—gefitinib (Iressa), sunitinib (Sutent)—targeting proangiogenic pathways have been approved by the FDA for various tumor types. Angiogenesis is implicated in different biologic stages of hematologic malignancies and solid tumors. Angiogenesis is likely to be involved in the early stages of carcinogenesis, when mutations in normal cells result in cancer cells (in situ) and later when further gene modulation, growth, and migration occur *(51)*. The molecular elements associated with angiogenesis are critical to a greater or lesser degree in a large number of human cancers, if not all, and thus are a prime focus of targeted anticancer therapy. It is possible for future adjuvant anticancer therapeutic approaches to include angiogenic inhibition.

2.6. Immune Modulation

Cancer immunotherapy has largely failed to meet our expectations *(52,53)*. Despite extensive research, progress, and a more complete understanding of this field, the immune recognition of human malignancy remains one of the greatest challenges in cancer medicine. Several immune-modulating approaches have been attempted, and many others are currently being investigated *(54)*. A significant obstacle to further understanding and developing immune-enhancing strategies is the lack of well validated immune monitoring assays *(53)*. Work by Allison and collaborators during the past decade demonstrated the importance of negative T-cell co-stimulatory molecules in human malignancy *(20)*. Among them, the cytotoxic T lymphocyte-associated antigen-4 (CTLA4) is an intracellular negative T-cell regulator expressed by T cells during their activation process *(55)*. Activation of cellular immunity requires an initial interaction between T cells, antigens, and antigen-presenting cells (APCs) (or tumors). The initial step includes the recognition of the antigen by the APCs and its presentation to naive T cells via a T-cell receptor and a major histocompatibility complex receptor. Subsequently, co-stimulatory receptors located on the surface of T cells and APCs interact to complete T-cell activation and expansion. Once the activation process begins, CTLA4 is expressed to the cellular surface of T cells and competes with CD28 (a positive regulator) for its ligands—B7.1 and B7.2 (CD80 and CD86)—located on the surface of APCs. However, a greater CTLA4 affinity for these ligands results in more avid CTLA4 binding and immune down-regulation *(56)*. Therefore, monoclonal antibodies targeting CTLA4 exert immune-enhancing effects by disrupting peripheral immune tolerance, a mechanism associated with carcinogenesis in immune-suppressed patients.

At present, two human monoclonal antibodies are under development: CP-675206 (Pfizer, Groton, CT, USA) and ipilimumab (Medarex-BMS, Princeton, NJ. USA). Both agents are in advanced steps of the approval process and have thus far proven relatively safe, with demonstrated efficacy in the treatment of human malignancies *(57,58)*. Clinical trials in earlier phases of development to test the antitumor activity of CTLA4 blockade in patients with prostate, ovarian, lymphoma, renal cell, and breast carcinoma are also underway *(59–61)*. Combinations of available agents with other immune-modulating strategies in the future will build further on our present knowledge and open new research avenues.

3. CHALLENGES ASSOCIATED WITH TARGETED ANTICANCER AGENTS

3.1. Drug-Related Challenges

Some of the attributes of an ideal targeted compound include optimal target selectivity, validation of the biologic target, a predictable pharmacokinetic profile (oral formulation or monthly/annual parenteral/subcutaneous administration), minimal toxicity, minimal drug–drug interactions, and a low cost-efficacy ratio. The physical properties of an agent are critical as they largely determine variables such as delivery and distribution. Because most targets are within the cell, efficient diffusion across cell membranes is also highly desirable, especially because inadequate intracellular drug concentrations may promote the rapid development of tumor resistance. Determining optimal target concentrations and intracellular drug levels is difficult and is not performed routinely *(62)*.

Modifying the physical properties of anticancer agents to improve their pharmacodynamic behavior is a continuous challenge. Several investigators have attempted to modify the parental drug; the success of these efforts is best exemplified by modulations including pegylation of agents such as growth factors and interferon. These modifications generally result in longer half-lives and at least similar efficacy (63,64). New pegylated agents may prove to be of greater benefit.

3.1.1. MONOCLONAL ANTIBODIES

Antibody-based compounds usually target surface receptors that, under pathologic conditions, drive cancer growth, prevent cell death, or suppress immune functions. Another option is to target antigens specific to cancer cells (e.g., anti-CD33, anti-CD20) directly, thereby killing the tumor population. Immunoglobulin G (IgG) constitutes approximately 75% of all human serum immunoglobulin and is the most commonly used class of antibodies. Its molecular weight is approximately 155 kDa, with a half-life of approximately 21 days (except for that of IgG3, which is 7 days). The large size of these compounds confers relatively slow diffusion across tissues, and their convective flows may be adversely affected by the high interstitial pressure of tumors (62). In fact, immunoscintigraphy studies demonstrate that under ideal circumstances only 0.01% to 0.10% of intravenously administered monoclonal antibodies reach and bind to parenchymal targets (65). Their structural and kinetic characteristics give these antibodies obvious advantages and disadvantages relative to small molecules.

Several types of antibody have been developed. At present, the fully humanized constructs are generally accepted as safe and predictable for use as platforms to target several surface proteins. A different construct, single-chain antibodies (scFv), are generally smaller, which allows greater tumor penetration and faster clearance rates.

When binding their target, monoclonal antibodies can induce antibody-dependent cell-mediated cytotoxicity (ADCC) or complement-dependent mediated cytotoxicity. Recent data suggest that the addition of cytotoxic agents to monoclonal antibody therapy results in enhanced ADCC (66). In this study, the authors demonstrated increased trastuzumab therapy-associated ADCC in 9 patients receiving trastuzumab in combination with paclitaxel compared with 19 patients receiving the antibody alone. A significant increment in the number of natural killer (NK) cells was found in association with the observed ADCC. These data shed further light on the augmented efficacy of antibodies when combined with chemotherapy. In addition to their intrinsic ability to induce cytotoxicity, antibodies can deliver toxins, radionuclides, cytokines, and other cytotoxins that kill cells through their internalization after binding to their target with exquisite specificity (67). Initial concerns about the induction of human anti-human antibodies have gradually dissolved with the emergence of fully humanized forms of these constructs. Production of monoclonal antibodies has improved rapidly and dramatically, and these agents have been proven efficacious in several diagnostic and therapeutic settings.

3.1.2. SMALL MOLECULES

Small-molecule compounds are characterized by a molecular weight < 1000 kDa and structural properties that clearly make them more attractive than their larger counterparts when used to target various structures inside the cell. Oral administration is possible for most of these compounds, and their pharmacologic profiles are well defined in most instances (68). Given that most small molecules target the ATP binding site in kinases, an initial challenge was to compete efficiently with high intracellular ATP concentrations (2–10 mM) and to attain drug specificity for the ATP-binding site, which is an evolutionarily well conserved region in nearly all kinases. However, small molecules have been developed against ligands, receptors, protein tyrosine kinases, phosphatase kinases, and other intracellular signaling molecules; and this well-funded concern was cleared over time. (For an excellent review, please see Arslan et al *(69)*). Several novel small molecules are currently in development or undergoing final steps for FDA approval for different indications.

3.1.3. Small Interfering RNAs

RNA interference is a protective mechanism employed by eukaryotic cells to suppress the expression of genes that are critical to vital cell functions. It is also a defense mechanism that shields the host's genome from the incorporation of viruses and other small living organisms. Small interfering RNAs (siRNAs) are effector molecules that, when introduced into cells, can silence specific genes and modulate intracellular signaling *(70)*. The process is driven by a dicer nuclease (RNase-III type, a member of the RNase III superfamily of bidentate nucleases), which cleaves double-stranded DNA into siRNA fractions, which are 21 to 23 nucleotides in size. The siRNA fraction is capable of forming RNA-induced silencing complexes (RISCs). Driven by the antisense strand of siRNA, the RISC recognizes and cleaves complementary mRNA in the cytoplasm via endoribonuclease.

siRNAs can be severalfold more efficient in catalyzing reactions than ribozymes or antisense oligonucleotides *(71)*. Despite its obvious advantages, this technology is not devoid of potential pitfalls: It appears that efficient, highly specific mRNA cleavage may require a high degree of complementarity. Other concerns are the potential induction of interferon responses through toll-like receptors, alerting the immune system of a potential "viral" attack, and off-target effects secondary to binding of "similar" mRNA sequences *(71)*. Thus far, preclinical studies are promising, and Phase I studies are underway.

3.1.4. Nanoparticles

Nanovectors are vehicles in the 1- to 1000-nm range (from a few atoms to subcellular size) capable of carrying anticancer drugs in their interior or attached to their surface. These compounds generally are composed of three parts: a core constituent material, a loaded therapeutic particle or imaging device agent, and a surface biologic modifier with the ability to target specific cellular molecules *(72)*. Nanovectors also can affect specific genes when used for tumor-specific gene delivery. siRNA-nanovectors can also be used to deliver siRNA efficiently to human tumors in vitro and in vivo. Liposomes are the most basic form of nanovectors. (For an excellent review, see Ferrari *(72)*). Perhaps the greatest advantage of this delivery technology lies in its ability to traverse anatomic and physiologic barriers (blood-brain barrier, reticuloendothelial system) and deliver its load. In theory, nanotechnology could potentially solve many of the present drug delivery challenges and substantially improve the imaging and early detection techniques currently available.

3.2. Target-Related Challenges

The ability of an agent to bind and modulate a selected target specifically has major therapeutic implications. Although specificity has been much desired, a lack of it has not necessarily represented a therapeutic disadvantage. The recruitment of neighbor molecules may block alternate signaling pathways or kill diverse cells in the local microenvironment, providing a wider range of therapeutic applications. An exacerbation of systemic toxic effects, however, is an obvious concern.

Several structural characteristics must be considered when designing targeted molecules. Among them, an important consideration is the shape of the protein–protein interface; this poses a challenge because the surface included in the interface is usually about 750 to 1500 Å *(2)*. Nonetheless, the entire surface is not necessarily included in the "hot spot"; and finding the specific site to bind may require substantial effort. Stoichiometry and the site of binding are additional concerns. These binding sites are adaptive and flexible, properties that may preclude satisfactory access to the target.

3.2.1. TARGET SPECIFICITY

Targeting highly specific molecular abnormalities requires validation of molecular markers and may restrict the patient population that can benefit from a specific approach (i.e., BCR-ABL). In contrast, successfully modulating less selective targets (either surface receptors or targets common to many biologic processes) will likely affect a large number of patients suffering from cancer and other disorders. Angiogenesis is common to most human cancers. A popular example of the success of this approach is bevacizumab, a fully humanized monoclonal antibody directed against vascular endothelial growth factor (VEGF), a prominent angiogenesis promoter. Bevacizumab combinations have been approved by the FDA for the treatment of patients with advanced colorectal, lung, and breast carcinoma. Furthermore, applications of antiangiogenesis strategies have extended to other disciplines and have positively affected the natural course of patients with macular degeneration or other vitreal disorders *(73,74)*. Understanding the selectivity of different targets and pathways and the impact their modulation will likely have on various physiopathologic processes will allow the reader to develop well designed clinical trials and programs to intervene in different cancer stages and other medical conditions (Table 1).

3.2.2. TARGET VALIDATION

Although target overexpression was initially thought to be necessary for the success of molecularly targeted therapies, recent data suggest that overexpression of the target in tumor tissues does not necessarily correlate with modulation of cellular functions after exposure to targeted agents. An example of this is the fact that epidermal growth factor receptor (EGFR) expression is not detectable in acute myeloid leukemia (AML) blasts, although exposure to gefitinib, an EGFR inhibitor, results in morphologic and genomic differentiation of AML cells in vitro. Furthermore, overexpression of a target does not necessarily translate to clinical benefit with treatment. A good example is the experience with gefitinib in patients with non-small-cell lung cancer, where mutations of the receptor were ultimately responsible for its activity *(75)*. Identification of these mutations is cumbersome and requires extensive investment and analysis of tumor tissues. However, the ultimate delineation of each agent's biologic effects will substantially narrow the target population and serve highly personalized approaches.

At the time targeted molecular therapies emerged in the clinical research arena, representatives of several clinical research committees and institutional review boards (myself included) critically reviewed protocols that included patients without known molecular abnormalities in the proposed target. Over time, responses were seen in several of these patients. Lack of target specificity was likely responsible for these fortunate outcomes. In other instances, the initially postulated target was only one among many modulated targets, albeit unknown. Agents with known biologic activity but little efficacy against diseases known to express the target were withdrawn from further development. A clear example is the farnesyltransferase inhibitors R115777, BMS-214662, and SCH 66336, agents that were developed to target malignancies with RAS mutations. The biologic targets were initially believed to be farnesyltransferases, a group of enzymes responsible for transferring a farnesyl group from farnesyl pyrophosphate to the pre-RAS protein. Farnesyl is necessary to attach RAS to the cell membrane; and if RAS does not attach, it is unable to transfer signals from membrane receptors. Inhibition of farnesyltransferases was documented in most trials. Only one of these agents continued development (R115777, tipifarnib, Zarnestra; Johnson & Johnson, Piscataway, NJ. USA). Subsequent research and clinical experience proved that farnesyltransferase was not, however, the main target affected by these agents and that RAS overexpression was not necessary for tumors to respond to this group of agents *(76)*. Similarly, geranylgeranyltransferase I, a related enzyme in charge of transferring a geranyl-geranyl group, a 20-carbon isoprenoid, to K- and N-RAS, was subsequently identified as another potential target. The ultimate FDA approval for farnesyltransferase inhibitors may be for the treatment of patients with myelodysplasia. Future studies in leukemia may combine these agents with dasatinib, a dual Src-Abl kinase inhibitor.

3.3. Tumor-Related Challenges

Human neoplasms involve well over 200 processes. Although some depend almost exclusively on the oncogenic activity of a protein mutation in its early stages of development, most malignant conditions accumulate molecular transformations that ultimately dictate the biologic nature of each process.

3.3.1. TUMOR RESISTANCE

Drug resistance and treatment-related toxicities are major obstacles to the development of cancer agents. Several mechanisms of tumor resistance have been identified during the last decade (Table 2). However, this conundrum remains a major obstacle to the success of various cancer therapies.

Among the mechanisms of drug resistance, drug–drug interactions, with host proteins and enzymatic processes, and the genomic response to their exposure remain of utmost importance. Extracellular and intracellular levels of cellular proteins play a substantial role in these physiologic processes, and their variation may result in drug inactivation. For example, more

Table 2
Mechanisms of Tumor Resistance

Mechanism	Reference
Mutation of target kinase	*(150,151)*
Amplification of target genes	*(13)*
Activation of alternate pathways and downstream elements (cross talk)	
Overexpression of the target (in response to a ligand or targeted agent)	
Epigenetic abnormalities	*(152)*
DNA repair	*(77)*
Drug inactivation	*(77)*
Activation of drug resistance genes (activation of drug efflux pumps)	*(77)*

than 80% of fluorouracil is metabolized by dihydropyrimidine dehydrogenase (DPD) in the liver. Hence, tumor overexpression of DPD has been demonstrated in association with tumor resistance to fluorouracil-based regimens *(77)*. Other examples of drug inactivation include the conjugation of platinum and its derivatives with glutathione (GSH) and subsequent inactivation *(78)*. Similarly, genomic and proteomic events governing influx and efflux cellular mechanisms are also responsible for the regulation of drug exposure and a known mechanism of tumor resistance. DNA repair is another largely responsible event involved in tumor death and resistance. (For an excellent review see Longley and Johnston *(77)*.)

The individual toxicities and efficacies of anticancer agents administered at similar doses to different individuals are well established. The field of pharmacogenomics will further establish the genetic factors associated with these differences, as liver and renal function alone do not sufficiently explain interindividual biologic differences in response to various therapeutic agents *(79)*.

DNA sequence abnormalities and the expression of mRNA molecules and proteins predict tumor response to cytotoxic drugs *(79,80)*. A good example of the importance of human genotype polymorphisms on treatment-related toxicities is CYP3A5 polymorphisms and their association with the severity of toxicities associated with irinotecan, a topoisomerase I inhibitor catalyzed by cytochrome P450 (CYP). One Phase III study compared systemic fluorouracil and leucovorin in one arm with a combination of irinotecan, fluorouracil, and leucovorin in another arm among 400 patients with high-risk stage III colorectal carcinoma after surgical resection of their primary tumor. Côté et al. recently studied the genotype profiles of 184 patients treated in this clinical trial and correlated their findings with the toxicities experienced by these patients. UGT1A1*28 homozygous patients experienced greater hematologic toxicities (50%) than UGT1A1*1 homozygous patients (16.2%, $p = 0.06$). This study supports the benefit of identifying UGT1A1 promoter polymorphisms before administering irinotecan-based therapies. Furthermore, the -3156G>A polymorphism in this population seemed to better predict hematologic toxicities than the UGT1A1 (TA)6TAA>(TA)7TAA polymorphism *(81)*. Because of situations like this, the incorporation of pharmacogenomic analysis early in drug development has gained great interest and is the subject of substantial investigation. Although limiting the number of agents that reach advanced levels of preclinical and clinical development, this discipline is likely to produce future safety benefits, leading to improved efficacy.

4. DRUG DEVELOPMENT PROCESS

4.1. Clinical Development and Marketing Approval

Drug development in cancer medicine is highly selective and costly. It is estimated that about 1 of every 5000 compounds investigated enters clinical testing. The expenditure of developing medications from the bench to the clinic has been estimated at between US $800 million and US $1.7 billion over a period of 7.3 years *(82,83)*. Finally, only 1 of every 20 agents for which an investigational new drug application is filed is ultimately approved by the FDA *(83)*.

Similarly, sophisticated refinements in biotechnologic modalities have exponentially increased the prices of the final products. An example commonly cited is the evolution of therapy-derived costs in colorectal cancer. In this setting, the price of therapeutic regimens has increased 340-fold during the last decade. The expenses associated with two courses of systemic therapy in the United States are on the order of US $40,000 per patient (including scans, laboratory studies, and infusion unit access) *(84)*. If not controlled, the financial burden on patients and health systems worldwide will make our new, targeted strategies accessible to only a few patients and may ultimately jeopardize cancer care even in the wealthiest societies.

4.2. Study Endpoints

The mechanisms for FDA approval of anticancer drugs have been recently modified *(85,86)*. In the past, to attain investigational new drug approval for a particular indication, a minimum of two well controlled, prospective, randomized trials were required. The outcome required a survival and/or quality of life benefit analysis prior to FDA approval. Improvement in overall survival was always regarded as the primary endpoint for these Phase III studies. The use of historical controls was, for the most part, unacceptable. However, alternative endpoints recently accepted by the FDA for drug approval include progression-free survival, time to tumor progression, quality of life, and of course overall survival *(87,88)*.

4.2.1. Endpoints Based on Tumor Assessment

Regardless of the endpoints selected for drug approval, the sponsor and the FDA must prospectively agree on each of the following prior to starting the approval process: study design, definition of disease progression, data to be captured in the case report forms, statistical analysis plan, methods employed to handle missing and deficient data, data sharing and censoring methodology, and operating procedures of an independent endpoint review committee *(89)*. Study endpoints based on tumor assessments include disease-free survival (DFS), objective response rate (ORR), time to progression (TTP), progression-free survival (PFS), and time to treatment failure (TTF). Compared with TTP, PFS is the preferred endpoint as it includes deaths and hence can better reflect overall survival.

4.2.1.1. Tumor Assessment Challenges. With the advent of newer therapies, our ability to induce long periods of tumor stability has substantially modified the way we assess patients after therapy and made us more cautious about defining clinical benefit. Unlike cytotoxic regimens, targeted therapies may be able to induce longer periods of disease stability and provide improved quality of life to our patients. With this premise in mind, our assessment of clinical benefit has to be tuned accordingly. The RECIST (response evaluation criteria in solid tumors) guidelines were developed in 2000 in an attempt to standardize tumor assessment, incorporating radiographic techniques available at the time *(90)*. Since their development, however, new technologies have emerged, and novel compounds repeatedly challenge our traditional approach to tumor evaluation. For example, another important lesson learned from the GIST/imatinib experience was that targeted therapies have the potential to induce objective responses even when initial radiographic evaluations are consistent with tumor growth *(91)*. Whereas this is a common phenomenon in immunotherapy, this situation had not previously been encountered with cytotoxic-based therapies. Although images of lesions during or after treatment may indicate growth of tumor tissue, this tumor growth is concomitantly characterized by central liquefaction of the tumor and necrosis, so the bulk of tumor subsequently regresses in size and eventually disappears. These observations are now more common with several other agents and pose an additional challenge in targeted drug development: the pitfalls of using existing tumor assessment guidelines in the setting of novel targeted therapies and their impact on the interpretation of antitumor responses and trial results.

Unfortunately, several of the newer radiographic techniques remain to be validated, and their incorporation into our standard tumor assessment guidelines is a slow but continuously evolving process. The validation and application of several techniques, such as positron emission tomography/computed tomography (PET/CT) imaging, dynamic contrast enhanced magnetic resonance imaging (DCE/MRI), and others, are much needed; and their contribution to the interpretation of cancer therapies in the future is exciting and potentially beneficial. It is quite likely that the incorporation of these techniques and other assessment tools (i.e., tumor markers, organ function measurements) to RECIST 2.0 criteria will improve the tumor assessment guidelines uniformly employed in clinical investigation. These issues are to be carefully considered when planning clinical trials critical to FDA approval of a given agent. Other promising technologies for the interpretation of therapeutic efficacy include surrogate markers and biomarkers as they may accurately predict patient populations likely to benefit from therapy.

5. CONSIDERATIONS OF POTENTIAL FUTURE APPROACHES

5.1. Imatinib Mesylate: Outlier or Precursor of a New Era of Successful Therapies in Cancer Medicine?

Although the CML experience of the last decade remains an example to emulate, I believe the complexity that most obstructs our success in the battle against cancer is *tumor heterogeneity*. To best understand the multiple challenges presented by targeted therapies, the reader must think of human malignancy as a dysfunctional biologic cellular cascade in which multiple molecular and genetic steps lead to degenerative and permanent modifications that affect vital functions such as growth, differentiation, migration, and survival. The deregulation of one of these processes (or several at one time) results in immortalized, uncontrolled cells that host highly sophisticated survival mechanisms. Certain tumors are classic examples of one specific dysfunctional mechanism, whereas others, indeed most solid tumors, result from a plethora of abnormalities that ultimately rule the vital functions of cancer cells.

The complexity of this process is much greater if we also concur with the notion that these independent cells have the ability to manipulate their microenvironment and surrounding tissues *(92)*. A simplistic view of this problem is, in my mind, best exemplified by CML. Early in the course of this disease, BCR-ABL is the dominant molecular abnormality. The BCR-ABL oncoprotein has constitutive tyrosine kinase activity secondary to oligomerization of $p210^{BCR/ABL}$ and deletion of the inhibitory part of ABL. Inhibition of the oncogenic activity of BCR-ABL with imatinib mesylate induces remission and controls the neoplastic process in the early stages of disease (chronic phase). In contrast, our ability to control the cellular growth at later stages (accelerated and blastic phases), when a larger number of new clones with acquired mutations have developed, is far more limited. The result is a larger number of treatment failures and tumor recurrence in advanced disease stages (Fig. 2).

Studies carried out by Schmitt and others in murine lymphomas support this concept. Transplanting mixed populations of Bcl-2–expressing murine stem cell virus-infected and uninfected cells derived from the same primary lymphoma into recipient mice, these investigators monitored the percentage of Bcl-2–overexpressing cells in the lymph node tumor cells of the recipient at baseline and after therapy with cyclophosphamide. As expected, the fraction of Bcl-2–overexpressing cells increased during tumor formation in vivo. Subsequent cyclophosphamide therapy produced homogeneous Bcl-2–overexpressing lymphomas within

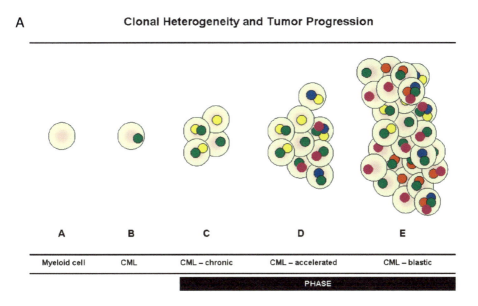

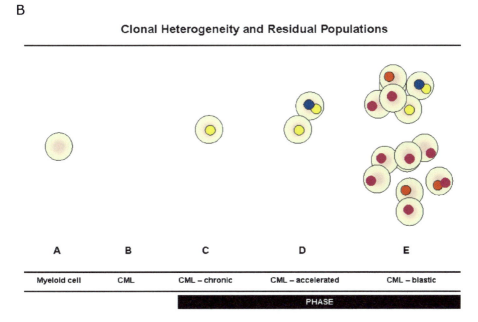

Fig. 2. A Clonal heterogeneity in chronic myeloid cells (CML). A, normal myeloid precursor. B, translocation of chromosomes 11 and 22 results in BCR-ABL with CML transformation. C, chronic phase CML. D, accelerated phase CML. E, blastic phase CML. Accumulation of molecular and genetic abnormalities results in modification of biologic behavior and overall resistance. **B** Treatment with imatinib mesylate results in inhibition of BCR-ABL (green dots) and control of cellular populations in which the oncogenic activity of BCR-ABL is responsible for the biologic behavior of the malignant clone. The accumulation of mutations and inhibition of sensitive clones unveils resistant cellular populations that maintain the biologic characteristics acquired over time. This model matches the clinical, hematologic, and molecular responses to imatinib therapy.

6 days. In other words, the treatment failure rapidly selected for pure Bcl-2–overexpressing tumors (resistant clones) from baseline heterogeneous tumor populations *(93)*.

5.2. Targeted Therapies Against Solid Malignancies: As Successful as Those Directed Against Their Hematologic Counterparts?

Hematologic malignancies and solid tumors differ greatly from a biologic and therapeutic standpoint. However, targeted therapies may close this gap. First, the easier access to tumor tissue for most hematologic neoplasms than for their solid counterparts is perhaps responsible for our much greater understanding of the morphologic and molecular features of hematologic cancers. This, in turn, has resulted in more comprehensive histologic and molecular classifications and even further treatment and research on these disorders *(94)*. Among the solid tumors, only breast and prostate cancers have reasonably effective treatments based on expression of molecular differences, namely tissue expression of hormonal receptors and, more recently, HER2. Identification of the latter had profound implications for the prognosis and therapy of breast cancer and has set the stage for ongoing and future investigations in other tumor types. For most other solid tumors, however, our understanding is still quite limited, and we continue to treat patients with regimens developed against malignancies on the basis of their organ of origin or their morphologic appearance.

While the ultimate goal of therapy is the same for all cancers, the historical approach to hematologic cancers is to destroy the majority of blood cells affected by cancer and to provide support until the host recovers fully. The hope then is to eradicate malignant cells and allow normal cells to regrow without malignant contamination. Hence, highly toxic therapies are accepted. For patients with solid neoplasms, on the other hand, the goal is to treat tumors with large populations of resistant cells while affecting the host as little as possible.

Despite these fundamental differences, the biology and clonal evolution of hematologic and solid malignancies are similar in many ways. Like hematologic neoplasms, solid tumors are the result of molecular mutations in normal cells. Early therapy controls these clones in most instances. However, the development of subsequent mutations and changes in the tumor microenvironment are responsible for cellular migration and tumor resistance. At that point, tumors are largely incurable, and patients usually die of their disease.

5.3. Combined Therapies

Combining agents directed against different targets is a natural option for bypassing therapeutic limitations such as tumor heterogeneity and multiple resistance mechanisms. In 1965, James Holland, Emil Frei, and Emil Freireich postulated that, like therapy for tuberculosis, cancer therapies should include combinations of medications with different anticancer mechanisms *(95)*. Historical examples of success with this approach are ABVD (adriamycin, bleomycin, vinblastine, dacarbazine) for Hodgkin's disease, CHOP (cyclophosphamide, doxorubicin, vincristine, prednisone) for lymphoma, MVAC (methotrexate, Velban, doxorubicin or cyclophosphamide) for bladder cancer, and BEP (bleomycin, etoposide, cisplatin) for testicular cancer. This treatment approach represented a major milestone in the cancer battle. However, although combination therapies result in higher response rates in most tumor types, there is greater toxicity and minimal or no impact on survival. This important concept attests to the fact that despite substantial progress in drug development and technology during the past four decades our challenges remain, to a large extent, unchanged.

Potential combinations of targeted therapies include agents affecting one or several mechanisms of action and individual or multiple signaling pathways through modulation of different molecular targets *(96)*. A rational design for these combinations requires extensive knowledge of tumor and molecular biology, integrating the particular toxic effects and interactions among these compounds. Potential avenues to explore include maximal inhibition of a pathway (inhibiting receptor and downstream elements), maximal inhibition of a target (antibody plus small molecule), inhibition of complementary pathways (e.g., inhibition of RAS and elements of the PI3K pathway), and targeting different biologic mechanisms (e.g., angiogenesis inhibitors plus mTOR or apoptosis elements). (For an excellent review, see Dancey and Chen *(97)*). Useful design strategies ideally integrate traditional cytotoxic agents or combinations thereof with targeted agents that have demonstrated biologic activity but low clinical efficacy when administered alone. An example of the importance of combining cytotoxic agents with targeted agents is in the setting of apoptosis. Whereas chemotherapy and/or radiation therapy induce cell death through modulation of elements in the intrinsic pathway, targeting tumor necrosis factor (TNF)-related apoptosis-inducing ligand (TRAIL) and its death receptors effectively alters signaling through the extrinsic pathway. Current research explores these approaches, which already are proving somewhat efficacious *(98)*.

The rapid availability of compounds directed against specific targets has become challenging to scientists, investigators, and regulatory agencies. Nonetheless, combining anticancer agents is once again identified as critical to making progress in the ongoing cancer treatment process and to the ultimate success of cancer research. This strategy is now possible, to a certain extent, through concerted efforts of the National Cancer Institute through the Cancer and Therapeutics Evaluation Program, industry, and independent groups of investigators during the early and late stages of drug development. Albeit theoretically reasonable, combining these agents may be hampered by their limited individual efficacies, intellectual property issues, and high treatment-related costs.

5.4. Tumor Tissue Banking

As tumor banks are developed and new technologies, such as microarrays, for the study of tumor tissues become readily available and less expensive, it is critical that large numbers of tumor specimens be collected and resources rigorously devoted to the analysis of their molecular profiles. More importantly, while strictly protecting the identity and rights of patients, the analysis of these tissue specimens should include correlation with clinical information and treatment outcomes.

We must also keep in mind that several fundamental principles of medicine were developed through postmortem examinations. However, the rate of autopsies has decreased dramatically over the past few decades *(99)* and the reasons are poorly understood. Multiple studies indicate attitude changes relating to factors such as patient age, the requesting physician, cause of death, and country of death. In any case, this phenomenon is worldwide, and little is being done to remediate it. The analysis of tumor and tissue material after participation in clinical trials must continue to be emphasized. Furthermore, these analyses may provide greater insight into tumor heterogeneity and tumor distribution. Nonetheless, prompt tissue recovery for molecular analysis makes this approach expensive and limited to few facilities.

5.5. *Prompt Access to Investigational Compounds*

The rapid availability of investigational compounds undergoing early clinical testing to patient populations in which a benefit has been demonstrated a priori should be strongly considered for several reasons *(100)*. First, and perhaps most important, is the fact that advanced cancer is a rapidly progressive process from which life span is seriously limited. Patients with metastatic cancer cannot afford to wait for the results of Phase III studies and subsequent FDA approval. Importantly, this particular patient population is usually not eligible for Phase II and III clinical trials because of the number of previous therapies, mild to moderate organ dysfunction from previous therapies, or administration of standard treatments containing one of the agents included in the comparison arm. A major challenge to consider when supporting prompt access to new compounds is the need to include patients with largely preserved organ function and performance. Failing to do so will result in greater treatment-related toxicities and a marginal risk-benefit ratio, further affecting the drug development process.

Second, the treatment of these patients and their tissue analysis will serve the scientific community and our society in general to better understand a given tumor type and metabolic differences between responders and nonresponders. Following these steps will considerably accelerate the drug development process and delineate future applications for each agent. In turn, the FDA and other regulatory agencies could reward sponsors adhering to this modus operandi by allowing the safety and scientific data obtained from these "compassionate cohorts" to be included in their approval packages. As data mature, the doses and schedules of these compassionate trials could be modified through timely amendments.

Third, the quickest route to personalized cancer medicine is early access to investigational new compounds that have known biologic effects on specific targets and adequate safety profiles identified in earlier studies. The concept of personalized cancer therapeutics is not a new one. In fact, it is a well known objective since the late 1950s *(101)*. However, the continuous discovery of existing molecular and biologic mechanisms in hosts and tumors has further heightened our hope to treat cancer patients with highly selective anticancer agents with low toxicity profiles. The recognition of pathway deregulation specific to tumor types and individuals is unfortunately not sufficient. A larger number of targeted agents are required to explore their efficacy when administered alone or in combination with other molecular modulators.

An alternative approach is to continue to develop drugs in a traditional fashion and to test the tumors of responders versus those who do not respond to therapy and characterize the specific target mutations likely responsible for the treatment outcome *(10,102)*. However, this approach has thus far proven lengthy and expensive. Notwithstanding, the mechanisms for drug testing, development, and approval have to rapidly adapt to the technologic advances and the ethical challenges presented by this rapidly evolving field.

6. CONCLUSIONS

The technological and scientific progress over the last three decades has had a dramatic impact on the approach to cancer therapeutics. Designed "targeted" molecular therapies require the application of specific biologic, molecular, and genomic knowledge in addition to the traditional "organ of origin" and morphologic features of human cancer. Moreover, these tailored molecular therapies are more "scientifically rational" and exhibit better safety profiles.

As in the era of cytotoxic agents, the accumulation of molecular abnormalities at different structural and functional levels accounts for rapid development of tumor resistance and treatment failure. We still have good opportunities to control malignant clones when fewer of these changes have occurred, and the growth and malignant biology of the tumor is in the control of one or few of these aberrant changes. However, in advanced tumor stages, when multiple metastatic implants carry large cell logs with innumerable molecular abnormalities, our task is more difficult and our chances of success fewer.

To decrease cancer mortality across all tumor types successfully, several objectives must be considered. First and foremost, we must develop generalized knowledge of the most common molecular abnormalities shared by different tumor types and a correlation between responders and nonresponders so we can identify the patient population that will most likely benefit from the targeted agents under development. That requires numerous clinical protocols that allow tumor biopsies once clinical responses are in progress.

The traditional sequential approach to drug development has changed substantially. For the initial anticancer compounds, findings of early in vitro experiments and data from in vivo models and animal toxicity studies were extensively reviewed before first-in-human clinical studies. However, animal models have historically demonstrated little, if any, ability to predict clinical outcome in humans *(103)*. Novel targeted therapies require highly reliable information regarding the biology and the potential biologic events resulting from modulation of the target. By the time a target is selected, information regarding its specificity to tumor tissues, its degree of expression or mutation in tumor cells, the role in cellular functions, or its importance to particular neoplastic processes is known. A subsequent series of studies involving advanced structural chemistry techniques takes place; and in most instances a series of analogues is evaluated comprehensively prior to the decision to move its development to the clinical setting. Nonetheless, toxicity data requirements have changed only minimally.

Despite these rapid advances in technology, we must not forget that the ultimate goal for tailored molecular therapies should be to address molecular signatures specific to each individual's disease process. This objective requires many more targeted agents and a faster drug development process.

A final but critical aspect to incorporate into our objectives is to understand that earlier access to human testing is necessary. Continued efforts and new mechanisms to promote clinical studies testing drug combinations in humans are most needed. Drastic modifications to the regulatory obstacles of our current drug development process must take place to reach patients with advanced cancer earlier, increase patient accessibility to novel compounds, and decrease the costs of drug development.

REFERENCES

1. Druker BJ, Tamura S, Buchdunger E, et al. Effects of a selective inhibitor of the Abl tyrosine kinase on the growth of Bcr-Abl positive cells. Nat Med 1996;2(5):561–6.
2. O'Brien SG, Guilhot F, Larson RA, et al. Imatinib compared with interferon and low-dose cytarabine for newly diagnosed chronic-phase chronic myeloid leukemia. N Engl J Med 2003;348(11):994–1004.
3. Van Oosterom AT, Judson I, Verweij J, et al. Safety and efficacy of imatinib (STI571) in metastatic gastrointestinal stromal tumours: a phase I study. Lancet 2001;358(9291):1421–3.
4. Demetri GD, von Mehren M, Blanke CD, et al. Efficacy and safety of imatinib mesylate in advanced gastrointestinal stromal tumors. N Engl J Med 2002;347(7):472–80.
5. Wyman K, Atkins MB, Prieto V, et al. Multicenter phase II trial of high-dose imatinib mesylate in metastatic melanoma: significant toxicity with no clinical efficacy. Cancer 2006;106(9):2005–11.
6. Vuky J, Isacson C, Fotoohi M, et al. Phase II trial of imatinib (Gleevec) in patients with metastatic renal cell carcinoma. Invest New Drugs 2006;24(1):85–8.

7. Gross DJ, Munter G, Bitan M, et al. The role of imatinib mesylate (Glivec) for treatment of patients with malignant endocrine tumors positive for c-kit or PDGF-R. Endocr Relat Cancer 2006;13(2):535–40.

8. Bond M, Bernstein ML, Pappo A, et al. A phase II study of imatinib mesylate in children with refractory or relapsed solid tumors: a Children's Oncology Group study. Pediatr Blood Cancer 2007 Jan 29; [Epub ahead of print].

9. Hirota S, Isozaki K, Moriyama Y, et al. Gain-of-function mutations of c-kit in human gastrointestinal stromal tumors. Science 1998;279(5350):577–80.

10. Heinrich MC, Corless CL, Demetri GD, et al. Kinase mutations and imatinib response in patients with metastatic gastrointestinal stromal tumor. J Clin Oncol 2003;21(23):4342–9.

11. Druker BJ. Imatinib: paradigm or anomaly? Cell Cycle 2004;3(7):833–5.

12. Heinrich MC, Corless CL, Duensing A, et al. PDGFRA activating mutations in gastrointestinal stromal tumors. Science 2003;299(5607):708–10.

13. Gorre ME, Mohammed M, Ellwood K, et al. Clinical resistance to STI-571 cancer therapy caused by BCR-ABL gene mutation or amplification. Science 2001;293(5531):876–80.

14. Sawyers CL. Research on resistance to cancer drug Gleevec. Science 2001;294(5548):1834.

15. Donato NJ, Wu JY, Stapley J, et al. Imatinib mesylate resistance through BCR-ABL independence in chronic myelogenous leukemia. Cancer Res 2004;64(2):672–7.

16. Shah NP, Nicoll JM, Nagar B, et al. Multiple BCR-ABL kinase domain mutations confer polyclonal resistance to the tyrosine kinase inhibitor imatinib (STI571) in chronic phase and blast crisis chronic myeloid leukemia. Cancer Cell 2002;2(2):117–25.

17. Shah NP, Tran C, Lee FY, et al. Overriding imatinib resistance with a novel ABL kinase inhibitor. Science 2004;305(5682):399–401.

18. Talpaz M, Shah NP, Kantarjian H, et al. Dasatinib in imatinib-resistant Philadelphia chromosome-positive leukemias. N Engl J Med 2006;354(24):2531–41.

19. Kantarjian H, O'Brien S, Cortes J, et al. Survival advantage with imatinib mesylate therapy in chronic-phase chronic myelogenous leukemia (CML-CP) after IFN-alpha failure and in late CML-CP, comparison with historical controls. Clin Cancer Res 2004;10(1 Pt 1):68–75.

20. Leach DR, Krummel MF, Allison JP. Enhancement of antitumor immunity by CTLA-4 blockade. Science 1996;271(5256):1734–6.

21. De The H, Chomienne C, Lanotte M, et al. The t(15;17) translocation of acute promyelocytic leukaemia fuses the retinoic acid receptor alpha gene to a novel transcribed locus. Nature 1990;347(6293):558–61.

22. Warrell RP Jr, de The H, Wang ZY, et al. Acute promyelocytic leukemia. N Engl J Med 1993;329(3):177–89.

23. Warrell RP Jr, Frankel SR, Miller WH Jr, et al. Differentiation therapy of acute promyelocytic leukemia with tretinoin (all-trans-retinoic acid). N Engl J Med 1991;324(20):1385–93.

24. Soignet SL, Maslak P, Wang ZG, et al. Complete remission after treatment of acute promyelocytic leukemia with arsenic trioxide. N Engl J Med 1998;339(19):1341–8.

25. Soignet SL, Frankel SR, Douer D, et al. United States multicenter study of arsenic trioxide in relapsed acute promyelocytic leukemia. J Clin Oncol 2001;19(18):3852–60.

26. He LZ, Tolentino T, Grayson P, et al. Histone deacetylase inhibitors induce remission in transgenic models of therapy-resistant acute promyelocytic leukemia. J Clin Invest 2001;108(9):1321–30.

27. Warrell RP Jr, He LZ, Richon V, et al. Therapeutic targeting of transcription in acute promyelocytic leukemia by use of an inhibitor of histone deacetylase. J Natl Cancer Inst 1998;90(21):1621–5.

28. Nan X, Ng HH, Johnson CA, et al. Transcriptional repression by the methyl-CpG-binding protein MeCP2 involves a histone deacetylase complex. Nature 1998;393:386–9.

29. Maslak P, Chanel S, Camacho LH, et al. Pilot study of combination transcriptional modulation therapy with sodium phenylbutyrate and 5-azacytidine in patients with acute myeloid leukemia or myelodysplastic syndrome. Leukemia 2006;20(2):212–7.

30. Gilbert J, Gore SD, Herman JG, et al. The clinical application of targeting cancer through histone acetylation and hypomethylation. Clin Cancer Res 2004;10(14):4589–96.

31. Gore SD, Baylin S, Sugar E, et al. Combined DNA methyltransferase and histone deacetylase inhibition in the treatment of myeloid neoplasms. Cancer Res 2006;66(12):6361–9.

32. Lo Coco F, Zelent A, Kimchi A, et al. Progress in differentiation induction as a treatment for acute promyelocytic leukemia and beyond. Cancer Res 2002;62(19):5618–21.

33. Soriano AO, Yang H, Tong W, et al. Significant clinical activity of the combination of 5-azacytidine, valproic acid and all-trans retinoic (ATRA) acid in leukemia: results of a phase I/II study. Blood 2006;108(11).

34. Burger JA, Kipps TJ. CXCR4: a key receptor in the crosstalk between tumor cells and their microenvironment. Blood 2006;107(5):1761–7.

35. Giles R, Loberg RD. Can we target the chemokine network for cancer therapeutics? Curr Cancer Drug Targets 2006;6(8):659–70.

36. Barber MA, Welch HC. PI3K and RAC signalling in leukocyte and cancer cell migration. Bull Cancer 2006;93(5):E44–52.
37. Peruzzi B, Bottaro DP. Targeting the c-Met signaling pathway in cancer. Clin Cancer Res 2006;12:3657–60.
38. Devine SM, Flomenberg N, Vesole DH, et al. Rapid mobilization of CD34+ cells following administration of the CXCR4 antagonist AMD3100 to patients with multiple myeloma and non-Hodgkin's lymphoma. J Clin Oncol 2004;22(6):1095–102.
39. Flomenberg N, Devine SM, Dipersio JF, et al. The use of AMD3100 plus G-CSF for autologous hematopoietic progenitor cell mobilization is superior to G-CSF alone. Blood 2005;106:1867–74.
40. Blank M, Shiloh Y. Programs for cell death: apoptosis is only one way to go. Cell Cycle 2007;6(6):686–95.
41. Danilov AV, Danilova OV, Klein AK, et al. Molecular pathogenesis of chronic lymphocytic leukemia. Curr Mol Med 2006;6(6):665–75.
42. Tsujimoto Y, Jaffe E, Cossman J, et al. Clustering of breakpoints on chromosome 11 in human B-cell neoplasms with the t(11;14) chromosome translocation. Nature 1985;315:340–3.
43. Adachi M, Tefferi A, Greipp PR, et al. Preferential linkage of bcl-2 to immunoglobulin light chain gene in chronic lymphocytic leukemia. J Exp Med 1990;171(2):559–64.
44. Schena M, Larsson LG, Gottardi D, et al. Growth- and differentiation-associated expression of bcl-2 in B-chronic lymphocytic leukemia cells. Blood 1992;79:2981–9.
45. Kitada S, Andersen J, Akar S, et al. Expression of apoptosis-regulating proteins in chronic lymphocytic leukemia: correlations with in vitro and in vivo chemoresponses. Blood 1998;91(9):3379–89.
46. Zapata JM, Krajewska M, Morse HC 3rd, et al. TNF receptor-associated factor (TRAF) domain and Bcl-2 cooperate to induce small B cell lymphoma/chronic lymphocytic leukemia in transgenic mice. Proc Natl Acad Sci U S A 2004;101(47):16600–5.
47. Lickliter JD, Cox J, McCarron J, et al. Small-molecule Bcl-2 inhibitors sensitise tumour cells to immune-mediated destruction. Br J Cancer 2007;96(4):600–8.
48. O'Brien S, Moore JO, Boyd TE, et al. Randomized phase III trial of fludarabine plus cyclophosphamide with or without oblimersen sodium (Bcl-2 antisense) in patients with relapsed or refractory chronic lymphocytic leukemia. J Clin Oncol 2007;25(9):1114–20.
49. Folkman J. Angiogenesis: an organizing principle for drug discovery? Nat Rev Drug Discov 2007;6(4):273–86.
50. Folkman J. Tumor angiogenesis: therapeutic implications. N Engl J Med 1971;285(21):1182–6.
51. Folkman J, Kalluri R. Cancer without disease. Nature 2004;427:787.
52. Rosenberg SA, Yang JC, Restifo NP. Cancer immunotherapy: moving beyond current vaccines. Nat Med 2004;10:909–15.
53. Rosenberg SA, Sherry RM, Morton KE, et al. Tumor progression can occur despite the induction of very high levels of self/tumor antigen-specific CD8+ T cells in patients with melanoma. J Immunol 2005;175(9):6169–76.
54. Ribas A, Butterfield LH, Glaspy JA, et al. Current developments in cancer vaccines and cellular immunotherapy. J Clin Oncol 2003;21:2415–32.
55. Chambers CA, Kuhns MS, Allison JP. Cytotoxic T lymphocyte antigen-4 (CTLA-4) regulates primary and secondary peptide-specific CD4(+) T cell responses. Proc Natl Acad Sci U S A 1999;96(15):8603–8.
56. Chambers CA, Kuhns MS, Egen JG, et al. CTLA-4-mediated inhibition in regulation of T cell responses: mechanisms and manipulation in tumor immunotherapy. Annu Rev Immunol 2001;19:565–94.
57. Phan GQ, Yang JC, Sherry RM, et al. Cancer regression and autoimmunity induced by cytotoxic T lymphocyte-associated antigen 4 blockade in patients with metastatic melanoma. Proc Natl Acad Sci U S A 2003;100(14):8372–7.
58. Ribas A, Camacho LH, Lopez-Berestein G, et al. Antitumor activity in melanoma and anti-self responses in a phase I trial with the anti-cytotoxic T lymphocyte-associated antigen 4 monoclonal antibody CP-675,206. J Clin Oncol 2005;23(35):8968–77.
59. Small EJ, Tchekmedyian NS, Rini BI, et al. A pilot trial of CTLA-4 blockade with human anti-CTLA-4 in patients with hormone-refractory prostate cancer. Clin Cancer Res 2007;13(6):1810–5.
60. Hodi FS, Mihm MC, Soiffer RJ, et al. Biologic activity of cytotoxic T lymphocyte-associated antigen 4 antibody blockade in previously vaccinated metastatic melanoma and ovarian carcinoma patients. Proc Natl Acad Sci U S A 2003;100(8):4712–7.
61. Peggs KS, Quezada SA, Korman AJ, et al. Principles and use of anti-CTLA4 antibody in human cancer immunotherapy. Curr Opin Immunol 2006;18(2):206–13.
62. Lankelma J. Tissue transport of anti-cancer drugs. Curr Pharm Des 2002;8(22):1987–93.
63. Dummer R, Garbe C, Thompson JA, et al. Randomized dose-escalation study evaluating peginterferon alfa-2a in patients with metastatic malignant melanoma. J Clin Oncol 2006;24(7):1188–94.

64. Green MD, Koelbl H, Baselga J, et al. A randomized double-blind multicenter phase III study of fixed-dose single-administration pegfilgrastim versus daily filgrastim in patients receiving myelosuppressive chemotherapy. Ann Oncol 2003;14(1):29–35.

65. Li KC, Pandit SD, Guccione S, et al. Molecular imaging applications in nanomedicine. Biomed Microdevices 2004;6(2):113–6.

66. Miura D, Yoneyama D, Furuhata Y, et al. Paclitaxel enhances antibody-dependent cell-mediated cytotoxicity of trastuzumab by a rapid recruitment of natural killer cells in Her-2 overexpressing breast cancer. J Clin Oncol 2007;25(18S):3503.

67. Bild AH, Yao G, Chang JT, et al. Oncogenic pathway signatures in human cancers as a guide to targeted therapies. Nature 2006;439(7074):353–7.

68. Peng B, Hayes M, Resta D, et al. Pharmacokinetics and pharmacodynamics of imatinib in a phase I trial with chronic myeloid leukemia patients. J Clin Oncol 2004;22(5):935–42.

69. Arslan MA, Kutuk O, Basaga H. Protein kinases as drug targets in cancer. Curr Cancer Drug Targets 2006;6(7):623–34.

70. Soutschek J, Akinc A, Bramlage B, et al. Therapeutic silencing of an endogenous gene by systemic administration of modified siRNAs. Nature 2004;432(7014):173–8.

71. Dykxhoorn DM, Palliser D, Lieberman J. The silent treatment: siRNAs as small molecule drugs. Gene Ther 2006;13(6):541–52.

72. Ferrari M. Cancer nanotechnology: opportunities and challenges. Nat Rev Cancer 2005;5(3):161–71.

73. Bashshur ZF, Bazarbachi A, Schakal A, et al. Intravitreal bevacizumab for the management of choroidal neovascularization in age-related macular degeneration. Am J Ophthalmol 2006;142:1–9.

74. Lynch SS, Cheng CM. Bevacizumab for neovascular ocular diseases. Ann Pharmacother 2007;41:614–25.

75. Lynch TJ, Bell DW, Sordella R, et al. Activating mutations in the epidermal growth factor receptor underlying responsiveness of non-small-cell lung cancer to gefitinib. N Engl J Med 2004;350(21):2129–39.

76. Alsina M, Fonseca R, Wilson EF, et al. Farnesyltransferase inhibitor tipifarnib is well tolerated, induces stabilization of disease, and inhibits farnesylation and oncogenic/tumor survival pathways in patients with advanced multiple myeloma. Blood 2004;103(9):3271–7.

77. Longley DB, Johnston PG. Molecular mechanisms of drug resistance. J Pathol 2005;205(2):275–92.

78. Siddik ZH. Cisplatin: mode of cytotoxic action and molecular basis of resistance. Oncogene 2003; 22(47):7265–79.

79. Efferth T, Volm M. Pharmacogenetics for individualized cancer chemotherapy. Pharmacol Ther 2005; 107(2):155–76.

80. Ferrando AA, Armstrong SA, Neuberg DS, et al. Gene expression signatures in MLL-rearranged T-lineage and B-precursor acute leukemias: dominance of HOX dysregulation. Blood 2003;102(1):262–8.

81. Cote JF, Kirzin S, Kramar A, et al. UGT1A1 polymorphism can predict hematologic toxicity in patients treated with irinotecan. Clin Cancer Res 2007;13:3269–75.

82. DiMasi JA, Grabowski HG. Economics of new oncology drug development. J Clin Oncol 2007;25(2): 209–16.

83. Schein PS, Scheffler B. Barriers to efficient development of cancer therapeutics. Clin Cancer Res 2006;12 (11 Pt 1):3243–8.

84. Schrag D. The price tag on progress—chemotherapy for colorectal cancer. N Engl J Med 2004;351(4):317–9.

85. Milsted RA. Cancer drug approval in the United States, Europe, and Japan. Adv Cancer Res 2007;96:371–91.

86. Visscher MB. New drugs: the tortuous road to approval. Science 1967;156(773):313.

87. Johnson JR, Temple R. Food and Drug Administration requirements for approval of new anticancer drugs. Cancer Treat Rep 1985;69:1155–9.

88. Beitz J, Gnecco C, Justice R. Quality-of-life end points in cancer clinical trials: the U.S. Food and Drug Administration perspective. J Natl Cancer Inst Monogr 1996;(20):7–9.

89. Guidance for Industry Clinical Trial Endpoints for the Approval of Cancer Drugs and Biologics. 2007. Accessed June 6, 2007, at http://www.fda.gov/cder/guidance/index.htm#clinical%20medicine/.

90. Therasse P, Arbuck SG, Eisenhauer EA, et al. New guidelines to evaluate the response to treatment in solid tumors; European Organization for Research and Treatment of Cancer, National Cancer Institute of the United States, National Cancer Institute of Canada. J Natl Cancer Inst 2000;92(3):205–16.

91. King DM. The radiology of gastrointestinal stromal tumours (GIST). Cancer Imaging 2005;5:150–6.

92. Fidler IJ, Kim SJ, Langley RR. The role of the organ microenvironment in the biology and therapy of cancer metastasis. J Cell Biochem 2007;101:927–36.

93. Schmitt CA, Rosenthal CT, Lowe SW. Genetic analysis of chemoresistance in primary murine lymphomas. Nat Med 2000;6:1029–35.

94. Harris NL, Jaffe ES, Diebold J, et al. The World Health Organization classification of neoplastic diseases of the haematopoietic and lymphoid tissues: report of the Clinical Advisory Committee Meeting, Airlie House, Virginia, November 1997. Histopathology 2000;36(1):69–86.

95. Frei E 3rd, Karon M, Levin RH, et al. The effectiveness of combinations of antileukemic agents in inducing and maintaining remission in children with acute leukemia. Blood 1965;26(5):642–56.

96. Hainsworth JD, Sosman JA, Spigel DR, et al. Treatment of metastatic renal cell carcinoma with a combination of bevacizumab and erlotinib. J Clin Oncol 2005;23:7889–96.

97. Dancey JE, Chen HX. Strategies for optimizing combinations of molecularly targeted anticancer agents. Nat Rev Drug Discov 2006;5(8):649–59.

98. De Vries EG, Gietema JA, de Jong S. Tumor necrosis factor-related apoptosis-inducing ligand pathway and its therapeutic implications. Clin Cancer Res 2006;12(8):2390–3.

99. Ahronheim JC, Bernholc AS, Clark WD. Age trends in autopsy rates: striking decline in late life. JAMA 1983;250:1182–6.

100. Groopman J. The right to a trial: should dying patients have access to experimental drugs? New Yorker 2006, pp 40–7.

101. Cortazar P, Johnson BE. Review of the efficacy of individualized chemotherapy selected by in vitro drug sensitivity testing for patients with cancer. J Clin Oncol 1999;17(5):1625–31.

102. Heinrich MC, Corless CL, Blanke CD, et al. Molecular correlates of imatinib resistance in gastrointestinal stromal tumors. J Clin Oncol 2006;24(29):4764–74.

103. Martin DS, Balis ME, Fisher B, et al. Role of murine tumor models in cancer treatment research. Cancer Res 1986;46(4 Pt 2):2189–92.

104. Nakayama T, Cho YC, Mine Y, et al. Expression of vascular endothelial growth factor and its receptors VEGFR-1 and 2 in gastrointestinal stromal tumors, leiomyomas and schwannomas. World J Gastroenterol 2006;12(38):6182–7.

105. Guidi AJ, Abu-Jawdeh G, Tognazzi K, et al. Expression of vascular permeability factor (vascular endothelial growth factor) and its receptors in endometrial carcinoma. Cancer 1996;78:454–60.

106. Ozdemir F, Akdogan R, Aydin F, et al. The effects of VEGF and VEGFR-2 on survival in patients with gastric cancer. J Exp Clin Cancer Res 2006;25:83–8.

107. Pisacane AM, Risio M. VEGF and VEGFR-2 immunohistochemistry in human melanocytic naevi and cutaneous melanomas. Melanoma Res 2005;15(1):39–43.

108. Wu Y, Hooper AT, Zhong Z, et al. The vascular endothelial growth factor receptor (VEGFR-1) supports growth and survival of human breast carcinoma. Int J Cancer 2006;119:1519–29.

109. Chung GG, Yoon HH, Zerkowski MP, et al. Vascular endothelial growth factor, FLT-1, and FLK-1 analysis in a pancreatic cancer tissue microarray. Cancer 2006;106(8):1677–84.

110. Puputti M, Tynninen O, Sihto H, et al. Amplification of KIT, PDGFRA, VEGFR2, and EGFR in gliomas. Mol Cancer Res 2006;4(12):927–34.

111. Grau SJ, Trillsch F, Herms J, et al. Expression of VEGFR3 in glioma endothelium correlates with tumor grade. J Neurooncol 2007;82(2):141–50.

112. Marshall J. Clinical implications of the mechanism of epidermal growth factor receptor inhibitors. Cancer 2006;107(6):1207–18.

113. Smith JS, Lal A, Harmon-Smith M, et al. Association between absence of epidermal growth factor receptor immunoreactivity and poor prognosis in patients with atypical meningioma. J Neurosurg 2007;106:1034–40.

114. Johnston JB, Navaratnam S, Pitz MW, et al. Targeting the EGFR pathway for cancer therapy. Curr Med Chem 2006;13(29):3483–92.

115. Downward J. Targeting RAS signalling pathways in cancer therapy. Nat Rev Cancer 2003;3(1):11–22.

116. Dahlberg PS, Jacobson BA, Dahal G, et al. ERBB2 amplifications in esophageal adenocarcinoma. Ann Thorac Surg 2004;78:1790–800.

117. Ramachandran C, Rodriguez S, Ramachandran R, et al. Expression profiles of apoptotic genes induced by curcumin in human breast cancer and mammary epithelial cell lines. Anticancer Res 2005;25(5):3293–302.

118. Wooster R, Futreal AP, Stratton MR. Sequencing analysis of BRAF mutations in human cancers. Methods Enzymol 2005;407:218–24.

119. Salh B, Marotta A, Matthewson C, et al. Investigation of the Mek-MAP kinase-Rsk pathway in human breast cancer. Anticancer Res 1999;19:731–40.

120. Mishima K, Yamada E, Masui K, et al. Overexpression of the ERK/MAP kinases in oral squamous cell carcinoma. Mod Pathol 1998;11(9):886–91.

121. Garavello W, Nicolini G, Aguzzi A, et al. Selective reduction of extracellular signal-regulated protein kinase (ERK) phosphorylation in squamous cell carcinoma of the larynx. Oncol Rep 2006;16(3):479–84.

122. Jinawath A, Akiyama Y, Yuasa Y, et al. Expression of phosphorylated ERK1/2 and homeodomain protein CDX2 in cholangiocarcinoma. J Cancer Res Clin Oncol 2006;132:805–10.

123. Bergqvist J, Elmberger G, Ohd J, et al. Activated ERK1/2 and phosphorylated oestrogen receptor alpha are associated with improved breast cancer survival in women treated with tamoxifen. Eur J Cancer 2006;42(8):1104–12.

124. Milde-Langosch K, Bamberger AM, Rieck G, et al. Expression and prognostic relevance of activated extracellular-regulated kinases (ERK1/2) in breast cancer. Br J Cancer 2005;92(12):2206–15.

125. Liu SY, Yen CY, Yang SC, et al. Overexpression of Rac-1 small GTPase binding protein in oral squamous cell carcinoma. J Oral Maxillofac Surg 2004;62(6):702–7.

126. Christensen JG, Burrows J, Salgia R. c-Met as a target for human cancer and characterization of inhibitors for therapeutic intervention. Cancer Lett. 2005 Jul 8;225(1):1–26. Epub 2004 Nov 11. Review.

127. Lee SH, Shin MS, Kim HS, et al. Somatic mutations of TRAIL-receptor 1 and TRAIL-receptor 2 genes in non-Hodgkin's lymphoma. Oncogene 2001;20(3):399–403.

128. Arai T, Akiyama Y, Okabe S, et al. Genomic organization and mutation analyses of the DR5/TRAIL receptor 2 gene in colorectal carcinomas. Cancer Lett 1998;133:197–204.

129. Pai SI, Wu GS, Ozoren N, et al. Rare loss-of-function mutation of a death receptor gene in head and neck cancer. Cancer Res 1998;58(16):3513–8.

130. Planas-Silva MD, Bruggeman RD, Grenko RT, et al. Overexpression of c-Myc and Bcl-2 during progression and distant metastasis of hormone-treated breast cancer. Exp Mol Pathol 2007;82(1):85–90.

131. Hellemans P, van Dam PA, Weyler J, et al. Prognostic value of bcl-2 expression in invasive breast cancer. Br J Cancer 1995;72(2):354–60.

132. Popovic B, Jekic B, Novakovic I, et al. Bcl-2 expression in oral squamous cell carcinoma. Ann N Y Acad Sci 2007;1095:19–25.

133. Tas F, Duranyildiz D, Oguz H, et al. The value of serum Bcl-2 levels in advanced lung cancer patients. Med Oncol 2005;22:139–43.

134. Ganigi PM, Santosh V, Anandh B, et al. Expression of p53, EGFR, pRb and bcl-2 proteins in pediatric glioblastoma multiforme: a study of 54 patients. Pediatr Neurosurg 2005;41:292–9.

135. Yoshino T, Shiina H, Urakami S, et al. Bcl-2 expression as a predictive marker of hormone-refractory prostate cancer treated with taxane-based chemotherapy. Clin Cancer Res 2006;12(Pt 1):6116–24.

136. Yee D. Targeting insulin-like growth factor pathways. Br J Cancer 2006;94:465–8.

137. Happerfield LC, Miles DW, Barnes DM, et al. The localization of the insulin-like growth factor receptor 1 (IGFR-1) in benign and malignant breast tissue. J Pathol 1997;183:412–7.

138. Cardillo MR, Monti S, Di Silverio F, et al. Insulin-like growth factor (IGF)-I, IGF-II and IGF type I receptor (IGFR-I) expression in prostatic cancer. Anticancer Res 2003;23:3825–35.

139. Adams SF, Hickson JA, Hutto JY, et al. PDGFR-alpha as a potential therapeutic target in uterine sarcomas. Gynecol Oncol 2007;104:524–8.

140. Hofer MD, Fecko A, Shen R, et al. Expression of the platelet-derived growth factor receptor in prostate cancer and treatment implications with tyrosine kinase inhibitors. Neoplasia 2004;6:503–12.

141. Casali PG, Messina A, Stacchiotti S, et al. Imatinib mesylate in chordoma. Cancer 2004;101:2086–97.

142. MacDonald TJ, Brown KM, LaFleur B, et al. Expression profiling of medulloblastoma: PDGFRA and the RAS/MAPK pathway as therapeutic targets for metastatic disease. Nat Genet 2001;29:143–52.

143. Lassus H, Sihto H, Leminen A, et al. Genetic alterations and protein expression of KIT and PDGFRA in serous ovarian carcinoma. Br J Cancer 2004;91:2048–55.

144. Burger H, den Bakker MA, Kros JM, et al. Activating mutations in c-KIT and PDGFRalpha are exclusively found in gastrointestinal stromal tumors and not in other tumors overexpressing these imatinib mesylate target genes. Cancer Biol Ther 2005;4:1270–4.

145. Carvalho I, Milanezi F, Martins A, et al. Overexpression of platelet-derived growth factor receptor alpha in breast cancer is associated with tumour progression. Breast Cancer Res 2005;7:R788–95.

146. Kitadai Y, Sasaki T, Kuwai T, et al. Expression of activated platelet-derived growth factor receptor in stromal cells of human colon carcinomas is associated with metastatic potential. Int J Cancer 2006;119:2567–74.

147. Golub TR, Barker GF, Lovett M, et al. Fusion of PDGF receptor beta to a novel ets-like gene, tel, in chronic myelomonocytic leukemia with t(5;12) chromosomal translocation. Cell 1994;77:307–16.

148. Cools J, DeAngelo DJ, Gotlib J, et al. A tyrosine kinase created by fusion of the PDGFRA and FIP1L1 genes as a therapeutic target of imatinib in idiopathic hypereosinophilic syndrome. N Engl J Med 2003;348:1201–14.

149. Singh A, Karnoub AE, Palmby TR, et al. Rac1b, a tumor associated, constitutively active Rac1 splice variant, promotes cellular transformation. Oncogene 2004;23:9369–80.

150. Tamborini E, Bonadiman L, Greco A, et al. A new mutation in the KIT ATP pocket causes acquired resistance to imatinib in a gastrointestinal stromal tumor patient. Gastroenterology 2004;127:294–9.

151. Kobayashi S, Boggon TJ, Dayaram T, et al. EGFR mutation and resistance of non-small-cell lung cancer to gefitinib. N Engl J Med 2005;352:786–92.

152. Feinberg AP, Ohlsson R, Henikoff S. The epigenetic progenitor origin of human cancer. Nat Rev Genet 2006;7:21–33.

20 Toward Personalized Therapy for Cancer

Sarah J. Welsh, BM Bch, PhD *and Garth Powis,* PhD

ABSTRACT

Personalized medicine is a model for the way medicine will evolve through the use of specific treatments and therapies best suited to an individual's genotype. It is driven by patient demand for safer and more effective medicines and therapies. This chapter focuses on the role of personalized medicine in cancer and explores its use in current clinical practice, its likely application in the future, and the challenges to be overcome to achieve this goal. Economic, social, and ethical considerations relating to personalized medicine are also discussed.

Key Words: Cancer, Personalized medicine, Individualized therapy, Pharmacogenomics, Targeted therapy, Molecular targets

1. INTRODUCTION

Personalized medicine models how medicine will evolve through the use of specific treatments and therapies tailored to each individual's genotype. It is driven by patient demand for safer and more effective medicines and therapies. It capitalizes on essential molecular processes in the body, such as cell cycle control, angiogenesis, and cell signaling. The concept of individualizing treatment is not a new one. Factors expressed through each person's specific genetic burden influence his or her response to specific drugs (pharmacogenetics). This is reflected in the scientific literature from the 1960s (reviewed in ref. 1). The number of new articles published remained constant until 1996 when technical developments, such as functional genomics and new insights into the highly complex nature of many diseases,

From: *Current Clinical Oncology: Targeted Cancer Therapy*
Edited by: R. Kurzrock and M. Markman © Humana Press, Totowa, NJ

resulted in pharmacogenomics (reviewed in ref. 2). Pharmacogenomics—the study of how an individual's genetic makeup affects the body's response to drugs—is closely related to pharmacogenetics. Pharmacogenetics is generally regarded as the study of genetic variation that gives rise to differing responses to drugs, whereas pharmacogenomics is the broader application of genomic technologies to new drug discovery and further characterization of older drugs. Pharmacogenomics emphasizes the influence of a whole set or complement of genes on the response to drugs, with the aim of improving drug efficacy rather than simply being concerned with drug safety. Subsequent growth in the new field of pharmacogenomics-based personalized medicine has been exponential, particularly in the area of cancer therapy.

The term "personalized medicine" is mainly used in the context of pharmacogenomics. Because this view can be rather narrow, personalized medicine also includes areas such as disease susceptibility and molecular traits and mechanisms underlying individual characteristics. Applications of personalized medicine range from personal risk profiles leading to personal preventative measures, such as vaccination, and personalized health planning leading to early diagnosis. It includes genetic counseling, databases, and decision support tools. This chapter focuses on the role of personalized medicine in cancer therapy and explores its use in current clinical practice, its likely application in the future, and the challenges still to be overcome to achieve ultimate efficacy.

2. WHY IS PERSONALIZED MEDICINE IMPORTANT IN CANCER?

Personalized medicine is more important for cancer patients than for those with other diseases for several reasons. First, cancer is a highly heterogeneous disease with significant molecular differences in the expression and distribution of tumor cell markers among patients with the same type and grade of tumor. Second, cellular mutations tend to accumulate as cancer progresses, further increasing tumor heterogeneity. Third, currently used cancer therapies at the doses employed are often toxic to normal cells, sometimes resulting in severe side effects rarely seen in other diseases. Finally, cancer patients often have a limited amount of time to try one kind of treatment and if it does not work to then try others until the optimal therapeutic regimen is found. Therefore, cancer therapy presents a unique example of personalized medicine in which an individual's genotype not only determines therapeutic and toxic responses to a drug (the pharmacogenotype), but also the nature of the specific tumor.

3. TO WHAT EXTENT IS CANCER MEDICINE ALREADY PERSONALIZED?

During the past two decades, we have amassed a plethora of information detailing the basic biologic processes in cancer that have become perturbed. We now know the key elements of growth factor binding, signal transduction, gene transcription control, cell cycle checkpoints, apoptosis, angiogenesis, and metastasis; and more than 350 mutated genes have been causally implicated in cancer development (3). Indeed, systematic sequencing of DNA corresponding to the coding exons of 518 protein kinase genes in 210 diverse human cancers showed that approximately 120 of the genes screened are estimated to carry mutations that drive the development of cancer by conferring a growth advantage on the cell in which they are active (4). The new paradigm for cancer therapy is to develop agents that target the precise molecular pathology driving the progression of individual cancers. Investment in genomics, genetics, and cytogenetic automation has already resulted in a large number of rationally designed anticancer drugs with a record number of novel compounds currently in clinical trials (reviewed in ref. 5). High profile drugs such as imatinib (Gleevec) *(6)*, trastuzumab (Herceptin) *(7)*, erlotinib (Tarceva) *(8)*, and bevacizumab (Avastin) *(9)* specifically target underlying molecular dysregulation and are in widespread clinical use. We are able to identify patients with precise molecular lesions that respond to the agents and by so doing have provided important proof-of-principle evidence for the benefits of targeted therapy in cancer, representing significant progress in actualizing the personalized medicine approach.

One of the consequences of using targeted therapy against a defined molecular lesion is that a move toward target-based, rather than disease-based, clinical drug development is required, as a defined molecular lesion can occur in more than one type of cancer. Imatinib is an example of the new agents approved for targeted therapy in cancer *(6)*. Imatinib was originally developed to target the Bcr-Abl receptor tyrosine kinase, which is formed from a reciprocal chromosomal translocation between the long arms of chromosomes 9 and 22 *(10)*. This process fuses the body of the Abelson tyrosine kinase (*abl*) gene on chromosome 9 with the breakpoint cluster region (*bcr*) gene on chromosome 22 to generate an oncogene that encodes the chimeric Bcr-Abl protein. The Bcr-Abl protein is a constitutively active, cytoplasmic form of the ABL kinase, which transforms primary myeloid cells to leukemic cells via ABL receptor tyrosine kinase activity *(11,12)*. This characteristic genetic abnormality, known as the Philadelphia chromosome, is present in the marrow cells of more than 90% of all patients with chronic myelogenous leukemia (CML) (reviewed in chapter 1) and in 15% to 30% of patients with acute lymphoblastic leukemia (ALL) (reviewed in Chapter 1) *(10)*. Imatinib selectively inhibits Bcr-Abl by occupying the ABL adenosine triphosphate (ATP) binding site, maintaining the protein in an inactive conformation, thereby inhibiting its tyrosine kinase activity *(13)*, resulting in 89% overall survival of patients after 5 years *(14)*. Subsequent analysis has also revealed activity against the tyrosine kinases associated with the c-Kit protein (stem cell factor receptor) and platelet-derived growth factor receptor (PDGFR) *(15–17)*.

Constitutive activation of the c-Kit tyrosine kinase has been shown to be critical in the pathogenesis of gastrointestinal stromal tumor (GIST), a rare neoplasm for which there had historically been no effective systemic therapy *(18)*. Indeed, activating mutations of c-*Kit* and/or PDGFR have been found in 88% and 5% of GISTs, respectively *(19)*, with 100% of GIST tumor specimens demonstrating positive immunostaining for the KIT protein *(20)*. Clinical trials subsequently demonstrated that imatinib is an effective therapy in GIST, with a 53.3% overall efficacy rate (complete response + partial response) and a 84.3% rate for disease control (complete response + partial response + stable disease) with a 1-year survival rate of 88% (reviewed in ref. 21). Imatinib is now approved for the treatment of GIST, demonstrating the importance of a target-based, rather than disease-based, approach for future clinical drug development.

To achieve the goal of personalized medicine, biomarker and imaging tests must be available to identify the molecular targets in a patient's tumor and the patient's pharmacogenotype in addition to developing drugs with defined molecular specificities. Biomarkers act as molecular signposts of the physiologic state of a cell and are determined by the genes, proteins, and other organic chemicals made by the cell *(22)*. The advantage of using biomarkers to identify patients who are likely to benefit from a particular treatment is demonstrated by the success of the humanized murine monoclonal antibody trastuzumab (Herceptin) in breast cancer *(7)* (see Chapter 3). Trastuzumab targets the human epidermal growth factor receptor 2 (HER2), which belongs to a family of four transmembrane receptor tyrosine kinases that mediate cell growth, differentiation, and survival of cells *(23)*. Overexpression of the HER2 protein, amplification of the *HER2* gene, or both occur in 15% to 30% of breast cancers. These events are associated with increased proliferation, decreased cell death, and increased metastasis *(24)*. HER2 overexpression is a marker of poor prognosis in patients with node-positive breast cancer and might predict resistance to endocrine therapy *(25–27)*. Trastuzumab therapy significantly improves response rates in women with HER2-overexpressing breast cancer, either alone or in combination with chemotherapy (25% and 50%, respectively *(28,29)*). However, trastuzumab therapy shows poor response rates in tumors expressing lower levels of HER2 (35% in HER2-overexpressing tumors versus 0% in tumors expressing lower levels of HER2) *(28)*. Given its implications for prognosis and treatment, as well as the costly nature of trastuzumab, the accurate identification of HER2 overexpression is of considerable importance. Patients likely to benefit from trastuzumab are selected through the use of immunohistochemistry test kits or fluorescence in situ hybridization (FISH) assays, which detect the presence of the HER2 protein *(30)*. Patients whose tumors do not express HER2/neu are spared futile treatment and potential treatment-related side effects and, instead, are offered alternative therapy, saving precious time and resources.

A related objective of using biomarker tests is the ability to monitor the effect of a defined drug on its molecular target and to assess early response so a nonresponding patient can be spared unnecessary treatment and can be offered alternative therapies. An example is the use of imatinib for treatment of CML *(6)*. Although clinical trials showed that imatinib was particularly effective in newly diagnosed chronic-phase CML *(14)*, patients with advanced CML are less sensitive to imatinib, with 24% and 66% of patients in accelerated and blastic phases, respectively, failing to achieve hematologic remission despite treatment with high doses of imatinib *(31)*. Additionally, responses to imatinib in patients with advanced disease are often transient, generally lasting less than 6 months *(31–36)*. Consequently, patients are regularly monitored using a number of parameters, including levels of Philadelphia chromosome-positive cells. Failure to achieve a hematologic response after 3 months of therapy, a cytogenetic response after 6 months, a major cytogenetic response (Philadelphia chromosome-positive cells reduced to < 35%) after 12 months, or a complete cytogenetic response after 18 months are indications for modifying imatinib therapy *(37)*. Modification includes treatment with higher doses of imatinib, imatinib combinations, new tyrosine kinase inhibitors (dasatinib *(38)* or nilotinib *(39)*), allogeneic stem cell transplantation, or investigational therapies. For patients who achieve a complete cytogenetic response, hematologic and cytogenetic assessments are continued, with regular molecular monitoring of Bcr-Abl versus ABL transcript levels as increasing levels of BCR-ABL transcripts are associated with the emergence of BCR-ABL mutants and resistance to imatinib *(40,41)*.

Biomarkers can also provide essential information about how much drug is needed to inhibit a particular molecular target in a tumor and whether there is a benefit in administering a higher drug dose. Ideally, these tests should be noninvasive as biopsying solid tumors is expensive and subjects patients to additional invasive procedures with associated risks. Although traditional sources such as serum or plasma are currently in routine use, advances in noninvasive techniques such as molecular imaging show potential for providing detailed functional and metabolic information (reviewed in ref. 42). There has been a major increase in the use of positron emission spectroscopy (PET), which allows dynamic, noninvasive measures of the three-dimensional distribution of a positron-labeled compound in the living body *(43)*. By labeling molecules of interest (e.g., drugs, metabolic substrates, peptides, antibodies) with positron-emitting isotopes such as ^{11}C, ^{18}F, ^{124}I or ^{13}N, pharmacokinetic and pharmacodynamic measurements can be performed in addition to evaluating the effect of novel therapeutics on generic and specific biologic endpoints (42). In studies that employ generic endpoints, PET has been used to monitor changes in cellular proliferation using ^{11}C-thymidine (43,44), tissue perfusion with ^{15}O-H_2O (45), glucose utilization with ^{18}FDG (46), and DNA synthesis using ^{18}F-fluorothymidine (47). Specific biologic endpoints have the potential to provide proof of principle for a proposed mechanism of action for existing or novel therapies. Examples include the detection of thymidylate synthase inhibition with ^{11}C-thymidine (48), detection of hypoxia using ^{18}fluoromisonidazole and other ^{18}F-labeled 2-nitroimidazoles (49,50), imaging of apoptosis using ^{124}I-annexin V (51), and visualization of the pharmacodynamics of HER2 degradation due to heat shock protein 90 (Hsp90) inhibition (52). Positron-labeled antibodies or peptides also offer the potential for noninvasive monitoring of receptor expression such as the detection of overexpression of Erb-B2 receptors with (68) Ga-labeled anti-Erb-B2 antibody (53).

However, although PET imaging has enormous potential advantages for use in drug development, not all compounds can be radiolabeled and each compound must be considered on an individual basis. Additionally, PET images have low anatomic resolution as well as a lack of chemical resolution, being unable to distinguish between the parental radiotracer and its labeled, or unlabeled, metabolites. Radiation exposure is also a potential limitation of PET radioisotopes, particularly if studies are performed on multiple occasions. Alternative methods include magnetic resonance imaging (MRI) and magnetic resonance spectroscopy (MRS) (reviewed in ref. 42). MRI is routinely used in the initial evaluation of tumor size, shape, and anatomic appearance; and changes in these parameters can be used to assess and quantify the pharmacodynamic effects of a drug (54). In addition, dynamic contrast-enhanced MRI (DCE-MRI) is proving increasingly useful for assessing pharmacodynamic endpoints, especially for changes related to the vasculature (54–58). Importantly, almost all major hospitals in the developed world have access to MRI for routine use.

Magnetic resonance spectroscopy is the only noninvasive in vivo method available for chemically distinguishing between, and measuring concentrations of, drugs and their metabolites (59). Although MRS does not provide an anatomic image, data are visualized in the form of a spectrum in which the peaks correspond to different cellular constituents (59). Thus, MRI can be used to define the volume in a tumor or normal tissue, and MRS can be used to measure the concentration of endogenous biochemical compounds or drugs in that volume in real time. The advantage of this approach is that only the drug is administered, no samples are taken, and no ionizing radiation is used. MRS has been shown to increase the level of diagnostic confidence in numerous situations in which conventional MRI may be unhelpful (reviewed in ref. 60). Additionally, studies have shown that MRS can be used to monitor response to chemotherapy in lymphomas, germ cell tumors, and gliomas (61–63). To date, pharmacokinetic studies using MRS in patients have been restricted to (1) fluorine-containing drugs such as 5-fluorouracil (5FU), its prodrug capecitabine, and gemcitabine using ^{19}F-MRS and (2) ifosfamide and cyclophosphamide using ^{31}P-MRS (reviewed in ref. 42). The elimination rate of 5FU from tumors in patients is associated with response, allowing early prediction of the likely success or failure of a treatment regimen (64). However, the value of MRS data is highly dependent on expert spectroscopists for acquisition, analysis, and interpretation of MR spectra. For that reason, MRS is not generally used in routine clinical practice outside of specialist centers. Because of the logistical and ethical issues associated with invasive measurements, MRS has great potential for satisfying the increasing requirement for minimally invasive assays to measure pharmacokinetic and pharmacodynamic target modulation in the future.

The newly emerging area of cancer phenomics can be used as a practical illustration of how genetic studies can be successfully integrated with phenotypic data to improve the specificity of personalized medicine (reviewed in ref. 65). Cancer phenomics refers to the systematic and detailed collection, objective documentation, and cataloguing of phenotypic data at many levels, including clinical, molecular, and cellular phenotype(s). Data are most mature for germline mutations in the receptor tyrosine kinase RET (rearranged during transfection). RET plays a crucial role in transducing growth and differentiation signals in tissues derived from the neural crest *(66,67)*. Germline mutations in RET, which lead to a constitutively active receptor tyrosine kinase or decreased specificity for its substrate, predispose to the cancer-associated syndrome multiple endocrine neoplasia-2 (MEN-2) *(68)*. MEN-2 is a clinical syndrome marked by a predisposition to developing medullary thyroid cancer and pheochromocytoma in addition to encompassing other endocrine, mucocutaneous, and skeletal features. MEN-2-associated tumors are most often bilateral and multifocal, and they occur at a much younger age than their sporadic counterparts. Meticulous characterization of RET phenomics at the clinical and biochemical levels has revolutionized the clinical management of families manifesting the MEN-2 syndrome *(65)*. When a mutation is identified in an individual, predictive testing can be performed on family members; and only those who carry the mutation require further MEN-2 management. The correlation between genotype and phenotype in MEN-2 has led experts to suggest individualized recommendations for the timing of prophylactic thyroidectomy (surgical removal of the thyroid gland) on the basis of the RET mutation genotype. For other mutations in *RET*, phenomics points to the wisdom of establishing a specific routine surveillance program for early detection as the most appropriate management route. Advances in noninvasive sampling techniques, such as the use of buccal cell isolates as a source of DNA, offer an acceptable sample collection method for such surveillance programs *(69)*. Knowledge of the molecular pathways that are dysregulated as a result of *RET* mutations will enable targeted therapies to be explored that might prove useful for treating tumors arising as a result of *RET* mutations.

4. FUTURE OF PERSONALIZED MEDICINE IN CANCER

The Human Genome Project and its successor the Cancer Genome Project and related activities are expected to identify most of the genes that are involved in the preponderance of common human cancers during the next 5 years. Together these projects will provide a vast repository of comparative information about normal and malignant cells. Instead of licensing drugs for empiric use in different types of cancer with relatively poor response, new therapies will require the identification of specific molecular lesions resulting in tailored therapies and improved response rates. Reduced toxicity due to increased selectivity will allow new therapies to be given over prolonged periods of time, in some cases for the rest of a patient's life, a concept unthinkable in the current setting of cytotoxic therapy. More complete knowledge of tumor biology and the role of target pathways in normal physiology will reduce the likelihood of unforeseen toxicities that can limit or even curtail a drug's usefulness. Unexpected cardiotoxicity in some patients treated with imatinib is an example *(70)*.

Detailed analysis of the differences between normal and malignant cells also allows the possibility of individual cancer risk assessment, leading to tailored prevention programs and specific screening programs to detect early cancer. Although cancer prevention now absorbs only a small fraction of the total funding for cancer care and research, this percentage is likely to increase in the postgenomic era *(71)*. Currently, it is accepted that more than 120 genes are associated with the development of various cancers *(4)*. However, the detection of polymorphisms in low-penetrance cancer-related genes—or a combination of changed genes—will allow people at increased risk to be identified, and the demand for prevention strategies will increase. It is predicted that within the next two decades most people will be genetically mapped and their information easily stored on a "smart card." *(72)* Thus, predisposition to some cancers will be found during early adult life with potential for correction well before manifestation of the disease.

Multiple technologies already exist for the goal of personalized treatment in cancer to be achieved. Molecular diagnosis can be established at multiple levels where molecular differences can be found between individuals with identical clinical manifestations. Currently available diagnostic procedures are insufficient to determine which patients can primarily benefit from rational tumor therapy. In the future, gaining information on individual morphology, genetic, proteomic, and epigenetic alterations will be essential to provide clinicians with relevant information to prescribe an individualized clinical treatment plan.

DNA microarray technology is the first approach close to being used in routine diagnosis (reviewed in ref. 73). Microarrays consist of a solid support, such as a silicon chip or glass slide, with thousands of immobilized complementary DNA molecules specific for individual genes (up to 20,000) or oligonucleotide probes (up to 65,000) arranged in a defined order. To analyze gene expression, target nucleic acids are extracted from tissue and most commonly labeled with fluorescent dye. A genetic expression profile indicating overexpression, underexpression, no change, or complete absence for each gene in the tissue sample is obtained by monitoring the amount of label that has hybridized to each location on the microarray. Patterns of gene changes or novel genes associated with disease development or clinical outcome of an individual tumor can then be identified by specialist bioinformatic programs that use statistical methods to evaluate the complex information and translate molecular information into clinically relevant data.

For example, microarray analysis has been used to classify acute leukemias *(74)*. By analyzing gene expression profiles in 38 acute leukemia samples, 1100 genes were identified that were differentially expressed between acute lymphoid leukemia (ALL) (reviewed in Chapter 11) and acute myeloid leukemia (AML) (reviewed in Chapter 2). By focusing on the 50 genes whose expressions were correlated most closely with disease type, a classification scheme was developed that was able to identify accurately new ALL or AML samples, as well as B-lineage or T-lineage ALL, among the ALL group samples. Subsequent work using oligonucleotide microarrays to analyze the gene expression patterns of more than 12,600 genes in leukemic blasts from 360 pediatric ALL patients identified all known prognostically significant leukemia subgroups *(75)*. Additionally, the study identified distinct expression profiles that predicted relapse with high accuracy within specific subtypes (no single gene could be used to predict the risk of relapse).

Microarrays can also be used to identify patients who are likely to benefit from a particular therapy and those who should be given additional therapy to increase their chances of survival. In a breast cancer study, microarrays were used to analyze 25,000 genes in 78 primary breast tumors from young women who were node-negative at the time of diagnosis *(76)*. Seventy representative genes were identified that accurately predicted subsequent metastatic status in 83% of patients. The set of 70 genes was then shown to predict accurately the future metastatic status in 17 of 19 additional independent breast tumors, showing that the predictive power of this indicator for clinical metastasis in node-negative breast cancer is much greater than standard approaches. In fact, using current criteria, 70% to 91% of breast cancer patients treated with surgery and radiotherapy would be advised to receive unnecessary adjuvant chemotherapy *(77)*. This approach was also able to identify women who appeared to need more aggressive therapy for their breast cancer.

Similar analysis of proteins as proteomic patterns also appears on the horizon (reviewed in ref. 78). It is estimated that our 40,000 genes may generate around 1 million distinguishable functional entities at the protein level due to differential splicing and translation and numerous posttranslational modifications. Therefore, although complex, the proteome offers a much richer source for the functional description of cancers and the discovery of diagnostic therapeutic targets than genomic analysis, especially given the dynamic nature of cancer. The main current applications of proteomics include protein expression profiling of tumors, tumor fluids, and tumor cells; protein microarrays; mapping of cancer signaling pathways; pharmacoproteomics; identification of biomarkers for diagnosis, staging and monitoring of the disease and therapeutic response; and profiling the immune response to cancer. The most clinically advanced of these applications is the use of protein microarrays, which are mainly employed for functional studies with antibodies that recognize posttranslational modifications. For example, screening of ovarian tumor cell lysates with phospho-specific antibodies for extracellular signal-regulated kinase 1/2 (ERK 1/2), AKT, and glycogen synthase kinase 3β (GSK-3β) suggested that in ovarian cancer signaling pathways may be activated in a patient-specific, rather than type- or stage-specific, pattern *(79)*. Thus, proteomic technologies, particularly when combined with genomic analyses, offer enormous potential for the delivery of personalized medicine, although their implementation in routine clinical medicine remains a challenge.

An alternative strategy for delivering personalized management of cancer via proteomics is phage display (reviewed in ref. 80). Phase display technology utilizes combinatorial libraries of proteins expressed on phage particles that can be selected for specific binding to cancer cells. Although phage display has yet to reach its potential in research and clinics, it has great promise for various applications, including identification of cell-specific targeting molecules; identification of cell surface biomarkers; profiling cell-specific delivery of cytotoxic agents, identification of cancer biomarkers, profiling of tumor specimens, and design of peptide-based anticancer therapeutics for personalized treatments. Importantly, phage display does not require any prior knowledge about cell surface targets for identification of cell-targeting molecules, nor does the target have to be immunogenic. Unlike traditional approaches applied to individualized cancer medicine, phage display offers the parallel development of anticancer therapeutics with companion diagnostics. Unfortunately, at the present time, only low numbers of samples can be processed, and a high throughput solution lies in the development of instrumentation for automation of key steps in the process. However, phage display has the necessary prerequisites to find a unique niche for improving personalized medicine in the future.

The development of high throughput methods for investigating the methylation status of DNA provides another level for obtaining pertinent information. Epigenetic modification of DNA by the addition of a methyl group to cytosine residues in CpG dinucleotides is one of the most important mechanisms of tumor suppressor gene inactivation known today *(81,82)*. Although a multitude of publications on high-throughput analysis of DNA methylation in tumor samples already exist, this technology needs further development to enter routine clinical practice (reviewed in ref. 73). Nevertheless, it is clear that, individually, neither genomic, proteomic, nor epigenomic analysis can provide all the information required for an efficient individualized approach. Therefore, a "multiplex" approach combining the various biologic levels of DNA, RNA, and protein may be necessary to classify malignant tumors functionally with the highest relevance for prognosis and therapy.

5. CHALLENGES FOR ACHIEVING PERSONALIZED MEDICINE

One of the major limitations to achieving personalized medicine is our incomplete knowledge of tumor biology. Our understanding will continue to be supplemented by data from the Human Genome Project and the Cancer Genome Project and their related activities. However, continued investment in technical developments and bioinformatics is necessary to develop special methods capable of detecting the entire spectrum of rate-limiting oncogenic pathways in tumors before and after therapy to identify patients who can benefit from novel therapies. The work needed includes broad profiling of human tissue for morphology, genetic, proteomic, and epigenetic alterations, as described above. Before such an integrated approach into daily routine cancer care can be established, extensive development is necessary to allow firm prediction of the activation of a certain pathway in clinical material.

More insidious challenges stem from the way cancer drugs are currently developed, the simplest being that currently drugs frequently enter clinical trials without a "validated" biomarker or imaging test to select patients most likely to respond to a given therapy or for identifying response to treatment. "Validated" means that the test is standardized and has been shown to be reproducible across institutions—if not in patients then at least in animal models. Instead of being an afterthought, these tests need to be developed early in the development of a drug so they are ready for use in clinical trials. Additionally, current requirements for disease-specific drug trials mean that responding patients must be identified by separate trials for each disease group. A move to target-based rather than disease-based clinical drug development requires a paradigm shift in how cancer drugs are identified.

We are still in the era of the "one drug fits all" mentality. The success of the pharmaceutical industry evolved from this philosophy, and it will be a difficult barrier to surpass. With the continuing focus on the search for "blockbuster" drugs having annual sales of $1 billion, there is a natural disinclination to subdivide the market, which is what personalized medicine apparently accomplishes. If only 10% of patients with a particular cancer can be shown to respond to a particular agent because only they possess the requisite molecular target(s) for a given drug, the market for this pharmaceutical agent is reduced by 90%. Of course the patients are likely to take the agents for longer periods of time, but this is not viewed as compensation for decreasing the size of the target market. The drug may also be active in subsets of patients with other cancers, so the total market could eventually attain "blockbuster" drug proportions. Imatinib, discussed previously, is an example because it is active in several small cancer subtypes. However, having such information about any given drug is by no means certain during the early stages of its development when important strategic decisions are being made. Therefore, at the moment, there is a perceived commercial risk in personalizing cancer therapy and testing patients for molecular targets.

What if we are wrong about the target? What if other, as yet unknown targets are responsible for or contribute to the therapeutic effect? These are legitimate concerns; but without well designed studies with validated tests, we will not know if the concerns are well founded. The increasing tendency to run clinical trials simultaneously at multiple institutions also augments the need to have properly validated tests that can be conducted by all institutions. This requires test validation to be built into a drug's development early on. In a risk-averse market, it is safer to stick to a "one drug fits all" approach; and after all, "better the devil you know than the devil you don't." Attempts are being made to develop alternate strategies to accompany personalized medicine, such as the use of therapeutic combinations, which it is hoped will make an inactive drug active in more patients but still treat all patients with a given disease with the drug. However, an apprehension is that the real goal in such an approach, ultimately, is obfuscation with the underlying intent to defuse the perceived threat of personalized medicine, thereby maintaining the current unsustainable commercial model. An alternative strategy could be to treat a molecular target, not a disease, and to design clinical trials that cut across tumor types, thus reducing the financial burden of testing a drug in essentially repetitive multiple disease-specific trials. This, of course, would necessitate a paradigm shift in how we think about and organize cancer treatment. Nonetheless, personalized medicine is proving its value in other diseases and has begun to do so in cancer. The ethics and cost to society and cancer patients who are treated with drugs to which they have little likelihood of response because they do not have its requisite target (as to the best of our ability we understand it) cannot be ignored.

A further challenge for drug development results from the likely need to administer the newer molecularly targeted drugs, which are nearly all cytostatic and arrest tumor growth, in combination with more conventional cytotoxic drugs that cause tumor shrinkage. This approach retains many of the toxic effects of current therapy. It may be that in the future we will accept time to disease progression rather than tumor shrinkage as the endpoint of therapy—if patients are able to live with their cancer under control—in the same way that individuals live with diabetes controlled by antidiabetic drugs. With more than 10 million survivors in America alone, cancer is evolving into another chronic disease. This reality would be one step toward the ultimate goal for cancer therapy, which is cure with complete eradication of all traces of a patient's tumor.

A rational way to develop molecularly targeted cancer drugs is to use combinations that attack different moieties in the same or parallel signaling pathways. However, the reluctance of pharmaceutical companies to test their experimental agents in combination with a competitor's agent is a frustration for many clinical investigators. A framework for providing intellectual property protection to companies that test drugs in combination has been provided by the National Cancer Institute Cancer Therapy Evaluation Program (CTEP), and a number of CTEP-sponsored drug combination studies are underway. This type of model must be extended and made more readily available in the future.

Other challenges for drug development include widespread frustration with the cost and time it takes to bring a new cancer drug to trial. Initiatives are in place to help speed up the drug development process, in both the drug discovery pipeline and the design of clinical trials. The implementation of chemical biology, which provides experimental techniques for linking together elements from all stages of what was previously viewed as a linear pathway from gene to drug, may help accelerate the drug development process. To encourage more rapid introduction of drugs into clinical trials, the FDA has introduced microdose exploratory studies, dubbed "phase 0," which utilize less than 1/100th of the dose calculated to yield a pharmacologic effect, thereby allowing the collection of human pharmacokinetic and bioavailability data earlier in the drug development process. These human data can then be combined with preclinical data to select the best drug candidates to advance to more expensive and extensive clinical development. However, much work needs to be done in this area to ensure that the concept of personalized medicine becomes a reality.

Finally, there has been much discussion about the economic, social, and ethical aspects of personalized medicine. Inevitably, conflicting demands will be placed upon available resources, particularly given the possibility that cancer could become a chronic disease within the next two decades owing to advances in understanding the fundamental biology of cancers and translation of this knowledge into impressive and efficacious therapies. The cost of treating a cancer patient is expected to quadruple by 2025 compared to 2005 *(72)*. The only way to reduce cancer care costs will be to ensure that expensive medicines are given only to patients who are predicted to benefit from them and to confirm their response as rapidly as possible.

As with all health issues, access will be determined by cost and political will. Politicians will be forced to consider the alignment between patients' requirements and "taxpayers" and "voters" wishes. For example, fewer than 50% of voters in the United Kingdom currently pay a tax, and the percentage of taxpayers is likely to decline as the population ages. The interests of voters may be very different from the interests of taxpayers. Additionally, whatever system is put in place to pay for cancer-related care, there is the prospect of a major socioeconomic division in cancer care. A small proportion of the elderly will have made suitable provisions for retirement, in terms of both health and welfare, but most will not be properly prepared. Policymakers need to start planning now. The most productive way forward is to start involving cancer patients and health advocacy groups in the debate to ensure that difficult decisions are reached by consensus.

The tools of genetic and molecular medicine are powerful, but so are the social and ethical risks. Personal values at stake are privacy, protection of minority populations, and prevention of discrimination. Early in the Human Genome Project it was recognized that the project also had ethical, legal, and social implications (ELSIs), and the ELSI program was established. Its goals remain key objectives in the vision for the future of genomics research *(83,84)*. One proposal about how to safeguard privacy advocates three major pillars on which to base protection for pharmacogenetic testing *(85,86)*: informed consent, trusted intermediaries, and legal protection. Informed consent is well known from clinical trials and is based on the assertion that the decision to carry out, continue, or stop an investigation rests exclusively with the patient. The patient also decides whether and to what extent he or she wishes to be informed of his or her medical condition and the results of the investigation *(87)*. Trusted intermediaries are proposed to act as "firewalls" between genetic tests and medical records to independently hold DNA samples and test results. The intermediary would release genetic information about a person only to those who need access to it and only when that person specifically has requested it. Legal protection has the aim of protecting human dignity and personality, of preventing improper genetic testing and improper use of genetic data, and of guaranteeing the quality of genetic tests and interpretation of their results. The basic principles of this legislation are prohibition of discrimination, informed consent, right of not knowing, protection of genetic data, and licensing of genetic testing.

A further important social concern is the protection of minority groups who are genetically prone to a specific condition. On one hand, they might strongly benefit from future drugs tailored to their specific genetic makeup. This same population is frequently underprivileged in the current "one drug fits all" era. A potential problem is, however, their risk of becoming therapeutic orphans, as it may be difficult to recruit sufficient patient numbers for trials *(88)*, and it may not be profitable for industry to develop special drugs for this population *(89)*.

Finally, a critical issue for the social acceptance of personalized medicine is the danger of discrimination on the grounds of the findings resulting from genetic testing *(90)*. Discrimination may result from decision-making on the basis of faulty or incomplete data or misinterpretation of the implications of genetic test results regarding morbidity or mortality (irrational discrimination) or that based on scientifically sound and empirically supported discrimination (rational discrimination) *(91)*. Although it is likely that irrational discrimination will be banned, rational discrimination is already in common use by insurers to classify risk based on age, sex, occupation, personal and family medical histories, serum cholesterol level, and alcohol and tobacco use. Personal genetic profiles are an extension of this risk evaluation, with profiling likely to become more precise in the future. However, it is often difficult to differentiate between rational and irrational discrimination, and the misuse of personal risk profiles is a real danger for the success of personalized medicine, which needs legal regulation.

6. CONCLUSION

We are in one of the most exciting times of modern cancer therapy, marked by the development of rational therapy and the move toward personalized treatment for cancer. The concepts to be tested are well established, and new drugs are becoming available. Novel emerging technologies in target identification, drug discovery, molecular markers, and imaging will make the goal of individualizing cancer treatment a reality. The era of personalized health planning, early diagnosis, and selecting optimal drugs for each patient with predictable side effects are developments directly in our sights.

REFERENCES

1. Yong WP, Innocenti F, Ratain MJ. The role of pharmacogenetics in cancer therapy. Br J Clin Pharmacol 2006;62(1):35–46.
2. Watters JW, McLeod HL. Cancer pharmacogenomics: current and future applications. Biochim Biophys Acta 2003;1603:99–111.
3. Futreal PA. A consensus of human cancer genes. Nat Rev Cancer 2004;4:177–83.
4. Greenman C, Stephens P, Smith R, et al. Patterns of somatic mutation in human cancer genomes. Nature 2007;446:153–8.
5. Collins I, Workman P. New approaches to molecular cancer therapeutics. Nat Chem Biol 2006;2:689–700.
6. Capdeville R, Buchdunger E, Zimmerman J, et al. (ST571, imatinib), a rationally developed, targeted anticancer drug. Nat Rev Drug Discov 2002;1:493–502.
7. Morris S, Carey L. Trastuzumab and beyond: new possibilities for the treatment of HER2-positive breast cancer. Oncology 2006;20:1763–71.
8. Cohen MH, Johnson JR, Chen YF, et al. FDA approval summary: erlotinib (Tarceva) tablets. Oncologist 2005;10:461–6.
9. Hadj Tahar A. Bevacizumab for advanced colorectal cancer. Issues Emerg Health Technol 2004;63:1–4.
10. Rowley JD. A new consistent chromosomal abnormality in chronic myelogenous leukemia identified by quinacrine fluorescence and Giemsa staining. Nature 1973;243:290–3.
11. Daley GQ, Van Etten RA, Baltimore D. Induction of chronic myelogenous leukemia in mice by the P210bcr/abl gene of the Philadelphia chromosome. Nature 1990;247:824–30.
12. Lugo TG, Pendergast AM, Muller AJ, et al. Tyrosine kinase activity and transformation potency of bcr-abl oncogene products. Science 1990;247:1079–82.
13. Schindler T, Bornmann W, Pellicena P, et al. Structural mechanism for STI-571 inhibition of abelson tyrosine kinase. Science 2000;289:1938–42.
14. O'Brian SG, Guilhot F, Larson RA, et al. Imatinib compared with interferon and low dose cytarabine for newly diagnosed chronic phase chronic myeloid leukemia. N Engl J Med 2003;348:994–1004.
15. Heinrich MC, Blanke CD, Druker BJ, et al. Inhibition of KIT tyrosine kinase activity: a novel molecular approach to the treatment of KIT-positive malignancies. J Clin Oncol 2002;20:1692–703.

16. Joensuu H, Roberts PJ, Sarlomo-Rikala M, et al. Effect of the tyrosine kinase inhibitor STI571 in a patient with a metastatic gastrointestinal stromal tumor. N Engl J Med 2001;347:481–7.
17. Apperley JF, Gardembas M, Mello JV, et al. Response to imatinib mesylate in patients with chronic myeloproliferative diseases with rearrangements of the platelet-derived growth factor receptor beta. N Engl J Med 2002;347:481–7.
18. Hirota S, Isozaki K, Moriyama Y, et al. Gain-of-function mutations of c-kit in human gastrointestinal stromal tumors. Science 1998;279:577–80.
19. Heinrich MC, Corless CL, Demetri GD, et al. Kinase mutations and imatinib response in patients with gastrointestinal stromal tumors. J Clin Oncol 2003;21:4342–9.
20. Sihto H, Sarlomo-Rikala M, Tynninen O, et al. KIT and platelet-derived growth factor receptor alpha tyrosine kinase gene mutations and KIT amplifications in human solid tumors. J Clin Oncol 2005;23:49–57.
21. Kubota T. Gastrointestinal stromal tumor (GIST) and imatinib. Int J Clin Oncol 2006;11:184–9.
22. Frank R, Hargreaves R. Clinical biomarkers in drug discovery and development. Nat Rev Drug Discov 2003;2:556–80.
23. Gschwind A, Fischer OM, Ullrich A. The discovery of receptor tyrosine kinases: targets for cancer therapy. Nat Rev Cancer 2004;4:361–70.
24. Slamon DJ, Clark GM, Wong SG, et al. Human breast cancer: correlation of relapse and survival with amplification of the HER2/neu oncogene. Science 1987;235:177–82.
25. Piccart-Gebhart MJ, Proctor M, Leyland-Jones B, al e. Herceptin Adjuvant (HERA) Trial Study Team: trastuzumab after adjuvant chemotherapy in HER-2 positive breast cancer. N Engl J Med 2005;353:1659–72.
26. Slamon DJ. Randomised phase III trial comparing AC-T vs AC-TH vs TCH in HER2 positive node positive or high risk node negative breast cancer. Presented at the San Antonio Breast Cancer Symposium, 2005.
27. Joensuu H, Kellokumpu-Lehtinen PL, Bono P, et al. Adjuvant docetaxol or vinorelbine with or without trastuzumab for breast cancer. N Engl J Med 2006;354:809–20.
28. Vogel CL, Cobeigh MA, Tripathy D, et al. Efficacy and safety of trastuzumab as a single agent in first-line treatment of HER2-overexpressing metastatic breast cancer. J Clin Oncol 2002;20:719–26.
29. Slamon DJ, Leyland-Jones B, Shak S, et al. Use of chemotherapy plus a monoclonal antibody against HER2 for metastatic breast cancer that overexpresses HER2. N Engl J Med 2001;344:783–92.
30. Leong TY-M, Leong AS-Y. Controversies in the assessment of HER2: more questions than answers. Adv Anat Pathol 2006;13(5):263–9.
31. Talpaz M, Goldman JM, Sawyers CL, et al. High dose imatitinib (STI571, Gleevec) provides durable long-term outcomes for patients (pts) with chronic myeloid leukemia (CML), in accelerated phase (AP) or myeloid blast crisis (BC): follow up of the phase II studies. Blood 2003;102:905a-6a. Abstract.
32. Druker BJ, Sawyers CL, Kantarjian H, et al. Activity of a specific inhibitor of the bcr-abl tyrosine kinase in the blast crisis of chronic myeloid leukemia and acute lymphoblastic leukemia with the Philadelphia chromosome. N Engl J Med 2001;344:1038–42.
33. Ottman OG, Druker BJ, Sawyers CL, et al. A phase 2 study of imatinib in patients with relapsed or refractory Philadelphia chromosome positive acute lymphoid leukemias. Blood 2002;100:1965–71.
34. Sawyers CL, Hochhaus A, Feldman E, et al. Imatinib induces hematologic and cytogenetic responses in patients with chronic myelogenous leukemia in myeloid blast crisis: results of a phase II study. Blood 2002;99:3530–9.
35. Talpaz M, Silver RT, Druker BJ, et al. Imatinib induces durable hematologic and cytogenetic responses in patients with accelerated phase chronic myeloid leukemia: results of a phase 2 study. Blood 2002;99:1928–37.
36. Silver M, Talpaz M, Sawyers CL, et al. Four years follow up of 1027 patients with late chronic phase (L-CP), accelerated phase (AP), or blast crisis(BC) chronic myeloid leukemia (CML) treated with imatinib in three large phase II trials. Blood 2004;104:10a. Abstract 23.
37. Baccarani M, Saglio G, Goldman JM, et al. Evolving concepts in the management of chronic myeloid leukemia: recommendations from an exert panel on behalf of the European Leukemia Net. Blood 2006;108:1809–20.
38. Talpaz M, Shah NP, Kantarjian H, et al. Dasatinib in imatinib-resistant Philadelphia chromosome-positive leukemias. N Engl J Med 2006;354:2531–41.
39. Weisberg E, Manley P, Mestan J, et al. AMN107 (nilotinib): a novel and selective inhibitor of BCR-ABL. Br J Cancer 2006;94:1765–9.
40. Mauro MJ, Deininger MW. Chronic myeloid leukemia in 2006: a perspective. Haematologica 2006;91:152.
41. Branford S, Rudzki Z, Parkinson I, et al. Realtime quantitative PCR analysis can be used as a primary screen to identify patients with CML treated with imatinib who have BCR-ABL kinase domain mutations. Blood 2004;104:2926–32.

42. Workman P, Aboagye EO, Chung Y-L, et al. Minimally invasive pharmacokinetic and pharmacodynamic technologies in hypothesis testing clinical trials of innovative therapies. J Natl Cancer Inst 2006;98(9): 580–98.

43. Gupta N, Price PM, Aboagye EO. PET for in vivo and pharmacokinetic and pharmacodynamic measurements. Eur J Cancer 2002;38:2094–107.

44. Eary JF, Mankoff DA, Spence AM, et al. 2-[C-11]thymidine imaging of malignant brain tumors. Cancer Res 1999;59:615–21.

45. Wilson CB, Lammertsma AA, McKenzie CG, et al. Measurements of blood flow and exchanging water space in breast tumors using positron emissio tomography: a rapid and noninvasive dynamic method. Cancer Res 1992;52:1592–7.

46. Findlay M, Young H, Cunningham D, et al. Non-invasive monitoring of tumor metabolism using fluorodeoxyglucose and positron emission tomography in colorectal cancer liver metastases: correlation with tumor response to fluorouracil. J Clin Oncol 1996;14:700–8.

47. Shields AF, Grierson JR, Dohmen BM, et al. Imaging proliferation in vivo with [F-18]FLT and positron emission tomography. Nat Med 1998;4:1334–6.

48. Wells P, Aboagye EO, Gunn RN, et al. 2-[11C]thymidine positron emission tomography as an indicator of thymidylate synthase inhibition in patients treated treated with AG337. J Natl Cancer Inst 2003;95:675–82.

49. Rasey JS, Koh WJ, Evans ML, et al. Quantifying regional hypoxia in human tumours with positron emission tomography of [18-F]fluoromisonidazole: a pre-therapy study of 37 patients. Int J Radiat Oncol Biol Phys 1996;36:417–28.

50. Barthel H, Wilson H, Collingridge DR, et al. In vivo evaluation of [18-F]fluoroetanidazole as a new marker for imaging tumor hypoxia with positron emission tomography. Br J Cancer 2004;90:2232–42.

51. Keen HG, Dekker BA, Disley L, et al. Imaging apoptosis in vivo using 124-I-annexin and PET. Nucl Med Biol 2005;32:395–402.

52. Smith-Jones PM, Solit D, Afroze F, et al. Early tumor response to HSP90 therapy using HER2 PET: comparison with 18F-FDG PET. J Nucl Med 2006;47:793–6.

53. Smith-Jones PM, Solit D, Akhurst T, et al. Imaging the pharmacodynamics of Her2 degradation in response to Hsp90 inhibitors. Nat Biotechnol 2004;22:701–6.

54. Padhani AR. Functional MRI for anticancer therapy assessment. Eur J Cancer 2002;38:2116–27.

55. Ostergaard L, Sorenson AG, Kwong KK, et al. High resolution of cerebral blood flow using extravascular racer bolus passages. Part II. Experimental comparison and preliminar results. Magn Reson Med 1996;36:726–36.

56. D'Arcy JA, Collins I, Rowland IJ, et al. Applications of sliding window reconstruction with cartesian sampling for dynamic contrast enhanced MRI. NMR Biomed 2002;15:174–83.

57. Leach MO, Brindle KM, Evelhoch JL, et al. The assessment of antiangiogenic and antivascular therapies in early-stage clinical trials using magnetic resonance imaging: issues and recommendations. Br J Cancer 2005;92:1599–610.

58. Leach M, Brindle KM, Evelhoch JL, et al. Assessment of antiangiogenic and antivascular therapeutics using MRI: recommendations for appropriate methodology for clinical trials. Br J Radiol 2003;76:S87–91.

59. Kurhanewiez J, Swanson MG, Nelson SJ, et al. Combined magnetic resonance imaging and spectroscopic imaging approach to molecular imaging of prostate cancer. J Magn Reson Imaging 2002;16:451–63.

60. Sibtain NA, Howe FA, Saunders DE. The clinical value of proton magnetic resonance spectroscopy in adult brain tumors. Clin Radiol 2007;62:109–19.

61. Murphy PS, Viviers L, Abson C, et al. Monitoring temozolamide treatment of low-grade glioma with proton magnetic resonance spectroscopy. Br J Cancer 2004;90:781–6.

62. Murphy PS, Dzik-Jurasz A, Baustert I, et al. Choline signal correlates with vascular permeability in human gliomas. Proc Int Soc Magn Reson Med 2000;8:393.

63. Schwarz AJ, Maisey NR, Collins DJ, et al. Early in vivo detection of metabolic response: a pilot study of ^{1}H MR spectroscopy in extracranial lymphoma and ERM cell tumors. Br J Radiol 2002;75:959–66.

64. Wolf W, Waluch V, Presant CA. Non-invasive ^{19}F-MRS of 5-fluorouracil in pharmacokinetics and pharmacodynamics. NMR Biomed 1998;11:380–7.

65. Zbuk KM, Eng C. Cancer phenomics: RET and PTEN as illustrative models. Nat Rev Cancer 2007;7:35–45.

66. Takahashi M. Cloning and expression of the RET oncogene encoding a receptor tyrosine kinase with two otential transmembrane domains. Oncogene 1988;3:571–8.

67. Nakamura T, Ishizaka Y, Nagao M, et al. Expression of the RET proto-oncogene product in human normal and neoplastic tissues of neural crest origin. J Pathol 1994;172:255–60.

68. Eng C, Mulligan LM. Mutations of the RET proto-oncogene in multiple endocrine neoplasia type 2 related sporadic tumors and Hirschsprung disease. Hum Mutat 1997;9:97–109.

69. King IB, Satia-Abouta J, Thornquist MD, et al. Buccal cell DNA yield, quality, and collection costs: comparison of methods for large scale studies. Cancer Epidemiol Biomarkers Prev 2002;11:1130–3.

70. Kerkela R, Grazette L, Yacobi R, et al. Cardiotoxicity of the cancer therapeutic agent imatinib mesylate. Nat Med 2006;12:908–16.

71. Bosanquet N, Sikora K. The Economics of Cancer Care. Cambridge, UK: Cambridge University Press; 2006.

72. Sikora K. Personalized medicine for cancer: from molecular signature to therapeutic choice. Adv Cancer Res 2007;96:345–69.

73. Dietel M, Sers C. Personalized medicine and development of targeted therapies: the up-coming challenge for diagnostic molecular pathology: a review. Virchows Arch 2006;448:744–55.

74. Golub TR, Slonim DK, Tamayo P, et al. Molecular classification of cancer: class discovery and class prediction by gene expression monitoring. Science 1999;286:531–7.

75. Yeoh EJ, Ross ME, Shurtleff SA, et al. Classification, subtype discovery, and prediction of outcome in pediatric acute lymphoblastic leukemia by gene expression profiling. Cancer Cell 2002;1:133–43.

76. Van't Veer LJ, Dai H, van de Vijer MJ, et al. Gene expression profiling predicts clinical outcome in breast cancer. Nature 2002;415:530–6.

77. Caldas C, Aparicio SA. The molecular outlook. Nature 2002;415:484–5.

78. Kolch W, Mischak H, Pitt AR. The molecular make-up of a tumor: proteomics in cancer research. Clin Sci 2005;108:369–83.

79. Wulfkuhle JD, Auino JA, Calvert VS, et al. Signal pathway profiling of ovarian cancer from human tissue specimens using reverse-phase protein microarrays. Proteomics 2003;3:2085–90.

80. Samoylova TI, Morrison NE, Globa LP, et al. Peptide phage display: opportunities for development of personalized anti-cancer strategies. Anticancer Agents Med Chem 2006;6:9–17.

81. Baylin SB, Esteller M, Rountree MR, et al. Aberrant patterns of DNA methylation, chromatin formation and gene expression in cancer. Hum Mol Genet 2001;10:687–92.

82. Jones PA, Baylin SB. The fundamental role of epigenetic events in cancer. Nat Rev Genet 2002;3:415–28.

83. Clayton EW. Through the lens of the sequence. Genome Res 2001;11(5):659.

84. Collins FS, Green ED, Guttmacher AE, et al. A vision for the future of genomics research. Nature 2003;422:835–47.

85. Robertson JA, Brody B, Buchanan A, et al. Pharmacogenetic challenges for the health care system. Health Aff (Millwood) 2002;21:155–67.

86. Robertson JA. Consent and privacy in pharmacogenetic testing. Nat Genet 2001;28(3):207–9.

87. Medical-ethical guidelines for genetic investigations in humans. Available at http://wwwsamwch/content /Richtlinien/e_Genpdf/, 1993.

88. Palmer LJ, Silverman ES, Drazen JM, et al. Pharmacogenomics of asthma treatment. In: Licinio J, Wong, ML (eds) Pharmacogenomics: The Search for Individualized Therapies. Weinham, Germany: Wiley-VCH; 2002.

89. Rothstein MA, Epps PG. Ethical and legal implications of pharmacogenomics. Nat Rev Genet 2001;2: 228–31.

90. Breithaupt H. The future of medicine: centralised health and genetic databases promise to increase quality of healthcare while lowering costs; but to get there, many legal and social obstacles will have to be overcome to prevent abuse. EMBO Rep 2001;2:465.

91. Anderlik MR, Rothstein MA. Privacy and confidentiality of genetic information: what rules for the new science? Annu Rev Genom Hum Genet 2001;2:401–33.

Index

Printed In The United States Of America